Comprehensive Review of Geriatric Psychiatry

Comprehensive Review of Geriatric Psychiatry

EDITED BY

Joel Sadavoy, M.D.
Lawrence W. Lazarus, M.D.
Lissy F. Jarvik, M.D., Ph.D.

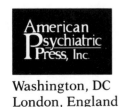

Washington, DC
London, England

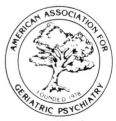

Sponsored by the
American Association
for Geriatric
Psychiatry

Note: The authors have worked to ensure that all information in this book is accurate as of the time of publication and consistent with standards of the general medical community. As medical research and practice advance, however, therapeutic standards may change. For this reason and because human and mechanical errors sometimes occur, we recommend that readers follow the advice of a physician who is directly involved in their care or the care of a member of their family.

Books published by the American Psychiatric Press, Inc. and the American Association for Geriatric Psychiatry represent the views and opinions of the individual authors and do not necessarily represent the policies and opinions of the Press, the American Psychiatric Association, or AAGP.

Copyright © 1991 American Psychiatric Press, Inc.
ALL RIGHTS RESERVED
Manufactured in the United States of America on acid-free paper.
First Edition

94 93 92 91 4 3 2

American Psychiatric Press, Inc.
1400 K Street, N.W., Washington, DC 20005

Library of Congress Cataloging-in-Publication Data
Comprehensive review of geriatric psychiatry / edited by Joel Sadavoy, Lawrence
   W. Lazarus, Lissy Jarvik. —1st ed.
      p.   cm.
   Includes bibliographical references and index.
   ISBN 0-88048-362-8 (alk. paper)
   1. Geriatric psychiatry.   I. Sadavoy, Joel, 1945–
II. Lazarus, Lawrence W., 1941–   .   III. Jarvik, Lissy F.
   [DNLM: 1. Geriatric Psychiatry.   2. Mental Disorders—in old age.
WT 150 C737]
RC451.4.A5C634   1991
618.97'689—dc20
DNLM/DLC
for Library of Congress   90-1203
                                                                                      CIP

British Cataloguing in Publication Data
A CIP record is available from the British Library.

Contents

List of Contributors

Robert Abrams, M.D. Associate Professor of Clinical Psychiatry, Cornell University Medical College, New York.

Marilyn S. Albert, Ph.D. Associate Professor of Psychiatry and Neurology, Harvard Medical School; Coordinator, Geriatric Neuropsycho-Behavioral Clinic, Massachusetts General Hospital, Boston.

Cathy A. Alessi, M.D. Fellow in Geriatric Medicine, Pritzker School of Medicine, University of Chicago Hospital.

Andre Allen, M.D. Clinical Associate Professor, Department of Psychiatry, Duke University Medical Center, Durham, NC.

Dan G. Blazer II, M.D., Ph.D. Professor of Psychiatry, and Director, Affective Disorders Program, Duke University Medical Center, Durham, NC.

Julia E. Bradsher, M.A. Graduate Research Assistant, Department of Sociology, University of Miami.

Stanley H. Cath, M.D. Medical Director, Family Advisory and Treatment Center, Tufts University Medical Center, Belmont, MA.

Christine K. Cassel, M.D. Chief, Section of General Internal Medicine, Pritzker School of Medicine, University of Chicago.

Carl Cohen, M.D. Professor of Psychiatry, Director of Geriatric Psychiatry, State University of New York.

David K. Conn, M.B. B.Ch Assistant Professor of Psychiatry, University of Toronto; Coordinator, Consultation-Liaison Service, Baycrest Centre for Geriatric Care, Toronto.

Sharon M. Curlik, D.O. Assistant Professor, Department of Psychiatry, Medical College of Pennsylvania; Staff Psychiatrist, Philadelphia Geriatric Center.

Carl Eisdorfer, M.D., Ph.D. Professor and Chairman, Department of Psychiatry, University of Miami, Director for the Center on Aging Adult Development, University of Miami.

Spencer Eth, M.D. Acting Chief of Psychiatry and Associate Chief of Psychiatry Inpatient Service, Veterans Administration Hospital, Los Angeles.

David G. Folks, M.D. Associate Professor of Psychiatry, and Director, Geriatric Psychiatry, University of Alabama School of Medicine at Birmingham.

Deborah Frazier, Ph.D. Director of Clinical Psychology, Philadelphia.

Marion Goldstein, M.D. Clinical Associate Professor of Psychiatry, and Director, Division of Geriatric Psychiatry, Erie County Medical Center, State University of New York at Buffalo School of Medicine.

Gary Gottlieb, M.D. Associate Professor of Psychiatry, and Director, Section of Geriatric Psychiatry, University of Pennsylvania; Senior Fellow, Leonard Davies Institute of Health; Wharton School of Economics, Philadelphia.

Barry Gurland, M.D. John E. Borne Professor of Clinical Psychiatry, Columbia University, New York; Director of Columbia University Center for Geriatrics and Gerontology.

M. Jackuelyn Harris, M.D. Assistant Professor of Psychiatry, University of California, San Diego, and San Diego Veterans Administration Medical Center.

Donald P. Hay, M.D. Associate Clinical Professor of Psychiatry, University of Wisconsin, Milwaukee.

Nathan Herrmann, M.D. Assistant Professor of Psychiatry, University of Toronto; Staff Psychiatrist, Department of Psychiatry, Sunnybrook Medical Centre, Toronto.

Leonard L. Heston, M.D. Professor of Psychiatry, Mental Illness Residents and Educational Institute, Western State Hospital, WA.

Lissy F. Jarvik, M.D., Ph.D. Distinguished Physician, Department of Veterans Affairs, West Los Angeles Veterans Administration Medical Center, Brentwood Division; Professor, Department of Psychiatry and Biobehavioral Sciences, University of California, Los Angeles; Chief, Section of Neuropsychogeriatrics, The

Neuropsychiatric Institute, University of California, Los Angeles; Chief, Psychogeriatric Unit, West Los Angeles Veterans Administration Medical Center, Brentwood Division, Los Angeles.

Michael Jenike, M.D.   Associate Professor of Psychiatry, Harvard Medical School, Director of the Obsessive-Compulsive Disorders Clinic and Research Unit, Massachusetts General Hospital.

Dilip V. Jeste, M.D.   Professor of Psychiatry and Neurosciences, University of California, San Diego, and San Diego Veterans Administration Medical Center, La Jolla, CA.

Ira R. Katz, M.D., Ph.D.   Professor, Department of Psychiatry, Medical College of Pennsylvania; Chairman, Department of Psychiatry, Philadelphia Geriatric Center, Philadelphia.

F. Cleveland Kinney, M.D., Ph.D.   Assistant Professor of Psychiatry and Anatomy, University of Alabama School of Medicine at Birmingham.

Pauline R. Langsley, M.D.   Assistant Professor of Psychiatry, Rush Medical School, Chicago.

Lawrence W. Lazarus, M.D.   Assistant Professor of Psychiatry, and Director, Geriatric Psychiatry Fellowship Program, Rush Medical School, Chicago.

Molyn Leszcz, M.D.   Assistant Professor of Psychiatry, University of Toronto; Head, Group Therapy Service, Mount Sinai Hospital and Baycrest Centre for Geriatric Care, Toronto.

Andrew Leuchter, M.D.   Assistant Professor of Psychiatry, University of California, Los Angeles; Co-Director, Geriatric Inpatient Ward, Los Angeles.

Elaine A. Leventhal, M.D., Ph.D.   Associate Professor, Medical Division of General Internal Medicine and Geriatrics, Robert Wood Johnson Medical School, University of Medicine and Dentistry of New Jersey, New Brunswick, NJ.

Charles F. Longino, Ph.D.   Professor, Department of Sociology, and Director of Center for Social Research in Aging, University of Miami.

Michael Manley, M.D.   University of California, San Diego, and San Diego Veterans Administration Medical Center.

Richard Margolin, M.D.   Assistant Professor of Psychiatry and Radiology, Director of the Division of Geriatric Psychiatry, Director of Geropsychiatry Clinic, Vanderbilt University Medical Center, Nashville, TN.

Barnett S. Meyers, M.D.   Associate Professor of Clinical Psychiatry, Cornell University Medical College; Chief, Geriatric Specialty Clinic, New York Hospital, Westchester Division, White Plains, NY.

Norman S. Miller, M.D.   Cornell University Medical College, The New York Hospital, Cornell Medical Center.

Leonard W. Poon, Ph.D.   Professor of Psychiatry, Director of Gerontology Center, University of Georgia, Athens, Georgia.

Stephen Read, M.D.   Assistant Professor, Department of Psychiatry, University of California Los Angeles Medical Center, Torrance, CA.

Domeena C. Renshaw, M.D.   Professor, Department of Psychiatry, and Director, Sexual Dysfunction Clinic, Loyola University, Chicago.

Charles F. Reynolds III, M.D.   Professor of Psychiatry, Director of Sleep Evaluation Center, University of Pittsburgh, Western Psychiatric Institute and Clinic, Pittsburgh.

Joel Sadavoy, M.D.   Associate Professor of Psychiatry, University of Toronto; Head, Department of Psychiatry, Baycrest Centre for Geriatric Care; and Consultant in Psychiatry, Mount Sinai Hospital, Toronto.

Robert L. Sadoff, M.D.   Clinical Professor of Psychiatry, and Director, Center for Studies in Social-Legal Psychiatry, University of Pennsylvania, Philadelphia.

Charles Shamoian, M.D., Ph.D.   Professor of Clinical Psychiatry, Cornell University Medical College, Director, Division of Acute Treatment Services, New York Hospital, Cornell Medical College.

Ilene C. Siegler, Ph.D., M.P.H.   Associate Professor of Medical Psychology, Department of Psychiatry, Duke University Medical Center, Durham, NC.

Ivan L. Silver, M.D.   Assistant Professor of Psychiatry, University of Toronto; Coordinator of Geriatric Psychiatry, Department of Psychiatry, Sunnybrook Medical Centre, Toronto.

Allan Steingart, M.D.   Assistant Professor of Psychiatry, University of Toronto, Coordinator, Psychiatry Day Hospital, Department of Psychiatry, Baycrest Centre for Geriatric Care, Toronto.

Marie-France Tourigny-Rivard, M.D.   Director of Geriatric Psychiatry, Royal Ottawa Hospital, Assistant Professor of Psychiatry, University of Ottawa.

Jeffrey I. Victoroff, M.D.   Department of Neurology, Reed Neurological Research Center, University of California Los Angeles, School of Medicine, Los Angeles.

George J. Warheit, Ph.D.   Professor of Psychiatry and Chairman, Department of Psychiatry, University of Miami, Coral Gables, FL.

Robert C. Young, M.D.   Associate Professor of Clinical Psychiatry, Cornell University Medical College, Associate Attending Psychiatrist, New York Hospital–Cornell Medical College and Westchester Division.

SECTION 1

The Aging Process

CHAPTER 1

Joel Sadavoy, M.D.
Lawrence W. Lazarus, M.D.
Lissy F. Jarvik, M.D., PH.D.

INTRODUCTION

New Clinical Perspectives on Aging

Geriatrics and geriatric psychiatry are at a historic turning point. Major growth in clinical interest and research activity in the area of aging have been catalysts for academic developments in geriatric psychiatry—indeed, in geriatrics as a whole (Rowe et al. 1987)—during the last quarter of the 20th century. Until then one could not find even a handful of medical schools in the United States offering specialized training in geriatrics. Prior to 1978, there had been only a single specialty training program in geriatric psychiatry; but in the following decade, the number of geriatric psychiatry specialty training programs grew to more than 30—including nearly one-fourth of the medical schools in the United States (Cohen 1989). Since the mid-1970s, three areas of significant conceptual growth have become particularly apparent: differentiating changes of normal aging from symptoms of illness in later life, the modifiability of illness in later life, and the modifiability of normal aging for better functioning.

Differentiating Changes of Normal Aging From Symptoms of Illness in Later Life

If one fails to distinguish illness from normal aging, then clinical symptoms are overlooked—dismissed as inevitable concomitants of the aging process; treatment options, then, fail to be considered. As the influence of gerontology became increasingly evident in the mid-1970s, challenging questions were raised about illness versus

3

normal aging. Nowhere is this occurrence better illustrated than in the case of Alzheimer disease (AD). Many saw senility as their fate in growing old, an unavoidable concomitant of aging. But two types of evidence began to throw into question that point of view. First, longitudinal psychometric data began to accumulate, documenting that many older persons maintained high levels of cognitive functioning. When speed was not a factor, some of them—especially those who were healthy—showed improvement in performance during their eighties. The second line of evidence came from neurochemistry and led to new hypotheses about a deficiency of the neurotransmitter acetylcholine in the brains of "senile" older adults (Cohen 1989), thus pointing to the presence of disease as opposed to a scheduled developmental event in one's later years. Concepts of depression similarly evolved—no longer viewed as going with the normal territory of aging—as did perspectives on other disorders in older adults.

The Modifiability of Illness in Later Life

Once clinicians and researchers began to recognize the role of illness in producing some of the mental changes of later life, the next step was to appreciate its modifiability, especially the modifiability of mental illness in late life. Growing clinical experience and new research methodologies showed that depression in elderly patients did respond to psychopharmacology and psychotherapy. Moreover, new views on treatment emerged even for AD with the awareness of the modifiability of excess disability states—including alterable, comorbid conditions (e.g., depression and delusions) that compound dysfunction (Group for the Advancement of Psychiatry Committee on Aging 1988).

Modifiability of Normal Aging for Better Functioning

The growth of understanding about how much functional decline in later life is attributable to disorder rather than to development has made it increasingly difficult to determine exactly what changes do indeed represent normal aging. However, in practical terms the distinction may no longer be important, because it is becoming apparent that even normal changes may be modified to enhance effective functioning in later life. For example, even though there is agreement among researchers that reaction time increases with aging, new data indicate that the rate of reaction in later life can be improved with practice. Thus, an investigation of the effects of videogame play on responses of elderly adults reported improvement in both the speed and the accuracy of responses following a 7-week training program (Clark et al. 1987). Such research should put to rest the negative stereotype about "old dogs and new tricks," and it is at the same time highly relevant to the development of interventions to promote mental health.

The Capacity to Change and the Significance of Time in Later Life

Particularly in the domain of psychiatric treatment, perspectives on time have a major influence on practitioner behavior. To the extent that the service provider feels that the patient has only a limited amount of time left, treatment planning may be compromised. Neither doubt about time left nor skepticism about the capacity to change in later life stands up to clinical experience. The significance of time and the capacity to change in old age are captured by Somerset Maugham in an observation on the behavior of the elder Cato approximately 20 centuries ago: "When I was young, I was amazed at Plutarch's statement that the elder Cato began, at the age of eighty, to learn Greek. I am amazed no longer. Old age is ready to undertake tasks that youth shirked because they would take too long" p. 297. With people aged over 85 representing the fastest growing age group, most older adults have much time left for both life and treatment in their later years. This optimism is reflected in the potential for change that is evident in geriatric patients who undertake psychodynamically oriented psychotherapy late in life (Sadavoy and Leszcz 1987).

The Special Knowledge of Geriatric Psychiatry

The special knowledge of geriatric psychiatry needs to be examined along two planes: 1) as it relates to elderly patients and 2) as it relates to aging per se (Cohen 1988; Lazarus 1988). From the perspective of elderly patients, the focus of geriatric psychiatry ranges from attention to special, later-life problems (e.g., late-onset schizophrenia and AD) to interventions (e.g., retirement counseling and geriatric psychopharmacology) and service settings (e.g., geriatric assessment units and nursing homes). The general perspective on aging of geriatric psychiatry, however, is less well appreciated. It is through this perspective that geriatric psychiatry makes contributions not only to older patients but to all age groups.

In any field, whenever a problem can be examined in a new light, the opportunity for new insights presents itself. The longitudinal view developed through research on the elderly has helped to shed new light on mental disorders affecting the young as well as the old. For example, why is it that the group of late-onset schizophrenics passes through so much of the life cycle before first developing psychosis? Moreover, by studying this group of individuals, new information may be gained about schizophrenia independent of age. What might be learned about schizophrenia, in general, by studying it in people who grow old with the disorder but experience an attenuation (burnout) of its symptoms with aging?

Another example comes from research in geriatric depression. An early theory of depression, the catecholamine hypothesis, stated that the mood disorder resulted from a central deficit in the neurotransmitter norepinephrine. Meanwhile, studies on the aging brain revealed that monoamine oxidase (MAO) levels *increased* with advancing years. Because MAO reduces norepinephrine levels, all older adults should be depressed, and increasingly so over time. But epidemiological studies showed that this was not the case.

These findings from research on aging, together with other evidence incompatible with the catecholamine hypothesis, have helped generate newer theories of depression, such as the "dysregulation hypothesis," which postulates disruption in mechanisms that regulate the activity of neurotransmitters rather than their levels (Siever and Davis 1985).

The 70-Year Follow-up

Much can be learned by following a given disorder over time to study its natural history. The problem for the researcher is that doing so takes time. The geriatric patient offers a modified shortcut in this process. If an older patient is being followed for major depression or chronic schizophrenia, one has the opportunity to look back, via the patient's history, to examine the course of the illness over a period of decades—at times, over a period of 70 or more years. This is a unique opportunity offered only by geriatric patients, who provide us the opportunity to expand our understanding of mental disorders across the life cycle.

Interaction of Mental and Physical Health Phenomena

A clinical dimension that distinguishes older patients, in general, from younger ones is the greater likelihood of experiencing more than one concurrent illness in later life, including coexistent mental health and physical impairments. Accordingly, geriatric patients provide one of the best windows on mechanisms underlying the influence of mental illness on physical condition and, conversely, on the influence of somatic disorder on mental condition. It is through the geriatric patient that one most commonly comes into clinical contact with that elusive "whole person" in a biopsychosocial context (Jarvik 1983).

Certificate of Added Qualifications in Geriatric Psychiatry

A certificate of added qualifications in geriatric psychiatry is now planned, with the first examination scheduled for April 1991. Several factors have led to the historic movement toward developing the first new area of special competence in American psychiatry (since child psychiatry) in nearly three decades.

The dramatic growth in numbers of people aged 65 and older—more than 12% of the population, over 30 million people—has resulted in a historically new challenge for society. Moreover, the 85-and-older age group is expected to increase sixfold to sevenfold by the middle of the 21st century, at which time it will number more than 15 million. Everyone who will be 85 in 2050 is alive today.

As the aging population has grown, so have the numbers of psychiatrists interested and specializing in care of the elderly. By the late 1980s the total number of American psychiatrists was approximately 35,000. A decade earlier, relatively few psychiatrists expressed interest in working with older adults. But formal surveys during the 1980s found more than 5,000 psychiatrists providing active treatment to elderly patients, with an indication of that number being on the rise (Cohen 1989). Moreover, the need for training in this area prompted a dramatic growth in the number of postresidency training programs in geriatric psychiatry.

With the dramatic growth between 1978 and 1988 in the number of postresidency specialty training programs in geriatric psychiatry, American psychiatry reached a critical mass of training programs consistent with subspecialization.

The number of research projects on mental health and aging has soared since the mid-1970s, significantly stirred in the United States by the establishment of the Center on Aging at the National Institute of Mental Health, and the National Institute on Aging—the latter with a budget of one-quarter of a billion dollars in 1990. By then, support in the United States for AD research alone had reached more than $130 million annually. Early in 1980 the growth of knowledge was marked by the publication of major texts on mental health and aging and on geriatric psychiatry; since then, separate texts have been written for almost every one of the chapters in the original comprehensive works (i.e., separate geriatric texts now exist on depression, schizophrenia, AD, psychotherapy, and psychopharmacology).

Medicare can be described as national health insurance for America's older adults. But for more than a generation since its inception—from the early 1960s to the late 1980s—Medicare provided very little coverage for outpatient services for community-dwelling, older adults, which group includes 95% of people aged 65 and older. Consequently patients were discouraged from using mental health services and practitioners were discouraged from providing them. Psychiatry's previous low visibility vis-à-vis elderly patients did not help in attempts to secure improved patient benefits. Psychiatry's new statement about interest, knowledge, and skills in the area of geriatric psychiatry, made by its movement toward developing added qualifications, in all likelihood influenced the granting of new psychiatric benefits under Medicare as the 1980s came to a close (see Chapter 34).

The American public has been growing increasingly sophisticated in its knowledge and expectations of geriatric health care. By so doing, it has been influencing the profession to pay greater attention to specialization, thereby, to a degree, responding to consumer demand. Public pressure is enhanced further when families themselves form organizations to better highlight need and focus attention in various areas. For example, the Alzheimer's Association in the United States, formed in 1980, now has more than 200 local chapters across the country.

The goal of the added qualifications process is to allow the general practitioner of psychiatry to add qualifications, not to establish a new guild within a guild. The added qualifications process in geriatric psychiatry is an attempt to strengthen both academic leadership and the capacity of the general psychiatrist to address mental illness in geriatric patients. It should strengthen both fellowship training in geriatric psychiatry and the development of geriatric psychiatry rotations in general residency training. A similar situation exists in both internal medicine and family practice. Ideally, this process will lead to significant growth of expert faculty in geriatric psychiatry; significant growth of research focused on mental health and mental illness in older adults; improved psychogeriatric skills of psychiatrists in general; improved psychogeriatric skills for practitioners in all fields who work with older patients; enhanced public awareness of the nature of mental illness in later life and its modifiability through the application of psychogeriatric interventions; and heightened awareness in policymakers of the state of the art in psychogeriatrics, leading to the development of increasingly effective policies addressing mental health needs of older persons (Cohen 1989).

The Beginning

The Bible described King David as having a depression (Psalms 31:9–12):

> Be gracious unto me, O Lord, for I am in distress;
> Mine eye wasted away with vexation, yea, my soul and my body.
> For my life is spent in sorrow, and my years in sighing;
> My strength faileth because of mine iniquity, and my bones are
>   wasted away.
> Because of all mine adversaries I am become a reproach, yea. . . .
> I am forgotten as a dead man out of mind;
> I am like a useless vessel.

Thus, we know that the history of geriatric psychiatry is rooted in biblical times.

The Maximes of PtahHaty described dementia (depressive pseudodementia) in the seventh century B.C. (Loza and Milad 1989):

> Sovereign my master the old age is here, senility has descended in me, the weakness of my childhood is renewed, so I sleep all the time. The arms are weak, the legs have given up following the heart that has become tired. The mouth is mute, it can no longer speak, the eyes are weak, the ears are deaf, the nose is blocked, it can no longer breathe. The taste is completely gone. The spirit is forgetful. It can no longer remember yesterday. The bones ache in the old age, getting up and sitting down are both difficult. What was nice has become bad. What causes senility in men is bad in every way.

Yet examples of good mental health in the elders of ancient Egypt also exist (Loza and Milad 1989). The statue of Nebenterou, son of the high priest of the Twelfth Dynasty (950–730 B.C.) bore the following engraving: "I have spent my life in happiness, without the worry of illness. . . . I have outlived my contemporaries. May this happen to you too."

Evidence of attempts to treat dementia have been found in the Edwin Smith papyrus, as well as the Magical Papyri.

During the Coptic Era (Loza and Milad 1989) (A.D. second to seventh centuries), Father Jean Cassien described a paranoid psychosis in a French monk in his book *Les Conférences des Pères du Desert*. The monk ultimately kills himself in a delusional state.

Plato observed that older people did not have an increasing anxiety about death. He believed that reductions in the power of impulses led to the sense of tranquility and greater freedom to pursue philosophy and intellectual endeavors. In 44 B.C., at the age of 62, Cicero wrote an essay on senescence (*De Senecute*) in which he described the problems and goals for older people. He acknowledged ageism in Roman society while stressing the value of older people in administrative and intellectual pursuits. Cicero echoed Plato's ideas about diminishing sexual pleasure and greater acceptance of death in old age. He also described the severe regression that can occur with dementia, a condition he viewed with abhorrence.

Modern Clinical Geriatric Psychiatry

In the Middle Ages, Esquirol differentiated dementia (loss of mental faculties) from amentia (mental retardation). However, he did not believe that dementia was an irreversible process. Berios differentiated depression and dementia in the 19th century based on his book, *Montpelier*.

In the early years of psychoanalysis, Freud was pessimistic about the application of psychoanalytic techniques to the treatment of "older people" (people aged over 40). When Freud was 42 he wrote *Sexuality in the Aetiology of the Neuroses* (Freud 1959), in which he stated as follows (p. 245): "With persons who are too far advanced in years, it [psychoanalytic method] fails because, owing to the accumulation of material, so much time would be required so that the end of the cure would be reached at a period of life in which much importance is no longer attached to nervous health." Subsequently, he recognized that his statements were based on his limited number of cases, predominantly of hysteria and obsessional neurosis.

Twenty years later, however, Abraham (1927) described his years of employing psychoanalytic techniques in the treatment of older people: "It would seem incorrect today to deny a priori the possibility of exercising a curative influence upon the neurosis in the period of involution and rather it is the task of psychoanalysis to inquire under what conditions the method of treatment can attain results in the later years."

Abraham described a successful treatment of a melancholic man aged 50 who had been institutionalized several times. This man was the first of several patients he treated who were in their middle years. He concluded that "the age at which the neurosis breaks out is of greater importance than the age at which treatment has begun" (Abraham 1927).

At around the same time, Sandor Ferenczi (1955) described psychodynamic changes in later life, which include a decreased ability to sublimate, increasing narcissism, and often a more negative and hostile approach to life. Ferenczi theorized that in old age there is a reversion to the discharge of pregenital impulses including voyeurism, exhibitionism, and a tendency to masturbate—which he termed "underdistinguished" anal and urethral eroticism.

In 1906, two revolutionary monographs were written. One was the classic description of dementia by Alzheimer (1906). The other was written by Gaupp (Barraclough 1989), who differentiated dementias from nondementias (mainly depression). Although some nondementias ended in dementia, Gaupp observed that most did not.

Hitler's ascension in Germany prompted the relocation to the United Kingdom of two very important individuals in the field of geriatric psychiatry. In the subsequent decades, Felix Post and Sir Martin Roth made major contributions to the field of geriatric psychiatry. Under the guidance and direction of Dr. Aubrey Lewis, Felix Post assumed the first geriatric psychiatric position in England in 1947 at the Bethlem Hospital. By 1950–51, Post had developed an entire ward of people over the age of 60. Among his trainees were David Kay, who made major contributions to the understanding of the epidemiology of mental disorders in late life, and Raymond Levy and Tom Arie, who have continued in Post's tradition. Levy is currently the first professor of the Department of Psychiatry of Old Age at Maudsley, while Arie chairs the Division of Health Care of the Aged in Nottingham.

Post, Roth, Kay, and B. Hopkins intensively studied older patients who were hospitalized in the 1950s and determined that there was no evidence that depressed patients without brain symptoms subsequently developed them (Barraclough 1989; Post 1965).

Roth's research, in distinguishing between affective and organic disorders, turned up a small group with paranoid symptoms (hallucinations and delusions) in otherwise well-maintained personality in late life (paraphrenia).

Around the same time, T. K. Henderson of Edinburgh and Duncan McMillan of Nottingham were working intensively with older people with mental disorders. McMillan focused on integration of services with a strong social-psychiatric approach. He played a major role in the development of respite care to meet the need of families who had depressed and demented patients living with them. McMillan emphasized the importance of ready access to appropriate levels and intensity of service based on the patient's and family's needs.

In the United States, the first relevant treatise on geriatric psychiatry was written by Benjamin Rush in 1805, entitled "An account of the state of the body and the mind in old age; with observation on its diseases and remedies" (Busse 1989).

Hall published *Senescence: The Last Half of Life* in 1922. One of his findings included the observation, based on questionnaires, that older people did not become more fearful of death. In 1914, Nascher published a textbook titled *Geriatrics: The Diseases of Old Age and Their Treatment*, thereby establishing a new name for the field. Nascher, who is considered the father of geriatrics in America, continued his interest in working in the field. His final paper, "The Aging Mind," published in 1944, described the characteristics of chronic brain syndrome. Nascher hypothesized that there was a genetic etiology of chronic brain syndrome.

Organized Geriatric Psychiatry

In the late 1930s, voices all over the world spoke of the need to establish a gerontological society. Prior to that time, a great deal of emphasis had been placed on how to extend the human life span, with little attention to careful and thoughtful study of the aging process. Shock (1988) and Busse (1989) wrote detailed reviews of the history of the International Association of Gerontology (IAG), established in Liège, Belgium, 1950. The IAG has supported regular, well-attended conferences all over the world addressing many gerontologic issues, including mental health and mental illness.

In the 1940s and 1950s, several other major national and international geriatric organizations were founded. The American Geriatric Society was founded in 1942 and began to publish a journal, *The Journal of the American Geriatric Society*, in 1953. The Gerontological Society of America was founded in 1945 and began to publish the *Journal of Gerontology* in 1946. At that time, however, the number of investigators involved in research on aging was extremely small.

Three other developments in geriatric psychiatry in the United States began in the 1950s and picked up momentum in the following decades.

The Group for the Advancement of Psychiatry (GAP) was founded in 1946 with goals "to collect and appraise significant data in the field of psychiatry, mental health and human relations; to re-evaluate old concepts and to develop and test new ones; and to apply the knowledge thus obtained for the promotion of mental health in group human relations" (GAP 1950, p. 6). *The Problem of the Aged Patient in the Public Psychiatric Hospital* was GAP's first geropsychiatric monograph, published in 1950 by the Committee on Hospitals (GAP 1950).

The GAP Committee on Aging was established in the early 1960s by Jack Weinberg, future president of the American Psychiatric Association (APA). A second treatise on "Psychiatry and the Aged: An Introductory Approach" was published in 1965 (GAP 1965). Other monographs addressed issues related to community mental health (GAP 1971), curriculum development (GAP 1983), and psychotherapy of Alzheimer's disease (AD) (GAP 1988).

In 1954 longitudinal studies on aging began at Duke University. These studies led to a series of books based on research findings, many taken from the longitudinal data (Busse and Pfeiffer 1969; Palmore 1970, 1974). Busse established the first geriatric psychiatry training program at Duke University Medical Center in 1965. In the late 1960s, Carl Eisdorfer, Eric Pfeiffer, Adrian Verwoerdt, and others began to make major contributions to the field of geriatric psychiatry, under the leadership of Ewald (Bud) Busse.

The Boston Society for Gerontologic Psychiatry (BSGP) was founded by a group of psychoanalytically oriented psychiatrists—Martin Berezin, Stanley Cath, David Blau, and Ralph Kahana among others—with a special interest in developmental issues related to aging. The BSGP's semiannual, half-day workshops became the primary source of intellectual stimulation for budding geriatric psychiatrists across the country. Papers from BSGP's symposia were published in three books in the 1960s (Berezin and Cath 1965; Levin and Kahana 1967; Zinberg and Kaufman 1963). Subsequently, BGSP created *The Journal of Geriatric Psychiatry* in 1967 and has continued this publication uninterrupted since that time. In the 1970s, the inspiration provided by BSGP stimulated similar groups in Chicago, Houston, New York, and greater Washington, DC.

The late 1950s and 1960s also witnessed the introduction of psychotropic medication, which provided unprecedented pharmacological relief from depression, anxiety, and psychosis. Chlorpromazine (Thorazine), lithium carbonate, imipramine hydrochloride (Tofranil), chlordiazepoxide hydrochloride (Librium) and diazepam (Valium) were introduced or developed.

In the mid-1960s, APA created a small component on aging, with particular interest in community geriatric psychiatry, under the leadership of Alexander Simon. It was not until 1979, however, that APA played a major role in the development of the field.

The 1960s also marked the inception of several Great Society programs, including Medicare and Medicaid, which allowed more older people to receive inpatient psychiatric services. Unfortunately, outpatient services were severely limited by a $250 annual cap, which remained until 1988.

The 1970s

The 1970s marked a significant worldwide increase in psychogeriatric services and training. In France, Jean-Marie Leger, professor and chairman of the Department of Psychiatry at the University of Limoges, started a psychogeriatric service that included community psychiatry, inpatient and outpatient psychiatric services, and an outreach program. All medical students rotated through the psychogeriatric service. Soon, newly trained French psychiatrists developed satellites with similar services in other parts of France. French geropsychiatrists have frequently divided into psychoanalytic versus organic camps. Doctor Henri Ey of Bonneval began to bridge this gap with an integrated approach.

In Switzerland, two psychogeriatric centers were established in French-speaking areas. After Junat established a substantial program in Geneva, Dr. Christian Mueller similarly established a service and academic component in Lausanne. The effects of aging on schizophrenia and other psychiatric disorders were studied by Luc Ciompi (1972), who found an unusually high percentage of dementia in elderly schizophrenics.

In the late 1960s, Kiloh emigrated from Newcastle in the United Kingdom to Sydney, Australia. Kiloh was a general psychiatrist with a special interest in electroencephalography. Dr. D. K. Henderson, a research psychiatrist, established a division of psychogeriatric research, while Edmund Chiu of Melbourne conducted research on dementias that are uncommonly seen. These three spawned a new generation of Australian psychogeriatricians.

The decade from 1965 to 1975 marked the establishment in the United States of three major federal agencies devoted to gerontology. In 1965, the new Administration on Aging was established with the specific purpose of developing and coordinating services and research initiatives for the elderly. In 1971, the second White House Conference on Aging took place, leading to specific recommendations that catalyzed the formation of the National Institute of Mental Health (NIMH) Center for Studies of the Mental Health of the Aging, as well as the National Institute on Aging (NIA) (White House Conference on Aging 1981). NIA was assigned responsibility for promoting, coordinating, and supporting research regarding normal aging, as well as pathology and problems of the aged. NIA's mandate from Congress included conducting research in behavioral and social sciences, as well as biological and biomedical sciences. Robert Butler, a geriatric psychiatrist with extensive clinical, research, and teaching experience, was NIA's first director. In its first decade, more than 100 new researchers were trained (Butler 1977).

NIMH had sponsored research on the mental health of the aging on a limited basis between 1960 and 1976 (U.S. Department of Health, Education, and Welfare [DHEW] 1977). Under the energetic and creative leadership of its first chief, Dr. Gene Cohen, the NIMH Center for Studies of the Mental Health of the Aging grew rapidly as it carried out its mandate to support and coordinate research, clinical training projects, and research training. Geropsychiatric training, fellowship programs, continuing education, demonstration curricula and training projects, and in-service training all flourished. In 1976, the Secretary of Health, Education, and Welfare appointed Eric Pfeiffer to establish an agenda on the needs of the mental health of older Americans. President Carter in 1977 established a task panel regarding mental health and mental illness in late life. Both reports were published in 1978 (HEW 1979a).

By 1978, there was a clear need for an American organization with a specific focus on geriatric psychiatry. Although the field had been developing significantly since the late 1940s, the increasing number of older people, the concomitant number of older persons with psychiatric disorders—particularly depressions and dementias—and the larger base of knowledge mandated the establishment of a forum in which to exchange ideas. The interest level of professionals regarding older people had significantly increased, with growing efforts to provide services to older people (Finkel 1979).

In late 1978, Sanford Finkel assembled a group of 15 nationally recognized leaders in the field of geriatric psychiatry to discuss the establishment of a national organization, the American Association for Geriatric Psychiatry (AAGP). This organizational meeting occurred at the 1978 annual meeting of APA, the theme of which centered on aging. The initial goals of the organization were as follows:

- To provide a focus for dissemination of information to the psychiatrists who care for the elderly. A primary mechanism would be the publication of a newsletter that would provide information regarding mental health issues and the elderly.
- To increase the attention of APA on the field of aging with particular reference to services, training, research, and policy development. AAGP also wished to advocate the establishment of a significant component on aging in APA.
- To encourage throughout the country the development of local societies concerned with mental health aspects of aging. The first AAGP newsletter included "A Rationale for the Establishment of an American Psychiatric Association Council on Aging" (Finkel 1978).

In its first year, AAGP accomplished its first and third goals, and AAGP representatives successfully solicited the assistance of Alan Stone, president-elect of APA, to support the establishment of an APA Council on Aging. On February 23, 1979, the APA created a Council on Aging, effective September 1979.

Also in 1979, Congress held the first national legislative conference on the mental health of older Americans.

The 1980s

In 1980, two major textbooks were published in the field of geriatric psychiatry: *The Handbook of Mental Health and Aging* and *A Handbook of Geriatric Psychiatry* (Birren and Sloane 1980; Busse and Blazer 1980). They appropriately reflected and started a veritable explosion in information and knowledge in the field of geriatric psychiatry.

The APA Council on Aging, working in close collaboration with AAGP, focused on several important issues of our time: psychiatric services, reimbursement options, AD, the interface of medicine and psychiatry in geriatrics, the White House Conferences on Aging of 1981 and 1991, postgraduate education, nursing homes, geriatric psychiatry in the public sector, minorities, forensic psychiatric issues, and psychotropic medication for older people (Baker et al. 1985; Finkel et al. 1981; Moak et al. 1989). Chairpersons of the council were Jack Weinberg, Charles Gaitz, Charles Wells, Sanford Finkel, Charles Shamoian, Gene Cohen, and Jerome Yesavage.

At the same time, AAGP was becoming a major force on the national scene. As the decade progressed, membership approached 1,000 psychiatrists. Its newsletter began publishing six times per year and a variety of new programs were instituted. Some of the major accomplishments of AAGP included an active advocacy role with the American Board of Psychiatry and Neurology to achieve "added qualifications" in geriatric psychiatry, with the first examination scheduled for 1991. This event followed the decision, 3 years earlier, of the American Board of Internal Medicine and the American Board of Family Practice to offer certificates of added qualifications in geriatrics in 1988. In anticipation of this major landmark event, AAGP edited and published a syllabus of geriatric psychiatry (Lazarus 1988). AAGP presidents in the 1980s included Sanford Finkel, Eric Pfeiffer, Alvin Levenson, Lissy Jarvik, Elliott Stein, Charles Shamoian, Lawerence Lazarus, and George Grossberg.

The 1980s also marked the substantial growth of lay organizations concerned with the elderly. In addition to the continued growth of the American Association for Retired Persons and the National Council on Aging, the Alzheimer's Disease and Related Disorders Association (ADRDA) was organized to meet an increasing human need and pursue the following goals:

- To better serve Alzheimer's patients and other patients with dementia and their families (ADRDA's goals included supporting research into diagnosis, therapies, causes and cures for AD).
- To aid and organize family support groups in their own localities so as to give assistance, encouragement, and education to afflicted families.
- To sponsor educational forums.
- To dispense information to both lay and professional people with AD.
- To advise government agencies (federal and state) of the needs of afflicted families as well as the need for extensive research on a nationwide scale.
- Most important, to offer assistance, when needed in any manner whatsoever, to those afflicted and their loved ones.

The cause of the demented and their families has been furthered substantially by the publication of *The 36-Hour Day*, written by Nancy Mace and geriatric psychiatrist Peter Rabins (Mace and Rabins 1981).

In 1980, child psychiatrist Arthur Kornhaber established the Foundation for Grandparenting. This group emphasizes the relationship between grandparent and grandchild as a meaningful, healthy, positive relationship. Among its accomplishments, the foundation has brought to the attention of legislators the need to establish the legal right for grandparents and grandchildren to maintain contact after the middle generation has divorced (Kornhaber and Woodward 1981).

The 1981 White House Conference on Aging established a number of sound recommendations based on the multi-disciplinary mini-conference on the Mental Health of Older Americans (White House Conference on Aging 1981). The action group to implement the recommendations did some careful research on community mental health centers and the general problems of underserving the elderly (Fleming et al. 1984). Further, the White House Conference recommendation to expand mental health benefits was finally implemented in 1988. At the end of the decade, outpatient psychiatric benefits increased from $250 a year to $1,000 a year (50% of $500 versus 50% of $2,200). Psychologists became eligible for reimbursement under certain conditions. Further, under the leadership of Margaret Heckler, Secretary of Health and Human Services, Alzheimer's centers in various sections of the country were created and psychiatrists treating demented patients were reimbursed without an annual maximum when providing medical therapy and medication to demented elderly.

Congress passed Public Law 99-660 in 1986, authorizing a Council on Alzheimer's Disease, as well as a panel on AD with a primary goal of creating a major services research program in the area of AD and related dementias. Meanwhile, research budgets for aging and mental health have increased annually in both NIA and the NIMH Center for Studies of the Mental Health of the Aging.

International activities have also grown rapidly. The World Psychiatric Association section on geriatric psychiatry increased its visibility with meetings in Europe and North America. In Sweden, much progress was made in diagnostic tests for AD and other dementias (Steen and Bucht 1988); and in Japan, dementia research has expanded with special emphasis on diagnosis, pathology, and caretaker support (Homma and Hasegawa 1989).

In 1988, the Royal College of Physicians in London created its first examination for a diploma in geriatric medicine. The examination was not for "geriatric specialists," but rather for physicians who are general practitioners and who wish to have special expertise in geriatric medicine. An extensive psychogeriatric program has been established in Nottingham, United Kingdom, under the leadership of Tom Arie, a geriatric psychiatrist who has developed a comprehensive system of training for medical students, physicians, nurses, and other geriatric health care professionals (Arie et al. 1985).

The Canadian Psychiatric Association developed a division on aging in the 1970s. The Canadian Geriatric Association also was active in the 1970s, and both groups continued their activities into the 1980s. The first Canadian division of geriatric psychiatry for the training of geriatric psychiatrists was established at the University of Toronto in 1978 under the leadership of Dr. Abraham Miller. In 1981, the Royal College of Physicians and Surgeons of Canada gave its first examination for certification in geriatric medicine, and in 1983 the college mandated that all psychiatric training programs include psychogeriatric experience (Reichenfeld 1987).

The World Health Organization (WHO) has had a long-standing interest in psychogeriatrics, having published an early monograph (1972) which elaborated the extent of the potential problems of psychopathology in later life, organizational services, research, epidemiology, and training (Henderson and MacFadyen 1985). WHO has made efforts to stimulate the production of self-help guides and has developed monographs on drugs and senile dementia as well as mental health care (WHO 1972, 1983, 1984, 1985). Other areas of exploration in psychogeriatrics include assessing mental health care needs in the community and attention to diagnostic classification. Currently, there is a great deal of interest in these dementias with focus on improving clinical drug evaluation and other therapeutic interventions.

The World Assembly on Aging met in Vienna in 1982 to determine an international policy on many issues related to aging, including psychogeriatrics (United Nations 1983).

The major thrust for international collaboration in psychogeriatrics in the 1980s came from the International Psychogeriatric Association (IPA). The fledgling organization began as the "Nottingham 1980 Club," following an annual 2-week psychogeriatric conference for geriatric psychiatrists, internists, and general practitioners engaged in psychogeriatric clinical work. The course was devised and supervised by Tom Arie. Shortly after the 1980 meeting, two Canadians, Imre Fejer and Hans Reichenfeld, sought to establish an international organization. After collaboration with

Dr. A. Ashour of Ain Shams Medical School in Egypt, Cairo became the site of the first meeting of the IPA: the International Conference for the Mental Health of the Elderly. As a result of the meeting, the Egyptian medical schools in Cairo incorporated geriatrics into their training, and the Egyptian Medical Association developed a special committee on geriatrics. The conference was marred by Mideast politics, and subsequently the small international group was temporarily divided by factions. However, unified support was established by the late 1980s. Under the strong leadership of Presidents Manfred Bergener, Gustav Bucht, and Kazuo Hasegawa, and with publication of a newsletter and later a journal (*International Psychogeriatrics*) and two annual conferences, the organization has grown significantly and has played a role in the founding of national psychogeriatric societies in Japan, Italy, and Sweden.

The 1980s also saw a rapid growth in the number of journals in geriatric psychiatry, including *The International Journal of Geriatric Psychiatry* (Elaine Murphy, editor), *International Psychogeriatrics* (Gene Cohen, editor), *Comprehensive Gerontology* (Alvar Svanborg, editor), *The Journal of Alzheimer's Disease and Related Disorders* (Lissy Jarvik, editor), and *The Journal of Cross-Cultural Anthropology* (Jay Sokolovsky, editor), to name but a few. Pharmaceutical companies have become increasingly interested and involved as the world's population ages. The Sandoz Research Awards in Gerontology were established in 1984, and the Bayer Psychogeriatric Research Awards were established in 1989. Sandoz, Bristol-Myers, Bayer, Hoffmann-LaRoche, Upjohn, Mead-Johnson, Charter Medical, and many others have sponsored educational and research activities.

Other ideas that grew up in the 1980s included the concept of the teaching nursing home (Schneider et al. 1985); age-associated memory impairment as a condition of "normal aging"; and new assessment scales, including the Global Deterioration Scale (Reisberg et al. 1982), the Geriatric Depression Scale (Sheikh et al. 1986), and a variety of brief mental status measurements (of which the Mini-Mental State Exam [Folstein et al. 1975] remains the most popular). The use of sophisticated equipment for diagnostic purposes (e.g., nuclear magnetic resonance, magnetic resonance imaging, positron emission tomography, single photon emission computed tomography, and position emission tomography) has risen rapidly in our technologically oriented world (Margolin and Daniel 1990). Further, the use of electronics and electronic gadgets has played an increasing role in supporting the mental health of the elderly (Lieff 1990; Stein 1990).

In the chapters that follow, the reader will be provided with state-of-the-art knowledge in the broad field of psychogeriatrics, as well as insights into future trends and possibilities in the years immediately ahead. One fact is abundantly clear: the amount of amassed knowledge and research activity in the field of geriatric psychiatry in the 1990s will, by itself, be greater than in all the history of psychogeriatrics before 1990.

References

Abraham K: The applicability of psychoanalytic treatment to patients at an advanced age, in Abraham, K. Selected papers on psychoanalysis. London, Hogarth Press, 1927, pp 312–317

Alzheimer A: A characteristic disease of the cerebral cortex, in The Early Story of Alzheimer's Disease. New York, Raven Press, 1906

Arie T, Jones R, Smith C: The educational potential of old age psychiatric services, in Recent Advances in Psychogeriatrics. Edited by Arie T. Edinburgh, Churchill Livingstone, 1985

Baker FN, Pen IN, Yesavage JY: An Overview of Legal Issues in Geriatric Psychiatry. Washington, DC, American Psychiatric Association, 1985

Barraclough B: Conversations with Felix Post: part II. Psychiatric Bulletin 13:114–119, 1989

Berezin MA, Cath SH (eds): Geriatric Psychiatry: Grief, Loss, and Emotional Disorders in the Aging Process. New York, International Universities Press, 1965

Birren J, Sloane B: Handbook of Mental Health and Aging. Englewood Cliffs, NJ, Prentice-Hall, 1980

Busse EW: The myth, history, and science of aging, in Geriatric Psychiatry. Edited by Busse EW, Blazer DG. Washington DC, American Psychiatric Press, 1989, pp 3–34

Busse EW, Blazer DG (eds): Handbook of Geriatric Psychiatry. New York, Van Nostrand Reinhold, 1980

Busse EW, Pfeiffer E (eds): Behavior and Adaptation in Late Life. Boston, MA, Little, Brown, 1969

Butler RN: Mission of the National Institution on Aging. J Am Geriatr Soc 25(30): 97–103, 1977

Ciompi L: The outcome of late life psychiatric disorders. J Geriatr Psychiatry 39:789–794, 1972

Clark JE, Lanphear AK, Riddick CC: The effects of videogame playing on the response selection processing of elderly adults. J Gerontol 4:82–85, 1987

Cohen GD: The Brain in Human Aging. New York, Springer, 1988

Cohen GD: The movement toward subspecialty status for geriatric psychiatry in the United States. International Psychogeriatrics 1:201–205, 1989

Ferenczi S: A contribution to the understanding of the psychoneuroses of the age of involution, in Selected Papers: Problems and Methods of Psychoanalysis, Vol III. Final Contributions to the Problems and Methods of Psychoanalysis. Edited by S. Ferenczi. New York, Basic Books, 1955

Finkel SI: The rationale for the creation of an American psychiatric council on aging. AAGP Newsletter 1:5, 1978

Finkel SI: Experience of a private practice psychiatrist working with the elderly in the community. Inst J Mental Health 8:147–172, 1979

Finkel SI, Borson S, Shamoian C, et al: The American Psychiatric Association Task Force Report on the 1981 White House Conference on Aging. Washington, DC, American Psychiatric Association, 1981

Fleming AS, Buchanan JG, Santos JF: Report on the Survey of Community Health Centers by the Action Committee to Implement the Mental Health Recommendations of the 1981 White House Conference on Aging. Chicago, The Retirement Research Foundation, 1984

Folstein, M, Folstein S, McHugh PR: Mini-Mental State: a practical method of grading the cognitive state of patients for the clinician. J Psychiatr Res 12:189–198, 1975

Freud S: Sexuality in the Aetiology of the Neuroses, in Freud Collected Papers. Edited by Ernest Jones, Vol I. London, Hogarth Press, 1948

Group for the Advancement of Psychiatry: Psychiatry and the Aged: An Introductory Approach. Vol 5, No 59. New York, GAP, 1965

Group for the Advancement of Psychiatry: Mental Health and Aging: Approaches to Curriculum Development, Vol 11, No 114. New York, Mental Health Materials Center, 1983.

Group for the Advancement of Psychiatry, Committee on Aging: The Aged and Community Mental Health: A Guide to Program Development, Vol VIII, No 81. New York, GAP, 1971

Group for the Advancement of Psychiatry: The Psychiatric Treatment of Alzheimer's Disease. Report No. 125, New York, Brunner/Mazel, 1988

Group for the Advancement of Psychiatry Committee on Aging: The Psychiatric Treatment of Alzheimer's Disease. New York, Brunner/Mazel, 1988

Group for the Advancement of Psychiatry: The problem of the aged patient in the public psychiatric hospital. No. 14, New York, GAP, 1950

Hall GS: Senescence: The Last Half of Life. New York, Appleton, 1922

Henderson JH, MacFadyen DM: Psychogeriatrics and the programmes of the World Health Organization, in Recent Advances in Psychogeriatrics. Edited by Arie T. Edinburgh, Churchill Livingstone, 1985

Homma A, Hasegawa K: Recent developments in gerontopsychiatric research on age-associated dementia in Japan. International Psychogeriatrics 1:31–50, 1989

Kornhaber A, Woodward KL: Grandparents/Grandchildren: The Vital Connection. Garden City, NY, Anchor Press/Doubleday, 1981

Jarvik L: The impact of immediate life situations on depression, illness, and loss, in Depression and Aging. Edited by Bresla D, Haig MR. New York, Springer, 1983

Lazarus LW (ed): Essentials of Geriatric Psychiatry. New York, Springer, 1988

Levin S, Kahana RJ: Psychodynamic Studies on Aging, Creativity, Reminiscing, and Dying. New York, International Universities Press, 1967

Lieff J: High technology and geriatric psychiatry, in Clinical and Scientific Psychogeriatrics. Edited by Bergener M, Finkel S. New York, Springer, 1990 pp 112–135

Loza N, Milad G: Old Age in the History of Ancient Civilization in Egypt. (submitted) 1989

Mace NL, Rabins PV: The 36-Hour Day. Baltimore, MD, Johns Hopkins University Press, 1981

Margolin R, Daniel D: Neuroimaging in geropsychiatry, in Clinical and Scientific Psychogeriatrics. Edited by Bergener M, Finkel S. New York, Springer, 1990

Maugham S: The Summing Up. London, William Heinemann Ltd., 1938

Moak GS, Stein EM, Rubin JEV: The Over-50 Guide to Psychiatric Medications. Washington, DC, American Psychiatric Association, 1989

Nascher IL: Geriatrics: The Diseases of Old Age and Their Treatment. Philadelphia, PA, P. Blokiston's Son, 1914

Nascher IL: The Aging Mind. Medical Record 157:669, 1944

Palmore E (ed): Normal Aging: Reports from the Duke Longitudinal Study, 1955–1969. Durham, NC, Duke University Press, 1970

Palmore E (ed): Normal Aging: II. Durham, NC, Duke University Press, 1974

Post F: The Clinical Psychiatry of Late Life. Oxford, Pergamon, 1965

Reichenfeld HF: Geriatric psychiatry north of the border. AAGP Newsletter 9:(3)11–12, 1987

Reisberg B, Ferris SH, DeLeon MJ, et al: The Global Deterioration Scale for assessment of primary degenerative dementia. Am J Psychiatry 139:1136–1139, 1982

Rowe JW, Grossman E, Bond E, The Institute of Medicine Committee on Leadership for Academic Geriatric Medicine: Academic geriatrics for the year 2000. N Engl J Med 316:1425–1428, 1987

Sadavoy J, Leszcz M: Treating the Elderly With Psychotherapy: The Scope for Change in Later Life. New York, International Universities Press, 1987

Schneider EL, Wendland CJ, Zimmer AW, et al: The Teaching Nursing Home—A New Approach to Geriatric Research, Education, and Clinical Care. New York, Raven, 1985

Sheikh JI, Yesavage JA, Brink PL: Geriatric Depression Scale (GDS): recent evidence and development of a short version, in Clinical Gerontology: A Guide to Assessment and Intervention. Edited by Brink TL. New York, Haworth Press, 1986

Shock NW: The International Association of Gerontology: A Chronicle—1950 to 1986. New York, Springer, 1988

Siever LJ, Davis KL: Overview: toward a dysregulation hypothesis of depression. Am J Psychiatry 142:1017–1031, 1985

Steen B, Bucht G: Psychogeriatrics in Sweden. IPA Newsletter 5(3):23–25, 1988

Stein E: Gadgets and other high-tech devices for use with the elderly, in Clinical and Scientific Psychogeriatrics. Edited by Bergener M, Finkel S. New York, Springer, 1990

United Nations, World Assembly on Aging: Vienna International Plan of Action on Aging. New York, United Nations, 1983

U.S. Department of Health, Education, and Welfare, Public Health Service: National Institute of Mental Health Research on the Mental Health of the Aging—1960–1976. (DHEW Publ No 79-397) Rockville, MD, 1977

U.S. Department of Health, Education, and Welfare, Federal Council on Aging: Mental health and the elderly—recommendations for action. The Reports of the President's Commission on Mental Health: Task Panel on the Elderly and the Secretary's Committee on Mental Health and Illness of the Elderly (DHEW Publ No 80-20960). Washington, DC, U.S. Government Printing Office, 1979

White House Conference on Aging: Report of the Mini-Conference on the Mental Health of Older Americans (Mer-16). Washington, DC, U.S. Government Printing Office, 1981

World Health Organization: Senile Dementia: Report of a Scientific Group. Geneva, World Health Organization, 1972

World Health Organization: Psychogeriatrics. Report of a World Health Organization Scientific Group. Technical Report Series No 507. Geneva, World Health Organization, 1972

World Health Organization: Mental Health Care of the Elderly: Report on a Working Group. Copenhagen, World Health Organization regional office for Europe, 1983

World Health Organization: Self Health Care and Older People: A Manual for Public Policy and Programme Development. Copenhagen, World Health Organization, 1984

World Health Organization: Drugs and the Elderly. Copenhagen, World Health Organization, 1985

Zinberg NE, Kaufman I: Normal Psychology of the Aging Process. New York, International Universities Press, 1963

CHAPTER 2

Barry Gurland, M.D.

Epidemiology of Psychiatric Disorders

Overview

Epidemiology can contribute to learning about psychiatric problems in relation to aging by the study of the variation in frequency of psychiatric problems between subgroups of aging persons. Frequency is usually expressed as prevalence (over a period of time or at a single point in time) or incidence (new cases or episodes during a period of time, usually a year). A more complex strategy of epidemiology is discovery of the current characteristics (e.g., age) or antecedent characteristics (e.g., previous personality) that are unique to persons with a given psychiatric problem.

Subgroups of persons can be delineated in any manner that offers promise of revealing variation in frequencies of psychiatric problems or of their associated characteristics. Analysis of the characteristics of those subgroups and their circumstances can identify public health challenges and can lead to an understanding of the forces that govern the origin and course of psychiatric problems.

Characteristics that are routinely used to define subgroups of persons or the associations of psychiatric problems include the setting (e.g., geographic region, community or institution, type of health services), demography (e.g., age, gender, race), and social context (e.g., marital status, income, education, occupation). Each of these characteristics can be measured crudely or can be refined (e.g., by detailing the social network) to allow the examination of a promising hypothesis. Other informative subgroups or associated characteristics may be derived from suspected risk factors, previous personality, life events, personal and family history of psychiatric problems, service utilization, physical health disorders, and the like. Correspondingly, psychiatric problems are typically taken to mean diagnostic groups but may be restricted to those meeting criteria in a nomenclature, such as DSM-III-R (American Psychiatric Association 1987), or may be expanded to refer to innovative categories, symptoms, or such nonspecific problems as the functional consequences of psychiatric disorder.

Epidemiology makes little sense if it is restricted to mustering subgroups and counting problems; it is the analysis of the circumstances surrounding variation that carries fundamental clinical and organizational implications for geriatric psychiatry.

Epidemiologic Issues That Span Psychiatric Problems

Given the protean applications of epidemiology and its ubiquitous relevance to psychiatric problems in aging, there is a likelihood of redundancy between this chapter on epidemiology and corresponding sections of the chapters on particular psychiatric problems. In order to minimize redundancy, I will concentrate in this chapter on epidemiologic issues that are best addressed by scanning across specific psychiatric problems. Some issues regarding psychiatric problems of the elderly that lend themselves to this approach are 1) estimating the extent and location of the need for treatment of problems; 2) scouting for opportunities to reduce the risk of onset, persistence, or relapse of problems; 3) gauging the effects of age on severity and course of problems; and 4) clarifying what it is about psychiatric problems that is specific to aging.

Estimating the Extent and Location of the Need for Treatment

The need for treatment of psychiatric problems in a defined population should be estimated with a level of accuracy that would guide (not mislead) policy and organization for services. This estimating requires knowledge of certain features of each problem: prevalence at a point in time by setting and demography; incidence of cases and episodes during the period of aging; potential for benefits from treatment; proportion of cases receiving inappropriate treatment; and contacts of cases with health care resources during the course of the problem, with possible sites of treatment or referral and availability of internal sources of care. In addition, it is desirable to know the extent to which disposition and treatment are determined by overlap between psychiatric problems and the frequency of types of comorbidity. Other informative facts that can guide estimates of need for treatment include the range of duration of the problem and the rates of recovery and relapse with and without treatment; the frequency and severity of consequences; and the size and location of high-risk groups. Moreover, barriers and resistances to access, extent of demand, compliance with treatment recommendations, quality and cost of care, and human resources considerations also have a bearing on estimations of fulfilled and unfulfilled needs for treatment.

These important epidemiologic indicators of need are incompletely documented. Nevertheless, it is evident from prevalence data that psychiatric problems are frequent during the period conventionally designated as old age (starting at age 65).

In the community elderly (i.e., samples representative of all noninstitutionalized persons aged 65 years or older in a geographic area), depressions conforming to DSM-III (American Psychiatric Association 1980) criteria (major depression, dysthymia, cyclothymic disorder, and atypical depression) are between 2% and 4% (Myers et al. 1984) of the population, with major depression accounting for less than 1% (Blazer et al. 1980); but if all persons with depressive symptomatology of clinical interest are included, the rates rise to between 10% and 15% (Blazer and Williams 1980; Gurland et al. 1983).

Active symptoms among schizophrenic individuals grown old and late-onset persistent paranoid states are noted in less than 0.5% of the population, although their obtrusive behavior may leave the impression of a more frequent presence (Kay 1972). With more sensitive measures, as much as 11% or more of the elderly are found to be paranoid (Lowenthal 1964; Savage et al. 1972).

About 7.5% of all elderly suffer from progressive dementias; about two-thirds of these reside in the community (Gurland and Cross 1982), although this proportion can drop to one-half or less where the capacity of long-term care facilities is large (Bland et al. 1988).

Anxiety disorders including panic, phobia, and obsessional and somatization disorders range from 4% upward, with the most common form being agoraphobias, especially in older women (Turnbull and Turnbull 1985); alcohol and drug dependence is about 1% to 2% (Bland et al. 1988; Kramer et al. 1985; Weissman et al. 1985).

Among short-stay psychiatric inpatients, depressions that meet DSM-III-R criteria are common. Often half of all admissions meet the criteria for major depression. A minority (about 10%) of first admissions to inpatient units after the age of 60 have late-onset symptoms closely related to schizophrenia (Kay and Roth 1961).

In long-stay psychiatric centers such as state psychiatric hospitals, there are a disproportionate number of elderly—as much as half the resident population (Goodman and Siegel 1986); a substantial proportion, if not a majority (35%–60%) of these elderly are first admitted during earlier adulthood with a diagnosis of schizophrenia. Many aged schizophrenic individuals are placed in nursing homes, especially if chronic medical problems have supervened. On average, about 3% of elderly nursing-home residents have a primary paranoid state. Half or more of the long-stay residents in nursing homes suffer from Alzheimer's disease (AD) or related dementia. Overall, the great majority of nursing home residents suffer from a psychiatric problem in the form of a disorder (mostly dementia) or a behavioral disturbance (Rovner et al. 1986); the need for suitably trained staff in these locations is pressing.

Some psychiatric problems of the elderly are encountered more frequently in medical than in psychiatric settings. In medical settings, anxiety and depressive disorders are common, especially atypical rather than major depressions (Sireling et al. 1985), and depressions accompanying acute and chronic medical disorder (Kukull et al. 1986). Affective and anxiety disorders are associated with both acute and chronic limitations of physical functioning (Wells et al. 1988). Confusional states occur in more than 25% of general medical inpatients (Knight and Folstein 1977) and rehabilitation inpatients (Garcia et al. 1984) and even more commonly in neurology service populations (DePaulo and Folstein 1978). Psychotropic medications such as sedatives and hypnotics are actively dispensed to the elderly, often by primary care physicians, who are often the sole providers of professional care for the patients with mental health problems (Ware 1986). Yet there are reports that medical residents often lack adequate knowledge of the recognition and treatment of comorbid depression (Rapp and Davis 1989). Furthermore, the elderly are less likely than younger patients to be evaluated and treated by a mental health specialist, even where there is contact with a health care center where specialist referrals are available and where the prevalence of psychiatric problems warranting conventional diagnosis is not decreased by age (Goldstrom et al. 1987).

Although the prevalence rate of dementia reaches 20% over age 80, the extent to which this scourge threatens the average person is better conveyed by the lifetime risk: about 1 in 3 for men who survive to 85 years (Sluss et al. 1981), and probably in the same range for women. Women are probably not more prone to develop dementia, but many more of them survive to extreme old age, where the risk is highest.

Rates of psychiatric problems relative to age suggest that depression plateaus after 65 years and then decreases with further aging (Comstock and Helsing 1976; Eaton and Kessler 1981; Frerichs et al. 1981; Gurland 1976; Myers et al. 1984; Robins et al. 1984). It may seem that the exceptionally high rate of suicide among elderly white males in this country stands in contradiction to the flat age variation curve of depression. Closer examination shows, however, that this rise in suicide rates with age is really a generational (cohort) phenomenon and is not due to aging (Cross and Gurland 1984); future groups of elderly white males will probably have lower rates of suicide as do current cohorts of females and nonwhites. Nevertheless, the elderly tend now to be deadly serious in their suicidal actions; their first attempt is likely to be their last.

Apart from cognitive impairment, the prevalence of most psychiatric disorders and overall prevalence decreases as older age supervenes (Bland et al. 1988; Kramer et al. 1985; Weissman et al. 1985).

Relative to younger age groups, the incidence rates for major depressive disorder, panic disorder, and drug abuse are lower in the elderly. However, the incidence of phobic disorders does not drop off with age, at least in males; obsessive-compulsive disorder may increase in elderly women, and alcohol abuse increases in the very old, especially in men (Eaton et al. 1989).

It is widely accepted that schizophrenia and conditions related to schizophrenia such as paranoid disorder (sometimes diagnosed as paraphrenia in Europe) may occur for the first time in late adulthood (45–64 years of age) or old age (Rabins et al. 1984; Volavka and Cancro 1986). Late-onset schizophrenia as a proportion of all schizophrenic individuals varies from about 10% (less for men and more for women) to as high as one-third of first admissions aged 45 to 64 years (Goodman and Siegel 1986). Manic states occur less commonly with advancing age but are often found—even in first episodes—to be associated with central nervous system lesions in this age group. Rates of dementia rise steeply with age and reach 20% over age 80. Incidence varies from less than 1% annually at age 70 to about 4% annually at age 85.

Epidemiologic data suggest higher rates of depression and dementia in certain socioeconomically disadvantaged elderly groups. However, at present this finding must be taken to refer to depressive symptoms and poor performance on measures of cognitive performance; the implications for diagnosis and the need for treatment are not clear.

Scouting for Opportunities to Reduce the Risk of Onset, Persistence, and Relapse

The discovery of precedents of a condition can suggest preventive interventions. In the instance of depression in old age, there is a strong clinical impression, and some research evidence (Murphy 1982), that negative life events such as bereavement often—some say usually—precipitate the episodes of symptoms. Persons without a significant other with whom they can share their thoughts and feelings and from whom they can gather encouragement and comfort appear to be particularly vulnerable. Diagnostic caution is necessary, however, in light of evidence presented by Zisook at the 1990 annual meeting of the American Association for Geriatric Psychiatry. In the examination of a sample of bereaved elderly, symptoms of self-limiting grief could not be distinguished from diagnostic symptoms of depression in the first 3 months after the loss.

These views gain some support from epidemiology. In a community study that included the elderly with disabilities, it was found that life events, chronic strain, and social support had independent effects on depression (Turner and Noh 1988). Caregivers of persons with dementia—especially those who seek help—are prone to develop clinically diagnosable depression (Gallagher et al. 1989). Life events have also been observed to influence the outcome of depression in the elderly (Murphy 1983). The outcome of depression is also altered by the size, functioning, and perceived helpfulness and warmth of the social network; the quality of social exchanges is more salient than the mere quantity of social interactions, however (George et al. 1989). Nevertheless, older subjects have fewer life events (Turner and Wood 1985), and life events may be less distressing to the elderly than to younger persons (Dean et al. 1980).

The correlation of depression in the elderly with physical illness or disability is especially striking (Revenson and Felton 1985; Turner and Noh 1988). This association holds true not only for the symptoms and syndromes of depression but also for depression diagnoses such as major depression (Hall et al. 1980; Kinzie et al. 1986); risk for depression in the physically ill elderly is increased up to threefold. An overlapping consideration is the frequency with which medication side effects lead to depression; more than one-third of major depressions found in one community study were associated with medication use (Kinzie et al. 1986). Lists of particularly depressogenic drugs and diseases are known (Ouslander 1982) and point to the need to avoid nonessential medications and optimize health. With some exceptions [e.g., depression following cerebrovascular lesions in specific regions of the brain, as described by Robinson et al. (1984)], the links between physical illness and depression are general and multiple rather than specific (Borson et al. 1986; Kukull et al. 1986).

The observation that coexistent depression slows recovery from physical illness suggests that treating the physical illness may be a means of secondarily preventing the prolongation of the depression. The converse aspect of prevention is also supported by epidemiologic data: depression impedes recovery of function in medical conditions such as ischemic heart disease (Morgan 1983), stroke (Feibel and Springer 1982), and disability from a variety of causes (Gurland et al. 1989). More broadly, there are data consistent with the possibility that mortality is increased in a number of psychiatric conditions (Granville-Grossman 1983), even allowing for the effects of suicide, accidental death, long-term psychiatric hospitalization, and maintenance medications (Sims and Prior 1978).

Longer-range possibilities for prevention of late-onset paranoid states (except those associated with cognitive impairment) are raised by epidemiologic findings. Most studies show that an abnormal personality (cold and querulous) and an unfavorable social milieu are a long prelude to the emergence of frank paranoid symptoms in old age (Christenson and Blazer 1984; Kay et al. 1976; Post 1966). Prior social isolation is common; the sufferers are often unmarried or have few children, although they usually manage in independent existence fairly well (Eisdorfer 1980). Even if these personal characteristics are prodromal signs of an eventual psychotic disorder, they offer a means of intervention for high-risk groups.

The role of deafness as a predisposing influence on late-life paranoid states is an epidemiologic finding (Cooper et al. 1976) that has tantalized investigators seeking to turn it to a useful clinical purpose. The data are consistent across long-stay and recently admitted psychiatric patients and community-residing elderly: deafness is more frequent, about threefold, in elderly persons with a late-onset paranoid disorder than in age-matched controls or patients with affective disorder. Hearing impairment, which affects receptive communication in social situations, is quite severe on audiometric testing. Most intriguing is that the deafness is the conductive type associated with the sequelae of middle ear disease, not the type induced by aging processes. By its nature and by report, the deafness seems to begin many years before the onset of paranoid symptoms, but not prior to the developmental stage of language acquisition. Deafness appears to predispose to paranoid disorder even in those without the typical vulnerable personality. The majority of recent studies are in line with these conclusions (Eastwood et al. 1985).

Although the dementias are for the most part not yet proven to be amenable to preventive strategies, consideration of the relative rates of the dementia subtypes and of conditions that can mimic dementia keeps the issue of prevention open. In a typical survey of a representative sample of the general elderly population, AD alone accounts for about 55% to 60% of cases of dementia, fewer than 10% to 15% are due to multi-infarcts or other cerebrovascular disorders, and in another 15% both are present and it is difficult to establish whether the pathology of AD or of multi-infarcts predominates. The residual group amounts to about 15% and includes dementias or states of cognitive impairment associated with well-recognized neurological diseases (e.g., Huntington's chorea or parkinsonism) and a variety of causes that may be treatable, for example, local or general increased intracranial pressure; systemic effects from metabolic, toxic, or anoxic conditions; and altered mood. In specialized services devoted to the diagnostic evaluation of cases suspected to be dementia, reversible or treatable conditions are found in the range of 10% to 20% of cases (Cummings 1983; Rabins 1985).

Also eminently treatable is delirium, which presents with symptoms distinguishable from dementia. Because delirium is usually caused by factors surrounding medical illness, it is common in acute medical settings (McCartney and Palmateer 1985).

Gauging the Effects of Age on Severity and Course of Problems

The fact that rates of major depression and probably other types of depression do not rise with advancing age implies that the elderly are able to cope well with physical illness and other age-related insults. The elderly are less prone to self-blame regarding their disability (Felton and Revenson 1987) and more likely to receive calmly the reality or possibility of life-threatening illness such as cancer (Cohen 1980; Mages and Mendelsohn 1979). The elderly may be viewed as a band of survivors who have learned to cope with adverse circumstances, perhaps because certain negative events are sufficiently common at this age to acquire a normative value (they are "on time") (Neugarten and Datan 1973). Events such as physical illness tend to be more chronic than acute, and perhaps less stressful, as age increases. On the other hand, individuals with earlier-onset depression may be vulnerable to premature death or institutionalization and hence do not enter the cohort of community-residing elderly, or—a more optimistic view—they receive treatment that prevents new episodes from occurring in later life. Possibly there are neurobiological changes with age that make the older person less vulnerable to depression with or without a stressor such as disability. It has been suggested, although there are many reservations about the evidence, that successive cohorts of elderly have shown progressively higher rates of depression and an earlier age of onset (Klerman et al. 1985).

Recovery rates in major depression are comparable between the elderly and younger age groups (Post 1972). However, high rates of relapse are the rule among elderly depressives. Although 90% recover initially, about 75% relapse over the long term unless maintained on pharmacological treatment (Post 1984). Among treated elderly depressives followed for a few years, approximately one-third stay well, one-third remain depressed, and one-third recover and relapse.

The majority of schizophrenic individuals will achieve old age despite the fact that they have a higher death rate than the general population (Allebeck and Wistedt 1986). Most will be left with impaired functioning, including about one-third of the whole cohort who will have chronic or relapsing symptoms. However, about one-third of the survivors to old age will have recovered virtually completely (Ciompi 1985).

Clarifying What It Is About Psychiatric Problems That Is Particular to Aging

Psychiatric problems in the elderly occur in the context of physical, mental, and social aging. Among the population aged 65 years and older, a majority have at least one chronic physical disorder but a minority are impaired in mobility or capacity to carry out the daily tasks of independent living: self-care and household chores. Only about 5% of all elderly need to live in highly sheltered residences such as nursing homes, although this percentage increases sharply over the age of 80. Although there are changes in the speed and style of intellectual activities and slowing of the rate of new learning, the great majority of elderly remain mentally active and competent. That is the normal standard against which the onset of disease is evaluated.

Comorbidity would be a feature of psychiatric disorders in old age even if there were no casual relationship involved. The increase of concurrent physical and mental problems, beyond chance, with respect to depression and acute or chronic physical disorder was mentioned earlier. This increase occurs for other psychiatric disorders such as manic states as well.

An important type of concurrence is that of depression and intellectual impairment. In general, depressive disorders in the elderly, such as major depressions, are quite distinct in nature and natural history from the dementias such as AD. Kay (1962) and Post (1972) found no increased risk of dementia in patients with late-onset depression. However, Reding and associates (1985) demonstrated that 57% (16 of 28) of the depressed, nondemented elderly subjects went on to develop frank dementia. Some investigators (e.g., Jacoby et al. 1980, 1983) have found brain changes (enlarged ventricles and reduced radiodensity) in late-onset depressions. These changes do not occur in age-matched early-onset depressions; moreover, the changes do not include the pathology typical of Alzheimer's or multi-infarct dementias (Tomlinson et al. 1968).

Yet depression and dementialike syndromes are found to occur together even when diagnoses are carefully established. Setting aside those DSM-III-R exclusionary criteria that bear on the presence of an organic etiology, major depression is found in cases of Alzheimer's and related dementias at high rates—20% to 30% in some series (Larson et al. 1985). In these mixed conditions, the cognitive impairment component usually follows a progressively deteriorating course despite improvement in depression in response to treatment (McAllister and Price 1982; Rabins 1984). In about 10% of major depressions a syndrome resembling dementia may arise that is resolved when the depression remits (Madden et al. 1952; Post 1975). Termed depressive pseudodementia by some, it comes under the wider rubric of treatable or reversible dementias.

The proportion of cases with this uncharacteristically poor outcome ranges from a minority of about 20% (Rabins 1985) to about half (Reding 1985), or even a large majority if follow-up is long enough (Kral 1983). A useful position to take is that depression in the elderly, if free of cognitive impairment, is no different in outcome than depressions at younger ages, although it is often more difficult to treat; but if cognitive impairment is concurrent, the prognosis is somewhat more guarded. As for short-term outcomes, depressions that are apparently primary in terms of their responsiveness to pharmacological interventions account for about 5% of cases referred for investigation of dementia and 20% of treatable dementia syndromes (Larson et al. 1985; Rabins 1985). These figures underline the necessity of a careful search for an underlying depression in all new cases of dementia.

The symptoms found in aging schizophrenic patients whose conditions began in earlier life tend to be less vivid and disturbing to the patient and others. When the symptoms result from a late-onset type of condition, a paranoid picture is likely to predominate (Larson and Nyman 1970).

Aging adds distinctive characteristics to the nature, presentation, and treatment of psychiatric problems but also to the social milieu, a vital aspect of treatment that is also illuminated by epidemiology. One-third of elderly people live alone, but regardless, most elderly have someone, usually a daughter, who will assist in the support and management of treatment.

Conclusion

Epidemiologic perspectives highlight the need for specially skilled treatment of psychiatric problems in the elderly, because treatable problems are frequently encountered and require age-relevant understanding for diagnosis, evaluation of causes, and administration of treatment, and because they offer opportunities for prevention. With proper treatment, prognosis in some conditions is as good as and sometimes better than for similar problems in younger persons. Even life-long conditions sometimes improve in old age.

The compelling importance of the field of geriatric psychiatry stems not only from the growing number and proportion of elderly (especially the very old—over 80) but equally from gains in longevity and active life expectancy. This change in the life span means that old age occupies a larger proportion (currently about 20%) of the average life. Consequently, the quality of life in old age and the impact of psychiatric problems on that quality are growing in relevance to the whole of a person's life.

References

Allebeck P, Wistedt B: Mortality in schizophrenia. Arch Gen Psychiatry 43:650–653, 1986

American Psychiatric Association: Diagnostic and Statistical Manual of Mental Disorders, 3rd Edition. Washington, DC, American Psychiatric Association, 1980

American Psychiatric Association: Diagnostic and Statistical Manual of Mental Disorders, 3rd Edition, Revised. Washington, DC, American Psychiatric Association, 1987

Bland RC, Newman SC, Om H: Prevalence of psychiatric disorders in the elderly in Edmonton. Acta Psychiatr Scand 77(suppl 338):57–63, 1988

Blazer D, Hughes DC, George LK: The epidemiology of depression in an elderly community population. Am J Psychiatry 137:4, 439–444, 1980

Borson S, Barnes RA, Kukull WA, et al: Symptomatic depression in elderly medical outpatients, I: prevalence, demography, and health service utilization. J Am Geriatr Soc 34:341–347, 1986

Christenson R, Blazer D: Epidemiology of persecutory ideation in an elderly population in the community. Am J Psychiatry 141:1088–1091, 1989

Ciompi L: Aging and schizophrenic psychosis. Acta Psychiatr Scand 71 (suppl 319):93–105, 1985

Cohen F: Coping with surgery: information, psychological preparation, and recovery, in Aging in the 1980s: Psychological Issues. Edited by Poon LW. Washington, DC, American Psychological Association, 1980, pp 375–382

Comstock, GW, Helsing KJ: Symptoms of depression in two communities. Psychol Med 6:551–563, 1976

Cooper AF, Garside RF, Kay DWK: A comparison of deaf and non-deaf patients with paranoid and affective psychoses. Br J Psychiatry 129:532, 1976

Cross PS, Gurland BJ: Age, period, and cohort views of suicide rates of the elderly, in Suicide and the Life Cycle: Proceedings of the American Association of Suicidology 15th annual meeting, New York, April 1982. Edited by Pfeffer C, Richman J., 1984, pp 70–71

Cummings JL: Treatable dementias. Adv Neurol 38:165–183, 1983

Dean A, Lin N, Mark T, et al: Relating types of social support to depression in the life course. Paper presented at the American Sociological Association, New York, 1980

DePaulo J, Folstein M: Psychiatric disturbances in neurological patients: detection, recognition, and course. Ann Neurol 4:225–228, 1978

Eastwood MR, Corbin S, Reed M, et al: Acquired hearing loss and psychiatric illness: an estimate of prevalence and co-morbidity in a geriatric setting. Br J Psychiatry 147:552, 1985

Eaton W, Kessler LG: Rates of symptoms of depression in a national sample. Am J Epidemiol 114:528–538, 1981

Eaton WW, Kramer M, Anthony JC, et al: The incidence of specific DIS/DSM-III mental disorders: data from the NIMH Epidemiologic Catchment Area Programs. Acta Psychiatr Scand 79:163–178, 1989

Eisdorfer C: Paranoia and schizophrenic disorders in later life, in Handbook of Geriatric Psychiatry. Edited by Busse EW, Blazer DG. New York, Van Nostrand Reinhold, 1980, pp 329–337

Feibel JH, Springer CJ: Depression and failure to resume social activities after stroke. Arch Phys Med Rehabil 63:276–278, 1982

Felton BJ, Revenson TA: Age differences in coping with chronic illness. Psychologizing and Aging. Aging 2:164–170, 1987

Frerichs RR, Aneshensel C, Clark VA: Prevalence of depression in Los Angeles County. Am J Epidemiol 113:1669–1699, 1981

Gallagher D, Rose J, Rivera P, et al: Prevalence of depression in family caregivers. Gerontologist 29:4, 449–456, 1989

Garcia C, Tweedy J, Blass J: Underdiagnosis of cognitive impairment in a rehabilitation setting. J Am Geriatr Soc 32:339–342, 1984

George LK, Blazer DG, Hughes DC, et al: Social support and the outcome of major depression. Br J Psychiatry 154:478–485, 1989

Goldstrom IG, Burns BJ, Kessler LG, et al: Mental health services use by elderly adults in a primary care setting. J Gerontol 42:147–153, 1987

Goodman A, Siegel C: Elderly schizophrenic inpatients in the wake of deinstitutionalization. Am J Psychiatry 143:204, 1986

Granville-Grossman K: Mind and body, in Handbook of Psychiatry, Mental Disorders, and Somatic Illness. Edited by Lader, MH. New York, Cambridge University Press, 1983, pp 5–13

Gurland B: The comparative frequency of depression in various adult age groups. J Gerontol 31:283, 1976

Gurland B, Cross P: The epidemiology of psychopathology in old age: some clinical implications. Psychiatr Clin North Am 5:11–26, 1982

Gurland B, Copeland J, Kuriansky J, et al: The Mind and Mood of Aging. New York, Haworth Press, 1983

Gurland BJ, Wilder DE, Golden R, et al: The relationship between depression and disability in the elderly, in Psychological Assessment of the Elderly. Edited by Wattis JP, Hindmarch I. London, Churchill Livingstone, 1988

Hall RCW, Gardner ER, Stickney SK, et al: Physical illness manifesting as psychiatric disease, II: analysis of a state hospital inpatient population. Arch Gen Psychiatry 37:989–995, 1980

Jacoby RJ, Levy R, Dawson JM: Computed tomography in the elderly, 3: affective disorders. Br J Psychiatry 137:70–275, 1980

Jacoby RJ, Dolan R, Levy R, et al: Quantitative computed tomography in elderly depressed patients. Br J Psychiatry 143:124–127, 1983

Kay DWK: Outcome and course of death in mental disorders of old age. Acta Psychiatr Scand 38:249–276, 1962

Kay DWK: Schizophrenia and schizophrenia-like states in the elderly. Br J Hosp Med 8:369, 1972

Kay DWK, Roth M: Environmental and hereditary factors in the schizophrenias of old age ("late paraphrenia") and their bearing on the general problem of causation in schizophrenia. J Mental Science 107:649, 1961

Kay DWK, Cooper AF, Garside RF, et al: The differentiation of paranoid from affective psychoses by patient's premorbid characteristics. Br J Psychiatry 129:207, 1976

Kinzie JD, Lewinsohn P, Maricle R, et al: The relationship of depression to medical illness in an older community population. Comp Psychiatry 27:241–246, 1986

Klerman G, Lavori PW, Rice J, et al: Birth-cohort trends in rates of major depressive disorder among relatives of patients with affective disorder. Arch Gen Psychiatry 42:689–693, 1985

Knight EB, Folstein MF: Unsuspected emotional and cognitive disturbance in medical patients. Ann Intern Med 87:723–734, 1977

Kral V: The relationship between senile dementia (Alzheimer type) and depression. Can J Psychiatry 28:304–306, 1983

Kramer M, German PS, Anthony JC, et al: Patterns of mental disorders among the elderly residents of eastern Baltimore. J Am Geriatr Soc 33:236–245, 1985

Kukull WA, Koepsell TD, Inui TS, et al: Depression and physical illness among general medical clinical patients. J Affective Disord 10:153–162, 1986

Larson C, Nyman G: Age of onset in schizophrenia. Human Heredity 20:241, 1970

Larson E, Reifler B, Sumi S, et al: Diagnostic evaluation of 200 elderly outpatients with suspected dementia. Gerontol 40:536–543, 1985

Lowenthal MF: Lives in Distress: The Paths of the Elderly to the Psychiatric Ward. New York, Basic Books, 1964

Madden JJ, Luhan JA, Kaplan LA, et al: Nondementing psychoses in older persons. JAMA 150:1567–1570, 1952

Mages NL, Mendelsohn GA: Effects of cancer on patients' lives: a personological approach, in Health Psychology. Edited by Stone GC, Cohen F, Adler NE. San Francisco, Jossey-Bass, 1979, pp 255–284

McAllister, TW, Price TR: Severe depressive pseudodementia with and without dementia. Am J Psychiatry 139:626–629, 1982

McCartney JR, Palmateer L: Assessment of cognitive deficit in geriatric patients. J Am Geriatr Soc 33:467–471, 1985

Morgan HG: General medical disorders, in Handbook of Psychiatry, Mental Disorders, and Somatic Illness. Edited by Lader MH. New York, Cambridge University Press, 1983, pp 14–36

Murphy E: Social origins of depression in old age. Br J Psychiatry 141:135–142, 1982

Murphy E: The prognosis of depression in old age. Br J Psychiatry 142:111–119, 1983

Myers JK, Weissman MM, Tischler GL, et al: Six-month prevalence of psychiatric disorders in three communities, 1980 to 1982. Arch Gen Psychiatry 41:959–967, 1984

Neugarten BL, Datan N: Sociological perspectives on the life cycle, in Life-Span Developmental Psychology: Personality and Socialization. Edited by Baltes PB, Schaie KW. New York, Academic, 1973, pp 53–69

Ouslander JG: Physical illness and depression in the elderly. J Am Geriatr Soc 30:593–599, 1982

Post F: The management and nature of depressive illness in late life: a follow-through study. Br J Psychiatry 212:393–404, 1972

Post F: Dementia, depression, and pseudo-dementia, in Psychiatric Aspects of Neurological Disease. Edited by Benson DF, Blumer D. New York, Grune & Stratton, 1975, pp 99–120

Post F: Affective psychoses, in Handbook of Studies on Psychiatry and Old Age. Edited by Kay DW, Burrows G. Elsevier Science, 1984, pp 277–278

Post F: Persistent Persecutory States of the Elderly. Oxford, Pergamon, 1986

Rabins P: The reversible dementias, in Recent Advances in Psychogeriatrics. Edited by Arie T. London, Churchill Livingstone, 1985

Rabins P, Pauker S, Thomas J: Can schizophrenia begin after age 44? Compr Psychiatry 25:290–293, 1984

Rapp SR, Davis KM: Geriatric depression: physician's knowledge, perceptions, and diagnostic practices. Gerontologist 29:252–257, 1989

Reding M, Haycox J, Blass J: Depression in patients referred to a dementia clinic: a three year prospective study. Arch Neurol 42:894–896, 1985

Revenson TA, Felton BJ: Patients' perceptions of the stressor of chronic illness. Paper presented at the meeting of the Gerontology Society of America, New Orleans, 1985

Robins L, Holzer J, Weissman M, et al: Lifetime prevalence of specific psychiatric disorders in three sites. Arch Gen Psychiatry 41:949–958, 1984

Robinson RG, Kubos KL, Starr LB, et al: Mood disorders in stroke patients: importance of location of lesion. Brain 107:81–93, 1984

Rovner BW, Kafonek S, Fillip L, et al: Prevalence of mental illness in a community nursing home. Am J Psychiatry 143:1446–1449, 1986

Savage RD, Gaber LB, Britton PG, et al: Personality and Adjustment in the Aged. New York, Academic, 1977

Sims A, Prior P: The pattern of mortality in severe neuroses. Br J Psychiatry 133:299–305, 1978

Sireling LI, Paykel ES, Freeling P, et al: Depression in general practice: case thresholds and diagnosis. Br J Psychiatry 147:113–119, 1985

Sluss TK, Gruenberg EM, Kramer M: The use of longitudinal studies in the investigation of risk factors for senile dementia-Alzheimer type, in Epidemiology of Dementia. Edited by Mortimer JA, Schuman LM. New York, Oxford University Press, 1981, pp 132–154

Tomlinson B, Blessed G, Roth M: Observations on the brains of non-demented old people. J Neurol Sci 7:331–356, 1968

Turnbull JM, Turnbull SK: Management of specific anxiety disorders in the elderly. Geriatrics 40:75–82, 1985

Turner RJ, Noh S: Physical disability and depression. J Health Soc Behav 29:23–37, 1988

Turner RJ, Wood DW: Depression and disability: the stress process in a chronically strained population, in Research in Community and Mental Health. JAI Press, 1985, 5:77–109

Volavka J, Cancro R: The late onset schizophrenic disorders, in Aspects of Aging. Edited by Busse E. Philadelphia, Smith Kline and French Laboratories, 1986

Ware JP: Use of outpatient mental health services by a general population with health insurance coverage. Hosp Community Psychiatry 37:1119–1125, 1986

Weissman MM, Myers JK, Tischler GL, et al: Psychiatric disorders (DSM-III) and cognitive impairment among the elderly in the U.S. urban community. Acta Psychiatr Scand 71:366–379, 1985

Wells KB, Golding JM, Burnam MA: Psychiatric disorder and limitations in physical functioning in a sample of the Los Angeles general population. Am J Psychiatry 145:712–717, 1988

CHAPTER 3

Leonard L. Heston, M.D.

Genetics of Geriatric Psychopathology

Analyses of traits shared within families are the classical foundation of human genetics, and they yield basic concepts important to clinical practice. However, over the past decade, the revolution of molecular genetics has been adding high-technology basic science to the structure. A working grasp of this science has become increasingly essential to clinicians.

Basic Genetics

Family Level

Genetic studies begin with *probands* (persons with an illness, through whom families are located). Most probands are highly selected because they must come to medical attention in order to become probands. As a result, on average, probands have dramatic illnesses, often unusually severe, and so are not representative of all persons with a given illness. This bias can be removed only if all affected persons in a population are equally likely to become a proband—generally an impossible condition to meet.

Probands' families are then studied to ascertain other affected persons or *secondary cases*. Relatives are nearly always grouped according to their degree of relationship to probands. On average, 50% of the genes of first-degree relatives (siblings, parents, and children) are identical to those of probands. Second-degree relatives (aunts, uncles, nieces, nephews, grandchildren) share 25%. Third-degree relatives (e.g., first cousins) and probands share, on average, 12.5%. Relatives' risks for recurrent disease are usually presented as age-specific incidences, the proportion of relatives of a specific type becoming affected with the proband's illness during a particular age interval. A correction is usually made, which allows for the risk remaining to unaffected persons who have lived through only part of the period of risk. Several available life-table methods are used for this purpose. A straightforward example can be found among the references.

These incidence estimates are called *empirical risks* because they are based on actual counts of relatives. For one disease to be considered, Huntington's disease (HD), the risk (50%) is a *genetic ratio* applicable to autosomal dominance. However, genetic ratios must be confirmed by empirical counts: repeated studies find that the proportion affected among first-degree relatives of probands with HD approaches 50% by age 70. But even for Huntington's, such summary estimates are misleading and age-specific incidences are much more informative.

Control populations are usually persons not at increased risk for the disease, but sometimes second- or third-degree relatives are used. These relatives can be especially useful controls because their genetic risk relative to first-degree relatives is known precisely from genetic theory, while they often share with probands ethnic, geographic, and socioeconomic factors. Genes are implicated in the etiology of illness when the risk to relatives significantly exceeds that of controls at specific ages.

Twinship is a special relationship that is most important in genetic research. Monozygotic (MZ) twins have all of their genes in common, whereas dizygotic (DZ) pairs, like nontwin siblings, share 50% of their genes. Significantly higher concordance for a trait among MZ compared to DZ pairs implicates genes. Concordance is usually reported as proband-wise. Given co-twins located through a proband-twin who has the condition of interest:

$$\text{concordance} = \frac{\text{number of co-twins with given disease} \times 100}{\text{number of co-twins at risk}}$$

In this analysis, both members of an affected pair may be probands if they are discovered in the same search. An alternate analysis, pair-wise concordance, divides the number of pairs in whom both have the illness by the total number of pairs ascertained. The proband-wise method is preferred when a total population cannot be surveyed.

Concordance provides an estimate of genetic resemblance. Discordance tells us that environment also contributes importantly to outcome—very importantly in most disease states. Differences between members of MZ pairs must be associated with environmental differences, or with stochastic processes such as gene inactivation. However, assiduous study of discordant pairs has not discovered precisely what environmental or stochastic factors are important and how they operate. This gap in our knowledge is an increasingly important one that is being highlighted by progress in the physical chemistry of deoxyribonucleic acid (DNA).

Molecular Level

We inherit DNA. DNA contains the information needed for life written in code: the genetic code. The coding components of DNA are four relatively small molecules, the nucleic acids (nucleotides), arranged in long strands and separated into packages, the chromosomes. Normally there are 46 chromosomes in each cell, 23 from the mother and 23 from the father. The order in which the four nucleic acids line up in DNA strands is inherited from the parents: half are arranged in sequences transmitted from the mother, half from the father. With exceptions unimportant for our purposes, each cell of the body contains about 6 billion nucleic acids.

DNA has several functions. As is well known, it can make exact copies of itself, thereby permitting reproduction. DNA also has two basic functions pertinent to psychiatric disease. First, the order of nucleic acids in DNA determines the structure of proteins. Second, DNA participates in regulating the amount of specific proteins produced at any given moment throughout life. Together, differences in protein structure and differences in regulation account for the range of biological diversity. This diversity includes disease.

A special property of DNA makes possible most of the applications of high-technology biology to clinical medicine. This property is the effectively invariant pairing of the nucleic acids that make up the coding segment of DNA. The four coding nucleic acids are adenine, cytosine, guanine, and thymidine, usually designated by their initials, A, C, G, and T. In nature and in the laboratory, A pairs with T and C pairs with G. Thus a sequence of bases like A-A-T-C-C anneals with T-T-A-G-G rapidly and with near perfect fidelity. Because of this property, a strand of DNA can be used as a *probe* to seek its complementary strand. This pairing forms the basis for much of molecular genetics and explains the origin of the term *recombinant DNA*. A *Northern blot* exposes DNA strands from two sources to each other to see if some strands anneal. The exposure takes place in an electrophoretic gel and is detected by autoradiography.

Structure of Proteins.   Some DNA segments code for specific amino acids to be linked together to form proteins. A sequence of three nucleic acids specifies one amino acid out of the 20 that make up our proteins. For example, A-C-G codes for threonine, T-T-T for phenylalanine. A segment of DNA some several thousand nucleic acids long contains the information needed to make one chain of amino acids. Such a chain may itself constitute a complete protein, but most are processed after manufacture, for example, being joined to other chains to make a more complex protein.

The overview thus far omits an important intermediate step: DNA does not directly code for proteins. It is first *transcribed* into ribonucleic acid (RNA), which is much like DNA except that 1) the nucleic acid uracil is substituted in RNA for thymine; 2) RNA is constantly turning over, whereas DNA is stable; and 3) RNA migrates from the nucleus to the cytoplasm, whereas DNA remains in the nucleus. In the cytoplasm, RNA is the template that determines the structure of proteins.

It is important to understand that RNA is processed after transcription. Long segments (exons) are excised, leaving introns, which are spliced together to form the final molecule of messenger RNA (mRNA). The details of this process are unimportant for our purposes, but it is important to realize that a segment of *genomic DNA* (i.e., the DNA of chromosomes) does not exactly correspond to a segment of mRNA that is translated into proteins. Many modern techniques involve inferring the structure of DNA from the structure of mRNA or proteins. But because only part of the DNA segment giving rise to the mRNA or protein can be deduced in this way, the resulting DNA is called *cDNA*, or *complementary DNA*. This feature of nature has also made the word "gene" ambiguous. "Gene" is increasingly used as a convenient shorthand term that is replaced by terms such as "DNA segment" in more exacting communication. RNA will also anneal to its complementary DNA; the result is a *Southern blot.*

Proteins, in their turn, are the stuff of life—its bricks, mortar, and tools. DNA supplies the information of life; proteins organize and perform its work. It helps understanding to think of two types of proteins. One type makes up the structure of the body. The *structural proteins* not only form our physical matrix, but they also manufacture nonprotein molecules such as hormones and neurotransmitters. Many structural proteins incorporate for use or transport small molecules such as minerals, fats, sugars, and vitamins. The second type of proteins is called *regulatory proteins*. They are coded for by regulatory DNA segments and interact with DNA that codes for structural proteins in order to increase or decrease production. Together, these types of proteins constitute the organizing framework of the body.

If, through a chance event (a mutation), one nucleic acid is substituted for another—say C for the second G in G-G-C, making G-C-C—then the amino acid alanine is substituted for glycine in the protein coded for by that DNA segment. This type of mutation is the simplest to describe. Others include deletion or addition of nucleic acids. Just where mutations occur is random. What effect it will have depends on where it occurs. A difference in protein structure that results from mutation may be entirely without practical effect on life; or it may alter the product of that segment just enough to make it slightly less efficient or more efficient, or enough to predispose to disease. In the foregoing example, the substitution of alanine for glycine in a specific protein is associated with phenylketonuria. Typical of what we are learning about the complexity of diseases, five other alterations in the same protein caused by different mutations are known to produce phenylketonuria. Also typical of disease, the effective treatment is the elimination of phenylalanine from the diet—an adjustment of environment. Without the environmental codeterminant, there is no disease.

Regulation of Protein Production. The second major function of DNA is to act in conjunction with other molecules to control the amounts of structural protein produced by specific DNA segments, given specific circumstances. Regulatory proteins, introduced earlier, are one such essential molecule, but nonprotein molecules such as hormones also regulate genes. Because these nonprotein molecules are themselves made or organized by proteins, it is apparent that DNA itself contains the information needed for its own regulation. Just exactly how this regulating is done mechanically is not known in detail, but the processes are rapidly being unraveled by research. In broad outline, some DNA segments are configured so as to provide sites for attachment of regulatory molecules. Such unions can decrease or increase decoding of specific DNA segments and hence lessen or augment production of particular products. The effects are finely graded, from complete blocking of production to massive increases. Like structural sites, regulatory sites on DNA are also subject to mutation with consequent change in functional capacity.

The substances that unite with DNA are, as described, the direct or indirect products of other DNA segments. Some may be produced in response to housekeeping demands, such as those imposed by internal timing or "clock" mechanisms. But many regulatory substances are produced in response to changes in the external environment. DNA is constantly finely modulating our responses to ongoing change in external environments, including memories stored in the brain and in the immune system. A useful example of these processes is provided by "heat shock proteins," which are produced by cells subjected to one or another of several noxious stimuli. The proteins coded for by heat shock genes are often called "stress proteins" or another similar name. They are produced by cells subject to one of several aversive stimuli: heat, for one (which explains the historical origin of the name), but also dozens of drugs, anoxia, hydrogen peroxide, and some endogenous hormones, among many others. Affected cells immediately slow or stop production of proteins appropriate to them under normal conditions and augment production by up to a hundredfold of several species of small heat shock proteins, some of which combine directly with DNA.

DNA and Disease. The first step in successful searches for the causes of genetic disease has been to locate roughly the disease-associated DNA segments on specific chromosomes. Then those DNA segments can be progressively delimited by locating markers on either side of them until eventually they are isolated. The next step is determining the nucleic sequence of that DNA segment. By working from the genetic code, the structure of any protein produced by that segment can be inferred. If all or part of the segment is regulatory and codes for no protein, the next steps are not so evident. Considerable trial-and-error research may be needed, but the technology now available certainly defines the relevant mechanisms. This step entails delimiting the environmental factors to which the regulatory mechanism responds, and what product it regulates in what direction—toward more or less of it—in response to change in that environment. Next, DNA segments associated with disease, the equivalent normal segments, and the products of each are directly compared. Finally, a way to bypass or neutralize the damage done by the defective segment is sought in order to provide effective treatments. This process has not yet been completed for any illness, but it is far along in some cases (e.g., cystic fibrosis), and there can be little doubt that psychiatric diseases can be approached in the same way.

Genetics of Aging Per Se

Progeroid Syndromes

Several genetic conditions feature apparent premature aging. In particular, progeria, Werner's syndrome, and Down's syndrome are often cited as models. However, for psychiatry, only Down's may provide a close analogy. The other conditions exhibit greatly advanced aging of specific tissues such as vasculature or integument, but the brain remains at its chronological age. Down's syndrome also features advanced aging of several tissues, but in this instance the brain is definitely affected with a specific age-related syndrome, Alzheimer's disease (AD), which is discussed at length later.

"Normal" Aging

In the broadest sense, the evidence for the influence of DNA on longevity is unequivocal. All differences between species are based on differences in DNA, and each species has a characteristic life span. Among human twins, the correlation of MZ pairs for length of life is twice that of DZ pairs, suggesting that genes are important in overall longevity in our species. However, no environmental factors have been defined that might be associated with survival. This area of research is likely to become a most important one. For example, the average difference in age at onset between MZ twins who both develop AD is about 10 years. Because genes are identical, the difference must be in chance (stochastic) factors or environment. And if 10 years, why not 20 or 40? Once the interaction between environment and DNA is understood, such questions will become pertinent.

Huntington's Disease

HD is the prototypical dementing illness. Children of affected persons start life with a 50% risk of developing the disease, with males and females equally at risk. The age at onset follows a normal distribution with a mean age of about 43 and 96% of cases having onset between ages 20 and 70. Age at onset introduces a prognostic concept essential to genetic counseling and to an overall grasp of the clinical implications of genetic disease. Suppose a normal male, age 43, has a parent affected with HD. What is the probability that he is a carrier of the Huntington's gene and will develop the illness? His risk at birth was 50%, but he has lived through half of the risk period. The offhand answer given by most people is 25%, but that is incorrect. Understanding the derivation of the actual risk (33%) will yield useful insights.

The probability is conditional and is estimated through application of Bayes's theorem. The easiest way to see this is to set up a table:

		Carrier	*Not carrier*
a.	Prior probability (probability knowing only that father had HD)	0.5	0.5
b.	Conditional probability (probability at age 43 of showing no clinical HD)	0.5	1.0
c.	Joint probability (probability that both a and b will occur)	$0.5 \times 0.5 = 0.25$	$1.0 \times 0.5 = 0.5$
d.	Posterior probability (joint probability of event [from c] divided by total joint probability)	$\dfrac{0.25}{0.5 + 0.25} = 0.33$	$\dfrac{0.5}{0.5 + .25} = 0.67$

These relationships are not intuitively obvious; readers unfamiliar with conditional probability will need to construct a few examples. The general formula is

prob carrier, given age attained = prob carrier × prob well at age if carrier/prob carrier × prob well at age if carrier + prob carrier × prob well at age if not carrier

In the foregoing example this is

$$\frac{0.5 \times 0.5}{0.5 \times .05 + 0.5 \times 1} = \frac{0.25}{0.25 + 0.5} = \frac{0.25}{0.75} = 0.33$$

The probability of attaining specific ages can be directly inferred from tables of ages at onset, which are readily available for most of the diseases to be considered.

HD is an example of the application of high-technology molecular genetics to clinical problems: today genetic counseling; soon to come, diagnosis; and tomorrow, treatment. Counseling is made possible through genetic linkage, essentially a method of marking chromosomes. This method is a complex procedure requiring a team of three or four specialists, but general clinicians will find a basic understanding of the process increasingly useful. In HD, the defective gene has been localized to chromosome 4, and several markers for the HD region are available. The gene itself is not marked, but DNA segments very close to it are so that, starting from embryonic tissues, the markers can identify a disease-carrying chromosome with probabilities approaching 99%.

The best current chromosome markers are fragments of DNA that vary in length from individual to individual. The fragments are produced by exposing DNA to endonucleases (enzymes present in bacteria, presumably to protect against invasion by foreign DNA). Each such enzyme—several dozen are known—splits DNA at a specific point identified by a sequence of six or so nucleic acids. Every time the enzyme recognizes its sequence, it cuts the DNA. If DNA from an individual is exposed to any one of the enzymes, it is split into millions of fragments. Because of mutations, every individual differs from every other individual in the number of DNA sequences that a particular enzyme recognizes and cuts. For example, if an enzyme recognizes T-G-G-T-A, it cuts the DNA chain, but if any of the nucleic acids are changed, say, A-G-G-T-A, the cut is not made. The result is that each of us is identified by the length of fragments produced. Because variation in DNA produces the different lengths, the polymorphism is inherited just like any Mendelian trait and can be traced from generation to generation. However, too many fragments are produced by treatment of the entire genome to be efficiently managed by current techniques. Therefore, practical use of the method depends on localizing DNA associated with a trait of interest to an area no greater than one chromosome. However, in the near future, genetic "maps" locating polymorphic markers very close to one another across the whole genome will be available and will make feasible screening searches for genes associated with any trait.

Fragment length polymorphisms (FLPs) mark chromosomes, making it possible to identify the ones carrying disease-associated genes. Again, the procedural details are not vitally important to clinicians, but clinicians should be able to estimate whether data available for a specific family are likely to be adequate to determine the carrier status of family members. The minimum requirements are these:

- DNA must be available for at least two persons—one affected and one nonaffected—who have lived through a large part of the age of risk. This number is the theoretical minimum; usually more family members are needed.
- DNA must be available for at least two generations.
- Phase must be potentially determinable.

The third requirement is usually the most problematic. "Phase," for our purposes, means determining which of the two chromosomes possessed by an individual carries the disease gene. Although phase is one of the variables solved for in the computer programs needed for adequate analysis, clinicians are called on to give initial feasibility estimates. This task is not prohibitively difficult. A basic understanding of what happens to chromosomes during gamete formation and careful study of several pedigrees should yield the needed intellectual tools.

Alzheimer's Disease

This dementing illness is distinctly age related. Its incidence increases steadily with age, with no definite plateau or decline, whereas the age at onset of most illnesses has a distribution about a mean so that incidence first increases, then decreases with age. The recurrence risk for AD among first-degree relatives is about five times that of control populations at ages from 50 to 80. Second-degree relatives have a risk about 2.5 times that of control populations. Males and females are equally at risk. After age 80 the evidence becomes hard to interpret because chronic diseases often associated with some compromise of mentation and AD itself both increase dramatically in the general population, confounding the results of family studies.

Among younger-onset cases (under 65), recurrent illness in families often follows an autosomal dominant pattern. With increasing age, this relationship weakens so that isolated cases begin to appear in families with many persons at risk. In all, about 50% of families studied have only one affected person. Some isolated cases are no doubt genetic, but segregating genes simply miss other family members. Also, some potentially affected family members doubtless die of other causes before the AD genotype is expressed. This likelihood would be exaggerated by selective factors operating on probands. Secondary cases, on average, are 8 years older than the proband through whom they were located. Thus the expected disease onset in relatives of a 70-year-old proband would be 78; and during such an 8-year interval, many deaths in gene carriers would be expected from causes other than AD. Again the evidence has led to different interpretations, but definitive conclusions await further evidence.

An understanding of the molecular genetics of AD has developed over the past 5 years. Two research paths were followed simultaneously. First, the amino acid sequence of amyloid [the 16-amino acid peptide that is one of the hallmarks of the neuropathology of the dementia of the Alzheimer type (DAT)] was determined. Based on this sequence, an oglionucleotide (the sequence of nucleic acids that must have been present in order to produce the peptide) was prepared. When exposed to single strands of DNA from chromosome 21, the oglionucleotide recognized and annealed to its complementary segment. The choice of DNA from chromosome 21 followed from the remarkable clue alluded to earlier: all (100% so far) cases of Down's syndrome who achieve early middle age and come to autopsy have been found to exhibit the neuropathology of AD. Of course, Down's is a trisomy of chromosome 21.

The second research pathway searched for linkage of FLPs from chromosome 21 to AD. A first positive report was followed by negative ones and more recently by further positive ones. At present, the evidence supports linkage to chromosome 21 in some families. There are no families in which linkage to other chromosomes has been proven, but the negative results leave open the possibility of genetic heterogeneity, which would not be surprising: so far most diseases known at the level of DNA have proven highly heterogeneous. One further result: the amyloid gene is not linked to the segment containing the putative AD gene.

Pick's Disease

Pick's disease is much rarer than AD in the population, but because its age distribution at onset is around a mean of age 54, its frequency is appreciable among younger dementia patients. The limited information available suggests a recurrence risk somewhat greater than AD—about 25% among first-degree relatives; data are insufficient to support useful age-specific incidences. Females may be at slightly higher risk than males.

Affective Illness

Geriatric onset of affective illness apparently reflects the tail of a distribution that begins during the adolescent years. That there is a genetic contribution to incidence has been well established, and that influence apparently extends through the life span. The incidence of unipolar illness does not increase in older age groups (although prevalence does, of course). The incidence of mania decreases so that onset after age 60 is rare and warrants a thorough search for other brain diseases.

Schizophrenia

As for affective illness, the incidence of schizophrenia is very low in older ages. However, a group of conditions variously named over the years—late-onset paraphrenia, paranoia, delusional disorder, and paranoid state are typical terms—appears with increased frequency in families of schizophrenics and, in the case of paraphrenia, also in families with affective illness. In a proportion of such cases, observation over time suggests that the outcome is typical schizophrenia with first-rank signs and chronic deficit state. However, most studies have found these relationships only weakly explanatory, and most instances of these diseases have no known genealogical connection to schizophrenia. Moreover, there is an excess of medical illness among such cases as compared to controls, again suggesting that a thorough search for a primary disease is warranted.

Suggested Reading

Bienz M, Pelham HR: Mechanisms of heat-shock gene actuation in higher eukaryotes. Adv Genet 24:31–72, 1987

Elandt-Johnson RC: Age-at-onset distribution in chronic diseases: a life table approach to analysis of family data. J Chronic Dis 26:529–545, 1973

Heston LL: Clinical genetics of dementing illnesses. Neurol Clin North Am 4:439–446, 1986

Heston LL, White JA, Mastri AR: Pick's disease: clinical genetics and natural history. Arch Gen Psychiatry 44:409–411, 1987

Kay DWK: Observations on the natural history and genetics of old age psychoses. Proc R Soc Med 52:791–797, 1959

Slater E, Cowie V: The Genetics of Mental Disorder. New York, Oxford

University Press, 1971 (Appendices C and D present simple life table methods. The book is still current with regard to psychiatric genetics.)

Weissman MM, Merikangas KR, Wickramaratne JK, et al: Family genetic studies of psychiatric disorders. Arch Gen Psychiatry 43:1104–1116, 1986

CHAPTER 4

Elaine A. Leventhal, M.D., PH.D.

Biological Aspects

Many theories have been advanced to account for aging. Although none has gained wide acceptance, some generalizations are agreed on by most investigators. Growth, development, and aging are the essences of biology. They are not static stages in a natural history but represent the continuously changing processes of the life cycle. "Normal" aging or senescence is associated with declines in actual numbers of active metabolic cells and in cellular functions over the life span. Decrements in overall reserve and declining ability to respond to stress and recover from illnesses represent losses in regenerative ability and deterioration in function that result eventually in death.

We can think of human aging in terms of multiple biological clocks that start to tick at conception and stop at death. Most cell proliferation peaks around birth, and virtually all growth ceases at puberty. A fraction of prenatal mitotic activity maintains homeostasis in the adult except at times of heightened physiologic demand caused by injury, infection, or other "stress insults." For some tissues (i.e., the ovary) the aging clock starts in utero, even though the fetal period is the time of most dramatic growth and cell division.

When growth stops, aging begins. It is characterized by different stem-cell-specific as well as gender-specific rates of decline that translate into loss of replicative and repair ability. The organism's innate biological plasticity and lifelong adaptive history allow for personalized patterns of accommodation to changes in the body's hierarchical regulation system. Thus aging also produces increasing heterogeneity among individuals as they age.

The emotional and behavioral components of illness become as atypical in their presentation in the aging individual as do physical illnesses. Therefore, it is important for the psychiatrist to understand the basic processes that determine how people behave as they age. The biological phenomena associated with senescence need to be understood in order to appreciate the remarkable degree of heterogeneity that is seen in clinical practice and to learn to treat those age-related behavioral changes that occur in both illness presentation and in the behaviors associated with illness and frailty.

General Aging

How a person ages physically and psychologically reflects his or her unique biology, that is, the genetic predisposition or relative resistance to certain chronic illnesses superimposed on their biological clocks. It also is a testimony to the effects of the individual's external environment and behaviors; of exposure to trauma, infections, and past diseases, and of the health and illness practices that the individual has adopted during the life span.

In biological senescence there is a quantitative loss of cells as well as changes in many of the enzymatic activities within cells. Most enzymatic syntheses continue, although some rates of production and clearance may decline and there may be diminished responsiveness to the demands for increased activity. Of the organ systems, the normal kidney, the lung, and the skin age much more rapidly than the heart and the liver in both sexes, whereas the musculoskeletal system and the gonads become atrophic at different times in the life span of males and females (Finch and Schneider 1985; Kenney 1989).

There are age-related changes in body composition with up to an 80% decrease in overall muscle mass and an average of 35% increase, as well as a significant redistribution, of body fat. Fat deposition accumulates around and within the viscera while there is a loss of fat on the surface. Thus older people lose "insulation" and are more sensitive to extremes of ambient temperature than younger people (Kenney 1989).

Skin

Aging of the skin is a reflection of physical changes, environmental exposures, and behaviors across the lifetime. The skin atrophies, with loss of the subcutaneous cushion of fat and the shrinkage of dermal appendages. There are fewer blood vessels in the skin and the rate of healing slows. The structural element elastin, responsible for the "stretch" in tissues, fragments with age. However, not all age-related changes represent cell or tissue loss or deterioration. Collagen accumulates, as evidenced by increased interstitial matrix formation. Examples of the effects of such age-related changes in elastin and collagen can be seen in wrinkling. Sun exposure accelerates fragmentation of skin elastin and encourages increased collagen deposition. The lifetime accumulation of the effects of solar exposure is accompanied by a loss of melanocytes, leading to a decrease in pigmentation in the skin and increased vulnerability to further sun damage. People with prolonged tanning exposure have more wrinkles at earlier ages as well as a greater incidence of malignancies related to solar damage (Kligman et al. 1985).

Cardiovascular System

The age-related decline in the cardiovascular system has been thought to be the major determinant of decreased tolerance for exercise and loss of conditioning and thus the major factor contributing to feelings of agedness and overall decline in reserve. However, there is much more than heart and blood vessel deterioration involved in the loss of energy reserve. There is a dependency, as well, on interactions between the musculoskeletal and pulmonary systems and the cardiovascular system. The biological complexities of these relationships become apparent when one examines the aging and gender differences in these particular organ systems.

In the heart, changes occur in the chambers, blood vessels, and valves. With time, the ventricular myocardium thickens, the ventricular cavities become smaller, and the amount of blood pumped per contraction decreases. Heart rate also slows with time. The decrease in rate may be related to "down regulation" or decreased responsiveness of adrenergic receptors on heart muscle even though synthesis and clearance of epinephrine do not change. There is also evidence that there are decreases in baroreceptor modulation of heart rate. Thus, the heart becomes incapable of generating high rates in response to increased activity and stress demands.

These anatomic changes in the vascular system affect function by causing declines in cardiac output and a decrease in response to work demands (Lakatta 1987; Morley and Reese 1989; Rodeheffer et al. 1984; Simpson and Wicks 1988). Blood vessels narrow as endothelial linings thicken and smooth muscle mass declines. Calcium may be deposited in vessel walls if intimal damage or medial necrosis is present. Thus, the blood vessels become more rigid, contributing to the slow elevation in blood pressure seen over time. In the absence of cardiovascular or renal disease, this condition may never reach the pathological range; an individual can be very old without hypertensive disease. When coronary artery disease is present along with normal cardiac aging, function is further compromised. Women appear to enjoy a slower rate of progression of arteriosclerotic disease before menopause while exposed to circulating estrogens. This advantage is reflected in the lower incidence of coronary artery disease in premenopausal women (Department of Health and Human Services 1982).

Respiratory System

The aging changes in the cardiovascular system are mirrored by an even more rapid rate of functional decline in the respiratory system. All parts of the pulmonary system age, including lung tissue as well as the muscles, ribs, and vertebral column of the thoracic cage. There is less work capacity as skeletal muscles of the chest wall, along with smooth muscles in bronchi, diaphragm, and chest wall, weaken; collagen is deposited and elastin fragments. The more rapid aging of the skeleton and the greater loss of muscle mass are important not only for diminished exercise capacity in females but also for the greater vulnerability of women to fractures and a greater possibility for immobilization. The most common form of loss of bone mass or osteopenia is calcium demineralization or osteoporosis, which can be especially prominent in the vertebral column of women and is important not only for posture but also for respiratory function. If the thoracic cage becomes smaller because of fractures of osteoporotic vertebrae, there is a decrease in chest capacity and thus in pulmonary function. (The bony changes are discussed further in the next section.) In the lung itself, the alveolar septae are critical as the exchange sites for the gases, oxygen, and carbon dioxide. Old lungs have scattered areas of fibrosis or disruptions in the septa that interfere with gaseous exchange (Kenney 1989). Even more than the functional changes in the cardiovascular system described previously, these manifestations of "senile" emphysema may limit the amount of exercise and energy that can be expended.

Moreover, it is difficult to determine how much of the decline in respiratory function that is observed is age related and how much is environmentally induced, because most individuals are exposed to some degree of air pollution. There are no studies of nonsmokers living in nonpolluted environments, but it must be expected that use of cigarettes or other inhaled substances exaggerates the aging changes previously described. Smoking produces an acceleration in fibrosis and septal damage leading to bullous formation. These disruptive changes in the alveolar walls result in decreased diffusion capacity, increased secretions, and an increased rate of chronic infection. Chronic bronchitis and emphysema mimic aging changes of senile emphysema, and thus there should be accelerated pulmonary aging in middle-aged smokers, which can be reversed or stabilized if smoking stops (Hermanson et al. 1988).

Aerobic exercise training has been shown to have significantly positive cardiovascular, pulmonary, and behavior effects on healthy older males and females (Blumenthal et al. 1989). After 4 months of training, these authors demonstrated an 11.6% improvement in directly measured peak Vo_2 and a 13% increase in anaerobic threshold (the amount of work tolerated before exercise-limiting ventilatory and metabolic change occurred). Anaerobic threshold is a reasonable reference for work involved in daily activities. In addition to increased aerobic fitness, they also found lower total and LDL cholesterol levels and increases in HDL levels. Changes in other physiological parameters that were found included lowered systolic and diastolic blood pressures and the suggestion that bone mineral might be increased in women at risk for fracture, although these latter data are not sufficiently convincing because of the relatively insensitive methodology used (single photon densitometry of the distal radius) and the short time covered by the study. The other major problem in extrapolating from this set of subjects to most elderly is that these study participants were healthy and had no concurrent diseases—a rare phenomenon in most older individuals. However, this study is interesting because its findings are similar to other exercise studies in the literature and because it also looked at the psychological effects of exercise. Although there were no measurable objective findings, subjects reported increased positive affect and feeling better physically.

Musculoskeletal System

Skeletal aging involving the bones, muscles, ligaments, and tendons probably generates most of the common symptomatology responsible for limitations of recreational activities and activities of daily living, as well as restrictions in job-related activities; the joint and muscle aches and stiffness of the arthritides are frequently ascribed to getting old. These symptoms also lead to use of both prescription and nonprescription analgesics, many of which can have significant psychotropic side effects such as depression.

Males maintain an advantage in greater musculoskeletal strength after pubescence, although with time they lose significant muscle mass, as do women. There are declines in skeleton mineralization at a rate of 0.8% to 1% each year over the life span for both men and women, but females show an increase in the rate of loss to between 8% and 10% per year around the menopause, and thus they are at risk for osteoporosis-related fractures. This difference represents an approximate 10-year advantage for males, although men may become osteoporotic because of concurrent disease.

The gender-specific rate of demineralization has a complex metabolic etiology that includes the permissive effect of circulating estrogens and progesterone on the maintenance of vertebral trabecular bone. Thus, postmenopausal women are more vulnerable to fractures of the vertebral spine than males of the same age. By contrast, calcium and vitamin D metabolism and weight-bearing activity may be critical for the remodeling of the cortical bones of the extremities. Although both men and women are at risk for fractures of the long bones, women are fracture prone 10 years earlier than men of the same age. Because of the role of exercise and diet in maintaining bone integrity, it would be expected that regimes that include increased calcium intake and weight-bearing exercise along with estrogen replacement should show some positive results in terms of bone density increases or slowing in the rate of demineralization. At this time, the evidence is controversial regarding the relationship to dietary intake of calcium and rates of bone loss or reversibility (Riggs et al. 1987), although there is much research activity directed at finding tolerable and efficient treatments. One of the better recent studies indicates that weight-bearing exercise may have a positive effect on mineral content of the axial skeleton (Dalsky et al. 1988). However, it is most likely that the critical times to preserve the skeleton for old age are in childhood, adolescence, pregnancy, and lactation (Raiz 1988; Raiz and Kream 1983).

Gastrointestinal Tract

In the oral cavity, aging changes are obvious. With time, the teeth show a reduction in dentine production, shrinkage and fibrosis of root pulp, gingival retraction, and loss of bone density in the alveolar ridges, especially after tooth loss. There is an increase in caries, especially of the root, that appears to be correlated with changes in bacterial content of the mouth and increased colonization with gram-positive facultative cocci replacing gram-negative anaerobic rods while the population of fusospirochetal organisms remains unchanged. There are no age changes in the salivary glands, and the xerostomia that is so common is a disease caused by such problems as obstructing nasal disease leading to mouth breathing, drugs, and autoimmune diseases such as Sjogren's syndrome (Baum 1988).

Primary aging is related to smooth muscle weakness and results in a decrease in the amplitude of peristaltic movements, although esophageal function is largely preserved. The stomach shows evidence of impaired secretory capacity with maximal stimulated gastric acid production decreasing by 5 milliequivalents per hour per decade. Levels of serum gastrin increase while levels of intrinsic factor decrease. Atrophic gastritis is common, appearing in 28% to 96% of elderly and often leading to vitamin B_{12} malabsorption. Gastric emptying appears to be impaired only slightly (Geokas et al. 1985; Minaker et al. 1988).

There is minimal change in the small intestine and only a marginal reduction in mesenteric and splanchnic blood flow in the absence of vascular disease. A significant decrease in absorptive surface area, with concomitant loss of microvilli of the brush border, has been observed and associated with a decrease in enzymatic activities. The overall weight of the small intestine decreases as the mucosal surface area declines, yet there are minimal overall decreases in levels of function. Xylose, iron, and folate absorption remains normal; although lipid and calcium absorption decline, the decline is probably related to decreases in vitamin D availability and activity. With decreases in gastric acid, the sterility of the tract is jeopardized and larger numbers of coliforms are seen. Although absorption is largely preserved, when poor intake and disease are involved, malnutrition may result (Geokas et al. 1985).

The large bowel experiences alterations in flora, but transit time is unchanged in normal aging individuals. Studies of transit time by ingestion of markers show that first markers will be passed in 3 days and 80% will appear by 5 days, with greater delays related to motility slowdown below the sigmoid (Geokas et al. 1985; Kenney 1989).

Liver

The liver decreases modestly in weight and size from 4% to 2% of total body weight. Hepatic blood flow shows a 1.5% fall per year, and there is a 50% reduction over the life span. All ingested drugs as well as metabolites absorbed from the small intestine and stomach pass through the liver. Some are unchanged, but others undergo metabolic detoxification by microsomal enzymes into water-soluble substances for renal excretion. With decreases in liver mass, losses in cellular microsomal enzyme activity (primarily cytochrome P-450) are seen; along with a decrease in blood flow, decreases in the rate of biotransformation occur. Thus, oxidation (phase 1 of hepatic microsomal enzyme synthesis) is the principal metabolic pathway that diminishes with age, particularly in men. These functional changes result in a prolongation in the half-life of those metabolites and drugs that are inactivated by the liver and thereby an increase in the bioavailability of those that undergo extensive first-pass hepatic metabolism. Conjugation or phase 2 remains largely unchanged, that is, glucuronidation is not altered (Geokas et al. 1985; Kenney 1989).

Endocrine System

Thyroid

The normal thyroid secretes a relatively inactive molecule—thyroxine (T_4)—which is converted peripherally to the active 3,5,3'-triiodothyronine (T_3). The secretory rate is under negative feedback control mediated by the secretion of thyroid-stimulating hormone (TSH) from the anterior pituitary. Thus, when insufficient T_4 is produced or there is inadequate conversion of T_4 to T_3 in the periphery, the pituitary responds by putting out more than normal amounts of TSH in an attempt to stimulate the thyroid to be more active. Contrary to earlier studies, new evidence indicates that there are no age-related changes in circulating hormone levels. TSH hypersecretion is reported to increase in persons over 60 years of age (Kabadi and Rosman 1986; Sawin et al. 1979). Because the thyroid does not respond by putting out more thyroid hormones, this finding suggests that possible age-related changes important for homeostasis may occur in the thyroid-pituitary axis.

Pancreas

The pancreas exhibits some moderate anatomic changes, with fat deposition and shrinkage of islets cells but no reduction in the amount or content of pancreatic fluid. Age-related impairment in glucose metabolism has been recognized for more than 60 years, but only recently have the mechanisms begun to be investigated. Most studies show that healthy elderly respond to oral or intravenous glucose challenges with modest impairments in glucose clearance. Insulin levels are equivalent or slightly higher than those from younger challenged individuals, although peripheral insulin resistance appears to play a significant role in carbohydrate intolerance. There is no evidence to support changes in basal hepatic glucose production or changes in insulin receptor numbers or affinity. The controversy now is focusing on the relative contributions of obesity, family history of diabetes, physical exercise, and the use of diabetogenic drugs in the development of senescent carbohydrate intolerance. Thus, it is reasonable to assume that the observed clearance abnormalities and insulin resistance in older people may be related to many factors other than biological aging and may be influenced substantially by diet or exercise (Marchesini et al. 1987; Pacini et al. 1988).

Kidneys

The kidneys, as one of the two major excretory systems, function by means of passive glomerular filtration, active tubular secretion and reabsorption, and passive tubular diffusion. All of these functions decline significantly with age. The decrements in renal function, unrelated to concomitant disease in other organ systems, occur because of a steady attrition due to sclerosis of nephrons over time. Of particular importance are the age-related changes in renal blood flow, glomerular filtration rate (GFR) and tubular secretion, as well as the kidney's ability to compensate for abnormalities of acid base, electrolyte and free water clearance declines by 40% to 50% in the lifetime. There is a modest reduction in the capacity to conserve sodium, with increased osmoreceptor sensitivity producing more vasopressin and water retention. Thus, the elderly are prone to develop the syndrome of inappropriate antidiuretic hormone secretion (Rowe et al. 1976; Wesson 1969). Although blood urea nitrogen (BUN) and creatinine may be elevated very late in life because of age-related declines in renal function, when circulating levels of BUN and creatinine rise before the ninth decade it may be assumed that the uremic individual either is exhibiting accelerated renal aging or has some significant pathology along with age-related changes in kidney function. If BUN is elevated alone, it may represent prerenal failure indicative of other illness-related pathology without obligatory renal dysfunction (Finch and Schneider 1985; Kenney 1989). This decline in renal function has serious implications for physicians' drug-prescribing patterns.

Immune System

Many studies have been directed toward understanding the impact of aging on the normal immune system and its autoregulation. It is useful to describe the system both anatomically and functionally in order to organize the frequently conflicting data in this area.

The immune system is organized into a pool of fixed and circulating cells—leukocytes, lymphocytes, monocytes, macrophages, and mast cells—which move in and out of, or are fixed in, various lymphoid organs such as spleen, lymph nodes, Peyer's patches, and thymus. Leukocytes may have a much more central role in immune function than previously assumed, but age-relevant studies are few; thus these subpopulations are not discussed here. The lymphocyte pool is made up of several subpopulations evolving from an ancestral stem cell in the bone marrow. These include the T-cell line of antigen-responsive cells and effector cells that can kill antigen-specific target cells on direct contact; the B-cell line of antigen-responsive cells and the immunoglobulin-producing plasma cells; and phagocytic mast cells fixed in tissues such as lymph nodes, lung, skin, and mucosa.

With increasing senescence, the total number of immune cells does not change, although there are increases in immature forms and decreases in germinal centers in lymph nodes. Increases of plasma cells and lymphocytes in the bone marrow probably occur because of redistribution. The total concentration of immunoglobulins is not altered, but there is a redistribution of immunoglobulin classes with increases in IgA and IgG and decreases in IgM in serum (Hallgren et al. 1973). Although well-controlled studies on "healthy" humans are infrequent and many of the data on aging and immune function are conflicting and extrapolated from animal models, there is agreement that the actual numbers of some immune cells decline with age. The result is a decline in cellular functions and a slowing of metabolic reactions (Hausman and Weksler 1985; Makinodan and Hirokawa 1985).

The major age-related cellular changes occur in the ratios of subpopulations of thymic-dependent cells, with increases in immature forms (OKT3) and T-helpers (OKT4) and declines in suppressor or cytotoxic (OKT8) cells and natural killer cells. There are less-vigorous delayed-sensitivity reactions to common skin antigens, decreased immunity to virus infections, and graft-versus-host reactions (Leventhal and Burns 1987; Makinodan and Hirokawa 1985).

B cells show little change in total number, but responsiveness to stimulation by T-cell-dependent antigens and to B-cell mitogens declines. Those B-cell functions that are not T-cell dependent are relatively preserved, and there are essentially no changes in the functioning of adherent cells (macrophages) and monocytes between young and old subjects (Antonaci et al. 1984; Kim et al. 1985).

Of the glandular components, the thymus is critical for immune function. It provides the microenvironment for T-cell differentiation and, as an endocrine organ, it produces in its stromal cells several hormones, including the thymosins and thymopoietic factor. Aging in the thymus is dramatic and plays a critical role in immunosenescence. The anatomic patterns in the thymus remain unaltered until approximately 9 years of age (prepuberty). By 11 to 13 years, the vasculature appears increasingly irregular, although parenchymal and perivascular nerves continue to be detectable in the capsule and proximal parts of the trabecula until age 25. The nonlymphoid structures remain intact in the involuted thymus, but the lymphocytic portions, particularly in the cortex, become almost nonexistent. The hormonal activity responsible for lymphocytic maturation resides in epithelial cells, which do not undergo involution, although these cells lose intimate contact with lymphocytes as the lymphoid elements atrophy. The decline in circulating levels of thymic hormone does not parallel the glandular lymphoid involution after puberty, and although hormonal levels peak prior to pubescence, they remain detectable until age 60 before becoming essentially unmeasurable beyond ages 60 to 70 (Goldstein et al. 1979).

There is also a humoral modulatory role for the sympathetic nervous system that appears to depend on sympathetic innervation of lymphoid organs augmented by plasma catecholamines of adrenal origin. Anatomic studies have demonstrated direct sympathetic innervation in fetal thymus as well as spleen. In both mice and humans, fibers are abundant in the adult thymus, around blood vessels and in the parenchyma, encircling or relayed on Hassal's corpuscles (Ghali et al. 1980; Williams and Felten 1981; Williams et al. 1981).

The anatomic linkages between neural and immune systems make clear that regulation and modulation of the immune system by the nervous system is extraordinarily complex. The linkages also indicate that there are many opportunities for disruption of intrasystem and intersystem regulatory mechanisms by various forms of internal and external stress throughout the lifetime. Thus, the regulatory function of the intrinsic compartments within the immune system may be influenced by, and dependent on, a variety of non-immune-system factors.

In one of the few longitudinal studies of the aging immune system, Goodwin and associates (1982) looked at 279 subjects, all over age 65 (mean age 72), on no treatment or over-the-counter drugs and without serious medical diagnoses. When they assayed delayed hypersensitivity, mitogen response, and autoantibody and circulating immune complexes, they found that mitogen responses and delayed hypersensitive skin tests were depressed in the healthy elderly population. Despite the theory that loss of T-suppressor function leads to increasing autoimmunoglobulin levels, there was poor correlation between the two assays, that is, no relationship between measures of cellular immunity and autoimmunity, and no significant correlation between circulating immune complexes and other autoantibodies. After excluding those subjects who developed serious illness, Goodwin continued to find, on the average, age-related decreases in cellular responses in repeat exams after 2 years. These clinical observations are compatible with findings that older T cells have a lower density and expression of surface markers and older B cells have fewer immunoglobulin markers and therefore declining function with age.

Gonads

Aging of the ovary begins in utero and continues throughout the life span. In the female, potential germ cells reach maturation in the ovaries during gestation and undergo massive attrition during the latter half of fetal development, declining from a population of 10×10^6 cells at the organogenesis of the ovary to 10^6 at birth. This steady decline in functional cell number continues until pubescence, when there remains a population of about 10,000 cells available for impregnation. The attrition of these cells continues, but at a slower rate, through the female reproductive period with its monthly cyclicity and interruptions for pregnancy (Nicosia 1983).

The maturation of germ cells and the production of hormones are controlled by a negative feedback loop between the brain and the gonads whereby hormones (leutinizing hormone [LH] and follicular stimulating hormone [FSH]) secreted by the anterior pituitary regulate the follicular ripening of ova and the production of the gonadal hormones, estrogen and progesterone. Follicles containing the mature ovum and capable of synthesizing estrogen and progesterone continue to decrease in number, so that at the climacteric there are too few remaining to produce adequate circulating hormones to stimulate the gonad-dependent end organs such as the breasts and genitalia (and trabecular bone of the vertebrae); nor are there enough to participate in the negative feedback cycling with the pituitary. As estrogenic stimulation declines further, females begin to experience the symptoms of hormonal deficiency including atrophy of the breasts and genitalia and vasomotor instability. The reduction in estrogen and progesterone results, finally, in the cessation of menstruation (menopause) and an uninhibited production of the pituitary gonadotropic hormones. All women show elevations in circulating pituitary gonadotropic hormones (LH and FSH) after they enter the perimenopausal period between the ages of 40 and 55, the physiologic significance of which is not clear (Barbo 1987; Mastroianni and Paulsen 1986). After the menopause, with loss of the protective effects of estrogen and progesterone, there is a greater vulnerability to stroke and coronary artery disease and the effects of osteoporosis.

Males, on the other hand, show minimal attrition of testicular structures or declines in hormonal synthesis and secretion. The potential sperm cells remain at a primitive level into adulthood, arrested in the testis at the spermatogonium stage. The process of maturation to mature sperm continues throughout the male lifetime, with declines occurring only very late in the seventh to eighth decades. Hormonal function also remains relatively stable, and in many men the negative feedback mechanisms with the anterior pituitary are unchanged until the eighth decade. Elevated gonadotropic hormones are rarely seen before the age of 70. In the normal population, a few individuals in their late forties and fifties have elevated levels of FSH, but the majority do not have increased levels until their seventies (Stearns et al. 1974).

Nervous System

One of the basic influences on the aging of the nervous system and subsequent loss of function is the selective degeneration of neurons. There are also differences in the patterns of aging between the central and the peripheral nervous system, presumably because of random demyelination of long tracts. Although there is constant cell loss, the recent study by Terry and associates (1987), using a large sample of healthy elderly, has clearly shown that age-related neuronal loss is minimal. The brain has enormous reserve, and very little cerebral function is lost over time, although greater functional decline is noted in the periphery. Cells disappear randomly throughout the cortex, but in other brain areas there is clustered loss, that is, there is a disproportionately greater loss of cells in the cerebellum, the locus ceruleus, the substantia nigra, and olfactory bulbs (Brody 1970, 1976a, 1976b). It may be that as a result of neuronal degeneration in these areas, some of the more characteristic aging behaviors such as mild gait disturbances, sleep disruptions, and decreased smell and taste perception are common. Yet, in the absence of disease, cognitive function remains intact although motor performance slows.

Neurotransmitter Distribution

There has been a great deal of attention to age-related changes in brain biochemistry, and many contemporary pharmacological interventions, such as dihydroxyphenylalanine (DOPA) replacement in Parkinson's disease, are directed at extending function in systems beset with irreversible anatomic changes and cell losses. The success of such interventions is dependent on understanding neurotransmitter metabolism and function. Although there are many identified neurotransmitters and much research on neuropeptides, behavior, and aging (Morley 1986), only the most age-relevant molecules are discussed here.

Acetylcholine

Acetylcholine (ACh) is widely distributed throughout the central and peripheral nervous system. It is synthesized from choline that is taken up at the presynaptic terminals and acetyl coenzyme A, which is synthesized in the mitochondria, in a reaction that is catalyzed by choline acetyltransferase (CAT). Choline uptake, the rate-limiting factor, shows significant decline with age, although whether the uptake decline reflects changes in number of septal or hippocampal neurons, or specific biochemical defects reflecting changes in structure or activity of binding site proteins, is not clear. In normals, data on CAT activity are inconsistent; however, levels of ACh consistently show no decline, reflecting probable concurrent decreases in release and metabolism at the time synthesis and precursor uptake are disappearing. Another method of assessing age-related changes in ACh function is to examine ACh inactivation by acetylcholinesterase (AChE). Again, there is much inconsistency in reported age-related changes in circulating levels of AChE, but there is reasonably good evidence that binding to cholinergic receptors declines with normal aging. This finding is independent of the cholinergic cell loss associated with dementia of the Alzheimer type (Finch and Schneider 1985; McGeer and McGeer 1975).

Dopamine

Dopamine (DA) is widely distributed in the central nervous system, primarily associated with medium-length projections (tuberoinfundibular, hypothalamic, and medullary periventricular systems) and long projections of the ventral tegmental and substantia nigra DA cell groups to neostriatal and limbic targets. DA is synthesized from dietary tyrosine by hydroxylation to DOPA catalyzed by tyrosine hydroxylase (TH) and then decarboxylated by DOPA decarboxylase. The activity of TH is reported to remain stable, whereas many studies suggest that DOPA decarboxylase declines with age, impairing synthesis of DA. This suggestion is consistent with findings that DA levels are decreased after mid-life in specific brain areas, that is, striatum (Rogers and Bloom 1985).

Plasma Catecholamines (Norepinephrine and Epinephrine)

Plasma norepinephrine (NE) represents a relatively small proportion of NE released from postganglionic sympathetic neurons, because most is taken up or degraded locally. Yet variations in circulating levels reflect biological responses to sympathetic nervous
system activity. For example, levels increase slightly with upright
posture and volume depletion, and greatly with severe exercise or
stress such as surgery or hypoglycemia. They decrease with spinal
anesthesia and drugs such as clonidine. NE shares several enzymes
of synthesis and catabolism with DA, thus the inconsistencies
in the literature on DA hold for NE as well. There are, however,
some human data that permit a few more definitive comments
about NE.

There is reasonably good evidence that NE receptor concentrations decline with aging (Schocken and Roth 1977). This decline
has been documented in the locus ceruleus, and beta-receptors
show some area-specific declines, that is, cerebellar Purkinje cells
and locus ceruleus (Brody 1976a, 1976b; McGeer and McGeer
1975). Yet NE from human cortex, striatum, hypothalamus, and
thalamus does not appear altered (Rogers and Bloom 1985).

Supine baseline levels of plasma NE increase as a function of
age, primarily in males, during stresses such as those previously
mentioned, providing evidence that sympathetic nervous system
activity increases with aging (Ziegler et al. 1976). There may be
several explanations for these findings. There is either increased
NE release from postganglionic sympathetic neurons or decreased
clearance; however, because metabolic clearance rate and half-life
are similar in young and old subjects, the variations noted may be
due to changes in synthetic rate and/or reduced receptor sensitivity in the elderly (Vestal et al. 1979).

No consistent findings of increased plasma levels of epinephrine with age are seen at rest or during sympathetic nervous system provocation. Although responses are similar across the age
range, there are some data that suggest that epinephrine clearance
is amplified, resulting in increased adrenomedullary release of epinephrine. Thus, there may be different effects of aging on the central nervous system regulation of postganglionic, sympathetic neurons and on adrenomedullary regulation (Lake et al. 1984).

In nonnervous tissues, declines in beta-receptors on lymphocytes, myocardium, and adipocytes have been demonstrated. However, other animal and human studies suggest that decreased responsiveness may represent declines in adenylate cyclase activity

rather than receptor-binding abnormalities (Bertel et al. 1980; Rogers and Bloom 1985; Zahniser et al. 1988).

Peripheral Nervous System

In the periphery, random disruption of the myelin sheaths of the long nerves is seen with aging. The slowing of motor function may reflect this loss, and nerve dysfunction may exaggerate myofibrillar losses. Thus, because of the interrelationship between nerves and muscles, muscle weakness may reflect not only myofibrillar loss but also disuse atrophy due to denervation. As neuronal numbers decline with age, lower levels of neurotransmitters are produced (Kenney 1989).

Sense Organs

Vision

There are minimal changes in the retina of the eye and thus minimal, neurally determined changes in light perception, although there is some shrinkage in the size and sensitivity of visual fields, which begins in the early forties (Burg 1968). The major changes that do occur are in the transparent portions of the ocular system, and cataract development is inevitable if the individual lives long enough for the following changes to occur. Pigment is laid down in specific patterns in the lens over time and is coupled with increased rigidity of the lenticular proteins. It is this alteration in the normal molecular alignment that results in the formation of cataracts (Benedek 1971; Spector et al. 1974). The rate of opacification is individually determined and may be accelerated by diseases such as diabetes mellitus, hypoparathyroidism, myotonic dystrophy, and Wilson's disease or the use of drugs such as chlorpromazine or corticosteriods. The world seen through a cataract is one of altered perception and sensory deprivation. Of importance as well for visual acuity is presbyopia, the standard marker of aging of the eye. It occurs as the muscles and ligaments supporting the lens become less taut and stretchable, compromising accommodation (Fisher 1973).

Audition

Another sensory area in which there is significant change is hearing. The ear, the receptor constructed to pick up vibrations and translate them into sounds, loses its sensitivity with aging. Prolonged exposure to loud noise or heavy sound pollution may accelerate the rate of permanent damage to the hair cells of the cochlea. There is also a genetic predisposition to hearing loss; thus the rates of decline in tone and speech discrimination may show significant individual variability. However, from the ages of 30 to 85, there is a dramatic decline in high-frequency perception in the very oldest individuals in comparison with young persons with presumed perfect hearing.

The hearing curves for women are less dramatic than those for males, although there still is significant falloff with age. Thus the assumption can be made that the gender difference may be related to occupational exposure (Belal 1975; Gacek 1975). What is important to recognize is that most studies have been done with an aged cohort that may have been exposed to significant noise in their youth. It may be that, in the next decade or two, frequency curves will show a less dramatic decrement over time in men and the gender differences may disappear. It is also interesting to speculate about what will happen to the hearing of the current cohort of adolescents who are constantly tuned into their portable cassette players or spend time in front of loud rock bands. They may have "old audiograms" in middle age.

Taste and Smell

There are significant increases in taste threshold because of decreases in taste sensitivity over the life span. At birth, there are taste buds lining the soft and hard palate and the buccal mucosa as well as the tongue. There is a slow attrition of taste buds during infancy, and at puberty palatal and buccal receptors are essentially lost. Taste perception becomes solely lingual and nasal; thus taste perception starts aging at adolescence. By 40 or 45 years of age, the tongue is an old organ.

Along with the deterioration of the olfactory bulbs and the accompanying loss in the "aromatic" component of taste perception, there is a decline in taste discriminations (Balogh and Lelkes 1961; El-Baradi and Bourne 1951; Schiffman et al. 1976). Hedonistic pleasure in eating and the aromas of cooking declines, bitter taste sensations predominate and greater use of sugar and excessive salting of foods is needed to stimulate taste experiences. The impact of loss of taste discrimination on overall nutritional status and disease is just beginning to be elucidated.

Touch

Anatomic studies have demonstrated a continuous decrease in organized receptors across the age span. Meissner and Pacinian corpuscles, involved in touch and vibration, decrease in number and show morphological changes, thus touch threshold increases as a function of age (Winkelmann 1965; Kenshalo 1977) and the number of touch spots per unit area of skin decreases by approximately 50% between the second and seventh decade (Rong 1943). In contrast, Merkel's corpuscles, the slowly adapting, low threshold mechanoreceptors, show no decline with time (Iggo 1966).

Proprioception

Aging results in degenerative changes and impaired postural reflexes, mild ataxias, and increased sway secondary to deficiencies in integrative function of the central nervous system with the cerebellum and the reticular formation along with disturbed perception of the vertical (Robinson and Conard 1986). This perceptual sense is vitally important for ambulation and balance because older individuals, more than young persons, attempt to monitor their movements by means of afferent feedback. Proprioceptive information facilitates stretch reflexes, which are necessary to convert limbs into fairly rigid pillars for support in walking and standing, as well as assuring awareness of limb orientation in space to guarantee proper foot placements (Isaacs 1983, 1985).

Studies of other non-central nervous system components vital for balance indicate that there is significant age-related decline in both active and passive motion detection thresholds (Skinner et al. 1984) and joint kinesthetics (Skoglund 1973). It also appears that such age-related changes are minimally apparent if movements under study are patient initiated, whereas constrained movements are less accurately performed by elderly subjects (Stelmach and Worringham 1985).

Pain

There is a large literature on pain, employing methodologies ranging from heat dolorimetry (Clark and Mehl 1971; Corso 1971; Sherman and Robillard 1960) to dental pain elicited by the application of electrical stimuli to the tooth pulp. These studies show increasing thresholds with age. Although histological studies indicate that free nerve endings are reformed continuously (Montagna and

Carlisle 1979), psychophysiological research has demonstrated that elderly persons have diminished pain acuity. Careful dissection of the complex components of pain perception, including both perception of stimuli intensities and interpretation of meaning and implications of painful stimuli, indicate that central integration and interpretation of sensory effects rather than receptor changes are implicated in rising pain thresholds (Harkins and Chapman 1977).

Summary

Significant biological changes occur at different rates in different organ systems. The response to stress on the system becomes compromised, yet in the absence of significant chronic disease, functional independence can be maintained well into the ninth decade. Specific aspects of senescence are particularly relevant for the psychiatrist who must appreciate the limited reserve yet the remarkable resiliency of the elderly "survivor," the fragility of the immune response, and the increased vulnerability to medications of all types—particularly psychoactive drugs.

References

Antonaci S, Jirillo E, Ventura MT, et al: Non-specific immunity in aging: deficiency of monocyte and polymorphonuclear cell-mediated functions. Mech Aging Dev 24:367–375, 1984

Balogh K, Lelkes K: The tongue in old age. Gerontol Clin 3:38–54, 1961

Barbo DM: The postmenopausal woman, in the Physiology of the Menopause. Med Clin North Am 71:11–22, 1987

Baum BJ: Oral cavity, in Geriatric Medicine, 2nd Edition. Edited by Rowe JW, Besdine RW. Boston, MA, Little, Brown, 1988, pp 157–166

Belal A Jr: Presbycusis: physiological or pathological. J Laryngol Otol 89:1011–1125, 1975

Benedek GB: Theory of transparency of the eye. Appl Optics 10:459–473, 1971

Bertel O, Buhler FR, Kiowski W, et al: Decreased beta-andrenoreceptor responsiveness as related to age, blood pressure, and plasma catecholamines in patients with essential hypertension. Hypertension 2:130–136, 1980

Blumenthal JA, Emery GF, Madden DJ, et al: Cardiovascular and behavioral effects of aerobic exercise training in healthy older men and women. J Gerontol 44(5):147–157, 1989

Brody H: Structural changes in the aging nervous system. Edited by Blumenthal HT. Interdisciplin Top Gerontol 7:9, 1970

Brody H: Aging of the vertebrate brain, in Development and Aging in the Nervous System. New York, Academic, 1976a

Brody H: An examination of cerebral cortex and brainstem aging, in Neurobiology of Aging. Edited by Terry RD, Gershon S. New York, Raven, 1976b, pp 177–181

Burg A: Lateral visual field as related to age and sex. J Appl Psychol 52:10–15, 1968

Clark WC, Mehl L: Thermal pain: a sensory decision theory analysis of the effect of age and sex on d', various response criteria, and 50% pain threshold. J Abnorm Psychol 78:202–212, 1971

Corso JF: Sensory processes and age effects in normal adults. J Gerontol 26:90–105, 1971

Dalsky GP, Stocke KS, Ehsani AA, et al: Weight-bearing exercise training and lumbar bone mineral content in postmenopausal women. Ann Intern Med 108:824–828, 1988

Department of Health and Human Services: Life Tables, Volume 2. Section 5. Vital Statistics of the United States. Washington, DC, U.S. Government Printing Office, 1982

El-Baradi A, Bourne GH: Theory of taste and odors. Science 113:660–661, 1951

Finch CE, Schneider EL. Handbook of Biology of Aging, Vol 2. New York, Van Nostrand Reinhold, 1985

Fisher RF: Presbyopia and changes with age in the crystalline lens. J Physiol (Lond) 228:765–779, 1973

Gacek RR: Degenerative hearing loss in aging, in Neurological and Sensory Disorders in the Elderly. Edited by Fields WS. New York, Stratton, 1975

Geokas MC, Conteas CN, Majumdar APN: The aging gastrointestinal tract, liver and pancreas. Clin Geriatr Med 1:177–206, 1985

Ghali WM, Abdel-Rahman S, Hagib M, et al: Intrinsic innervation and vasculature of pre- and post-natal human thymus. Acta Anat (Basel) 108:115–123, 1980

Goldstein AL, Thurman GB, Low TLK, et al: Relationship of thymus development and function with life span and disease. Agi Ser:Physiol Cell Biol Agi 8:51–60, 1979

Goodwin JS, Searles RP, Tung KSK: Immunological responses of a healthy elderly population. Clin Exp Immunol 48:403–410, 1982

Hallgren HM, Buckley CE, Gilbersten VA, et al: Lymphocyte phytohemagglutinin responsiveness, immunoglobulins and autoantibodies in aging humans. J Immunol 111:1101–1107, 1973

Harkins SW, Chapman RC: Age and sex differences in pain perception, in Pain in the Trigeminal Region. Edited by Anderson DJ, Matthews B. Amsterdam, Elsevier North-Holland, 1977, pp 435–445

Hausman PB, Weksler ME: Changes in the immune response with age, in Handbook of the Biology of Aging, 2nd Edition. Edited by Finch CE, Schneider EL. New York, Van Nostrand Reinhold, 1985, pp 414–432

Hermanson B, Omenn GS, Kronmal RA, et al: Beneficial six-year outcome of smoking cessation in older men and women with coronary artery disease. N Engl J Med 24:1365–1392, 1988

Isaacs B: Falls in old age, in Hearing and Balance in the Elderly. Edited by Hinchdiff R. New York, Churchill Livingstone, 1983, pp 373–388

Isaacs B: Clinical and laboratory studies of falls in old people: prospects for prevention, in Falls in the Elderly: Biological and Behavioral Aspects, Clinics in Geriatric Medicine. Edited by Radebauch TS, Hadley E, Suzman R. 1:513–524, 1985

Kabadi UM, Rosman PM: Thyroid hormone indices in adult healthy subjects: no influence of aging. J Am Geriatr Soc 36:312–316, 1986

Kenney AR: Physiology of Aging: A Synopsis, 2nd Edition. Chicago, Year Book Medical, 1989

Kim YT, Siskind GW, Weksler ME: Plaque-forming cell response of human blood lymphocytes, III: cellular basis of the reduced immune response in the elderly. Isr J Med Sci 21:317–322, 1985

Kligman AM, Grove GL, Balin AK: Aging of human skin, in Handbook of Biology of Aging, Vol 2. Edited by Finch CE, Schneider EL. New York, Van Nostrand Reinhold, 1985, pp 820–841

Lakatta EG: Cardiovascular function and age. Geriatrics 42:84–94, 1987

Lake CR, Chernow B, Feuerstein G, et al: The sympathetic nervous system in man: its evolution and the measurement of plasma NE, in Norepinephrine. Edited by Ziegler MG, Lake CR. Baltimore, Williams & Wilkins, 1984, pp 1–26

Leventhal EA, Burns EA: Immune dysfunction in the elderly and the occurrence of cancer: aging and the insults of a lifetime of living, in Tumor Immunology and Immunoregulation by Thymic Hormones. Edited by Dammacco F. Milan, Masson, 1987, pp 41–56

Makinodan T, Hirokawa K: Normal aging of the immune system. Edited by Johnson HA. Aging Series: Relations Between Normal Aging and Disease; 28:117–132, 1985

Marchesini G, Cassarani S, Checchia GA, et al: Insulin resistance in aged man: relationship between impaired glucose tolerance and decreased insulin activity on branched-chain amino acids. Metabolism 36:1096–1100, 1987

Mastrioanni I, Paulsen CA: The Climacteric. New York, Plenum, 1986

McGeer EG, McGeer PL: Age changes in the human for some enzymes associated with metabolism of catecholamine, GABA, and acetylcholine. Adv Behav Biol 16:287, 1975

Minaker KL, Bonis P, Rowe JW: Gastrointestinal system, in Geriatric Medicine, 2nd Edition. Edited by Rowe JW, Besdine RW. Boston, MA, Little, Brown, 1988, pp 495–512

Montagna W, Carlisle K: Structural changes in aging human skin. J Invest Dermatol 73:47–53, 1979

Morley JE: Neuropeptides, behavior and aging. J Am Geriatr Soc 34:52–62, 1986

Morley JE, Reese SS: Clinical implications of the aging heart. Am J Med 86:77–86, 1989

National Center for Health Statistics, unpublished data on 15 leading causes of death, 65 years of age and older in 1979, 1982

National Center for Health Statistics: Current Estimates from the National Health Interview Survey, United States, 1982. Vital Health Stat, Series 10, No. 150. Washington, DC, U.S. Government Printing Office, 1985

Nicosia SV: Morphological changes in the human ovary throughout life, in The Ovary. Edited by Serra GB. New York, Raven, 57–81, 1983

Pacini GM, Valerio A, Beccaro F, et al: Insulin sensitivity and beta-cell responsivity are not decreased in elderly subjects with normal OGTT. J Am Geriatr Soc 36:317–323, 1988

Raiz LG: Local and systemic factors in the pathogenesis of osteoporosis. N Engl J Med 318:818–828, 1988

Raiz LG, Kream BE: Regulation of bone formation. N Engl J Med 309:29–33, 83–89, 1983

Riggs BL, Wahner HW, Melton JL, et al: Dietary calcium intake and rates of bone loss in women. J Clin Invest 80:979–982, 1987

Robinson BE, Conard C: Falls and falling, in Geriatric Medicine Annual. Edited by Ham RJ. Oradell, NJ, Medical Economics Company, 1986, pp 198–212

Rodeheffer RJ, Gerstenblith G, Becker LC, et al: Exercise cardiac output is maintained with advancing age in healthy human subjects: cardiac dilatation and increased stroke volume compensate for a diminished heart rate. Circulation 69:203–213, 1984

Rogers J, Bloom FE: Neurotransmitter metabolism and function in the aging central nervous system, in Handbook of the Biology of Aging. Edited by Finch CE, Schneider EL. 1985, pp 645–691

Rong H: Altersveranderungen des beruhrungssinnes. Acta Physiol Scand 6:343–352, 1943

Rowe JW, Andres R, Tobin JD, et al: The effect of age on creatinine clearance in man: a cross-sectional and longitudinal study. J Gerontol 31:155–163, 1976

Sawin CT, Chopra D, Azizi F, et al: The aging thyroid: increased prevalence of elevated serum thyrotropin levels in the elderly. JAMA 242:247–250, 1979

Schiffman SS, Moss J, Erickson RP: Thresholds of food odors in the elderly. Exp Aging Res 2:389–398, 1976

Schocken DD, Roth GS: Reduced beta-adrenergic receptor concentrations in aging man. Nature 26:856–858, 1977

Sherman ED, Robillard E: Sensitivity to pain in the aged. Can Med Assoc J 83:944–947, 1960

Simpson DM, Wicks R: Spectral analysis of heart rate indicates reduced baroreceptor-related heart rate variability in elderly persons. J Gerontol 43:M21–M24, 1988

Skinner HB, Barrack RI, Cook SD: Age-related decline in proprioception. Clin Orthop 184:208–211, 1984

Skoglund S. Joint receptors and kinaesthesis, in Handbook of Sensory Physiology. Vol 2 Edited by Iggo A. 1973, pp 111–136

Spector A, Li S, Sigelman J: Age dependent changes in the molecular size of human lens proteins and their relationship to light scatter. Invest Ophthalmol 13:795–798, 1974

Stearns EL, MacDonnell JA, Kaufman BJ, et al: Declining testicular function with age. Am J Med 57:761–766, 1974

Stelmach CE, Worringham CJ: Sensorimotor deficits related to postural stability: implications for falling in the elderly, in Falls in the Elderly: Biological and Behavioral Aspects, Clinics in Geriatric Medicine. Edited by Radebaugh TS, Hadley E, Suzman R. 1:679–694, 1985

Terry RD, De Teresa R, Hansen LAS: Neocortical cell counts in normal adult aging. Ann Neurol 21:530–539, 1987

Vestal RE, Wood AJJ, Shand DG: Reduced beta-adrenoreceptor sensitivity in the elderly. Clin Pharmacol Ther 26:181–186, 1979

Wesson LG: Physiology of the Human Kidney. New York, Grune & Stratton, 1969

Williams, JM, Felten DL: Sympathetic innervation of murine thymus and spleen: a comparative histofluorescence study. Anat Rec 199:531–542, 1981

Williams JM, Peterson RG, Shea PA, et al: Sympathetic innervation of murine thymus and spleen: evidence for a functional link between the nervous and immune systems. Brain Res Bull 6:83–94, 1981

Zahniser NR, Parker DC, Bier-Laning CM, et al: Comparisons between the effects of aging on antagonist and agonist interactions with beta-adrenergic receptors on human mononuclear and polymorphonuclear leukocyte membranes. J Gerontol 43:M151–M157, 1988

Ziegler MG, Lake CR, Kopin JJ: Plasma noradrenaline increases with age. Nature 261:333–335, 1976

CHAPTER 5

Stanley H. Cath, M.D.
Joel Sadavoy, M.D.

Psychosocial Aspects

> From hour to hour we ripe and ripe,
> And from hour to hour we rot and rot,
> And thereby hangs a tale.
>
> —William Shakespeare

Introduction

Normal psychosocial aging may be conceptualized most completely from the interactive perspective. Elements beyond the control of the individual, both physical and environmental, impinge on the already-formed personality and psychological structure of the individual. These processes have been investigated from a variety of perspectives—the sociological, the intrapsychic, and the observable psychological—and from the cross-sectional and longitudinal-developmental points of view.

Theories on aging abound, but regardless of which sources one taps, certain themes recur. Primary among these are the themes of loss, including physical, psychological, sociological, and interpersonal losses; narcissistic trauma with associated psychological impact; the relationship of the elderly to awareness of mortality and death; the effect of early life on late-life development; and the basic stability of personality throughout the life cycle. Significant data may be derived from the intensive examination of individuals. Information on normal aging in individuals is often derived from psychoanalytic and other psychodynamic studies of the aging person, which may be criticized for lack of rigor. But, as Busse and Blazer (1980, p. 18) suggested, "as a method of investigation, the psychoanalytic method is ideal for observing a relationship between biological and social factors and their effect upon the individual." It is the only system to take into account the vital significance of unconscious needs that form transference and counter-transference.

Many people awaken to their aging with a start, as if it had not been there at all. Where have roots and familiar relationships gone and why has time not stood still? The rate of recognition of an altered, senescent self is quite variable, even though the "events" signaling depletion, deterioration, disease, and decay in ourselves and in significant others increase over time. One must constantly adapt to and mourn for all kinds of normative and unexpected losses. The intensity of the denial and disavowal often inherent in dealing with losses highlights how very painful is the psychological struggle to accept one's own and one's parents' destiny; for no matter how well we age—and some do so beautifully and creatively—from mid-life on, a little bit dies, then a little bit more, and on and on until there is no more dying to do.

The depleting processes of aging may be balanced by accumulated ego strengths or resiliency, that is, the capacity to accept change in the idealized self and others; to tolerate loss of autonomy when it is needed; to be alone when "accompanying others" such as spouses are lost along the way; and to care for the self.

Definitions of Aging

Biological

In that all kinds of people become old, their destinies in the last third of the life span are tremendously variable. It is not surprising that no scientist to date has satisfactorily defined aging. Some medical scientists subscribe to the concept that aging is an intrinsic, universal process of progressive and deleterious biological change, usually correlated with the passage of time. In this model, aging is associated with a decrease in viability and an increase in vulnerability, terminating invariably in the death of the individual. Kirkwood and Busse (1978) separated aging into 1) primary— that is, biological processes rooted in hereditary (inborn and inevitable) detrimental changes that are time related but etiologically relatively independent of stress, trauma, and acquired disease; and 2) secondary—defects and disabilities resulting from trauma and disease.

Eight biological theories of aging may be cited (Busse 1989):

1. The exhaustion theory: the body contains a fixed amount of energy, which is gradually dissipated—unwound like a watch spring.
2. The accumulation theory: deleterious material that kills cells (e.g., lipofuscin or hirano bodies) develops late in life.
3. The biologic programming theory: cells are genetically programmed to live for a specific period of time, leading to inevitable death.
4. The error theory: with senescence, alterations occur in the structure of the deoxyribonucleic acid (DNA) molecule; when the errors are transmitted to messenger ribonucleic acid, there is a buildup of defective enzymes leading ultimately to cell and organismic death.
5. The cross-linkage or eversion theory: there is a change in the linkages holding together the polypeptide strands of collagen, thus rendering collagen less permeable and elastic and therefore less capable of sustaining normal life.
6. The immunologic theory: with time, there is a reduction in the protective mechanisms of the immune system, which may become autoaggressive, leading to destruction of the body tissue.
7. The "aging clock" theory: this "clock" is said to reside in the hypothalamus. The hypothalamus is central to a variety of brain and endocrine functions, and cell loss in this site has a particularly important role in decline of homeostatic mechanisms with age.
8. The free radical theory: DNA damage, cross-linkage of collagen, and the accumulation of age pigments are caused by free radicals (molecules with unpaired electrons that exist normally in the body, as well as being produced by ionizing radiation, ozone, and chemical toxins).

Despite the various theories, a unified, satisfactory, and empirically demonstrated theory of aging does not yet exist (Busse 1989).

Sociological

As Hall (1984) stated, there has been little satisfactory, systematic theory development to explain the complex and widely divergent modes of aging. However, attempts have been made to explain the basic factors in aging. Atchley (1989) proposed a continuity theory: while the basic structure of the individual remains intact over time, a variety of adaptive changes may take place. In making adaptive choices, aging individuals attempt to preserve existing internal and external structures; that is, aging individuals are motivated toward inner psychological continuity and external continuity of social behaviors. Continuity theory consists of general adaptive principles that aging individuals may be expected to follow, and explanations of how the principles work. This theory is valid for normal aging but, according to Atchley, is not very helpful in understanding the external realities of pathological aging, wherein external continuity (e.g., in residence, activities, and roles) breaks down and the strategies that promote healthy continuity cannot be employed.

Internal continuity is motivated by four factors, according to Atchley: 1) to meet the needs of self-esteem preservation; 2) to preserve ego integrity (similar to the concept of vital involvement of Erikson et al. [1986]); 3) to meet important needs, for example, the maintenance of social interaction and social support; and 4) to provide a foundation for effective day-to-day decision making (i.e., continuity of cognitive function).

Internal continuity is necessary to the preservation of the individual's concepts of self and identity. The evidence is strongly in favor of the maintenance, over time, of inner continuity in the global aspects of self and identity (Kaufman 1987). Kaufman found that older people reinterpret their current experiences so that old values can take on new meanings in keeping with present circumstance. Lieberman and Tobin's work (to be described more fully later in this chapter) also indicated that internal self-concepts and beliefs are not readily vulnerable to environmental change (Lieberman and Tobin 1983). Similarly, external continuity in skills, activities, roles, and relationships remains remarkably stable through the fifties to the seventies (Bengston and Black 1973; Gordon et al. 1976; Lawton 1983).

Cummings and Henry (1961) proposed that disengagement is a pivotal component of aging, that is, disengagement from friends, activities, and roles is an inevitability in aging and a normative preparation for death. However, there have been many critics of this theory. For example, cross-cultural studies such as that of Simmons (1970) have shown that, in the presence of societal acceptance of the elderly, engagement may increase rather than decrease with age. Hence, the concept that disengagement is a normal adaptive mechanism explanatory of the observed phenomena of old age does not stand up to scrutiny.

Roscow (1967), whose activity theory bears some resemblance to that of Atchley (1989), suggested that social integration is the prime factor in determining psychosocial adaptation in later life. Social integration refers to how the individual is tied into the web of both life and action in his or her society. Such integration is dependent on social values, formal and informal group memberships, and social roles. When group membership and social role are altered by changes in health, finances, family ties, and so on, integration is weakened, leading to alienation. In this theoretical concept, disintegration is not a natural, inevitable decline, but rather a result of lost roles. Ideally an aging individual will try to anticipate and prepare for these difficult life changes. However, as Becker and Strauss (1956) suggested, when the passages of status are not subject to an orderly sequence, as they often are not in modern society, there can be no preparation for entering them. The result is that mature, anticipatory defenses (i.e., adaptation to future or imminent life change through anticipation) are difficult to employ, leading to confrontation with sudden change and profound loss. Interestingly, Hall (1984) noted that voluntary relinquishing of roles may lead to a kind of revitalization when new activities are undertaken, whereas involuntary role loss leads to depletion. Social disintegration results from failure to adapt to role loss.

Miller (1965) proposed an alternate explanation for social alienation in old age. In his model, alienation specifically arises from the loss of the identity that comes from work. In his view, leisure roles are unable to replace work roles as a source of personal identity. Atchley (1970) argued that "identity continuity" may be maintained if aging is accompanied by sufficient supplies of friends and money to enable the formation of a self-sustaining culture. Although Atchley's views have some face validity, Vaillant and Vaillant (1990) have shown that maintenance of family, especially sibling, ties (as opposed to friends and social ties) is an important factor in psychosocial adaptation with increasing age.

Individual

Unfortunately, as Baltes and Willis (1977) stated, all existing theories of psychological aging and development are incomplete. They pointed out that personality theories of aging are influenced by the fact that, as they traverse life experiences, people become increasingly different (although in extreme old age, the very elderly show considerable similarity in certain characteristics).

Freud (1898), in his early forties, wrote that the analysis of patients over 50 was contraindicated, doomed to failure because of the amount of material to deal with and the time required to deal with it. He said, "They have reached such an age that an improvement of their mental health would be of no real value." Six years later he reiterated this view by speaking of the inelasticity of mental processes and the ineducability of the older patient. Despite

Freud's genius and frequent wisdom, in this area of understanding his vision was limited and has subsequently been proved wrong.

An early view dissenting from this pessimistic perspective was expressed by Abraham (1965), who initially had agreed with Freud's views and thought that the mind at 40 might be too cluttered to change. Based on the degree of success he obtained in his treatment of older melancholics, however, he subsequently hypothesized that a long period of successful and social functioning after puberty was a favorable indicator of successful adaptation and that the duration of the neurosis was probably more important than the age of the patient in determining outcome of psychoanalytic treatment at advanced age.

Therapeutic optimism about old age and the clearly implied retention of a capacity to work through intrapsychic conflict and thereby change have been evident in a body of clinical literature. Kaufman (1963) reported on analysis with patients aged over 50 in long-term follow-up. Alexander (1944) similarly reported on two older men whom he had determined analyzable, not on the basis of their age, but on their personality characteristics.

Schaie (1977–1978) postulated four stages of cognitive development: 1) acquisitive (childhood and adolescence), 2) achieving (young adulthood), 3) responsible and executive (middle age), and 4) reintegrative (old age). These stages are not unlike those of Erikson (1959), who described the basic life tasks of a mature ego. His schema presents a series of eight bipolar stages, beginning with the normative prevailing of trust over mistrust in infancy, leading to the achievement of autonomy, industry, independent identity, and the capacity for a productive generativity. By old age, the birth of wisdom is derived from the triumph of integrity over despair. Integrity is based on the individual's acceptance of his or her successes and failures, with an internal feeling of peace. The person has gained a sense of the nature of life and a willingness to accept it. Such a sense of integrity permits the individual to deal with loss without being overcome by profound despair. Integrated older persons do not appear to be common, although data on this aspect of normative development are scarce.

King (1980) postulated that many of the conflicts associated with aging derive from the need to reexperience and work through adolescent trauma relating to problems of dependence and independence, the breakdown of old defenses leading to an identity crisis, and concomitant changes in self-image and narcissistic mortifications.

Tasks of Aging

Loss and Grief

For some, even when they are alone, there is remarkable peace of mind as well as an ease in retaining significance in other's lives in some creative or meaningful way, be it in work, as parents or grandparents, or as contributors to science or humanity. Such individuals have grieved well for previous losses and have been liberated by the maturation-mourning process (Pollock 1987). Pollock described the ability of some individuals to reach out to life with joy and enthusiasm throughout a long life span. He characterized the capacity to attain this level of adaptation in old age as deriving from a successful mourning-liberation process, saying that the painful internal detachment from ideals, goals, and objectives, and from individuals who no longer exist, results in an acceptance of the reality principle of functioning. With this accomplishment, freedom to view the world and oneself in it, serves as a stimulus for regeneration. Pollock further asserted that mourning is a process that goes on throughout life, often unnoticed. Those who are most successful at being able to adapt earlier in life will similarly cope with the loss and subsequent grief inherent in aging with a greater degree of adaptation.

Some individuals who have less inner reserve and lack the capacity to grieve effectively or tolerate depression may be shattered by separation from a sustaining other. Although inner strength, personality cohesion, and adaptative capacity are prime determinants of adaptation in late life, the sources and chances for refueling from the available surround also may be determined by various degrees of serendipity, for example, finding a late-life friendship or mentor relationship. Adaptation is further enhanced if the losses associated with aging occur intermittently, leaving enough time for restitution and reintegration in between. Unfortunately, the omniconvergence or summation of crises may lead to a cascade of disasters without time enough in between to mourn and recover (Cath 1965). Neugarten (1979) has shown that expected events occurring at a "normative" stage of life are less stressful and better managed than unexpected events occurring at unexpected times. Unfortunately, the aging individual has little control over the sequence or timing of undesirable events, which, if they occur in unfavorable sequence or quantity, may overwhelm even the strongest individual.

Attachment and Disengagement

Although normative aging does not appear to require inevitable disengagement—contrary to Cummings and Henry (1961)—it is apparent that loss of and alterations in relationships (including friendships, marriage, and family relationships) as well as giving up of various role-based activities in society, makes dealing with attachment and disengagement a central task of old age. Kalish and Knutson (1976) proposed that an appreciation and understanding of attachments provide an explanation for psychological changes in elderly people. This view is supported by the work of Lowenthal and Haven (1968), who showed that having a confidant was the greatest single factor discriminating those who would remain in the community from those who were institutionalized. The need for meaningful interpersonal contact is further supported by clinical data arising out of individual psychodynamic psychotherapy. Grotjahn (1940, 1955), for example, in a series of papers in the 1940s and 1950s, drew a parallel between the analytic situation seen with older patients and that seen with children, namely, the analyst serves more as a real object. This concept arises repeatedly in clinical reports of therapy with the aged.

A variety of metapsychological theories arising from psychoanalytic work supports and is supported by the empirical work on attachment. Winnicott (1965), Kohut (1971), Sander (1985), and Stern (1985) all suggest that the core self is created through a series of attachments to important others whose self-regulating characteristics facilitate the formation of internal structures. Individuals expect to serve and to be served by them in mutual, gratifying, and ongoing relationships. Erikson (1986) stressed the lifelong need for affirmation from a glowing face: The infant's instinctual smiles seems to predispose to the wakening of a generous breast and parental care. Sander (1985) similarly stressed the need to define derailments of feedback loops in the vital "nodal" interactions that create the logic of organization and from which the internalization of self-regulating, self-connecting, and self-righting systems emerge. Whatever model we use, there is one consistent finding: intrapsychic adaptation at any age includes the ongoing need for accompanying, affirming "others" in living, loving, and relating, either in the real mental-representational or the transitional worlds.

Acceptance of others and control of envy as an important task of aging is a recurring theme. Klein (1963) concentrated on the attenuation of excessive feelings of envy as a requirement for relatively normal adaptation to old age. Similarly Myers (1984) pointed out that one must accept one's past and not suffer too great a degree of envy if one is to navigate the aging period successfully. Indeed, the relationship between the aging individual and younger people is a frequently encountered related theme. Neugarten (1970), in studying mid-life transitioning into old age, commented on the fact that individuals sponsor their children or younger colleagues in various forms of mentorships. Kernberg, as described by Myers (1984), pointed out that narcissistic individuals not only devalue objects as a defense against envy but also often use younger people to restore their lost grandiosity. Such individuals envy, rather than take pleasure in, the growth and success of their children. Needing others to depend on leads to excessive shame and humiliation in these individuals, a particular danger imposed by the assaults of old age.

Kohut's (1971, 1977) appreciation of the need for others, mentally configured as selfobjects, is instructive. He emphasized the lifelong need for archaic selfobjects—those objects experienced not intrapsychically in their own right, but as mere extensions of the self. The loss of these affirming relationships in later life, coupled with other assaults to sources of narcissistic gratification, leave the elderly at greater risk to the depression, anger, disappointment, and withdrawal associated with narcissistic blows. Indeed, it appears to be an important but often unappreciated ego function of late life to maintain a capacity to recall evocative images that revitalize the self and give meaning to current existence.

Interestingly, however, Cath (1990) has observed that many elders with considerable core depletion (i.e., early-life failures in emotional development) have not only led integrated lives but also become increasingly competent as they age, for reasons difficult to define.

Kernberg (1980) pointed out that individuals who cannot recharge or revitalize themselves based on internalized value systems are vulnerable to the development of a pathological, grandiose personality. Such individuals are not prepared for loss, failures, crisis, or the inevitable aging process and must therefore suffer. Frequently these individuals experience no gratitude for what they received in the past, experience the past as a loss, wish they had it now, and are painfully resentful of its having ceased to be available. Such individuals are unprepared to acknowledge the passage of time and lack the accumulation of an internal life that would provide sustenance and compensation for the later losses and failures that are inevitable.

Maintenance of Self-Identity

Several authors have asserted that self-concept and self-image remain stable and do not become impoverished or negative in old age (e.g., Monge 1975; Richard et al. 1962). Vaillant and Vaillant (1990), in studying a "favored" sample of healthy men from age 18 through to age 65 (n = 173), found that the factors that favored good psychosocial adjustment in later life were sustained family relationships (especially prior closeness to siblings); maturity of defenses (as assessed prior to age 50, including sublimation, suppression, anticipation, altruism, and humor); absence of alcoholism; and absence of depressive disorder.

Schaie and Parham (1976) studied adults aged 22 to 77 before and after a 7-year interval. When studied longitudinally, the group showed little change. In cross section, the older group was more conservative and conscientious. Increased age was associated with increased excitability, decreased suspiciousness, and greater practical-mindedness.

Costa and McCrae (1978), in their cross-sectional evaluation, also found increased conscientiousness with age but no age-associated changes when the sample was examined longitudinally over 10 years. But they found increased liberalism and tender-mindedness, unlike Schaie and Parham. Siegler and associates (1979) found no differences among age groups whether examined cross-sectionally or longitudinally.

Although Lieberman and Tobin (1983, p. 240) reiterated that the "conventional wisdom is that, in spite of a plethora of changes in later life, each of us remains the same to ourselves," they also suggested that "neither systematic change nor stability is reflected in our current state of knowledge." They studied the stability and changes in the self and the processes that individuals employ in their quest to maintain self-identity. Their assumption was that the assaults associated with aging (i.e., losses of people and roles, denigration by society, and confrontation with bodily disintegration and personal death) cause "de-selfing."

They developed a 48-item questionnaire to assess self-concept in the elderly and contrasted the responses of 40 individuals who had already been institutionalized with 16 community controls and 22 elderly who were facing radical change in their "life space" by virtue of imminent institutionalization. Their results showed that the elderly are remarkably capable of retaining a persistent self-concept when confronting instability. The analysis of the data showed that the subjects maintained this stable self-concept through use of the generalized past for self-validation, for example, as indicated by use of the phrase "That's how I have always been" (rather than use of a specific example of behavior from the past—a mechanism employed infrequently by this population—for self-validation). An interesting finding was that adolescents are almost exclusively bound to the happenings of the present for self-validation, in contrast to the use of the generalized past by the elderly. These investigators concluded that the elderly use the past to validate self-image in the present. Those who turn to less adequate evidence from the past in order to maintain their sense of identity are the very ones whose ability to weather severe stress appears limited. The evidence and the conclusions are in broad support of clinically based assertions and sociologically based theories of aging.

Reminiscence is an often-stated, normative process of aging that may be related to the maintenance of identity and self-concept. Butler (1963) proposed that the process of reminiscence is a component of an inevitable life-review function in old age. Erikson (1959) also highlighted the role of dealing with the past, suggesting that reconciliation of the past is the method for achieving the goal of the last stage of development, that is, integrity. Lieberman and Tobin (1983) asked whether there is a specific, psychological dynamic for reminiscence, or whether reminiscence derives from failures in the current situation; that is, is it provoked by loss of relevant others and reference groups, and by failures of the body and so on, to provide adequate self-validation? Some clinicians (e.g., Sadavoy and Robinson 1989) have commented on the early prevalence of reminiscence in group therapy, apparently as a medium for social exchange between individuals who do not yet know each other well, noting that reminiscence gradually fades and is replaced by more current interactional discussions once group cohesion is established.

In his last book, *Vital Involvement in Old Age,* Erikson (Erikson et al. 1986) pointed to a fascinating late-life shift arising in the reminiscence process. Women who had previously reported dissatisfying relationships—for example, nothing in common with oppressive husbands with whom they had incessantly quarreled— by their eighties seemed to have a great need to believe it had been otherwise. The images transitioned into statements like, "The fact that we were so alike is one of the strongest ties" or "For 60 years we did everything together." General clinical experience tends to support this observation; for example, many children regard a parent's assertions of marital bliss as most unrealistic, if not postmortem fabrication. But such phenomena do warn that the human capacity to create narrative truth out of historical untruth needs to be respected (Cath 1972).

There are conflicting views on whether reminiscence is a universal process. Romaniuk (1978) suggested that it is, based on what he interpreted as positive answers in 80% of the institutionalized population. Coleman (1974) and McMahon and Rhudick (1967) indicated that it is not universal. However, the work of McMahon and Rhudick and of Coleman suggests that the presence of reminiscence seems to be associated with a greater degree of life satisfaction in old age.

Lieberman and Tobin (1983) undertook a structured analysis of reminiscence using three questionnaires: a life history interview, an evaluation-of-life questionnaire, and what they termed an on-memory questionnaire. The data gathered from these three structured interviews permitted them to examine three issues: 1) the importance of the past, 2) the presence of reconciliation (i.e., reworking and reorganizing memories, indicating that life review work is accomplished), and 3) the construction of the past as myth or drama rather than reality. In this study, they examined four groups: 25 middle-aged controls, 40 institutionalized elderly, 22 elderly facing critical life change, and 16 "normal," community-residing elderly.

The results showed that the past served as a powerful source of gratification and interpersonal attention for the elderly, thereby supporting the self-enhancing functions of reminiscence and its normative presence in old age. However, they could not substantiate the view that "life review" occurs in most elderly as a restitutive phenomenon.

Self-Esteem and Narcissism

Issues of self-esteem and narcissism associated with the maintenance of self-identity have been highlighted by many authors. Meerloo (1953) underlined the problem of self-esteem regulation in aging patients, their increased sense of loneliness, and their fear of death. Cath (1963), in a series of papers starting in 1963, expanded on some of the changes that occur in the middle years and that become so relevant to what follows in subsequent decades. He focused on changes leading to a loss of narcissistic gratification, describing the transition from creator and doer to progenitor and observer, and the need to integrate all of these transitions within the self and family image. He developed a schema of loss and restitution, as well as a framework for therapeutic intervention related to depletion and loss in five basic anchorages: the body, the family, the social networks, economic resources, and meaningful purposes to life. He found that losses in these five spheres may all converge and called the phenomenon "omni-convergence." He emphasized that the depletion of biological and psychological resources in the older individual may be compensated for by projective identification (i.e., rebuilding self-esteem through idealization of children).

Hanna Segal (1958), reporting on the analysis of an aging patient, commented on the patient's capacity to begin to work through his ambivalence toward his love objects. The patient ended the treatment feeling that his life had been worth living, was able to see younger people as more separate—to be loved for themselves—and to enjoy the thought of their living on and prospering after his own death.

Levin (1963) stated a classical economic position in noting that normal aging is dependent to a considerable degree on the capacity to redistribute libido to new objects and new aims. Berezin (1963) also noted the problems with loss of love objects and highlighted the difficulties in withdrawing and retiring from a meaningful lifelong occupation. Fromm-Reichman (1950) stressed the complex relationship between actual and fantasized relationships with others and the dread of loneliness. In her view, the objective, increasing loneliness of old age activates much earlier, psychologically primitive fears of loneliness.

Kohut (1971, 1977) emphasized the lifelong need of the individual for sustaining interactions with others (who function in part as selfobjects) and with environmental sources of narcissistic gratification. Lazarus (1987) reported Kohut's comment that it is more appropriate to focus on the elderly person and his or her environment as a unit rather than focusing only on the failures of the aged and on the defects of the self.

Meissner (1976) supported the idea that the greatest problem in late life is narcissistic loss. Lazarus (1980) suggested that normatively aging individuals possess adequate amounts of self-esteem and confidence and are thereby able to achieve wisdom, acceptance of mortality, and ability to share with and take pleasure in younger people.

Despite clinical support for the centrality of narcissistic assault on both normal and vulnerable personalities (Kernberg 1980; Sadavoy 1987), empirical data are scarce.

Dealing With Death

Becker (1973, p. ix) said, "The idea of death, the fear of it, haunts the human animal like nothing else; it is a mainspring of human activity—activity designed largely to avoid the finality of death, to overcome it by denying in some way that it is the final destiny for man."

Death is indeed central to aging. Gutman (1979), for example, suggested that older people may be better conceptualized as "terminating" rather than aging. Several authors have commented on the normative importance of facing one's death. For example, Sandler (1978) confirmed Freud's epigrammatic observation "To endure life, one must prepare for death," and Cath (1990) stated that mourning for the aging and death of one's parents is an excellent preparation for one's own later years.

However, despite the face validity of the association of death and death anxiety with old age, various clinical contributions suggest a need to modify this concept. Jaques (1970) proposed that the mid-life crisis arises as a result of the growing conscious awareness of eventual death accompanied by an increasing acknowledgment of the existence of hate and of the destructive impulses in each person. He described the explicit recognition of these two features as an essential aspect of this period of life. He suggested that a normative developmental task of middle age (rather than old age) is to begin to mourn eventual death. Such working through is possible if the primal object is sufficiently well-established in its own right and not excessively idealized or devalued. Meerloo (1953) underlined the problem of self-esteem regulation in aging patients, their increased sense of loneliness, and their fear of death. He believed the attempt to deny the imminence of death was to be found in dreams of older people.

Empirical data are sparse and perhaps somewhat contradictory. Holmes (1978) investigated the response of individuals suffering from chronic obstructive pulmonary disease ($n = 40$), whom he followed for 4 years. He noted that when invalidism, as a result of the pathology, became chronic and death approached, patients' preoccupation with dying was common but death was not feared. Rather, death was experienced as a goal that is both relevant and appropriate to the situation. He further pointed out that, although fear was expressed by some, the main source of distress for the patients was expressed in a power struggle and in conflicts with medical staff and families.

Lieberman and Tobin (1983, p. 203) attempted to examine empirically the relationship of aging and death. They pointed out that death is central to the psychology of aging and said, "Awareness of finitude is seen as an organizing concern for the aged." They attempted to study this concept prospectively, examining an institutionalized sample every 3 to 4 weeks using standardized measures. Two groups emerged: a "death-near" group (those who died a mean of 5.4 weeks after the study began) and a "death-far" group (those who died at least 1 year after completing the test).

It is not surprising that the results showed that cognitively the death-far group functioned better. Lieberman and Tobin concluded that impending death was associated with cognitive decline. But it is interesting that data regarding direct statements about death did not reveal extensive preoccupation and awareness of death in the spontaneous comments of the patients. However, the projective testing, as it emerged through use of the Thematic Apperception Test, (Murray 1943) did show evidence of death themes.

The conclusion of this component of Lieberman and Tobin's work suggested that there is decreased ego functioning as death approaches, as well as a loss of cognitive function. "It appears that many if not most elderly people approaching death are able to contain the experience and thereby limit conscious pain" (p. 228). In summarizing their results, they stated that the view of death as an overriding psychological factor in aging is not supported. Death anxiety in the elderly appears to be an "invention of the young" (Munnichs 1966).

Conclusion

Let us return to a more dynamic and more balanced understanding of the meaning of aging, depletion, dying, and death in both the conscious and unconscious awareness of aging people. Beyond the middle of the journey through life, the rate of recognition of an altered, senescent self and the issue of approaching mortality is quite variable even though the events signaling depletion, deterioration, disease, and decay in ourselves and in significant others increase over time. We are in constant mourning for all kinds of paradises lost. The intensity of the denial and disavowal reveal how very painful the psychological struggle to accept one's present human destiny and mourn for the past usually is as time goes by. Loss, depression, and creative restitution are inherent in human development and senescence.

It may be Washington Irving (1962, p. 49) who most closely approximated the complexity of this experience in his description (p. 49) of Rip van Winkle's awakening:

> He looked for his gun, but in place of the clean well-ordered fowling piece, he found an old fire lock lying by him, the barrel incrusted with rust, the lock falling off, and the stock worm-eaten.

Just as humans have done through the ages, Rip in his maturity awakes to his own aging and begins a frantic search for his roots and familiar relationships. Where have they gone? Why has time not stood still? And by subtle indication, where did he go wrong? But the time limit of human parts of the self and its connections is evident at birth and becomes a part of the uniquely human psychology of aging.

References

Abraham K: The applicability of psychoanalytic treatment of patients at an advanced age, in Selected Papers of Karl Abraham. Edited by Bryan D and Strachey A. London, Hogarth Press, pp 312–317

Alexander S: The indications for psychoanalytic therapy. Bull NY Acad Med, Second Series 20:6:319–332, 1944

Atchley RC: Retirement and leisure participation: continuity or crisis. Gerontologist:13–18, 1970

Atchley RC: A continuity theory of normal aging. Gerontologist 29:183–190, 1989

Baltes PB, Willis SL: Toward psychological theories of aging and development, in Handbook of the Psychology of Aging. Edited by Birren JE, Schaie KW. New York, Van Nostrand Reinhold, 1977, pp 128–150

Becker E. The Denial of Death. New York, Free Press, 1973, p ix

Becker HS, Strauss A: Careers, personality, and adult socialization. American Journal of Sociology:253–267, 1956

Bengston VL, Black D: Intergenerational relations and continuities in socialization, in Life-Span Developmental Psychology: Personality and Socialization. Edited by Baltes PB, Schaie KW. New York, Academic Press, 1973

Berezin MA: Some intrapsychic aspects of aging, in Normal Psychology of the Aging Process. Edited by Ainsberg NE. New York, International Universities Press, 1963, pp 93–117

Busse EW: The Myth, history, and science of aging, in Geriatric Psychiatry. Edited by Busse EW, Blazer DG. Washington DC, American Psychiatric Press, 1989, pp 3–34

Busse EW, Blazer DG: The theories and process of aging, in Handbook of Geriatric Psychiatry. Edited by Busse EW, Blazer DG. New York, Nostrand and Reinhold, 1980, pp 3–27

Butler R: The life review: An interpretation of reminiscence in the aged. Psychiatry 26:65–70, 1963

Cath SH: Some Dynamics of Middle and Later Years. Smith College Studies in Social Work. New York, International Universities Press, 1963, 33:2 pp 97–126

Cath SH: Some dynamics of middle-later years: a study of depletion and restitution, in Geriatric Psychiatry: Grief, Loss, and Emotional Disorder in the Aging Process. Edited by Berezin M, Cath SH. New York, International Universities Press, 1965, pp 21–72

Cath SH: The institutionalization of a parent: a nadir of life. Geriat Psychiatry 1(5):25–46, 1972

Cath SH: The awareness of the nearness of death and depletion and the senescent cell antigen: a reconsideration of Freud's death instinct on the new frontier between psychodynamic theory and biology, in New Concepts of Adult Development. Edited by Nemiroff R, Colarusso C. New York, Basic Books, 1990

Coleman PG: Measuring reminiscence characteristics from conversations as adaptive features in old age. Int J Aging Hum Dev 5:281–294, 1974

Costa PT, McCrae RR: Objective personality assessment, in The Clinical Psychology of Aging. Edited by Storandt M, Siegler IC, Elias MF. New York, Plenum, 1978, pp 119–143

Cummings E, Henry WE: The Process of Disengagement. New York, Basic Books, 1961

Erikson EH: Identity and the Life-Cycle: Psychological Issues. New York, International University Press, 1959

Erikson EH, Erikson JM, Kivnick HQ: Vital Involvement in Old Age. New York, WW Norton, 1986

Freud S: Sexuality in the aetiology of the neuroses (1898), in The Standard Edition of the Complete Psychological Works of Sigmund Freud, Vol 3. Translated and edited by Strachey J. London, Hogarth Press, 1962, pp 261–285

Fromm R: Principles of Intensive Psychotherapy. Chicago, University of Chicago Press, 1950

Gordon C, Gaitz CM, Scott J: Leisure and lives: personal expressivity across the life-span, in Handbook of Aging and the Social Sciences. Edited by Binstock RH, Shanas E. New York, Van Nostrand Reinhold, 1976

Grotjahn M: Psychoanalytic investigation of a seventy-one-year-old man with senile dementia. Psychoanal Q 9:80–87, 1940

Grotjahn M: Analytic psychotherapy with the elderly. Psychoanal Rev 42:419–427, 1955

Gutman D: The clinical pathology of later life: developmental paradigms. Paper presented at the West Virginia Gerontology Conference on Transition of Aging, May 1979.

Hall BA: Theories that explain psychosocial adjustment in aging, in Mental Health and the Elderly. Edited by Hall BA. Orlando, FL, Grune & Stratton, 1984

Holmes TH: Death and dying, in Usdin G, Hofling CK. New York, Brunner/Mazel, 1978, pp 166–183

Irving W: Rip Van Winkle/The Legend of Sleepy Hollow. New York, Washington Square Books, 1962

Jaques E: Work, Creativity, and Social Justice. New York, International Universities Press, 1970

Kalish RA, Knutson FW: Attachment versus disengagement: a life span conceptualization. Hum Dev 19:171–181, 1976

Kaufman SR: The Ageless Self: Sources of Meaning in Late Life. Madison, WI, University of Wisconsin Press, 1963

Kernberg O: Internal World and External Reality: Object Relations Theory Applied. New York, Jason Aronson, 1980

King PHM: The life-cycle as indicated by the nature of the transference in the psychoanalysis of the middle-aged and elderly. Int J Psychoanal 61:153–159, 1980

Kirkwood BC, Busse EW: Aging Research: review and critique, in Aging: The Process and the People. Edited by Usdin G, Hofling CK. New York, Brunner/Mazel, 1978, pp 129–165

Klein M: Our Adult World. New York, Basic Books, 1963

Kohut H: The Analysis of the Self. New York, International Universities Press, 1971

Kohut H: The Restoration of the Self. New York, International Universities Press, 1977

Lawton MP: Environmental and other determinants of well-being in older people. Gerontologist 23:348–357, 1983

Lazarus LW: Self psychology and psychotherapy with the elderly: theory and practice. J Geriatr Psychiatry 13:69–88, 1980

Lazarus LW: Psychological aspects and disorders associated with aging, in Psychogeriatrics: An International Handbook. Edited by Bergener M. New York, Springer, 1987, pp 75–95

Levin S: Libido Equilibrium in Normal Psychology of the Aging Process. Edited by Ginberg N and Kaufman I. New York, International Universities Press, 1963, pp 160–168

Lieberman MA, Tobin SS: The Experience of Old Age. New York, Basic Books, 1983, pp 240–241

Lowenthal MF, Haven C: Interaction and adaptation: intimacy as a critical variable, in Middle-Age and Aging. Edited by Neugarten BL. Chicago, IL, University of Chicago Press, 1968, pp 390–400

McMahon AW, Rhudick PJ: Reminiscing in the aged: an adaptational response, in Psychodynamic Studies on Aging: Creativity, Reminiscence, and Dying. Edited by Levin S, Kahana RJ. New York, International Universities Press, 1967

Meerloo JAM: Contributions of psychoanalysis to the problems of the aged, in Psychoanalysis and Social Work. Edited by Heimann M. New York, International Universities Press, 1953

Meissner WW: Normal psychology of the aging process revisited, 1: discussion. J Geriatr Psychiatry 9:151–159, 1976

Miller SJ: Social dilemmas of the aging leisure participant, in Older People and Their Social World. Edited by Rose AP, Peterson WP. Philadelphia, PA, F.A. Davis, 1965

Monge RH: Structure of the self-concept from adolescence through old age. Exp Aging Res 1:281–291, 1975

Munnichs JM: Old age and finitude: a contribution to psychogerontology. Bibliotheca Vita Humana No.4, 1966

Murray HA: Thematic Apperception Test Manual. Cambridge, Harvard University, 1943

Myers WA: Dynamic Therapy of the Older Patient. New York, Jason Aronson, 1984, pp 1–13

Neugarten BL: Dynamics of transition of middle age to old age: adaptation and the life cycle. J Geriatr Psychiatry 4:71–87, 1970

Neugarten B: Time, age and the life cycle. Am J Psychiatry 136:887–894, 1979

Pollock GH: The mourning liberation process: ideas on the inner life of the older adult, in Treating the Elderly With Psychotherapy. Edited by Sadavoy J, Leszcz M. New York, International Universities Press, 1987, pp 3–29

Richard S, Levison F, Petersen PG: Aging and Personality: A Study of Eighty-Seven Older Men. New York, Wiley, 1962

Romaniuk M: Reminiscence and the elderly: an exploration of its content, function press and product. Doctoral dissertation, University of Wisconsin at Madison, 1978

Roscow I: Social Integration of the Aged. New York, Free Press, 1967

Sadavoy J: Character disorders in the elderly: an overview, in Treating the Elderly in Psychotherapy: The Scope for Change in Later Life. Edited by Sadavoy J, Leszcz M. New York, International Universities Press, 1987

Sadavoy J, Robinson A: Psychotherapy with the organically impaired elderly, in Consequences of Brain Disease in the Elderly: Focus in Management. Edited by Conn D, Grek A, Sadavoy J. New York, Plenum, 1989

Sander LW: Toward a logic of organization in psychobiological development, in Biologic Response Styles: Clinical Implications. Edited by Klar H, Siever LJ. Washington, DC, American Psychiatric Press, 1985, pp 19–36

Sandler AM: Problem in the psychoanalysis of an aging narcissitic patient. Geriatr Psychoanal 11:5–36, 1978

Schaie KW: Toward a stage theory of adult cognitive development. Aging Hum Dev 8:129–138, 1977–1978

Schaie KW, Parham IA: Stability of adult personality traits: fact or fable? J Pers Soc Psychol 34:146–158, 1976

Segal H: Fear of Death: Notes on the Analysis of an old man. Int J Psychoanalysis 39:178–181, 1958

Siegler IC, George LK, Okun M: Cross-sequential analysis of adult personality. Developmental Psychology 15:350–351, 1979

Simmons LW: Aging in pre-industrial societies, in Handbook of Social

Gerontology. Edited by Tibbitts C. Chicago, University of Chicago Press, 1970

Stern D: The Interpersonal World of the Infant. New York, Basic Books, 1985

Vaillant G, Vaillant CO: Natural history of male psychosocial health, XII: a 45-year study of predictors of successful aging at age 65. Am J Psychiatry 147:31–37, 1990

Winnicott DW: The Maturational Process and the Facilitating Environment. New York, Washington Square Books, 1962, p 49

CHAPTER 6

George J. Warheit, PH.D.
Charles F. Longino, PH.D.
Julia E. Bradsher, M.A.

Sociocultural Aspects

Introduction

Aging and old age increase the risk of developing a variety of physical and mental health problems. Some of these are noted in this chapter, and detailed accounts of them are presented elsewhere in this text. Concurrent with biologically based changes in health, old age also brings many important socially induced changes, some of which have the potential for negative effect on both the physical and mental well-being of older persons. These social changes include altered statuses related to marriage and family patterns, living arrangements, work behaviors, retirement, economic stability, and sex roles (Rosow 1974; Streib 1984). In short, one of the major assumptions underlying the materials presented in this chapter is that getting old and being old in our society have social and psychological consequences as well as biological ones.

Throughout this chapter, aging is conceptualized as a process without fixed beginning or end. Old age, on the other hand, is arbitrarily defined as being older than 65. This chronological marker was chosen because it represents the age at which the majority of persons in our society can retire with full Social Security and other pension benefits. We recognize the limitations inherent in this rationale; we are also aware of the arbitrariness of all definitions of older age: the frail old, the old-old, and other similar categories.

Social and Demographic Characteristics

Age and Aging

America is growing older, and it is doing so at an accelerated rate. Evidence of this growth is provided by the U.S. Bureau of the Census, which reported that in the past two decades the number of persons aged 65 and older grew by 56% while the under-65 age group increased only 19%. Since the 1980 census, approximately 170,000 persons a month in the United States have reached their 65th birthday (U.S. Bureau of the Census 1987a). These data are even more remarkable when viewed in a historical context. In 1900 only 4% of this country's population was aged 65 or older. By the mid-1980s, about 12% of the population was 65 or older. In total numbers, the Bureau of the Census estimated in 1986 that there were 29.2 million Americans at least 65 years of age and that there were nearly 12 million persons aged 75 or older (Siegel and Davidson 1984; Spencer 1984; U.S. Bureau of the Census 1987a). Researchers estimated that there were about 32,000 persons 100 years of age or older in 1984 (Spencer et al. 1987).

The total number and overall percentage of Americans aged 65 and older will continue to increase into the 21st century. As those born during the baby boom years (1946–1964) move into older age early in the 21st century, 20% of the country's population will be 55 years or older. By the year 2010, approximately 25% of the population will be 55 or older and nearly 15% of all Americans will be 65 or older. In the year 2030, it is projected that one-third of the population will be 55 or older and that about one-fifth will be 65 or older (Spencer 1984; Aging in America 1987).

While the overall population of the United States is aging at an increasing rate, not all sex, race, and ethnic groups are equally represented in the total population of older persons. Women continue to live longer than men, and there are more whites aged 65 and older than blacks or Hispanics. (References to Hispanics throughout this chapter include persons of all racial groups within this very heterogenous population, because the Bureau of the Census combines all Hispanics in most of their reports and because these reports provide most of the reliable estimates concerning population patterns and trends.)

In 1986, there were 17.4 million women aged 65 or older but only 11.8 million men. And this disparity is growing, especially in the upper-age groups. In 1986, there were only 83 men for every 100 women in the 65–69 group, and in the 85-and-older cohort there were only 40 men for every 100 women (U.S. Bureau of the

Census 1987a). The same census report indicated that whites live longer than their black and Hispanic counterparts, although there is growing evidence that these differences are decreasing as a consequence of the lowering of infant and maternal death rates and by slight increases in survivorship among minorities aged 65 and older.

At present, there is a larger percentage of whites aged 65 and older than of blacks or Hispanics. In 1986, 13% of the white population was 65 or older; the rate for blacks was 8%; for Hispanics it was only 5%. These race-ethnic differences can be attributed in part to the higher fertility rates found among black and Hispanic populations and to the greater longevity rates among whites of both sexes.

In 1986, approximately 88% of the country's total population aged 65 and older was white, 9% was nonwhite, and approximately 3% was Hispanic. The approximate proportions of these groups in the total population were whites, 80%; nonwhites, 13%; and Hispanics, 7%. However, it is estimated that the proportion of older nonwhites and Hispanics will grow rapidly in the decades ahead. Projections indicate that although the white, non-Hispanic population 65 and older will increase by about 100% between 1985 and 2030, the rate of increase for nonwhites will be 165% and for Hispanics it will be 530%. Despite these increases among nonwhites and Hispanics, whites will still have a larger percentage of their total number aged 65 and older (24%) than will nonwhites (16%) or Hispanics (13%) (Spencer 1984, 1986).

The overall aging of the U.S. population is, of course, highly related to increased life expectancy. A child born in 1900 had a life expectancy of 47.3 years; in 1960, this figure had grown to 69.6 years and in 1985 it was 74.4 years. The increases in life expectancy during the first five decades of this century were due largely to decreased infant mortality and to reduced mortality from infectious diseases. By contrast, the increases in life expectancy over the past three decades have resulted largely from lower mortality among those in the middle-aged and older cohorts. Persons who became 65 years of age in 1985 could expect to live, on average, an additional 16.8 years. White females now have the longest life expectancy and black males the shortest (Health, U.S., 1986).

Work and Retirement

As people live longer, they spend more time in both work and retirement. Retirement was the domain of a privileged few earlier in

this century, but at present it has become more of an institutionalized expectation and there appears to be increasing acceptance of
it as a social status (Atchley 1984). In 1900, when the life expectancy of men was 46.3, their average work life was 32.1 years. They
could expect only 1.2 years in retirement or work at home. By 1950,
the life expectancy for men had increased to 65.6 years, of which
41.5 years were spent in work and 10.1 years were devoted to retirement or work at home. The data for 1980 showed that the life
expectancy for men had grown to 70.0 years, with the time in the
labor force decreasing to 38.8 years and the length of retirement
increasing to 13.6 years.

The labor force and retirement activities of women between
1900 and 1980 also showed remarkable changes. Life expectancy
rose from 48.3 in 1900 to 77.4 in 1980. And the labor force participation of women increased dramatically, rising from 6.3 years in
1900 to 30.6 years in 1980. Since 1900, the percentage of a woman's
lifetime spent in the labor force has increased from 13% to 38%,
and during the same period the percentage of time spent in retirement or work at home decreased from 60% to about 40% (Smith
1985).

In 1986, 55% of the men and 33% of the women aged 60 to 64
were in the labor force, but by age 70 only about 10% of men and
4% of women were employed (U.S. Department of Labor 1987).
These statistics reflect that a larger percentage of Americans of
both sexes are living longer and that many of them are retiring
earlier. A 1978 survey conducted by Harris showed that about two-
thirds of a national sample had left their jobs before age 65 and
that the median age at retirement was 60.6 years. Of those reported being retired, 81% were unemployed, 8% were working
part-time, and only 5% indicated they were working full-time
(Harris 1979). In addition, there is evidence from the research findings reported by Fields and Mitchell (1983) that strongly suggests
that changes in the age of eligibility for full Social Security benefits from age 65 to age 67 by the year 2027 will raise the average
retirement age by only about 3 months. These investigations also
determined that recent federal legislation eliminating mandatory
retirement at age 70 for most occupations is likely to have little
effect on the trend toward earlier retirement. The reasons given
most often for the increasing pattern of early retirement include
health problems, Social Security and other pension benefits, social
expectations, and long-held plans (Fields and Mitchell 1983).

Although retirement is becoming more of an institutionalized
status in our society than it once was, and although a larger per-

centage of Americans is retiring at earlier ages than ever before, unemployment still remains a serious problem for many who want to remain in the labor force. Also, people aged 65 or older who are without work tend to have longer periods of unemployment or underemployment than younger persons. And they frequently must take entry-level salaries and work for employers who offer few, if any, employee benefits. The U.S. Department of Labor reported that in 1986 there were 273,000 persons aged 60 and older who were unemployed and that approximately 91,000 of them were 65 or older. Because those who are not working but who have ceased looking for employment are not counted as unemployed, the statistics on unemployment among older persons are low estimates. If all non-labor force participants 60 and older were included, the total number would be approximately 459,000. This figure represents about 5.8% of all persons in this age cohort (U.S. Department of Labor 1987).

Economic Resources

Persons aged 65 and older in America tend to have lower incomes than those under 65. Moreover, the median income decreases with increasing age. In 1985, the median income of families with a head of household aged 25 to 64 was $30,504. For those with a head of household 65 or older it was $19,117, or about one-third less. Furthermore, income differentials increase as age differences increase. For example, persons in family units with a head of household 85 and older had median incomes in 1985 of $15,111. This amount is about one-half that of family units with a head of household aged 25 to 64 (U.S. Bureau of the Census 1987b).

From the viewpoint of cash income alone, older age is usually accompanied by a significant reduction in economic resources. As a consequence, older people are more likely than younger people to be at or near the poverty level. In 1986, 12.4% of people aged 65 and older were living in poverty versus 10.8% of people aged 18 to 64. The elderly were also more likely than the nonelderly to have incomes near the poverty level: 28% of all persons in families headed by someone aged 65 years or older were between poverty and 149% of poverty. By comparison, 22% of those living in families with the head of household younger than 65 were in poverty or between poverty and 149% of poverty (U.S. Bureau of the Census 1987b).

The same 1986 census report indicated that women aged 65 and older were poorer than men in the same cohort. Approximately

14.1% of the men 65 and older were below poverty or between poverty and 124% of the poverty level. The comparable rate for women in the same age cohort was 24.7%. In 1986, the median income of women was $6,425; for men it was $11,544. The oldest women (85 and older) are the poorest subgroup of the elderly; 20% of them were in poverty in 1986. And, although women accounted for only about 60% of the noninstitutionalized elderly in 1986, they comprised 71.8% of the elderly poor. It is also worth noting that when income data were analyzed for marital status groups, older women of every marital status in 1986 had lower incomes than their male counterparts. These low incomes are due, at least in part, to the consequences of long-term dependence on the incomes and pensions of men (U.S. Bureau of the Census 1987b).

The Bureau of the Census has also reported that blacks and Hispanics have lower incomes than whites. This point is true for all age groups including those 65 and older. The median income for older black men was only about one-half that of older white men in 1986, and the median income of black women was one-third less than that of white women. The median income of Hispanics was very similar to that of blacks. These income differences are reflected in the poverty rates for the three largest ethnic groups in the United States. The poverty rate for older whites in 1986 was 10.7%, for Hispanics it was 22.5%, and for blacks it was 31%. Almost one-half of the black elderly and one-third of the older Hispanics had incomes below 125% of the poverty level. By comparison, the percentage for older whites was 18.3%. Almost two-thirds of all black women 72 or older who lived alone had incomes below the poverty level in 1986 (U.S. Bureau of the Census 1987b).

It is not surprising that the relative disparity in income between younger whites, blacks, and Hispanics carries over into old age. The personal and social problems encountered by racial and ethnic minorities in our society are numerous, but perhaps none have more serious consequences for their overall health and social well-being than those associated with low socioeconomic status.

Other Economic Assets

There is a commonly held notion that the low income levels found among older persons are offset by the possession of other assets. As a subgroup, people aged 55 and older do tend to have more assets than people under 55. However, in 1983, about two-thirds of the net worth of all households with a householder 55 or older was in home equity, and nearly one-half of those persons' net worth (including the equity in their homes) was less than $50,000. Furthermore, about 40% had a net worth of less than $10,000 when home equity was excluded (U.S. Bureau of the Census 1986).

The data indicate that a great many older persons in the United States have very limited economic assets of any kind. Although the financial well-being of those 55 and older is generally much better than it was a generation ago, the cash available to most older Americans is still quite modest. Moreover, recent discussions concerning changes in the determination of cost-of-living adjustments may reduce future Social Security benefits. If this reduction occurs, or if the subscriber's cost for catastrophic health care coverage under Medicare increases, some of the recent economic gains made by the nation's elderly may be slowed or reduced.

Marital Status, Family Patterns, and Living Arrangements

The marital status, family patterns, and living arrangements of people aged 65 and older vary greatly for men and women. A 1984 survey revealed that most older men lived in family settings, whereas most women did not. About 75% of the men 65 and older were living in households where a spouse was present; the percentage for women was much lower: 38.3%. One-half of all women 65 and older were widows; among those 75 and older the percentage was 67%. Approximately 8.3 million persons 65 and older were living alone in 1986. Most were women; they comprised 80% of the overall total (6.6 million). Among all the noninstitutionalized elderly, only 15% of the men lived alone, whereas the overall rate for women was 40% (National Center for Health Statistics 1987a; U.S. Bureau of the Census 1987–1988).

Physical Health

Health Characteristics

Authors of other chapters in this text outline in detail the physical health characteristics and behaviors of older people in the United States. Therefore, only a brief mention of the physical well-being of older persons is made here. From a sociocultural perspective, there is no need to document what is a well-known fact, namely, that morbidity rates for most chronic illnesses increase in a linear fashion with age. Heart disease, cancer, and stroke (three of the leading causes of death in the United States) are most prevalent among people aged 65 and older. Older age is frequently accompanied by a higher risk for a variety of acute and infectious diseases as well.

Research has shown that 80% of all persons aged 65 and older have at least one chronic condition and that multiple disorders are commonplace (Lawrence and McLemore 1983). In a cross-sectional study of 2,115 randomly selected adults in north central Florida, Warheit and his colleagues (1986) found higher rates of physical health problems and prescription drug use among the 1,076 respondents in the sample who were aged 60 and older than they found among respondents under 60. When asked if they had taken any medicine prescribed by a doctor in the past year, 76.4% of the men and 81.1% of the women aged 60 and older responded affirmatively. When queried about prescription drug use at present, 85.9% of the men and 93.3% of the women aged 60 and older responded yes. Among men in this age cohort, 28.2% were taking two or three prescribed drugs on the day they were interviewed. The rate for women was 41.3%. About one-fifth of both sexes were taking four or five prescribed drugs on the day they were being interviewed (19.7% for men and 18.3% for women), and 8.5% of the men and 8.7% of the women were taking between six and ten prescribed medications. Overall, there was a linear relationship between older age and increased drug use (Warheit 1986).

Despite the prevalence of multiple chronic disorders and the high rates of prescribed drug use, it is erroneous to conclude on the basis of these facts alone that most Americans 65 and older experience serious, debilitating physical health problems on a daily basis. Although it is obvious that illness, functional loss, and disability are highly associated with the aging process, the results of a 1984 survey designed to obtain information on the prevalence of functional limitations among the elderly indicated that only about one in four persons 65 and older had any problems associated with taking care of themselves or managing their households. More women than men reported one or more problems related to the activities of daily living or home management tasks. The higher rates of problems for women are undoubtedly correlated with the older average age of women in the 65-and-older population. Functional loss was, in fact, most pronounced among those 85 and older: 14.9% of the men and 21.1% of the women in this age cohort reported four to seven personal care dysfunctions, and 17.8% of the men and 27.0% of the women reported between four and six home management problems (Dawson et al. 1987).

The number of days spent in bed during a year is another good indicator of poor health, functional loss, and disability. Data from the National Health Interview Survey show wide variations among older Americans. Almost two-thirds of people aged 65 to 74 indicated they had not been confined to bed at any time in the year prior to being interviewed, and only 7.8% reported being bedfast for a month or more. By contrast, 13.4% of those 85 and older had been confined to bed for a month or more, and 3.4% said they were in bed constantly. Overall, however, only 1.4% of all persons 65 and older reported being in bed all the time (Dawson et al. 1987).

The data on functional limitations, including confinement to bed, reveal that in spite of increased chronic health problems, most persons aged 65 and older living in community settings are able to take care of their personal needs and manage their households. These data also indicate that only a minority of older, community-residing persons, even among those 85 and older, had long periods of confinement in bed during the course of one calendar year.

Physical Health Self-Assessments

Additional data from the National Health Interview Survey reinforce the overall positive view of the health status of older persons. When asked to make self-assessments of their physical well-being, nearly three-fourths (70%) of those aged 65 and older reported that their health was excellent, very good, or good. The other 30% listed their health as fair or poor (National Center for Health Statistics 1987b). Similarly, Warheit and his colleagues found that 70.8% of the men and 66.8% of the women 60 and older rated their physical health as excellent or good. Another 15.5% of the men and 22.2% of the women indicated their health was fair. Only 13.8% of the males and 11.1% of the women responded that their health was poor or very bad (Warheit et al. 1986).

Both of the field surveys just cited also found that there was a general linear relationship between positive self-assessment of physical health and higher income. It is important to note, however, that these results are from research conducted with random samples of the general population and therefore do not include elderly persons residing in institutional environments. Nonetheless, the findings presented are good indicators of the positive overall health status of most older persons living in community settings.

Results from a small longitudinal study (LaRue et al. 1979) indicate persistence of this positive attitude, 62% of 69 survivors rating their health status as "excellent" or "good" at a median age of 84 years (range 77–93). Moreover, in this sample, physicians' ratings based on medical data correlated significantly with self-ratings of health, and both were predictive of survival time in those under the age of 85.

The results of earlier epidemiologic studies conducted in the southeastern United States by Warheit and his colleagues (n = 4,202) are also relevant at this point (Warheit et al. 1986). All respondents in a series of field surveys were asked to rate their physical health; at the same time, the mental health status of respondents was objectively determined by a number of psychiatric symptom and dysfunction scales including the Health Opinion Survey (HOS), developed by Macmillan (1957) using the Stirling County Study (Leighton 1963). Factor analysis of the HOS items conducted by Warheit and his colleagues revealed three main clusters: depression, anxiety, and psychophysiologic complaints. When the investigators analyzed the responses to the question "How would you rate your physical health at present?" and compared them to scores on the HOS and several of the Florida Health Study (Warheit et al. 1986) mental health measures, they found highly significant associations between negative physical health self-assessments and high psychiatric symptom scores. For example, among respondents who reported their physical health as excellent, only 2.5% had a "caseness" score on the HOS. [As used in the Stirling County Study and the research of Warheit and his colleagues, a "caseness" score on the HOS indicated that the individuals so identified had a very high probability of being diagnosed as having a psychiatric disorder were they to be evaluated by a qualified psychiatrist (Leighton 1963).] By contrast, 76% of those reporting their physical health as poor, and 86.5% of those reporting it as very bad, had scores in the "caseness" range. Similar relationships were found for physical health self-reports and the Florida Health Study depression, anxiety, and psychosocial dysfunction scales (Warheit et al. 1986).

It is recognized that there is disagreement in the literature about the validity of self-reported physical health and mental health problems, especially specific ones. Nonetheless, we believe that respondents in our surveys generally provided valid self-reports concerning their overall physical and mental health status. Evidence to support this belief is provided by a number of multivariate analyses. For example, when physical health self-rating scores were entered as a first-order term in a regression equation along with age, race, sex, and socioeconomic status, the self-ratings explained more of the total variance for the psychiatric symptom-dysfunction scale scores than all the social and demographic variables combined. Taken together, the sociodemographic variables explained 10.2% of the total variance for HOS scores. When the self-rating of physical health was added as a predictor variable, the explained variance tripled to 32.6% (Warheit et al. 1975). Similar results were found for all psychiatric symptom and dysfunction measures. Given these facts, the question "How would you rate your physical health at present?" appears to be an excellent one to ask very early during the taking of a psychiatric history.

The foregoing data are useful in demythologizing many of the commonly held beliefs concerning the health and social functioning of the elderly living in community settings. Succinctly stated, older individuals in community settings report far fewer functional limitations than common stereotypes lead one to believe. Parenthetically, it is also important to note that the social definitions attached to older age and the personal and social behaviors expected of older persons in our society may contribute to the development of some of their physical limitations and functional losses. That is, the physical inactivity of many older persons may be reflections of the social expectations placed on them. Although some of these expectations may have had a factual basis in our earlier history, many of them appear to be residual stereotypes of a bygone era. Because old age is a social as well as a biological phenomenon, professionals treating the elderly should keep in mind that persons of all ages respond to the social and behavioral expectations made of them by significant others, especially those who occupy positions of trust and authority.

Mental Health and Psychosocial Well-Being

Epidemiologic Findings

The most definitive research on the prevalence of psychiatric disorders in the general population has been produced by the Epidemiologic Catchment Area (ECA) projects conducted under the aegis of the National Institute of Mental Health. A full description of the ECA research is found in Eaton and Kessler (1985). Briefly, the ECA findings are based on a probability sample of 18,571 persons aged 18 and older residing in five different sites in the United States. Inasmuch as those 65 and older were overrepresented in the sample, data were obtained on 5,702 persons in this age cohort. The ECA projects obtained DSM-III diagnoses (American Psychiatric Association 1980) by means of the Diagnostic Interview Schedule (DIS) (Robins et al. 1981).

The 1-month prevalence rates for the ECA samples have been reported by Regier and associates (1988). The findings indicate that 15.4% of the total sample had at least one DIS/DSM-III-diagnosed disorder. People aged 65 and older had the lowest life-time rates of any of the age groups. They also had the lowest 1-month prevalence rates for all individual disorders. The one exception was severe cognitive impairment. The rate of severe cognitive impairment for all respondents 65 and older was 4.9%. For those aged 65 to 74, it was 2.9%; and for those aged 85 and over, it was 15.8%. Women of all age groups had higher rates than men for most disorders. The major exceptions were alcohol and drug abuse and dependence.

It is important to note that the ECA diagnoses based on DIS and DSM-III were determined using exclusionary criteria. Respondents whose psychiatric symptoms and dysfunctions were due to physical illness, accidents, drug use (licit or illicit), or alcohol use or abuse were not identified as meeting the criteria for a psychiatric diagnosis. The diagnoses of drug and alcohol abuse and dependence were made independently. The ECA rates do not, therefore, include the prevalence of a variety of mental health problems, including depression and anxiety, which may be dysfunctional for individuals but not severe enough to meet the criteria for a DSM-III diagnosis. For example, depressive symptoms resulting from physical health problems (a not uncommon condition among the elderly) would not, in most instances, lead to a diagnosis of major depression; nor would depressive symptoms arising from the heavy use of prescribed drugs. As a consequence, the rigidity associated with the making of a DIS/DSM-III diagnosis may mask the existence of mental health conditions that do not meet the DSM-III criteria but that nonetheless warrant professional treatment and care.

The ECA results generally confirm those reported earlier by researchers using measures that identify a variety of mental health problems but do not provide the specificity required to make a DSM-III diagnosis. For example, in their study of the general population, Warheit and colleagues (1986) found that people aged 60 and older had lower depression and psychosocial dysfunction scores than those in all age cohorts under 60. Only on the anxiety scale was older age associated with higher scores. Approximately 15% of those 60 and older had depression scores high enough to be regarded as clinically significant, whereas 18.9% of those aged 60 to 69, and 23% of those 70 and older had anxiety scale scores in the clinically significant ranges. The ECA researchers also found anxiety disorders to be much more prominent than depression among those 65 and older (Regier et al. 1988).

Epidemiologic field studies of the general population are based on subsamples of survivors at all age levels. Therefore, the overall lower rates of psychiatric problems and disorder among people aged 65 and older may be influenced by age-cohort survivor effects. In addition, most epidemiologic field surveys have not included institutionalized patients or residents of nursing homes. It has been estimated that in 1985 about two-thirds of the 1.3 million older residents in nursing homes were disoriented or memory impaired to the point of being unable to care for themselves (Dawson et al. 1987). Although including institutionalized populations of older persons in epidemiological field studies would increase the overall reported rates of mental disorders among the elderly and yield some increase in depressive diseases, the increase would be accounted for largely by those with severe cognitive impairment.

Use of Mental Health Services

On the basis of a great body of empirical data, it is reasonable to conclude that approximately 12% to 20% of those 65 and older residing in noninstitutional settings have a psychiatric disorder or mental health problem severe enough to warrant professional mental health services. However, findings from the ECA projects and from the research of other investigators indicate that the elderly are among the least likely to seek professional psychiatric assistance for their mental health problems.

Leaf and his colleagues (1985) also reported ECA data revealing that one of the best predictors for the use of mental health services among those identified as having a diagnosed psychiatric disorder was their mental health self-assessment. Moreover, Warheit and associates (1975) reported earlier that mental health self-assessments were excellent indicators of both the existence of a mental health problem (as determined by the HOS and the Florida Health Study depression, anxiety, and psychosocial dysfunction scales) and of health services.

The findings that show that mental health self-assessment is significantly correlated with objectively derived psychiatric diagnoses and/or the presence of other mental health problems, and with the use of mental health services, are important to professionals who are providing psychiatric care for the elderly. Answers to the questions "How would you rate your mental health?" and "How would you rate your physical health?" can provide strong clues to the mental health status of the respondents.

Psychosocial Well-Being

Our knowledge regarding the psychosocial well-being of the elderly is fragmented, ambiguous, and often filled with stereotypes drawn from history and perpetuated by both the print and electronic media. Frequently the elderly are presented as being feeble, impotent, lonely, afraid, socially isolated, and victimized by con artists and other criminals. Some indicators show that the elderly are at undue risk for some personal traumata. Serious illness and widowhood are found more often among the elderly than the young, and suicide rates are higher among aged 65 and older than among younger age cohorts. However, it must be noted that much of this excess mortality is due to the very high rates for older white men. In 1984, the suicide rate for the general population was 11.6 per 100,000. The rate for white men 65 years of age and older was 41.6, nearly four times higher than the national rate. The rate for older white men was three times that for older black men, six times that for older white women, and 24 times that for older black women (Health, U.S., 1986). Apart from these higher suicide rates for older white men, there are data showing that, at a general level, people aged 65 and older are remarkably similar in overall psychosocial well-being to those under 60. A field survey conducted in north central Florida by Warheit and his colleagues (1986) included a series of questions designed to elicit information on the psychosocial well-being of respondents aged 18 and older. A list of the indicators and a summary of the findings are presented in Table 6-1.

As can be seen, the differences between age groups are minimal in most instances, and for many of the items, those under 60 had a greater percentage of negative responses than those 60 and older. Overall, the data indicated that the great majority of older persons in the sample did not feel powerless, socially isolated, or lacking in social support. Similarly, the vast majority reported very low levels of suicidal ideation and behaviors. Most indicated they did not fear living alone and most said they were not afraid of bodily harm. A very small percentage reported having been a victim of a crime, and nearly 9 out of every 10 respondents aged 60 and older indicated that they were very or fairly satisfied with their lives in general.

Table 6-1. Indicators of Psychosocial Well-Being Among a Community Sample ($N = 2115$)

Item	60 + ($N = 1076$)		18–59 ($N = 1039$)	
	M	F	M	F
1. Close relative nearby to help if needed (% yes)	91	96	94	93
2. Close friend nearby to help if needed (% yes)	86	87	87	87
3. Friend nearby to talk to about fears, hopes, problems (% yes)	65	75	78	81
4. Could count on family if had real problem (% yes)	93	96	96	96
5. Feelings of loneliness (% never)	79	70	70	57
6. Feel alone and helpless (% never)	73	62	66	54
7. Feel people don't care what happens to you (% never)	77	72	67	61
8. Thought about suicide (% never)	95	96	87	88
9. Attempted suicide (% never)	98	98	98	93
10. General life satisfaction (% very/fairly satisfied)	89	87	87	87
11. Fear of bodily harm (% never)	92	76	86	75
12. Fear of living alone (% never)	85	80	86	78
13. Fear someone breaking into home (% never)	65	59	60	49
14. Been victim of crime (% yes)	5	6	16	8

Although more research is needed before definitive conclusions can be reached, the data from north central Florida cast doubts on many of the popular perceptions regarding the psychosocial well-being of the elderly in the United States as long as elderly is defined as above age 60 or 65, and not as above 85 or 90.

Summary

The information presented in this chapter is intended to provide a broad overview of the sociodemographic and sociocultural context within which older persons live in our society, and to provide data on ratings of their mental health and psychosocial well-being. The data presented reveal that, overall, today's elderly are more socially advantaged than their parents were. Longevity has been dramatically extended, retirement years have increased, economic resources are more abundant and secure, and health care is now available for most persons aged 65 and older. The data also indicate that although racial and ethnic minorities still lag behind whites in most indicators of physical and social well-being, some changes that are occurring have the potential to reduce the current discrepancies in life expectancy and years in retirement. However, in other areas, especially those associated with economic resources, large disparities continue to exist and to perpetuate many of the differences in health and health-related behaviors between racial and ethnic groups in the United States.

Most older Americans perceive their physical health as good or excellent; these perceptions are confirmed by objective data on personal and social functioning and by information on numbers of days spent in bed. Further, both physical and mental health self-assessments have been found to be very good predictors of the mental health status of older persons and of their use of mental health services as well.

The self-perception of mental health and psychosocial well-being of the vast majority of older persons has been found to be positive. However, many of the elderly living in community settings have mental health problems severe enough to require assistance from mental health professionals. Yet only a small percentage of those in need receive treatment and care. The recognition of mental health problems by primary physicians, accompanied by referrals to mental health specialists, would increase service rates and improve the psychiatric status of many older persons.

Finally, many of the data outlined in this chapter call into question a great number of false stereotypes and myths associated with the aging process and the age group over 65 in the United States. Few data are as yet available for the age groups over 80, the old-old. They are being gotten at this time.

References

Aging in America: Trends and projections, 1987–88 edition, Washington, DC: Prepared by U.S. Committee on Aging, American Association of Retired Persons, and U.S. Commission on Aging, 1987

American Psychiatric Association: Diagnostic and Statistical Manual of Mental Disorders, 3rd Edition. Washington, DC, American Psychiatric Association, 1980

Atchley RC: The process of retirement: comparing women and men, in Women's Retirement. Edited by Szinovacz M. Beverly Hills, CA, Sage, 1984

Dawson D, Hendershot G, Fulton J: Aging in the eighties: functional limitations of individuals 65 and older. Advance data No. 133, National Center for Health Statistics, June 1987

Eaton W, Kessler L (eds): Epidemiologic Field Methods in Psychiatry: The NIMH Epidemiologic Catchment Area Program. New York, Academic Press, 1985

Fields G, Mitchell O: Restructuring Social Security: How Will Retirement Ages Respond? Washington, DC, National Commission on Employment Policy, 1983

Harris L: Study of American Attitudes Toward Pensions and Retirement. New York, Johnson and Higgins, 1979

Health, United States, 1986. (DHHS Pub. No. (PHS) 87-1232). Washington, DC, Dec. 1986

LaRue A, Bank L, Jarvik L, et al: Health in old age: how do physicians' ratings and self-ratings compare. J Gerontology 34:687–691, 1979

Lawrence L, McLemore T: National ambulatory medical care survey. Advance data No. 88, National Center for Health Statistics, March 1983

Leaf PJ, Livingstone MM, Tischler GL, et al: Contact with health professionals for the treatment of psychiatric and emotional problems. Medical Care 23:1322–1337, 1985

Leighton D: The Character of Danger. New York, Basic Books, 1963

Macmillan A: The health opinion survey: technique for estimating prevalence of psychoneurotic and related types of disorder in communities. Psychol Rep 3:325–339, 1957

National Center for Health Statistics: Advanced reports on final marriage statistics, 1984. Monthly Vital Stat Rep Vol 36, No. 2, Supplement (2), June 1987a

National Center for Health Statistics: Estimates from the National Health Interview Survey, U.S. 1986. Vital Health Stat, Series 10, No. 164, October 1987b

Regier DA, Boyd JH, Burke JD, et al: One month prevalence of mental disorders in the United States. Arch Gen Psychiatry 45:977–986, 1988

Robins LN, Helzer, SE, Croughan J, et al: National Institute of Mental Health Diagnostic Interview Schedule: its history, characteristics, and validity. Arch Gen Psychiatry 38:381–389, 1981

Rosow I: Socialization to Old Age. Berkeley, CA, University of California Press, 1974

Siegel J, Davidson M: U.S. Bureau of the Census. Demographic and socioeconomic aspects of aging in the U.S. Current Population Reports Series P-23, No 138, August 1984

Smith S: Revised worklife tables reflect 1979–1980 experience. Monthly Labor Review, Vol 108, No 8, August 1985

Spencer G: U.S. Bureau of the Census. Projections of the population of the U.S. by age, sex and race: 1983–2080. Current Population Reports Series P-25, No 952, May 1984

Spencer G: U.S. Bureau of the Census. Projections of the hispanic population: 1983–2080. Current Population Reports Series P-25, No 995, Nov. 1986

Spencer G, Goldstein A, Taeuber C: America's Centenarians: Data From the U.S. Census. Washington, DC, National Institute on Aging and the U.S. Bureau of the Census, June 1987

Streib GF: Socioeconomic strata, in Handbook of the Aged in the United States. Edited by Palmore EB. Westport, CT, Greenwood Press, 1984

U.S. Bureau of the Census. Current Housing Reports Series H-150-83. Annual Housing Survey: 1983, part C, December 1984

U.S. Bureau of the Census: Household wealth and asset ownership: 1984. Current Population Reports Series P-70, No 7, July 1986

U.S. Bureau of the Census: Estimates of the population in the U.S. by age, sex, and race: 1980–1986. Current Population Reports Series P-25, No 1000, February 1987a

U.S. Bureau of the Census: Money income and poverty status of families and persons in the U.S.: 1986. Current Population Reports Series P-60, No 157, July 1987b

U.S. Bureau of the Census: Unpublished data from the March 1986 Current Population Survey. 1987–1988

U.S. Dept. of Labor, Bureau of Labor Statistics. Employment and Earnings, Vol 34, No 1, January 1987

Washington, DC, U.S. Committee on Aging, American Association of Retired Persons, and U.S. Commission on Aging: Aging in America: Trends and Projections, 1987–88 edition.

Warheit G: Florida Health and Family Life Study, Gainesville, Florida. Unpublished working paper No. 5. Epidemiology Research Unit, University of Florida, 1986

Warheit G, Robbins L, Swanson E, et al: A Review of Selected Research on the Relationships of Sociodemographic Factors to Mental Disorders and Treatment Outcomes: 1968–1974. Rockville, MD, National Institute of Mental Health, 1975

Warheit G, Bell R, Schwab J: An epidemiologic assessment of mental health problems in the Southeastern U.S., in Community Surveys of Psychiatric Disorders. Edited by Weissman M, Myers J, Ross C. Brunswick, NJ, Rutgers University Press, 1986

CHAPTER 7

Leonard W. Poon, PH.D.
Ilene C. Siegler, PH.D., M.P.H.

Psychological Aspects of Normal Aging

In this chapter we review findings in three domains within the psychology of aging: 1) experimental and cognitive psychology, 2) personality and social psychology, and 3) health and behavior.

These domains have been chosen to reflect the interactive nature of age-related changes and differences in behavior. The reader should note that most, if not all, psychological findings should be interpreted within the context of the sample characteristics studied. The notion of individual difference is emphasized in this chapter to highlight the dynamic nature of a person's psychological states. From this perspective, background information from which findings are abstracted have been included whenever possible. Owing to the number and complexity of concepts reviewed in this chapter, other relevant review sources are recommended for the reader as part of the introduction.

Approaches to "Age" in the Psychology of Aging

There are two approaches to the study of the developmental psychology of aging: 1) experimental aging research versus developmental research and 2) a psychology of aging versus a psychology of the aged.

We acknowledge research and editorial assistance from Deborah J. Welke in compiling the manuscript. Dr. Poon's work is partially supported by grant MH-43435 from the National Institute of Mental Health. Dr. Siegler's work is partially supported by AG-03188 and AG-05128 from the National Institute on Aging and HL-36587 from the National Heart, Lung and Blood Institute.

In experimental aging research, the goal of the research is to examine age-related differences in specific processes (e.g., memory) by comparing the performance of younger persons to older persons (cross-sectional studies). There is no intent to infer the developmental processes that would explain the observed differences. By contrast, developmental aging research examines age-related changes. Developmental researchers contend that longitudinal observations of changes over time for the same person must be carried out in order to infer stages of development for a specific person. Longitudinal studies assume that the birth cohorts of the individuals and the actual times of measurement do not influence the processes observed.

When the elderly person is studied without reference to the life span or developmental processes, we have, in essence, a psychology of the aged rather than of aging. By contrast, the psychology of aging or the life-span view emphasizes the continuity of patterns of behavior across the life cycle and is consistent with the case history approach in psychiatry. In areas where cohort variation (social and historical trends) is important, the best predictors of the behavior of a group of older persons may well be their own behaviors measured at an earlier point in time. To the extent that future generations of elderly are influenced by social change, the current psychology of the aged will become increasingly dated. However, both aspects, psychology of aging and of the aged, have generated important data, and findings from both areas will be reviewed.

Review Handbooks

The following periodic reviews and handbooks will help the reader to keep up with the rapid growth of information on basic mechanisms in the psychology of aging. Most notable are the *Handbook of the Psychology of Aging* (Birren and Schaie 1990), the *Annual Review of Gerontology and Geriatrics* (Maddox and Lawton 1988), and the *Handbook for Clinical Memory Assessment of Older Adults* (Poon 1986). The new journal *Psychology and Aging* represents a growing maturity of interest in geropsychology within the psychology community. Further, recent reviews of memory, personality, clinical psychology, health behavior, and policy issues may be found in a series of edited Masters Lectures presented at the meeting of the American Psychological Association (Storandt and VandenBos 1989).

The encyclopedia of aging (Maddox et al. 1987) provides short, efficient reviews on many topics in the psychiatry and psychology of aging. The findings from pertinent longitudinal studies of aging are summarized in two volumes: One review (Schaie 1983) covers 7 studies, and another (Mednick et al. 1984) reviews 31 studies of adolescents and adults in normal and clinical populations.

Experimental and Cognitive Psychology

The term *cognition* subsumes the range of human intellectual functioning, including perception, memory, reasoning, decision-making, problem solving, and formation of complex structures of world knowledge. Our knowledge of these cognitive processes and their limitations, together with the changes they undergo with normal and abnormal aging, can have a profound impact on the quality of life of older persons. For example, the knowledge can be used to improve human factor and environmental design, policies on work and retirement, accuracy of clinical assessment, and effectiveness of remediation and rehabilitation when they are warranted.

In examining the literature comparing cognitive performances among age groups, it is useful to keep in mind that the level of cognition can be affected by a number of individual, environmental, and task characteristics regardless of chronological age (Hultsch and Dixon 1990; Poon 1985). Depending on the task and the situation, some individuals tend to excel in certain types of performance and not in others. For example, in some cognitive tasks, some adults with high intelligence and education will show minimal decline in performance with increasing age, while adults with lower intelligence and education show significant decline (Bowles and Poon 1982; Poon and Fozard 1980). For those tasks, intelligence and education rather than chronological age are the important determinants of performance. In some cognitive tasks that are well practiced, the amount of age-related decline tends to be small or nonexistent (Salthouse 1982a). Cognition and aging research thus far has concentrated on differences between age groups in cognitive performance; however, more attention is being placed on identifying the effects of the individual, the environment, and the task characteristics in addition to chronological age to better understand cognitive differences among age groups (Poon et al. 1989).

Memory Functioning

Although all cognitive processes are intimately interrelated, age-related changes in memory functioning have received by far the largest share of research effort. For recent comprehensive reviews see Salthouse (1982a, 1985); Poon (1985); Poon et al. (1989); and Hultsch and Dixon (1990). Two reasons could account for the large share of attention focussed on memory performance and aging: 1) memory decline is one of two major concerns articulated by community-dwelling elderly adults (the other being loss of energy) (Lowenthal et al. 1967), and 2) memory dysfunction is a key behavioral benchmark in neuropsychopathology, for example, dementia of the Alzheimer type (Kaszniak et al. 1986). The investigation of memory functioning in both normal and abnormal aging has garnered a significant amount of research resources over the years.

Poon (1985) listed 20 reviews on memory and normative aging published since 1980 and demonstrated the prevalence of the information-processing model in examining age-related differences in memory components, stages, and processes. The information-processing model postulates that information flows from input to output through a series of stages—registration, primary memory, secondary memory, and tertiary memory. Registration is sensory memory, a preattentive and highly unstable system. Primary (short-term) and secondary (long-term) memory (Waugh and Norman 1965) are responsible for the acquisition and retention of new information. Primary memory is conceptualized as a limited-capacity store in which information is still "in mind" as it is being used. If the information is not rehearsed instantaneously so that it can be stored in secondary memory, it will be lost. Secondary memory is the repository of newly acquired information, while tertiary memory is the repository for well-learned and personal information.

It is important to note that this "linear" model is only one of several theoretical models of memory functioning (for example, episodic/semantic memory model [Tulving 1972], explicit/implicit memory model [Schacter 1987], and level of processing model [Craik and Lockhart 1972]). However, this model has been used extensively to gather the largest amount of data in the study of normal aging and in abnormal memory functioning (see Kaszniak et al. 1986 for a review). Findings on age-related differences in memory have been robust, and only a brief review will be attempted here.

A global summary of normal age-related changes in memory is presented in Tables 7-1 and 7-2. Table 7-1 shows that there is a general age-related decline in speed of retrieval from the various theoretical memory stores, and Table 7-2 shows that the most robust data indicate that age-related decline in memory capacity is found

Table 7-1. Cross-sectional experimental evidence for age-related slowing of memory processes

Component affected	Memory store				
	Sensory	Primary	Secondary	Working	Tertiary
Perceptual motor	Positive	Positive	Positive	—	Positive
Decision making	—	Positive	Positive	Positive	Negative

Note. Reprinted with permission from Fozard (1980).

Table 7-2. Evidence for age-related declines in memory capacity

Type of study and type of evidence	Memory store				
	Sensory	Primary	Secondary	Working	Tertiary
Cross-sectional studies					
Anecdotal	—	Positive	Positive	Positive	Positive
Psychometric	—	Negative	Positive	—	Negative
Experimental	Positive	Negative	Positive	Positive	Negative
Longitudinal studies					
Anecdotal	—	—	—	—	—
Psychometric	—	Negative	Positive	—	Negative
Experimental	—	—	Positive	—	—

Note. Reprinted with permission from Fozard (1980).

in secondary memory (Fozard 1980). Thus, although sensorimotor slowing appears to be inevitable with aging, the studies are not consistent in demonstrating decline in the capacities of sensory, primary, or tertiary memory. Aging, however, exerts a profound effect on the acquisition and retrieval of new information in secondary memory.

As described in the previous sections, a significant amount of recent research has been vested in examining the effects of individual, situational, and task differences that contribute to age differences in the acquisition and retrieval of information. The exploration of memory functioning in naturalistic, compared to laboratory, settings; the use of world knowledge; and the use of training strategies, mnemonics (memory aids), and practice all contribute to a more comprehensive view of memory and aging.

Intellectual Functioning

Research on intellectual functioning has one of the longest and most productive records in the psychology of aging (Birren et al. 1983; Jarvik et al. 1973; Schaie 1990; Siegler 1980).

The findings on intellectual functioning over the adult life span have been highly robust. Three general patterns of findings can be described: 1) Hertzog and Schaie (1986) reported on a new analysis of data from the Seattle Longitudinal Studies, which involved two longitudinal sequences of 162 persons tested in 1956, 1963, and 1970; the second sample was tested in 1963, 1970, and 1977. The data show a high degree of regularity in intellectual functioning across the adult age span. 2) There are two robust patterns of intellectual performance across the life span. Crystallized abilities, or knowledge acquired in the course of the socialization process, tend to remain stable over the adult life span. Fluid abilities, or abilities involved in the solution of novel problems, tend to decline gradually from young to old adulthood (Schaie 1990). For example, McCrae et al. (1987) reported consistent declines in divergent thinking (a component of creativity) in cross-sectional, longitudinal, and cross-sequential analyses. 3) Disease and pathology exert profound effects on intellectual functioning. Manton et al. (1986) evaluated cognitive performance in the Duke Longitudinal Study population. The data indicated clear relationships between poorer physical health (from heart disease or dementia) and declining cognitive performance, but interestingly not between depression ratings and cognitive performance.

Understanding and Remembering Written Information

Earlier studies of verbal memory and aging, employing serial or paired-associated learning procedures, found substantial age-related deficits (see Hultsch and Dixon 1990, Poon 1985, and Siegler 1980 for reviews). Several investigators have asked whether these findings also accurately predict the processing of written or spoken information in everyday life (Poon et al. 1989). These questions initiated several recent research programs investigating age differences in "discourse," "text," or "prose" processing—the acquisition of written or spoken communications.

The first generation of research on text processing presented contradictory and conflicting findings. Some studies found clear-cut age deficits (Cohen 1979; Gordon and Clark 1974; Zelinski et al. 1980) whereas others found no age differences (Harker et al. 1982; Meyer and Rice 1981; Taub 1979; Walsh 1982). To address these conflicting results, the second generation of research examined in detail the possible contributions of individual differences, the properties of the text to be processed, and the task demand on the observed processing performance (for detailed reviews see Hartley 1989 and Meyer and Rice 1989). For example, faster presentation rates compromise the comprehension and recall performance of the elderly more than young adults (Hartley 1989). This set of results seems to support the finding of cognitive slowing with increasing age so that the difficulty of a task would affect more the recall performance of older than of young adults.

The level of education and verbal intelligence could account for a significant portion of the age effects on text recall performance (Meyer and Rice 1989). Age deficits in prose recall were found to be significant for adults with average and low verbal ability. High verbal (measured by Wechsler Adult Intelligence Score [Wechsler 1981] vocabulary scores), old adults appear to utilize text structure as well as young adults (Meyer and Rice 1989) and take advantage of organized structures to facilitate their processing. On the other hand, low verbal, old adults show less sensitivity to text structures that could assist them in the processing task.

Current research programs are seeking answers to questions that could help us understand the impact of everyday processing demands on older learners. The research could also furnish clues for facilitating better acquisition and retention of prose information. One important conclusion from research on the acquisition of more meaningful information is that age-related differences are not as large as those indicated by earlier studies of age-related differences in serial or paired-associate learning.

Speech Comprehension

Written material can be scanned and reviewed during processing, but spoken speech can only be processed in a serial manner. While older adults have been shown to suffer from deficits in auditory processing (see Olsho et al. 1985 for a review) and speed of processing (Poon 1985), older adults do not seem to have obvious disproportionate problems in processing everyday conversations or spoken input from television or radio.

Several studies have found clear deficits in the ability of older adults to process spoken speech (Cohen 1979; Cohen and Faulkner 1982). For a review, see Stine et al. (1989). One of the major contributions to age-related peripheral hearing decline is presbycusis, which includes the loss of sensitivity to higher auditory frequencies, an increased probability of recruitment, and an increased probability of phonemic regression or decreased speech intelligibility. An important question for current research programs is how peripheral hearing deficits interact with available cognitive resources and experiences of older persons. This is an important question for both the understanding of speech comprehension by older individuals and for the design of methods to compensate for observed deficits.

In an experiment in which subjects must detect predictable or not predictable target words presented in varying levels of noise, Cohen and Faulkner (1983) found that elderly listeners made increasing use of the word-sentence context as the noise level increased. Similar findings were reported by Nickerson et al. (1981), who found that elderly subjects actually detected more target words embedded in cocktail-party noise than younger subjects. The finding suggested that older adults use the word-sentence context to compensate for their peripheral hearing deficits.

In another experiment reported by Wingfield et al. (1985), young and elderly subjects processed lists of words presented at varying speeds that varied in linguistic redundancy. While the performance of all subjects was affected by speech rate and the degree of redundancy, the performance of the elderly group was differentially depressed by increasing speech rate and by decreasing linguistic constraints. In other words, the results suggested that the older listeners rely on both the redundancy of language and linguistic constraints to maintain an acceptable level of performance. Taken together, these preliminary results suggest that the older listeners can compensate for peripheral hearing decline and that therapeutic procedures should take into account the individual's cognitive strengths and experiences.

Spatial Cognition

Are older adults particularly compromised in spatial compared to verbal functioning? This is a question that is drawing increasing research attention, but relatively few data sets are available. The limited research produced to date is contradictory. Reviews of psychometric and neuropsychologic literature (Albert and Kaplan 1980; Klisz 1978) support the notion of greater decline in right, compared to left, hemisphere function, whereas controlled laboratory experiments (e.g., Park et al. 1983) found minimal or no age differences.

Current research addressing problems of spatial orientation has begun to examine the relationship between individual spatial abilities, adaptive processes, and situational demands (for a review, see Kirasic 1989). While still in its infancy, this direction of research could point to the common and unique contributions of spatial and verbal abilities to different sets of everyday spatial demands. For example, Walsh et al. (1981) reported that spatial abilities were significant predictors of neighborhood knowledge, and in turn, neighborhood knowledge was a significant predictor of the use of goods and services in the neighborhood.

From a clinical evaluation perspective, tests of right-hemisphere functioning do not always predict everyday, spatially related problems. In a study examining the efficiency of shopping routes in supermarkets, Kirasic (1981) reported that an individual's psychometric spatial abilities seemed to be poor predictors of shopping efficiency for any age group. It would be important to pursue how spatial and other cognitive abilities interact in various situational demands for successful adaptation for the community-dwelling aged.

Problem Solving

A series of recent studies (e.g., Denney 1989; Hartley 1989) has examined age-related differences in problem solving from both the standard psychometric tradition and tests imitating problems encountered in everyday situations. Three sets of general observations can be made from these studies: 1) tests of performance in everyday problem-solving tasks show that although middle-aged adults can, in some situations, perform better than young adults, performance decline is still evident for the aged adults (Denney 1989); 2) traditional laboratory-based, problem-solving tasks seem to be predictive of everyday problem-solving performances for older adults; and 3) a significant amount of research remains to be done to understand changes in problem-solving styles and strategies in view of declining physical and cognitive abilities of older persons.

Applications

Research on the cognitive psychology of aging helps to answer the question of how middle-aged and older adults perform in the workplace and in other situations where learning of new information is required (Cross 1981; Stagner 1985). The question has changed from "Can older persons learn?" to "What is the most effective way to teach older persons the things they want to learn?" Willis (1985) reviewed the literature and concluded that older persons' learning capacities are greater and more plastic than had been realized.

Bates et al. (1986) tested subjects 60–86 years old who participated in a short-term (10-session) training session on the improvement of fluid abilities. Improvement of those older persons who had the training was highly significant and related to the degree of similarity of the abilities practiced in the training program to the abilities required to do well on the intelligence tests. The ability of an individual to transfer training from one task to another was found to be relatively specific, indicating that training programs should be guided toward the specific skills that older persons need to learn. The authors interpret their findings as suggesting a higher degree of reserve in fluid intellectual capacity for the elderly than had been shown previously. Training enhanced the ability to solve more difficult problems and increased the accuracy at all levels of performance.

Willis and Schaie (1986) evaluated the effects of cognitive training in panel members of Schaie's Seattle Longitudinal Study. Individuals with a mean age of 72.8 (range 64–95) were classified as stable or decliners over a 14-year period on measures of inductive reasoning and spatial orientation. Over the 107 subjects, 46.7% were stable, 15% to 16% declined on one measure, and 21.8% declined on both measures. A program was devised to provide training on the ability that had declined. Both stable and decliner groups benefited equally and significantly from training. Decliners returned to their original levels and the stable group improved beyond their original levels of performance. These results convincingly indicate that target training on complex tasks can be effective even for old persons. The implication of these findings is that an older individual past the current retirement age could entertain the option of staying in the work force if he or she wished to do so and obtain the proper training.

Issues of productivity and age remain important. Sterns and Alexander (1987) present a state-of-the-art review of industrial gerontology and point out that plant closings, reductions in the work force, and the introduction of new technologies will continue to challenge the role of the older employee in the workplace. While the Age Discrimination in Employment Act (ADEA) offers individuals protection, they must be willing to file suit to ensure their rights (see Edelman and Siegler 1978 for a history of the act). Older persons appear less likely to be willing to file discrimination complaints (Siegler 1979).

Personality and Social Psychology

Patterns of Personality Development

The findings on patterns of adult personality development are complex and controversial owing to differing conceptualizations of personality constructs by different investigators.

Bengston et al. (1985) present a unique approach to a review of the personality literature because they focus on the self and self-concept. Their analysis of the literature suggests the following trends: 1) Greater stability in personality across the adult life cycle is seen when it is measured with objective tests than when subjective measures of personality (such as ratings from psychiatric interviews) are used. 2) Self-esteem is maintained at adult levels in later life. 3) Different personality typologies adapt or respond differently to life events. 4) Gender differences are generally found. Not all personality patterns have the same consequences. Better adjusted patterns earlier in life may well lead to more positive outcomes later in life.

There have been important new reports from major studies of adult personality. Kelly and Conley (1987) reported new analyses from Kelly's longitudinal study of 300 engaged couples. The couples were born between 1905 and 1915 and were in their twenties when first studied. They were recruited between 1935 and 1938 and were followed for 45 years to study the relationship between couples' personality and their marital compatibility. Data on the couples' personality came from peer ratings by five acquaintances in 1935–1938 on the Personality Rating Scale. This scale has four traits: neuroticism, social extraversion, impulse control, and agreeableness. Additional data were collected in 1954–1955 and 1980–1981. The two criterion variables, marital stability and marital satisfaction, were assessed in 1980–1981. Data were available on 199 couples who remained married and 50 couples who divorced. Results of a regression analysis indicated that husband's neuroticism, wife's neuroticism, and husband's impulse control accounted for 14.8% of the variance in outcome. An additional 10% of the variance was accounted for by 14 marriage-attitude variables. These data are interesting because the respondents (those now aged 75–85 years) provide a window on the development of their cohort and suggest a different role for the husband's personality than for the wife's personality.

Vaillant (1983, 1984) describes the Study of Adult Development at Harvard Medical School. Two very different samples, undergraduates from Harvard College and adolescent boys from Boston (selected as nondelinquent controls), have been followed for 40 years in two prospective studies. The differences in socioeconomic status of the two samples, but general similarity of design make them excellent companion studies. Vaillant and Milofsky (1980) evaluated Erikson's theory of adult development by categorizing each man's developmental stage at age 47. They tested three propositions: different stages will be reached at different ages, the model should be independent of social class and education, and the stages should be sequential. Their conclusions were most interesting. There were no specific age linkages to achievement of the developmental stages, thus disproving the first hypothesis; development was relatively independent of social status as predicted; and the developmental tasks that Erikson suggested were observed in an ordered sequence as predicted.

The warning that development is a process and not a series of tasks to be completed is a useful one. Data from prospective studies assist in understanding how developmental processes work even if the respondents are not yet elderly. Long and Vaillant (1984) examined the current status of 456 adults who entered the study when they were inner-city Boston adolescents aged 14 and older in 1940. Ratings of the childhood families of the men (from chronically dependent to nonproblem but poor) served as the major predictor variable. The results indicated that by middle age, these childhood variables did not differentiate in terms of adult social class, income, employment record, number of sociopathic symptoms, and health/mental health. Only time in jail was more frequent for those who had come from multiproblem families. An analysis of individual differences in the sample of those who had the best and worst outcomes as adults suggested that high childhood IQ and good childhood coping skills were correlated with upward mobility, while those who remained in the lower classes or drifted downward in class from their parents were, as adults, alcoholic or mentally ill. The results of this study underscore the importance of using prospective data to make causal attributions about development. Long and Vaillant point out that all the subjects were white males selected for nondelinquency and that the time period from 1940 to 1975 provided an opportunity structure different from both earlier and later periods. Thus the implications of these findings for today's troubled youth need to be interpreted in the construct of opportunity for achievement later in the life cycle.

Caspi and Elder (1986) defined successful aging as high life satisfaction. The focus of their research is inherent in the question,

"Why do similar misfortunes lead one person toward bitterness and another toward satisfaction?" Using data on 79 women from the Berkeley Guidance Study, they examined the impact of adaptive resources in young adulthood (intellectual ability and emotional health) in interaction with social class (middle vs. working class) during the Great Depression (deprived were people who lost > 35% of 1929 assets and income vs. nondeprived who lost < 35%) in order to predict life satisfaction in 1970. Their results indicated different relationships for different social classes. For middle-class women, emotional health in early adulthood was related to life satisfaction in old age. For working-class women, intellectual ability in young adulthood mediated through social involvement was related to life satisfaction. The impact of deprivation was opposite. Middle-class women who were deprived during the depression had higher levels of life satisfaction in old age, whereas deprived working-class women had lower life satisfaction in old age. This thoughtful study begins to suggest a maturity in sociopsychological research that can begin to deal with the complexities of human development in an appropriate way. Given that many of today's elderly were influenced by the economic depression of the 1930s, these findings may help explain current levels of morale.

Levinson (1986) summarizes his view of the life cycle as a life structure with alternating periods of structure building and structure changing (transitions), and he provides a nice conceptualization of his thoughts on adult development. He argues that the biographical model of data collection is an important way to understand the content of adult lives. The most controversial aspect of Levinson's work has been the stress on relatively tight age linkages to the stages of adulthood.

Roberts and Newton (1987) reported the findings from four doctoral dissertations of 39 women aged 28–53 who were interviewed with a biographical interview similar to Levinson's study of 40 men. Support was found by Roberts and Newton for Levinson's theory that similar age ranges and themes were evident, even though the content was different. All in all, Levinson's major themes were supported. This concept of a life structure could be applied to the lives of elderly persons, and might provide new insight into personality development in the elderly.

Haan et al. (1986) reported on stability and change in Q-sort descriptions of personality from data collected over a 50-year period in the Institute of Human Development Studies at Berkeley. No evidence was found for stage theories of development. There was considerable variability in developmental patterns. Six major dimensions of personality were studied: self-confident/victimized; assertive/submissive; cognitively committed; outgoing/aloof; dependable; and warm/hostile. These dimensions were measured from age 6 to age 54–61. The findings were extremely complex and interesting. Some of the important general observations were: 1) Developmental trends were most evident in age-adjacent analysis (over short, rather than long, time periods). 2) Childhood and adolescence were times of stability and individual predictability. 3) The transition from adolescence to adulthood was the most unstable. Females changed more dramatically than males, and gender differences were large and striking. Because the findings are presented for the group over time, rather than as individual lives, it is hard to make direct comparisons with a biographical approach such as Levinson's. Haan et al. and Levinson give very different descriptions of personality development. The critical study—using the group approach of Haan and the biographical approach of Levinson has yet to be done.

Cooper and Gutmann (1987) compared the ego mastery styles of 50 middle-aged (43–51 years old) women in two groups: 25 who had children living at home (at least one child under age 18 who was financially dependent) and 25 whose children were independent and expected to remain so. All 50 women were currently employed teachers. They evaluated group differences in the Thematic Apperception Test (TAT) measures of ego mastery (where stories told to standard drawings are scored for content), a paper and pencil measure of androgyny, and interview measures of gender identity. The TAT measures indicated more "masculine" responses from the women no longer engaged in parenting although there were no group differences on the paper and pencil measure of androgyny. While this design controls for cohort effects in the two groups of women, the traits for the women whose children were launched may have been, in part, responsible for the effect. The design does not allow a clear interpretation.

Costa et al. (1986) report data from the National Health and Nutrition Examination Survey (NHANES 1) follow-up in order to evaluate stability and change in normal personality. The original survey was conducted in 1971–1975 and was a stratified probability sample of the non-institutionalized civilian population aged 1–74 years. The first follow-up was conducted in 1981–1984 on 14,407 adults aged 32–88 years at follow-up. Essentially, the findings indicate an extraordinary degree of stability in these data, replicating other longitudinal findings (Costa and McCrae 1986, 1989; McCrae and Costa 1984).

Caspi and Elder (1986) argued that stability of personal dispositions such as those studied by Costa and McCrae may depend on stability of social conditions and that life in the middle class may lead to greater stability by providing more stable conditions for behavioral continuity. However, the replication of stability of personality with the national data as shown by Costa et al. (1986) argues against the class interpretation, as do the prospective findings of Long and Vaillant (1984). By contrast, individual life histories studied by Levinson (1986) (and those who use retrospective biographical methods) may provide a picture of change because they are studies of the role of the self in various changing contexts. Retrospective studies are able to cover the full duration of the subjects' memories, accounting for part of the discrepancy. Costa and McCrae's (1989) review chapter on personality in adulthood focuses on the implications for clinical practice as well. Overall, the Costa and McCrae (1989) arguments that favor stability of adult personality are persuasive. Studies of personality continuity in the very old have not been done.

Social Interactions and Attributions

Studies of social interaction have examined interpersonal behaviors (Lachman 1986a, 1986b), social support (Cohen and Syme 1985), attribution paradigms (Lachman and McArthur 1986), and health psychology (Siegler and Costa 1985). Research on the stress/illness paradigm, life events and models of coping continue to be major contributors to understanding developmental patterns in middle and later life. An excellent review and approach to understanding social factors in health and aging can be found in Felton and Revenson (1990).

A number of the studies confirmed the expectation that a strong social support system is related positively to physical and mental health of the aged. The following is a description of select studies and their findings.

Social Support and Interaction. Because social interactions are influenced by stereotypes, it is important to examine the current stereotypes of the aged person. Research by Schmidt and Boland (1986) indicates that both positive and negative stereotypes of older persons are much more complex than had been thought. For example, their data did not support the idea that the myth of the generalized "older adult" is a societal stereotype, at least among educated university students aged 18–33. Lachman and McArthur

(1986) studied causal attributions made by young (mean age 19.3) versus old (mean age 74.9) male and female subjects. The two age groups made attributions for their own age group and also for the opposite age group, related to performance on cognitive (memory and problem solving), social (independence and nurturance), and physical domains (strength and speed). The investigators asked the subjects to rate three possible causes for performance: internal stable causes (ability), internal unstable causes (effort), and external causes. Lachman and McArthur findings were more positive than those of previous studies. Older as well as younger persons seemed to hold realistic views of the cause of variabilities on task performance for both themselves and the others.

There has been a developing interest in the role of social support as a moderating variable in the lives of middle-aged and older persons. Studies show a strong relationship between the presence of social support and health (Brodhead et al. 1983). Schulz and Rau (1985) reviewed the evidence on social support across the adult life course. They evaluated the effect of social support on coping with a variety of normative and non-normative life events. They concluded that over the life span the size of the social-support network remains relatively constant (8–15 persons) and that in non-normative events a large network is helpful. Diverse networks appear to be helpful in coping with normative but off-time events; and stability in the network can mean that negative as well as positive effects persist.

Minkler (1985) reviewed the evidence on social support of the elderly. She notes that even though networks tend to be smaller after the age of 70, most of the elderly have a basic support network; and furthermore that relationships between social support and other variables appear to be similar for older and younger age groups. The difference seems to lie in the problems they face rather than in the way that social support operates.

Pilisuk et al. (1987) evaluated medical care utilization in older (40- to 72-year-olds, mean age 49) members of a health maintenance organization (HMO) for a 5-year period. Social support was measured by a 65-item schedule of social functioning yielding three factors: spouse/family support, friend support, and positive network orientation (nonparanoid/trustful). Results indicated that utilization of health services increased as a function of older age, higher stress, and lower social support. Rook (1987) reviewed five studies which compared the role of social support and companionship. Under conditions of high stress, social support was helpful, whereas in low-stress situations, support had negative effects. Companionship produced a generally positive effect. Krause (1987) found that older persons who gave and received more social support had fewer depressive symptoms under conditions of financial strain, arguing for the role of social support as a buffer between depression and financial strain. Social support does not always produce a positive effect. A reciprocal relationship exists between the provider and the receiver of care in that the provider may also experience stress and depression (Rook 1987).

Larson et al. (1986) compared family and friends as sources of psychological well-being of the older person. Ninety-two retired adults carried pagers for 1 week and filled out self-reports when they were signaled on the pagers. They were randomly signaled once every 2-hour time block between 8 A.M. and 10 P.M. As a group, 76% of the pages were answered providing 3,412 self-reports of activity and affect. Data for married and unmarried groups were analyzed separately. The married spent their time with their spouse (41.5%) or alone (38.9%). The unmarried spent 65.8% of their time alone. Children occupied 6.8% of the unmarried's time and 2% of the married (+ 4% with children and spouse together). Friends occupied 14.2% of the time of the unmarried and 5.2% of the married (+ an additional 2.8% for spouse and friends). There were substantial differences in subjective state that varied as a function of the companion. Being with friends was consistently reported to have a higher positive effect than being with family for both the married and the unmarried. For the married, spouse plus friends had the highest effect. There are two variables Larson et al. did not measure: 1) the arena of choice that is present with friends and not with family, and 2) that social support is reciprocal with friends and may not be with family. These factors may play an important role in developing an understanding of how and why social support affects health.

The impact of social change on older persons as members of families was found to be significant. The psychological impact of divorce and step-parenting on the grandparent generation is an emerging research topic (Datan et al. 1987). The current trend toward reduced birthrate suggests that the next generation of elders will need to find nonfamilial relationships (Aizenberg and Treas 1985) to replace the networks now formed by family. Research on friendship networks among the elderly will become increasingly important as larger numbers of persons in nontraditional family structures survive into old age.

Health and Behavior

As life expectancy increases it becomes clear that very different subgroups exist among the elderly (Siegler 1989). Variations in health, rather than age, are responsible for a large portion of expected age differences (Siegler and Costa 1985). The frail, impaired elderly appear to have very little in common with their more robust age peers. Similarly, the data are beginning to show that, even in the middle years, premature morbidity and mortality may be lessened by modification of risk factors (Schoenbach 1985). Thus, attention to behavioral factors and their relationship to health is important for practical as well as theoretical reasons. In this section we will review research findings on risk factors, health behaviors, and interventions with older patient populations. For comprehensive reviews of behavioral, clinical, and neuropsychological assessment, the reader is referred to Poon et al. (1986).

Behavioral Medicine

Behavioral medicine is the study of the role that behavioral factors can play in our understanding of the causes and consequences of disease (Rodin 1987). The area of behavioral medicine is an outgrowth of the tradition in psychosomatic medicine. It is particularly useful in the study of aging because so many diseases of the elderly have behavioral components and because the elderly respond to behavioral treatment approaches. Similarly, there has been an increase in attention to the elderly as targets of public health interventions (Philips and Gaylord 1985).

Risk Factors. Behavioral factors have been shown to be important in the prediction of coronary heart disease (CHD) (Friedman and Booth-Kewley 1987; Williams et al. 1980, 1985) and in the treatment of arthritis (Verbrugge 1987) as well as diabetes (Surwit et al. 1982). Little is known about the role of behavioral factors in the etiology of stroke, dementia (Mortimer and Schumann 1981), or cancer (Fox 1978).

The Type A behavior pattern appears to be an independent risk factor for CHD. However, recent studies have reported that the relationship between Type A personality and disease is more likely to be an important predictor of *premature* (under the age of 50–55) mortality and morbidity than CHD later in life (see Anderson 1987; Siegler et al. 1985; Williams et al. 1986). The reasons for the relationships are unclear. The strongest arguments to date are for selection bias, that is those who are high on the Type A behavior pattern are those who are selected out by death and/or disease. Those who survive are therefore, as a group, more likely to be Type Bs. It is interesting that in their excellent meta-analysis of psychological predictors of CHD, Booth-Kewley and Friedman (1987) pay little attention to age as a mediator except to report that in prospective studies that controlled for other risk factors (age, smoking, serum cholesterol, blood pressure, or education), none of the risk factors was an important mediator between Type A and CHD.

Health Behaviors.   Leventhal et al. (1985) review the evidence of preventive health behaviors across the life cycle. They focus on specific health and risk behaviors. T. R. Prohaska, M. Keller, E. Leventhal, et al. (unpublished observations) asked 390 adults aged 20–34, 35–49, and over age 50 about the practice of 20 health habits. Respondents over 50 years old were significantly more likely to report avoiding harmful health habits than were younger respondents. Those over age 50 were less likely to engage in strenuous exercise and more likely to get medical check-ups. Prohaska et al. (unpublished observations) also asked their respondents to rate the efficacy of the health behaviors. There were no age differences in perceived effectiveness of the health behaviors. Older people were more likely than younger people to believe that specific modifications were effective for particular diseases. Leventhal et al. (1985) argue that a major mechanism of older persons for engaging in health preventive behaviors and in coping with illness is due to this belief system. This mechanism is similar to the view of Lazarus and his colleagues (Folkman et al. 1987), that emotion-focused coping was effective in dealing with chronic health problems. George and Siegler's (1985) findings on coping with stressful life events by older persons support the view that emotion-focused coping is particularly effective for coping with health events that cannot be modified. Felton and Revenson (1987) studied middle-aged and older persons with hypertension, rheumatoid arthritis, diabetes, and cancer. Coping was measured by six factor-analytically derived scales from the Lazarus Ways of Coping Scale. The resulting interactions of age, coping strategy, and the measure of illness tested underscore the complexity inherent in determining age relationships in this area.

Students of health behaviors are often oriented toward intervention strategies. Leventhal et al. (1985) argue that increased primary prevention efforts should be made with the elderly. However, a major barrier to the success of such efforts is that elderly persons are quite adept at accepting the distress of daily life as normal and coping by psychological reorganization.

Rodin (1986) reviewed the evidence relating health, locus of control, and aging. She argues that the elderly are particularly vulnerable to health-control issues because the role of stress is increased by experiencing more stress-inducing events and/or environmental challenges as well as having an increased physiological vulnerability to the effects of stress. She reports on some preliminary data from a community sample of older persons (aged 62–91). Baseline measures of immunocompetence were derived from 24-hour urine samples, and indices of B, T4, and T8 cell function were correlated with age, health, life satisfaction, major life events, expectation of stressors, and sense of control. Recency of life events and effects of these events on the respondents' sense of control were the major psychosocial predictors of immune function. These data begin to present the outlines for potential mechanisms whereby stress can be seen to influence health in the elderly.

Cicerelli (1987) studied health locus of control in elderly patients in a general hospital setting. He found that those who were highly external (believed that outcomes were controlled by powerful others) were better adjusted to the high-constraint setting of the inpatient hospital.

Woodward and Wallston (1987) studied 119 adults aged 20 to 99 and evaluated the relationship between older persons' desire for control of their health, age, and self-efficacy. They measured desire for control of health care, which is specific to situation, desire for information, and general desire for control. Self-efficacy was the respondent's degree of confidence in their ability to handle a situation. A health care self-efficacy scale was designed to measure the individual's level of self-confidence in each of the items in the health locus of control and health information scales. Three age groups were 20–39, 40–59, and 60–99. While the young and middle-aged groups were generally similar, together they were different from the older group on all health locus of control and self-efficacy measures. Individuals over age 60 had a lower desire for control over their health, as well as lowered self-efficacy. Because health events are generally uncontrollable, these results may also be seen as realistic.

Siegler and Gatz (1985) evaluated older persons' locus of control for causing an event to happen versus their locus of control for the handling of an event. They found that people took more responsibility for how they handled the event than for causing it to happen.

Lachman (1986b) has reviewed the evidence for stability and change in locus of control and found that the literature is contradictory. Lachman noted that elderly persons acknowledge the increasing importance of external sources of control in their lives while simultaneously maintaining their own sense of internality. Baltes and Reisenzein (1986) reviewed evidence on dependency in the elderly. Behaviors of both elderly persons and children were observed in institutional settings. Their results indicate that dependent behaviors of older persons are often followed by attention from other persons in the institutional setting.

Behavioral treatments are beginning to be applied to nursing home populations as well. Moran and Gatz (1987) reported increases in psychosocial competence among nursing home residents after short-term group therapy. As more and more older persons survive with disabilities, the role of rehabilitation becomes more critical and a greater part of the rehabilitation literature becomes concerned with geriatrics (Kemp 1985). Stephens et al. (1987) evaluated psychosocial factors in the rehabilitation of 48 elderly stroke patients with moderate levels of expressive and receptive speech. Individuals were interviewed about positive and negative interactions with members of their social networks in their homes (12.5% were discharged to nursing homes) and their overall adjustment. Persons who reported higher positive social interactions had higher cognitive scores and those with higher negative social interactions had poorer morale. These results are noteworthy, but the directionality of the interactions cannot be evaluated properly in the study's cross-sectional design. Similarly, as the data base develops on the effect of psychotherapeutic interventions with a wide variety of older patients in a variety of clinical settings, the efficacy of treatment is seen to follow principles for successful treatment that are generalizable across the life span and provide an optimistic view of the role of therapeutic interventions in enhancing the quality of life of older persons (Gatz et al. 1985).

Longevity, Successful Aging, and Thoughts for the Future

Longevity and successful aging are two distinct constructs. These constructs are seldom addressed together in the literature. However, aging is often measured with one of these common yardsticks and they are convenient positive endpoints for aging research. In evaluating factor analytic studies of psychological well-being, Okun and Stock (1987) conclude that three factors are adequate to describe the phenomenon: positive affect, negative affect, and cognition. Older persons tend to cognitively manipulate their perceptions to maintain appropriate psychological well-being in the face of imperfect circumstances. This tendency is supported by the longitudinal analysis performed by Costa and McCrae (1989) who found stability of mean levels in psychological well-being across the ages 25–74.

The purpose of this chapter is to provide a brief overview of the theory and data in the psychology of aging and the aged. We have reviewed data on how an individual's education, expertise, social and environmental support, and chronological age could influence cognitive performances and self-perception, as well as relationships with others. Current research is attempting to answer questions about how these factors affect an individual's health, coping mechanisms, work productivity, life satisfaction, and long-term care issues. Increasingly, research focusing on the behavior of middle-aged and older persons and diagnostic and treatment issues for older persons have made this a particularly interesting time to review the literature in psychology of adult development and aging for clinical applications.

References

Aizenberg R, Treas J: The family in late life: psychosocial and demographic considerations, in Handbook of the Psychology of Aging, 2nd Edition. Edited by Birren JE, Schaie KW. New York, Van Nostrand Reinhold, 1985

Albert MS, Kaplan E: Organic implications of neuropsychological deficits in the elderly, in New Directions in Memory and Aging: Proceedings of the George Talland Memorial Conference. Edited by Poon JL, Fozard LS, et al. Hillsdale, NJ, Lawrence Erlbaum, 1980

Anderson NB: Coronary prone behavior, in Encyclopedia of Aging. Edited by Maddox GL, Atchley RC, Poon LW, et al. New York, Springer, 1987

Baltes MM, Reisenzein R: The social world in long-term care institutions: psychosocial control toward dependency, in The Psychology of Control and Aging. Edited by Baltes MM, Baltes PB. Hillsdale, NJ, Lawrence Erlbaum, 1986

Baltes PB, Dittman-Kohli F, Kliegl R: Reserve capacity of the elderly in aging-sensitive tests of fluid intelligence: replication and extension. Psychology and Aging 1:172–177, 1986

Bengston VL, Reedy MN, Gordon C: Aging and self-conceptions: personality processes and social contexts, in Handbook of the Psychology of Aging, 2nd Edition. Edited by Birren JE, Schaie KW. New York, Van Nostrand Reinhold, 1985

Birren JE, Schaie KW (eds): Handbook of the Psychology of Aging, 3rd Edition. New York, Academic, 1990

Birren JE, Cunningham, WR, Yamamoto K: Psychology of adult development and aging, in Annual Review of Psychology. Edited by Rosenzweig MR, Porter LW. Palo Alto, CA, Annual Reviews Inc, 1983

Booth-Kewley S, Friedman HS: Psychological predictors of heart disease: a quantitative review. Psychol Bull 101:343–362, 1987

Bowles NL, Poon LW: An analysis of the effect of aging on recognition memory. J Gerontol 37:212–219, 1982

Brodhead E, Kaplan BH, James SA, et al: The epidemiologic evidence for a relationship between social support and health. Am J Epidemiol 117:521–537, 1983

Caspi A, Elder GH: Life satisfaction in old age: linking social psychology and history. Psychology and Aging 1:18–26, 1986

Cicerelli VG: Locus of control and patient role adjustment of the elderly in acute-care hospitals. Psychology and Aging 2:138–143, 1987

Cohen G: Language comprehension in old age. Cognitive Psychology 11:412–429,1979

Cohen G, Faulkner D: Memory for discourse in old age. Discourse Processes 4:253–265, 1982

Cohen G, Faulkner D: Word recognition: age differences in contextual facilitation effects. Br J Psychol 74:239–251, 1983

Cohen S, Syme SL (eds): Social Support and Health. Orlando, FL, Academic, 1985

Cooper KL, Gutmann DL: Gender identity and ego mastery style in middle-aged, pre-, and-post-empty nest women. Gerontologist 27:347–352, 1987

Costa PT Jr, McCrae RR: Cross-sectional studies of personality in a national sample, 1: development and validation of survey measures. Psychology and Aging 1:140–143, 1986

Costa PT Jr, McCrae RR: The Adult Years: Continuity and Change. Edited by Storandt MK, VandenBos GR. Washington, DC, American Psychological Association, 1989

Costa PT Jr, McCrae RR, Zonderman AB: Cross-sectional studies of personality in a national sample, 2: stability in neuroticism, extraversion, and openness. Psychology and Aging 1:144–149, 1986

Craik FIM, Lockhart RS: Levels of processing: a framework for memory research. Journal of Verbal Learning and Verbal Behavior 11:671–684, 1972

Cross KP: Adults as Learners. San Francisco, CA, Jossey-Bass, 1981

Datan N, Rodeheaver D, Hughes F: Adult development and aging, in Annual Review of Psychology. Edited by Rosenzweig MR, Porter HW. Palo Alto, CA, Annual Reviews Inc, 1987

Denney NW: Everyday problem solving: methodological issues, research findings, and a model, in Cognition in Everyday Life. Edited by Poon LW, Rubin DC, Wilson BA. New York, Cambridge University Press, 1989

Edelman CD, Siegler IC: Federal Age Discrimination in Employment

Law: Slowing Down the Gold Watch. Charlottesville, VA, Mitchie Company, 1978

Felton BJ, Revenson TA: Age differences in coping with chronic illness. Psychology and Aging 2:164–170, 1987

Felton BJ, Revenson TA: The psychology of health: issues in the field with special focus on the older person, in Aging Curriculum Content for Education in the Social-Behavioral Sciences. Edited by Parham IA, Poon LW, Siegler IC. New York, Springer, 1990

Folkman S, Lazarus RS: An analysis of coping in a middle age community sample. Journal of Health and Social Behavior 21:291–239, 1980

Folkman S, Lazarus RS, Pimley S, et al: Age differences in stress and coping processes. Psychology and Aging 2:171–184, 1987

Fox BH: Premorbid psychological factors related to cancer incidence. J Behav Med 1:45–133, 1978

Fozard JL: The time for remembering, in Aging in the 1980's: Psychological Issues. Edited by Poon LW. Washington, DC, American Psychological Association, 1980

Friedman HS, Booth-Kewley S: The "disease-prone personality": a meta-analytic view of the construct. Am Psychol 42:539–555, 1987

Gatz M, Popkin SJ, Pino CD, et al: Psychological interventions with older adults, in Handbook of the Psychology of Aging, 2nd Edition. Edited by Birren JE, Schaie KW. New York, Van Nostrand Reinhold, 1985

George LK, Siegler IC: Stress and coping in later life, in Normal Aging III. Edited by Palmore E, Busse EW, Maddox GL, et al. Durham, NC, Duke University Press, 1985

Gordon SK, Clark WC: Application of signal detection theory to prose recall and recognition in elderly and young adults. J Gerontol 29:64–72, 1974

Haan N, Millsap R, Hartka E: As time goes by: change and stability in personality over fifty years. Psychology and Aging 1:220–232, 1986

Harker JO, Hartley JT, Walsh DA: Understanding discourse—a life-span approach, in Advances in Reading/Language Research. Edited by Hutson BA. Greenwich, CT, JAI Press, 1982, pp 155–202

Hartley JT: Memory for prose: perspectives on the reader, in Cognition in Everyday Life. Edited by Poon LW, Rubin DC, Wilson BA. New York, Cambridge University Press, 1989

Hertzog C, Schaie KW: Stability and change in adult intelligence, 1: analysis of longitudinal covariance structures. Psychology and Aging 1:159–171, 1986

Hultsch DF, Dixon RA: Learning and memory in aging, in Handbook of the Psychology of Aging, 3rd Edition. Edited by Birren JE, Schaie KW. New York, Academic, 1990

Jarvik L, Eisdorfer C, Blum JE (eds): Intellectual Functioning in Adults. New York, Springer, 1973

Kaszniak AW, Poon LW, Riege W: Assessing memory deficits: an information-processing approach, in Handbook for Clinical Memory Assessment of Older Adults. Edited by Poon LW. Washington, DC, American Psychological Association, 1986

Kelly EL, Conley JJ: Personality and compatibility: a prospective analysis of marital stability and marital satisfaction. J Pers Soc Psychol 52:27–40, 1987

Kemp B: Rehabilitation and the older adult, in Handbook of the Psychology of Aging, 2nd Edition. Edited by Birren JE, Schaie KW. New York, Van Nostrand Reinhold, 1985

Kirasic KC: Studying the "hometown advantage" in elderly adults' spatial cognition and spatial behavior. Paper presented at a meeting of the Society for Research in Child Development, Boston, MA, July 1981

Kirasic KC: Acquisition and utilization of spatial information by elderly adults: implications for day-to-day situations, in Cognition in Everyday Life. Edited by Poon LW, Rubin DC, Wilson BA. New York, Cambridge University Press, 1989

Klisz D: Neuropsychological evaluation in older persons, in The Clinical Psychology of Aging. Edited by Storandt M, Siegler IC, Elias MF. New York, Plenum, 1978

Krause N: Chronic financial strain, social support, and depressive symptoms among older adults. Psychology and Aging 2:185–192, 1987

Lachman ME: Locus of control in aging research: a case for multidimensional and domain-specific assessment. Psychology and Aging 1:34–40, 1986a

Lachman ME: Control: change and cognitive correlates, in The Psychology of Control and Aging. Edited by Baltes MM, Baltes PB. Hillsdale, NJ, Lawrence Erlbaum, 1986b

Lachman ME, McArthur LZ: Adult age differences in the ability to cope with situations. Psychology and Aging 1:127–132, 1986

Larson R, Mannell R, Zyzanek J: Daily well-being of older adults with friends and family. Psychology and Aging 1:117–126, 1986

Leventhal H, Prohaska TR, Hirschman RS: Preventive health behavior across the life-span, in Preventing Health Risk Behaviors and Promoting Coping With Illness. Edited by Rosen JC, Solomon LJ. Hanover, NH, University Press of New England, 1985

Levinson DJ: A conception of adult development. Am Psychol 41:3–13, 1986

Long JVF, Vaillant GE: Natural history of male psychological health, XI: escape from the underclass. Am J Psychiatry 141:341–346, 1984

Lowenthal MF, Berkman PL, Beuler JA, et al: Aging and Mental Disorder in San Francisco. San Francisco, CA, Jossey-Bass, 1967

Maddox GL, Lawton MP (eds): Annual Review of Gerontology and Geriatrics, Vol 8. New York, Springer, 1988

Maddox GL, Atchley RC, Poon LW, et al (eds): Encyclopedia of Aging. New York, Springer, 1987

Manton KG, Siegler IC, Woodbury MA: Patterns of intellectual development in later life. J Gerontol 41:486–489, 1986

McCrae RR, Costa PT: Emerging Lives, Enduring Dispositions. Boston, MA, Little, Brown, 1984

McCrae RR, Arenberg D, Costa PT Jr: Declines in divergent thinking with age: cross-sectional, longitudinal, and cross-sequential analyses. Psychology and Aging 2:130–137, 1987

Mednick S, Harway M, Finello K: Handbook of Longitudinal Research. New York, Praeger, 1984

Meyer BJF, Rice GE: Information recalled from prose by young, middle, and old adults. Exp Aging Res 7:253–268, 1981

Meyer BJF, Rice GE: Prose processing in adulthood: the text, the learner, and the task, in Cognition in Everyday Life. Edited by Poon LW, Rubin DC, Wilson BA. New York, Cambridge University Press, 1989

Minkler M: Social support and health of the elderly, in Social Support and Health. Edited by Cohen S, Syme SL. Orlando, FL, Academic, 1985

Moran JA, Gatz M: Group therapies for nursing home adults: an evaluation of two treatment approaches. Gerontologist 27:588–591, 1987

Mortimer JA, Schumann LM (eds): The Epidemiology of Dementia. New York, Oxford University Press, 1981

Nickerson RS, Green DM, Stevens KN, et al: Some experimental tasks for the study of the effects of aging on cognition, in Design Conference on Decision Making and Aging Journal Supplemental Abstract Service. Selected Documents in Psychology. Edited by Poon LW, Fozard JL. Washington, DC, American Psychological Association, 1981

Okun MA, Stock WA: Correlates and components of subjective well-being in the elderly. J Appl Gerontol 6:95–112, 1987

Olsho LW, Harkins SW, Lenhardt ML: Aging and the auditory system, in Handbook of the Psychology of Aging, 2nd Edition. Edited by Birren JE, Schaie KW. New York, Van Nostrand Reinhold, 1985

Park CD, Puglisi JT, Sovacool M: Memory for pictures and spatial location in older adults: evidence for pictorial superiority. J Gerontol 38:582–588, 1983

Phillips HT, Gaylord SA (eds): Aging and Public Health. New York, Springer, 1985

Pilisuk M, Boylan K, Acredolo C: Social support, life stress, and subsequent medical care utilization. Health Psychol 6:273–288, 1987

Poon LW: Differences in human memory with aging: nature, causes, and clinical implications, in Handbook of the Psychology of Aging, 2nd Edition. Edited by Birren JE, Schaie KW. New York, Van Nostrand Reinhold, pp 427–473, 1985

Poon LW (ed): Handbook for Clinical Memory Assessment of Older Adults. Washington, DC, American Psychological Association, 1986

Poon LW, Fozard JL: Age and word frequency effects in continuous recognition memory. J Gerontol 35:77–86, 1980

Poon LW, Gurland BJ, Eisdorfer C, et al: Integration of experimental and clinical precepts in memory assessment: a tribute to George Talland, in Handbook for Clinical Memory Assessment of Older Adults. Edited by

Poon LW. Washington, DC, American Psychological Association, pp 3–10, 1986

Poon LW, Rubin DC, Wilson BA (eds): Cognition in Everyday Life. New York, Cambridge University Press, 1989

Roberts P, Newton PM: Levinsonian studies of women's adult development. Psychology and Aging 2:154–163, 1987

Rodin J: Health: control and aging, in The Psychology of Control and Aging. Edited by Baltes MM, Baltes PB. Hillsdale, NJ, Lawrence Erlbaum Associates, 1986

Rodin J: Behavioral medicine, in Encyclopedia of Aging. Edited by Maddox GL, et al. New York, Springer, 1987

Rook KS: Reciprocity of social exchange and social satisfaction among older women. J Pers Soc Psychol 52:145–154, 1987

Salthouse TA: Adult Cognition: An Experimental Psychology of Human Aging. New York, Springer-Verlag, 1982a

Salthouse TA: A Theory of Cognitive Aging. Amsterdam, North-Holland, 1985

Schacter D: Implicit memory: history and current status. Journal of Experimental Psychology: Learning Memory Cognition 13:501, 1987

Schaie KW (ed): Longitudinal Studies of Adult Psychological Development. New York, Guilford Press, pp 501–518, 1983

Schaie KW: Intellectual development in adulthood, in Handbook of the Psychology of Aging, 3rd Edition. Edited by Birren JE, Schaie KW. New York, Academic, 1990

Schmidt DF, Boland SM: Structure of perceptions of older adults: evidence for multiple stereotypes. Psychology and Aging 1:255–260, 1986

Schoenbach VJ: Behavior and life style as determinants of health and well-being in the elderly, in Aging and Public Health. Edited by Phillips HT, Gaylord SA. New York, Springer, 1985

Schulz R, Rau MT: Social support through the life course, in Social Support and Health. Edited by Cohen S, Syme SL. Orlando, FL, Academic, 1985

Siegler IC: Attitudes about age discrimination. Paper presented at Gerontological Society of America, San Diego, November 1979

Siegler IC: The psychology of adult development and aging, in Handbook of Geriatric Psychiatry. Edited by Busse EW, Blazer DG. New York, Van Nostrand Reinhold, 1980

Siegler IC: Developmental health psychology, in The Adult Years: Continuity and Change. Edited by Storandt MK, VandenBos GR. Washington, DC, American Psychological Association, 1989

Siegler IC, Costa PT Jr: Health behavior relationships, in Handbook of the Psychology of Aging, 2nd Edition. Edited by Birren JE, Schaie KW. New York, Van Nostrand Reinhold, 1985

Siegler IC, Gatz M: Age patterns in locus of control, in Normal Aging III: Reports from the Duke Longitudinal Studies, 1975–1984. Edited by E Palmore, EW Busse, GL Maddox, et al. Durham, N.C., Duke University Press, 1985

Siegler IC, Nowlin JB, Blumenthal JA, et al: Type A behavior pattern in later life. Paper presented at the meetings of the International Association of Gerontology, New York, July 1985

Stagner R: Aging and industry, in Handbook of the Psychology of Aging, 2nd Edition. Edited by Birren JE, Schaie KW. New York, Van Nostrand Reinhold, 1985

Stephens MAP, Kinney JM, Norris VK, et al: Social networks as assets and liabilities in recovering from stroke in geriatric patients. Psychology and Aging 2:125–129, 1987

Sterns HL, Alexander RA: Industrial gerontology, in Annual Review of Gerontology and Geriatrics, vol. 7. Edited by Schaie KW. New York, Springer, 1987

Stine EL, Wingfield A, Poon LW: Speech comprehension and memory through adulthood: the role of time and strategy, in Everyday Cognition in Adulthood and Late Life. Edited by Poon LW, Rubin DC, Wilson BA. New York, Cambridge University Press, 1989

Storandt M, VandenBos GR (eds): The Adult Years: Continuity and Change. Washington, DC, American Psychological Association, 1989

Surwit RS, Scovern AW, Feinglos MN: The role of behavior in diabetes care. Diabetes Care 5:337–342, 1982

Taub HA: Comprehension and memory of prose materials by young and old adults. Exp Aging Res 5:3–13, 1979

Tulving E: Episodic and semantic memory, in Organization of Memory. Edited by Tulving E, Donaldson W. New York, Academic, 1972

Vaillant GE: The Natural History of Alcoholism: Causes, Patterns and Paths to Recovery. Cambridge, MA, Harvard University Press, 1983

Vaillant GE: The study of adult development at Harvard Medical School, in Handbook of Longitudinal Research. New York, Praeger, 1984

Vaillant GE, Milofsky E: Natural history of male psychological health, IX: empirical evidence for Erikson's model of the life cycle. Am J Psychiatry 137:1348–1359, 1980

Verbrugge LM: Sex differences in health, in Encyclopedia of Aging. Edited by Maddox GL, Atchley RC, Poon LW. New York, Springer, 1987

Walsh DA, Krauss IK, Regnier VA: Spatial ability, environmental knowledge and environmental use: the elderly, in Spatial Representation and Behavior Across the Life Span. Edited by Liben L, Patterson A, Newcomb N. New York, Academic, 1981

Waugh NC, Norman DC: Primary memory. Psychological Review 72:89–104, 1965

Wechsler D: Wechsler Adult Intelligence Scale—Revised. San Antonio, TX, Psychological Corporation, 1981

Williams RB, Barefoot JC, Shekelle RB: The health consequences of hostility, in Anger, Hostility and Behavioral Medicine. Edited by Chesney MA, Rosenman RH. New York, Hemisphere/McGraw-Hill, 1985

Williams RB, Barefoot JC, Haney TL, et al: Type A behavior and angiographically documented coronary atherosclerosis in a sample of 2,289 patients. Paper presented at the American Psychosomatic Society Meetings, Baltimore, March 1986

Williams RB, Haney TL, Lee KL, et al: Type A behavior, hostility and coronary atherosclerosis. Psychosom Med 42:539–549, 1980

Willis SL: Towards an educational psychology of the older adult learner: intellectual and cognitive bases, in Handbook of the Psychology of Aging, 2nd Edition. Birren JE, Schaie KW. New York, Van Nostrand Reinhold, 1985

Willis SL, Schaie KW: Training the elderly on ability factors of spatial orientation and inductive reasoning. Psychology and Aging 1:239–247, 1986

Wingfield A, Poon LW, Lombardi L, et al: Speed of processing in normal aging: effects of speech rate, linguistic structure and processing time. J Gerontol 40:579–585, 1985

Woodward NJ, Wallston BS: Age and health care beliefs: self-efficacy as a mediator of low desire for control. Psychology and Aging 2:3–8, 1987

Zelinski EM, Gilewski MJ, Thompson LW: Do laboratory tests relate to self-assessment of memory ability in the young and old? in New Directions in Memory and Aging: Proceedings of the George Talland Memorial Conference. Edited by Poon LW, Fozard JJ, Cermak LS, et al. Hillsdale, NJ, Lawrence Erlbaum, 1980

SECTION 2

Principles of Evaluation and Diagnosis

CHAPTER 8

Ivan L. Silver, M.D.
Nathan Herrmann, M.D.

History and Mental Status Examination

Introduction

The ability of the geriatric psychiatrist to solve clinical problems is directly related to the comprehensiveness and depth of the data obtained from patients and their families. Historically, little attention has been paid to the psychiatric examination of elderly patients, although protocols for the cognitive assessment are available (Strub and Black 1985). In this chapter we present a guide for taking the psychiatric history, performing a functional assessment, and examining the mental status of the geriatric patient. Although numerous clinical examples are presented, the specific phenomenology of geriatric mental disorders has yet to be confirmed by careful experimental studies. More specific details about developmental inquiry, special tests, neuroimaging, and medical-legal issues are discussed in other chapters.

The geriatric history and mental status examinations are potentially long and complex because the patients have lived many years and many of them suffer from the comorbidity of neurological and medical illness. Emphasis on different aspects of the history will vary depending on the patient's problems. For instance, a corroborative history and a detailed cognitive assessment are priorities in patients with progressive dementing disorders and delirium. The family and past history are important for all patients but particularly essential for patients with affective or personality disorders.

The goals of the history and of the functional and mental status examinations are to 1) establish a provisional diagnosis and differential diagnoses; 2) develop an etiological formulation that traces the biological, psychological, and social factors that have predisposed, precipitated, and now perpetuate the patient's current mental illness; and 3) establish each patient's capacity to function independently.

General Considerations

There are several issues that a geriatric psychiatrist must consider before the assessment begins.

First, where should the patient be seen? Geriatric assessments may be undertaken in a variety of settings: at the bedside, in an outpatient office, at home, in an institution, in a day hospital, or in a specialized clinic. Where the clinician sees the patient may be critical because it can determine the quantity and quality of the data collected. For example, generally, one cannot expect to assess fully the capacity of a patient with dementia to remain at home by completing the assessment in an outpatient office. This assessment often requires observation and monitoring in the home environment. On the other hand, a workup to rule out reversible causes of dementia requires the facilities of a clinic or hospital setting.

Second, who should participate in the assessment? A basic tenet in geriatric assessment is that, whenever possible, a patient's spouse, caregiver, and family are seen for corroborative information, with appropriate regard for issues of confidentiality. This principle is critically important in the assessment of patients with cognitive impairment, but it may be equally important in patients who are cognitively intact. When mental disorders interfere with insight into the nature and quality of the illness, interviewing family members often provides a truer picture of the person's mental disorder. Historical events are verified and, in many cases, the diagnosis rests with the family members' ability to relate a coherent history. A family member often is the best person to describe the premorbid personality of the patient. This information is valuable because premorbid personality traits may change or become exaggerated in the context of a variety of geriatric mental illnesses, including dementia, affective disorders, and paranoid disorders.

Third, how should the interview be conducted? All psychiatric interviews should allow for a free exchange of information in an atmosphere of mutual trust, which leaves patients with the feeling that they are being understood. Particular attention should be paid to the capacity of the patient to tolerate a psychiatric interview. Long, detailed interviews are not tolerated well by severely disturbed or cognitively impaired patients. Brief interviews with active engagement and reassurance facilitate the process.

Consideration must be given to the common sensory impairments seen in some geriatric patients. Patients with poor hearing and vision may require special intervention. With deafness, turning on the hearing aid or speaking in a steady, low-pitched voice into the "good ear" may help. At times a sound-amplifying device may be necessary. For the visually impaired, sitting closer to the patient or ensuring that the patient is wearing his or her corrective lenses is helpful.

The appropriate use of touch may also reassure the patient and help facilitate the psychiatric interview.

Psychiatric History Assessment

A schema for the psychiatric assessment is suggested in Table 8-1. It is meant only as a tool to organize the data and not as a checklist for the examiner. Several detailed guides to the assessment of younger adults are available (Ginsberg 1985; Leff and Isaacs 1978; Waldinger 1984). The following discussion is meant as a guide to adapting the traditional psychiatric history to the needs of the geriatric population.

Identifying Data

The identifying data can be amended by adding the name of the primary caregiver, whether in or out of the home. If the patient lives in a residential setting, the type of institution is specified.

Table 8-1. Schema for the geriatric psychiatric assessment

Identifying data	Drug and alcohol history
Reliability of informant	Physical examination
Chief complaint	Functional status
History of presenting illness	Mental status
Past psychiatric history	Etiological formulation
Family history	Provisional diagnosis
Family psychiatric history	Differential diagnoses
Personal history	Investigations
Medical history	Comprehensive management plan
Current medications	

History of Presenting Illness

The purpose of the history of presenting illness is to document the events and arrange them in the order in which they happened. It is important to record all recent changes in the person's life, either environmental or physical. Environmental events and physical illness may precipitate mental illness in the elderly. For example, recent losses, separations, moves, and changes in support networks may be associated with the onset of affective and paranoid disorders or the exacerbation of cognitive disability. The cognitively impaired, frail elderly are particularly predisposed to superimposed delirium when relatively minor toxic, metabolic, or infectious disease intercedes. Certain physical disorders seem to precipitate specific mental disorders. For example, cerebrovascular accidents have been associated with depression and mania (Starkstein and Robinson 1989).

In order to focus the inquiry, the examiner must be familiar with the natural history and symptomatology of the common mental illnesses in the elderly. This knowledge is important because some mental disorders, particularly affective disorders, may present differently in old age. Many elderly depressives, for example, do not present with the classic sad and tearful demeanor (Post 1962). Common geriatric presentations include the hypochondriacal, agitated depressive who importunes the family in fits of desperation. The patient's frantic pleas for help may look "hysterical" to the observer and feel "manipulative" to the family. Depression may present with negativistic behavior such as refusal to move, eat, or drink. A suicidal gesture may herald the presence of this disorder. The recent onset in old age of phobias, obsessions, or compulsive behavior may signal the beginning of depression.

Vegetative symptoms of depression in the elderly include sleep, appetite, weight, and energy disturbance; loss of sexual drive; and diurnal variation in mood. Because the normal aging process can affect sleep, appetite, and energy, the clinician should note abrupt changes in these functions. Weight loss may be quantified by changes in dress or belt size.

When a cognitive disorder is suspected, interviewing a family member is essential. In this case, the clinician may have to elicit the entire history of the presenting illness from the family. Cognitive disorders affect memory, language, perception, mood, thinking, personality, and the person's capacity to function independently in his or her environment. For example, early in the course of Alzheimer's disease, patients misplace their belongings, have trouble with the names of familiar people, have trouble remembering new information, and show word-finding difficulties. Personality traits may become exaggerated and depressive symptoms or stealing delusions may coexist. Patients may give up their usual household activities, have trouble handling their finances, and rely increasingly on a single person, "the primary caregiver." The primary caregiver is in the best position to provide the clinician with this necessary information.

Past Psychiatric History

The record of past treatment successes and failures can aid in the development of a management plan for the current illness. The natural history of a patient's mental illness and the prognosis emerge from these data.

Family History

The parents of most geriatric patients are deceased; siblings may be deceased also. The cause of death, age at death, and the health of siblings can sometimes give clues about the patient's current problems. Similarly, a family psychiatric history provides valuable clues to the patient's diagnosis and may implicate genetic vulnerability. The past relationship of the patient to his or her parents often determines the quality of ensuing family and interpersonal relationships. Because the geriatric patient often relies on support for continuous good functioning, it is helpful to know about the quality of the patient's relationships with his or her spouse or primary caregiver, adult children, grandchildren, and friends.

Personal History

It is sometimes difficult to decide which events in an elderly patient's past are relevant to current problems and circumstances. Although the birth, developmental, childhood, and adolescent data are important, they are difficult to verify and corroborate through others. Knowledge of the patient's past almost always sheds light on the vulnerabilities and strengths of the patient and why some patients develop psychiatric symptomatology at particular points in their life. A review of the patient's life cycle establishes his or her premorbid capacity to adjust to important life events such as starting school, leaving home, establishing a career, getting married, the birth of children, death of parents, children leaving home, death of siblings, retirement, and death of a spouse.

The personal history should also include an inquiry into the person's activities, religious affiliation, hobbies, and connections with community resources. This information is useful in assessing each individual's social vulnerabilities and strengths.

Documenting a patient's premorbid personality provides a longitudinal view of the patient's characteristic personality function and helps avoid erroneous diagnostic conclusions based on cross-sectional examination. Although this type of information should be elicited from the patient, corroborative history from family or friends is often necessary.

A sexual history is often omitted in the elderly. This omission may be due to lack of knowledge or misconceptions of the examiner about sexuality in old age. A history of sexual orientation, activities, and practices and how the mental disorder has affected these functions is essential. For example, some elderly patients are very troubled by the anorgasmic side effects of many psychotropics. Developing a comfortable atmosphere for patients to raise these concerns during the assessment can be extremely therapeutic. This subject is dealt with in detail in Chapter 21.

Medical History, Medications, and Drug and Alcohol History

The clinician should carefully document all the past and current medical problems, with the dates of onset and treatment. The comorbidity of physical and mental illness, especially depression, is common in the elderly (Post 1969). Several physical illnesses, including Parkinson's disease and cerebrovascular disease, can precipitate a mood disorder or paranoid disorder. A variety of medications can precipitate psychiatric disorders such as delirium and affective and paranoid disorders (Johnson 1981). A list of all medications with dosage and date of onset is essential. (See Chapter 22.) Drug and alcohol abuse is often underestimated in the elderly (Brown 1982). Over-the-counter medications need to be included in this survey because many are neurotoxic even in moderate doses (e.g., bromides, aspirin, antihistamines).

Functional Assessment

Functional status consists of everyday behaviors in the home and community (Rubenstein et al. 1989). The capacity of an elderly person to remain independent is often jeopardized by the coexistence of physical and mental disability (Lawton 1988). This point

Table 8-2. Activities of daily living, for functional assessment

Physical (self-care) activities of daily living

Bathing	Eating
Dressing	Transferring
Grooming	Toileting

Instrumental activities of daily living

Using the telephone	Doing household chores
Shopping	Driving
Preparing food	Traveling
Using tools	Managing medication
Doing laundry	Managing money

is especially relevant in cognitively impaired and medically frail patients. The functional assessment is directed at quantifying how well patients can perform important tasks and maintain their independence. Ideally, it is completed in the patient's residence by careful observation of the person's functioning; otherwise, an interview with the primary caregiver is essential. Lawton and Brody (1969) and Katz and associates (1970) have divided the functional assessment (see Table 8-2) into two kinds of activities: physical activities of daily living and instrumental activities of daily living. The purpose of completing this assessment is to document the patient's functional strengths and vulnerabilities so that appropriate in-home supports for the caregiver and patient can be organized and the patient's progress can be monitored over time.

Mental Status Examination

The mental status examination is a cross-sectional assessment of the mental state of the patient at the time of the psychiatric interview. In an office setting, the examination begins as soon as the clinician meets the patient and family in the waiting room. While still greeting the patient, the clinician may note the following: How has the patient greeted the examiner? Does the patient know why she or he is being seen? How did the patient arrive for the assessment? Does the patient defer to the family for explanations? These observations often determine whether the clinician sees the patient or the family first. Much of the mental status examination is completed during the history taking. The skilled clinician uses appropriate moments in an interview to explore the phenomenology associated with the mental disorder. One challenge for the clinician examining an impaired elderly patient is to be able to ask about phenomena the patient is experiencing in words the patient can understand. A schema for the geriatric mental status examination is suggested in Table 8-3.

Appearance and Behavior

Geriatric patients' general appearance and behavior are often suggestive of the underlying psychiatric diagnosis. For example, an elderly patient sitting quietly, looking vacantly into space, dressed in ill-fitting, stained clothes with buttons missing and smelling of urine, suggests the possibility of a cognitive disorder although depressed patients also can present in that fashion when they lose motivation to take care of their appearance. Patients who greet the clinician with hesitation and furtive glances and who do not want the clinician to see their family suggest paranoid symptomatology. Posture, facial appearance, and movement can reflect mood and thinking disturbances and be affected by a variety of neurological conditions and psychotropic medications. For example, the shuffling, tremulous, elderly man who does not look at the examiner when he speaks and who will not get out of bed may have both Parkinson's disease and depression.

Speech

The rate, quantity, and quality of speech and the presence or absence of speech defects can offer clues to the diagnosis. For example, in geriatric depression the spontaneity, volume, and quantity of speech are often reduced. Depression also affects the capacity to express emotion (dysprosodia). In this case, speech sounds flat and monotonous.

Table 8-3.   Schema for mental status examination

Appearance and behavior	Perception
Speech	Obsessive-compulsive symptoms
Affect	Phobic symptoms
Subjective	Anxiety symptoms
Objective	Insight and judgment
Suicide potential	Competence
Thought	Mental
Process	Financial
Content	Cognitive assessment

Affect

Clinicians should elicit and describe the subjective affective disturbance of the patient. These subjective complaints may mislead the
examiner. For example, as many as one-fifth of elderly depressives
do not complain about being sad or depressed (Post 1972). Instead,
these patients may express their subjective distress as "bad
nerves," "funny feelings all over my body," or just feeling "sick." The
examiner makes note of the predominant affect expressed during
the interview and of the range, appropriateness, and control of affect. Disturbance in each of these functions may signal a different
underlying etiology. For example, incongruous, unrestricted affect
may be associated with multi-infarct dementia.

The geriatric patient requires a careful review of suicidal ideation and intent. The accuracy and depth of the inquiry are aided
by asking first about suicidal ideation and passive death wishes
and then (if appropriate) about specific intent, methods, and plans.
Additional risk factors in the elderly include poor physical health,
past history of suicide attempts, family history of suicide attempts
and completions, concurrent alcoholism or depression, presence of
command hallucinations, and social isolation.

Thought

The purpose of this section of the assessment is to describe the patient's thought content and process. The clinician should note the
specific preoccupations of the patient and the presence or absence
of delusions. For example, preoccupations in depression include
somatic and hypochondriacal concerns especially with the gastrointestinal, musculoskeletal, and nervous systems. These patients may worry that their health is deteriorating. These worries
may replace the subjective complaint of "depression."

If delusions are present, they should be described in detail preferably in the patient's own words. Mood-congruent delusions in severe geriatric depression can include delusions of poverty, sin,
guilt, nihilism, and hypochondriasis. Hypochondriacal delusions
are common and often center around the functions of the bowel
and brain. For example, a patient may believe there is a blockage
or tumor in the bowel and subsequently stop eating.

Delusions associated with dementia are common (Drevets and
Rubin 1989) and include delusions about stealing and persecution,
delusional jealousy (involving spouse), misidentification syndromes (involving caregiver or spouse), and reincarnation delu-

sions (involving dead relatives). More complex and systematized persecutory delusions may be present in paranoid patients with apparently intact cognition. Themes sometimes seen in these patients include fears about drug dealers, criminals, and prostitutes operating in nearby homes. These patients may fear that they are being constantly monitored and observed. Ideas of reference are often associated.

In elderly patients with intact cognition, thought process abnormalities are less common than in a younger-adult psychiatric population (Post 1967). Tangentiality and looseness of associations may be seen in dementias. Flight of ideas is common in mania of old age. Circumstantiality may be associated with an obsessional personality.

Perception

Perceptual disturbances include illusions, hallucinations, derealization, and depersonalization experiences. In the elderly, terrifying visual illusions and hallucinations are common in severe delirium. Olfactory and auditory hallucinations are seen in a variety of geriatric disorders including paranoid and affective disorders.

Obsessive-Compulsive, Phobic, and Anxiety Symptoms

There is little evidence that obsessive-compulsive or phobic symptoms commonly arise de novo in old age. When they do, it is most often in the context of a depressive disorder or in the early stages of a dementing disorder. The significance of anxiety disorders in the elderly is still not well described.

Judgment and Insight

Using information obtained in the history, the clinician determines whether the patient's mental illness interferes with judgment to the extent that it could jeopardize the health and safety of the patient or others. More subtle alterations in judgment include the inability to make and carry out plans and inappropriate behavior in social situations. Traditional tests of judgment that ask patients what they would do in imaginary situations are not very helpful because these tests are not sensitive to the subtle alterations in judgment seen in many geriatric disorders.

Insight refers to the degree of awareness and understanding patients have of their illness and the need for treatment. Does the patient realize that certain events may have predisposed or precipitated, or be perpetuating, the illness? In the elderly, judgment and insight are often affected by dementias, paranoid disorders, and affective disorders with delusions.

Competence

Geriatric psychiatrists are often required to assess a patient's capacity to make decisions. This assessment can involve evaluating the patient's ability to make or change a will, give power of attorney, or consent to treatment. Competence in each area should be tested separately. Competence is best viewed as a task-specific assessment. One of the more common competence assessments involves the capacity of the patient to give consent for medical treatment (Applebaum and Grisso 1988). The clinician can use the following questions as a guide: Is the patient aware he or she is suffering from a mental illness? Does the patient understand the nature of the proposed treatment? Does the patient understand the need for treatment and the implications of refusing treatment? Does the mental illness interfere with judgment and reasoning so much that it accounts for refusal of treatment?

Geriatric mental illness can interfere with capacity to manage one's finances (Lieff et al. 1984). The following questions can be used to complete this assessment: Does the person have knowledge of his or her current assets? Does the person have knowledge of his or her monthly expenses and bills? Does the person know where his or her assets are located and are being managed? Can the person complete simple calculations? Does the person suffer from delusions that would interfere with the capacity to manage his or her finances (e.g., delusions of poverty)? Is the person suffering from memory impairment sufficient to interfere with his or her capacity to remember recent and past financial transactions? Is the person's judgment so affected that his or her finances would be jeopardized (e.g., in a manic episode or in dementia)?

Cognitive Assessment

Purpose. The assessment of cognitive function is a crucial component of the geriatric mental status examination. The purpose of this portion of the comprehensive examination is to allow the clinician to answer the following questions.

First, is cognitive impairment present or absent? Traditionally this question has been phrased, "Is the illness functional or organic?" In psychogeriatrics, however, there is often an interplay between these two elements that challenges the validity of this diagnostic dichotomy. For example, the patient with depression who presents with what appears to be pseudodementia might be classified as having a "functional" illness, yet these symptoms may actually be the earliest signs of a bona fide dementing illness (Kral and Emery 1989). Conversely, a patient whose depression follows a left frontal cerebrovascular accident may be classified as having an "organic" illness; however, the affective component may respond well to the same somatic modalities as the "functional" illness (Starkstein and Robinson 1989). The question of whether cognitive impairment is present or absent is crucial in the determination of etiology, as well as in the formulation of a treatment plan.

Second, what is the pattern of the cognitive dysfunction? The pattern of cognitive impairment can reveal important clues about the etiology of the illness. It is not expected that the exact localization of a lesion will be elicited by the screening examination, but the examiner should be able to determine whether the lesion is diffuse (as in Alzheimer's disease) or localized (as in a right parietal lobe tumor).

Third, what is the quantity or severity of the cognitive impairment? When examinations of cognitive function are performed longitudinally, the answer to this question helps to determine the course and prognosis of the illness. The assessment of the quality and quantity of cognitive impairment, as well as a functional assessment, are essential to determine how much care or supervision these patients require.

Fourth, is a more elaborate neuropsychological examination necessary? Although much can be learned from a relatively brief screening examination, more detailed testing helps to establish a more accurate diagnosis when the findings are extremely subtle or when the clinician suspects an underlying dementia or neurological illness. When the diagnosis of dementia is likely, more detailed testing establishes areas of weakness and strengths in the various cognitive domains, in order to organize a comprehensive rehabilitation program. The examination should also help guide the choice of other investigations, such as electroencephalogram and neuroimaging, required to further elaborate the diagnosis.

Principles. The cognitive examination begins immediately with history taking. The examiner should be able to comment on such aspects as attention, concentration, memory, and language, simply by listening to how the patient relates the details of the history. These "passive" observations can be supplemented by subtle, in-context questioning throughout the history (e.g., asking patients the exact date of their anniversary while they talk about their marriage, asking patients to name all their grandchildren, or asking what day of the week they were admitted to the hospital).

The cognitive assessment should be carefully documented. For example, a clinician seeing a patient with Alzheimer's disease 2 years after initial diagnosis is better able to compare findings if the first examiner recorded "could recall 3 out of 4 objects after 5 minutes" than if he or she wrote "short-term memory fair."

Another important principle is that the examination be acceptable to both patient and examiner. For the examiner the tests should be easily administered, use minimal equipment, and take a short period of time. For the patient the tests must be nonthreatening and should not be unduly arduous, particularly if they follow a lengthy history.

The formal assessment should always begin with a short explanation to the patient (e.g., "I would now like to ask you some questions to see how well you can concentrate and remember things"). Elaborate explanations and use of the word "test" only serve to heighten the patient's anxiety, whereas being apologetic (e.g., "Some of these questions may seem a little silly") reduces the legitimacy and importance of the exam.

The examination is organized in a hierarchical fashion from basic functions to the more complex (see Table 8-4); for example, attention and concentration need to be assessed prior to any valid testing of memory. The examiner also has to demonstrate a certain degree of flexibility, depending on the clinical situation (e.g., comprehension needs to be tested early in any patient with a suspected aphasia). This hierarchical approach is also extended to assess tasks within a given cognitive domain. For example, a patient with suspected concentration impairment might first be asked to count backwards by ones from 100, prior to being asked serial sevens from 100. The former test is simpler and less threatening, the latter

Table 8-4. Format of the cognitive assessment

Attention and concentration	Memory
Language	Recent
Spontaneous speech	Remote
Comprehension	Constructional ability
Naming	Praxis
Orientation	Frontal systems

is more likely to demonstrate mild impairment, but may over-whelm patients if they have not had the opportunity to warm up to the testing procedures. Along with the recording of scores on individual tasks, the examiner should note the quality of the responses. "I don't know" responses, confabulations, lack of effort, and perseveration are all qualitative comments that provide useful diagnostic information.

Attention and Concentration.   Traditionally, attention has been tested using the task of repeating a string of digits forward and backward, and concentration has been measured with the serial sevens task. Although both tests can provide useful information, elderly persons often feel threatened when confronted with tasks involving numbers or arithmetic. The serial sevens subtraction test, in particular, may be more dependent on a patient's premorbid intellectual capacity and education than on an underlying impairment of concentration. A simple test to assess attention consists of reading a series of random letters to patients and asking them to indicate (tap or say yes) every time they hear the letter A. This task can be scored for errors of omission, commission, or perseveration. Simple tests of concentration include asking patients to state the days of the week backward, followed by months of the year backward. It is suggested that if they perform these two tasks flawlessly, patients can then be asked to do serial sevens from 100.

Language.   Although the exact characterization of an aphasia may be beyond the scope of a screening examination of cognition, the examiner does assess some aspects of a patient's expressive and receptive language function. Following the history, the examiner should be able to comment on many aspects of spontaneous speech such as articulation (presence of dysarthria), melody (prosody), the presence of word-finding difficulties, and evidence of specific aphasic errors (e.g., paraphasias). Paraphasias can include substitution of an incorrect word, referred to as a verbal or semantic paraphasia (e.g., "I cut meat with a pen"), or substitution of a syllable, called a phonemic or literal paraphasia (e.g., "I cut meat with a fife").

Comprehension can be tested by asking the patient to point to certain objects in the room. The test can be graded in difficulty by increasing the number of objects in a single command (e.g., "Point to the ceiling, the wall, and then the door") or by proceeding from the concrete (e.g., "Point to the light") to the more abstract (e.g., "Point to the source of illumination"). Alternatively, the examiner can pose a series of questions and ask the patient to respond yes or no. The examiner should pose the questions so that the yes/no responses vary randomly, in order to detect perseveration. This task is graded by varying the complexity of the question (e.g., "Is snow white?" vs. "Does a stone float on water?" vs. "Do you put on your shoes before your socks?"). Comprehension tests involving asking a patient to perform one-, two-, or three-stage commands can be useful, but may be difficult to interpret if the patient has a motor problem or apraxia.

Naming difficulties (anomia), which often occur in aphasic patients, can also be found in dementia such as Alzheimer's disease, as well as in toxic metabolic encephalopathies and in conditions with raised intracranial pressure (Cummings 1985). Naming is tested by pointing to a series of objects and asking the patient to name them (confrontation naming). The objects should include different categories (e.g., colors, body parts, clothing) and both high-frequency words (e.g., blue, red, mouth, hand, shirt, tie) and low-frequency words (e.g., purple, knuckles, watch crystal).

Orientation. Orientation is a function of memory, with both long-term (orientation to person) and short-term (orientation to place and time) components. Orientation to person, place, and time is tested sequentially. Patients are first asked their full name, age, and date of birth. Orientation to place is tested by asking where they are, as well as the city, state, and country they are in. They can also be asked their home address and more details of their current location (e.g., hospital floor, ward, room). Orientation to time includes asking the day, date, month, and year, as well as the time of day. If patients respond incorrectly to any of the above, they can be corrected and retested later in the interview as a test of ability to learn new information.

Memory. The testing of memory can be extremely complicated if all its dimensions are tested individually: immediate, recent, remote, recall, recognition, verbal, and visual. For the purpose of the cognitive screen, memory can be assessed quickly and simply in order to determine if more elaborate testing is indicated. The examiner begins by telling the patient to remember four words that he or she will be asked to recall in several minutes. Although any four unrelated words can be used, the examiner should use the same series of words for every patient in order to ensure consistency and ease of administration. Immediate recall is tested by asking the patient to repeat the four words immediately after the examiner's first recitation. The patient may require several trials to learn all four words, and the number of trials should be recorded. Recent memory is examined by asking the patient to recall the four words after 5 minutes. The examiner should record the number of words recalled spontaneously, as well as those recalled with the use of hints. Two kinds of hints or "cues" include semantic cues—hints related to the category of the object (e.g., "One word was a kind of animal")—and phonemic cues—given by progressively reciting the individual sounds or syllables of the word (e.g., "b . . . bl . . . bla . . . black").

Remote memory is assessed by noting patients' knowledge of the details of their personal history as well as by asking several questions of historical or political fact (e.g., names of the president and past president, dates of World War II). The performance on this task is dependent on the patient's premorbid intelligence and education and should be modified to account for sociocultural factors (e.g., asking a recent immigrant from England the names of prime ministers instead of presidents).

Constructional Ability. Constructional ability is assessed by asking the patient to draw or copy two- and three-dimensional figures. Although difficulty on these tests may indicate nondominant parietal lobe impairment, these tasks involve extensive cortical areas and in fact can be quite sensitive to subtle changes in overall cognition (Strub and Black 1985). For proper evaluation the clinician must ensure adequate light and vision (glasses are worn if necessary) as well as appropriate motor ability (no gross evidence of weakness or incoordination). Paper should be unlined so as not to produce "interference," and the patient should be given a pencil or a pen that writes easily, even at odd angles.

Constructional ability can be tested by asking the patient to draw freehand as well as copying figures. The patient can be asked to draw a circle, a cross, and a cube (in order of ascending difficulty). If the patient experiences any difficulty, the examiner draws the figure and asks the patient to copy it. Another simple, useful test of constructional ability is to hand patients a sheet of paper with a predrawn circle, and ask them to write in the numbers to make the circle look like the face of a clock. If they do this task correctly, they can be asked to draw in the hands to make the clock read three o'clock (a relatively easy task) or 10 minutes past 11 (a relatively difficult task). Clock drawing has been shown to be a good screening tool that correlates well with overall cognitive functioning (Shulman et al. 1986). It can also be used to demonstrate unilateral neglect and perseveration, and it is useful in following the progression of an illness (e.g., relative improvement in a resolving delirium, or worsening with a dementia).

Praxis. Ideomotor praxis involves the ability to perform volitional actions on command, in mime, without props (Cummings 1985). Testing involves limb, whole-body, and buccal-lingual commands. For the assessment of limb commands, the patient can be asked, "With your left hand, show me how you would comb your hair." Other limb commands could include brushing teeth, turning a key, or using a saw. Both hands should be tested separately. Common errors include performing the actions awkwardly, using the hands as the object instead of pretending to hold the object, and needing to use both hands or verbalizing the task first (Taylor et al. 1987). Whole-body commands include asking the patient to stand like a boxer or swing a bat like a baseball player. For buccal-lingual commands patients can be asked to pretend to lick crumbs off their lips, blow out a candle, or suck through a straw. Impairment of this kind of praxis (i.e., ideomotor apraxia) is usually related to dominant, parietal lobe dysfunction.

Frontal Systems Tasks. Frontal systems tasks are used to screen for dysfunction of the frontal lobes as well as their interconnected, subcortical structures. These tests are useful for assessing patients with frontal lobe pathology such as occurs in Pick's disease, as well as for assessing the cognitive functioning of patients with extrapyramidal disorders such as Parkinson's disease. In the latter, dysfunction in the basal ganglia, with its multitude of connections to the frontal lobes, can lead to a pattern of cognitive impairment referred to as subcortical dementia, which is quantitatively and qualitatively different from cortical dementias (Cummings and Benson 1983). The frontal lobes oversee many cognitive functions including attention, concentration, verbal fluency, abstraction, insight, and judgment. For the purposes of the cognitive screen, the following tests have been chosen because they tend to elicit two important signs associated with frontal lobe dysfunction, namely, perseveration and concrete thinking. (The assessment of attention, concentration, insight, and judgment has been described previously.)

Perseveration (the pathological repetition of speech or actions) may already be obvious from the history and previous testing, but it can also be assessed by presenting the patient an alternating sequence diagram or a drawing of several multiple loops (see Figure

8-1) and asking the patient to copy the diagrams exactly and continue the pattern across the page. Perseverative errors include drawing consecutive squares or triangles with the alternating sequence diagram and adding extra loops to the multiple loops. For another test, patients can be asked to tap once (with their hands on their knee or a desk) when the examiner taps twice, and twice when the examiner taps once. The examiner, while tapping randomly once or twice, observes whether patients can learn the correct response ("get into set"), how many errors are committed, and whether the errors are perseverative (e.g., continuing to tap twice every time the examiner taps twice). The task can then be made more difficult when the examiner "switches set" and asks the patient to tap twice every time the examiner taps once, but not to tap at all if the examiner taps twice. Particular attention is paid to whether the patient perseverates on the first series of instructions and continues to tap once every time the examiner taps twice.

Tests to elicit concrete thinking involve testing patients' ability to think abstractly. The results of these tests need to be interpreted cautiously, for they are highly dependent on educational level and cultural background. The patient can be asked to interpret metaphorical speech such as "he's blue," "she's yellow," "a heart of gold," or "heavy-handed." Patients can also be asked to interpret some common proverbs such as "Don't cry over spilled milk" (low difficulty) or "A stitch in time saves nine" (higher difficulty).

Concrete thinking can also be elicited by using a similarities task. The patient is asked to describe how two objects are alike. The task begins with a simple stimulus such as "How are an apple and an orange alike?" The response "They are both round" may be indicative of concrete thinking, but the examiner should explain that he or she was looking for the response "They are both fruit" and then proceed with the next stimulus. The stimuli are arranged in order of ascending complexity (e.g., orange/apple, shirt/pants, table/chair, airplane/bicycle). Continued responses that emphasize minute individual characteristics rather than the group or cate-

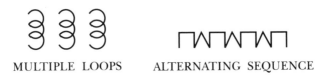

MULTIPLE LOOPS   ALTERNATING SEQUENCE

Figure 8-1. Perseveration can be assessed by asking patients to copy the multiple loops drawing or the alternating sequence diagram and continue the pattern across the page.

gory to which the objects belong are indicative of concrete thinking.

Standardized Cognitive Exams.   In recent years there has been a proliferation of brief, standardized, easily administered screening examinations for cognitive impairment. Such instruments include the Short Portable Mental Status Questionnaire (Pfeiffer 1975), the Blessed Dementia Index (Blessed et al. 1968), and the Clifton Assessment Schedule (Pattie and Gilleard 1976). One of the more widely accepted of these scales is the Mini-Mental State Exam (Folstein et al. 1975). The Mini-Mental State Exam provides a reliable, valid measure of cognition that includes tests of orientation, memory, concentration, language, and constructional ability. It is easy to administer and requires only about 10 minutes. It is particularly useful for research and educational purposes. Medical students, physicians other than psychiatrists, and allied mental health professionals can all be taught to use these measures, thus elevating their awareness of the necessity to consider cognitive function in all elderly patients. For the geriatric consultant, however, the more elaborate testing outlined previously can provide more information and allow for greater flexibility in testing the individual cognitive functions.

Conclusion

All geriatric patients require an appropriate physical examination with special attention directed to the neurological system. These areas are discussed in detail in Chapters 9 and 10.

With the history, functional, medical, and mental status assessments completed, the clinician can propose a provisional diagnosis and differential diagnosis, develop an etiological formulation, and establish the capacity of each patient to function independently.

The provisional and differential diagnoses will direct the clinician in planning for an orderly series of investigations and tests that will either confirm or refute the provisional diagnosis or the specific diagnoses in the differential.

By reorganizing the salient features of the assessment into an etiological formulation, the clinician will have developed a working hypothesis of the factors that make this patient vulnerable to developing a mental illness at this particular time. Knowing the biopsychosocial vulnerability of each patient is necessary to individualize the case management. Knowledge of the current capacity of the person to function in his or her environment will aid in determining what specific social supports must be provided to allow a person to continue living there. A comprehensive management plan including biological, psychological, and social therapies follows logically from the results of this assessment.

References

Applebaum PS, Grisso T: Assessing patients capacities to consent to treatment. N Engl J Med 319:1635–1638, 1988

Blessed G, Tomlinson BE, Roth M: The association between quantitative measures of dementia and of senile change in the cerebral gray matter of elderly subjects. Br J Psychiatry 114:797–811, 1968

Brown BB: Professionals' perceptions of drug and alcohol abuse among the elderly. Gerontologist 22:519, 1982

Cummings JL: Clinical Neuropsychiatry. New York, Grune & Stratton, 1985

Cummings JL, Benson DF: Dementia: A Clinical Approach. Boston, MA, Butterworths Publishers, 1983

Drevets WC, Rubin EH: Psychotic symptoms and the longitudinal course of senile dementia of the Alzheimer type. Biol Psychiatry 25:39–48, 1989

Folstein MF, Folstein SE, McHugh PR: Mini-Mental State: a practical method for grading the cognitive state of patients for the clinician. J Psychiatr Res 12:189–198, 1975

Ginsberg GL: Psychiatry history and mental status examination, in The Comprehensive Textbook of Psychiatry. Edited by Kaplan HI, Sadock BJ. Baltimore, MD, Williams and Wilkins, 1985

Johnson DAW: Drug-induced psychiatric disorders. Drugs 22:1, 57–69, 1981

Katz S, Downs TD, Cash HR, et al: Progress in development of the index of ADL. Gerontologist 10:20–30, 1970

Kral VA, Emery OB: Long term follow-up of depressive pseudodementia of the aged. Can J Psychiatry 34:445–446, 1989

Lawton MP: Scales to measure competence in everyday activities. Psychopharmacol Bull 24:609–614, 1988

Lawton MP, Brody EM: Assessment of older people: self-maintaining and instrumental activities of daily living. Gerontologist 9:179–186, 1969

Leff JP, Isaacs AD: Psychiatric Examination in Clinical Practice. Oxford, Blackwell Scientific Publications, 1978

Lieff S, Maindonald K, Shulman K: Issues in determining financial competence in the elderly. Can Med Assoc J 130:1293–1296, 1984

Pattie AH, Gilleard CJ: The Clifton Assessment Schedule—further validation of a psychogeriatric assessment schedule. Br J Psychiatry 129:68–72, 1976

Pfeiffer E: A short portable mental status questionnaire for the assessment of organic brain deficit in elderly patients. J Am Geriatr Soc 23:433, 1975

Post F: The significance of affective symptoms in old age. London, Oxford University Press, 1962

Post F: Aspects of psychiatry in the elderly. Proc R Soc Med 60:249–254, 1967

Post F: The relationship to physical health of the affective illnesses in the elderly. Proceedings of 8th International Congress of Gerontology, Washington, vol 1. 1969, pp 198–201

Post F: The management and nature of depressive illness in late life: a follow-through study. Br J Psychiatry 121:393–404, 1972

Rubenstein LV, Calkins DR, Greenfield S, et al: Health status assessment for elderly patients. J Am Geriatr Soc 37:562–569, 1989

Shulman KI, Shedletsky R, Silver IL: The challenge of time: clock-drawing and cognitive function in the elderly. International Journal of Geriatric Psychiatry 1:135–140, 1986

Starkstein SE, Robinson RG: Affective disorders and cerebrovascular disease. Br J Psychiatry 154:170–182, 1989

Strub RL, Black FW: The Mental Status Examination in Neurology. Philadelphia, PA, F. A. Davis, 1985

Taylor MA, Sierles FS, Abrams R: The neuropsychiatric evaluation, in The American Psychiatric Press Textbook of Neuropsychiatry. Edited by Hales RE, Yudofsky SC. Washington, DC, American Psychiatric Press, 1987, pp 3–16

Waldinger RJ: Psychiatry for Medical Students. Washington, DC, American Psychiatric Press, 1984

CHAPTER 9

Cathy A. Alessi, M.D.
Christine K. Cassel, M.D.

Medical Evaluation and Common Medical Problems

Introduction

Medical issues are important in the care of the older psychiatric patient. Medical illness may exacerbate psychiatric disorders or interfere with appropriate therapy. In addition, medical illness may present with symptoms that can be mistaken for primary psychiatric disease. Finally, signs and symptoms of medical illnesses may be subtle and nonspecific in the older patients and hence go unrecognized or are erroneously ascribed to "normal aging."

A large body of literature describes the distinction between physiologic changes due to normal aging and those due to disease. An awareness of both types of changes is important in the care of the older patient. Changes with normal aging impair the body's homeostatic mechanisms and result in decreased ability to deal with acute insult. Changes due to disease are also common; approximately 80% of people aged older than 65 have at least one chronic disease or disability (Soldo and Manton 1985).

Psychiatric Manifestations of Medical Illness in the Older Patient

Psychiatric symptoms can occur with practically any physical illness that has systemic involvement, can cause metabolic disturbance, or have direct central nervous system (CNS) effects. In addition, a variety of drugs can cause psychiatric symptoms at toxic doses, at normal therapeutic levels, or during periods of withdrawal (Abramowicz 1986). In fact, older patients may have several coexisting conditions or be taking several medications that could potentially explain or contribute to their psychiatric symptoms.

Physical illness in older patients can present as any of several psychiatric syndromes, such as dementia, delirium, depression (see Table 9-1), or anxiety (see Table 9-2). Each of these syndromes has multiple potential physical etiologies, as illustrated (Alexopoulos et al. 1988; Consensus Conference 1987; Cummings 1985; Cummings and Benson 1984; Lipowski 1989; Ouslander 1982; U'Ren 1989; Woodcock 1983). These syndromes are discussed in other chapters.

Several important clinical clues can alert the geriatric psychia-

Table 9-1. Physical disorders associated with depression in the older patient

Neurologic	Endocrine and metabolic
Parkinson's disease	Hyperthyroidism, hypothyroidism
Stroke	
Alzheimer's disease	Hyperparathyroidism, hypoparathyroidism
Subdural hematoma	
Temporal lobe epilepsy	Cushing's disease
Amyotrophic lateral sclerosis	Addison's disease
Multiple sclerosis	Hyperkalemia, hypokalemia
Normal pressure hydrocephalus	Hypernatremia, hyponatremia
	Hypercalcemia, hypocalcemia
Malignancy	Hyperglycemia, hypoglycemia
Brain tumor (primary or secondary)	Hypomagnesemia
	Hypoxemia
Leukemia	Vitamin B_{12} deficiency
Pancreatic	
Lung (particularly oat cell)	**Drugs**
Bone metastasis with hypercalcemia	CNS drugs (e.g., benzodiazepines, alcohol, levodopa, major tranquilizers)
Organ failure	Antihypertensives (e.g., beta-blockers, clonidine, reserpine, methyldopa, prazocin, guanethidine)
Renal failure	
Liver failure	
Congestive heart disease	
	Steroids (e.g., prednisone, estrogen)
Anemia	
Infections	Chemotherapy (e.g., vincristine, L-asparaginase, interferon)
Viral illness	
Chronic central nervous systems (CNS) infections	Cimetidine
	Digoxin

Table 9-2. Physical disorders associated with anxiety in the older patient

Neurologic	Cardiac
Early dementia	Coronary artery disease
Transient ischemic attack and stroke	Cardiac arrhythmias
Seizure disorder	Mitral valve prolapse
Endocrine	**Pulmonary**
Hypoglycemia	Recurrent pulmonary emboli
Hyperthyroidism	Chronic lung disease
Hypoparathyroidism	**Other**
Pheochromocytoma	Chronic pain
Cushing's disease	Anemia
Drugs	
Thyroid replacement	
Barbiturates	
Steroids	
Stimulants	
Vasodilators	
Caffeine	
Withdrawal from benzodiazepines, alcohol, barbiturates, neuroleptics, antidepressants	

trist to the possibility of an underlying physical illness (Ouslander 1982; Vickers 1988; Woodcock 1983):

- Abnormal cognitive function.
- Abnormal level of consciousness.
- Atypical age of onset of symptoms.
- Lack of expected family history of psychiatric illness.
- Symptoms more severe than expected.
- Coexisting physical illnesses that can cause psychiatric symptoms.
- Poor response to psychiatric treatment.
- Abrupt personality change followed by psychopathology.

Medical Evaluation of the Older Psychiatric Patient

The evaluation of the older psychiatric patient includes a thorough history and physical examination, cognitive screening, mental status examination, functional assessment, and appropriate screening laboratory tests.

The initial history and physical examination of the older patient is usually a lengthy process, particularly for patients with an extensive past medical history, several current physical complaints, or physical limitations that interfere with the examination. This initial evaluation frequently requires more than one visit, particularly for frail patients who fatigue easily from the examination process. For a review of history taking and the initial physical examination, the reader may refer to a geriatric medicine text (e.g., Calkins and Davis 1986; Cassel et al. 1989; Kane et al. 1989; Rossman 1986; Rowe and Besdine 1988). Psychiatric evaluation of the older patient is essential, but is discussed elsewhere in this text.

Screening laboratory tests are commonly ordered (see Table 9-3) for older psychiatric patients to rule out physical illness, particularly in patients with psychiatric symptoms that are of recent onset, severe, or resistant to therapy. Which screening tests are ordered is determined by the patient's clinical presentation. One study of older patients admitted to a psychiatric unit found only the following screening tests useful in the detection and treatment of an illness: midstream urine collection, chest X ray, vitamin B_{12} assay, electrocardiogram, and blood urea nitrogen (Kolman 1984).

Common Medical Problems

Although the medical conditions of old age that are most relevant to psychiatrists are covered in the following section, a discussion of all medical disorders of old age is beyond the scope of this text. The reader is referred to one of the above-mentioned geriatric medicine texts for additional reading.

Table 9-3. Laboratory screening tests in older psychiatric patients

Complete blood count	Syphilis serology
Blood glucose	Vitamin B_{12} and folate assays
Serum electrolytes	Urinalysis
Blood urea nitrogen and creatinine	Electrocardiogram
Liver enzymes	Chest X ray
Thyroid function tests (thyroxine level, free thyroxine index, thyroid-stimulating hormone level)	

Arthritis. The most common chronic condition among persons aged 65 and older is arthritis; it affects nearly 50% (Soldo and Manton 1985). Painful or stiff joints in older patients are usually due to osteoarthritis, which involves deterioration and abrasion of the articular cartilage. One-third of older patients have significant symptoms of joint discomfort, and approximately 10% have significant limitation due to osteoarthritis. The joints usually involved include the hands (proximal and distal interphalangeal), hips, knees, feet (first metatarsal-phalangeal), and the cervical and lower lumbar spine. The diagnosis is suggested by symptoms in one or more of these joints combined with evidence of degenerative changes on plain X rays. X-ray evidence of degenerative disease does not necessarily correlate with symptom severity. There are no diagnostic blood tests for osteoarthritis. An elevated erythrocyte sedimentation rate, weight loss, or constitutional symptoms suggest another disease process. Treatment of osteoarthritis is symptomatic, primarily with aspirin and nonsteroidal anti-inflammatory drugs; caution is indicated when the latter are used because they can cause severe gastric mucosal injury and even life-threatening gastric ulceration, or renal insufficiency in susceptible patients. Small doses of codeine may be useful in patients with severe symptoms who cannot tolerate other agents, with careful attention to the risk of addiction. Severe limiting symptoms in carefully chosen patients may be best treated with surgical joint replacement.

The other major rheumatologic diseases in older patients with joint discomfort include gout, pseudogout, polymyalgia rheumatica (with or without temporal arthritis), rheumatoid arthritis, and infectious arthritis (Moskowitz 1987; Sorenson 1989).

Hypertension. The second most common chronic condition, affecting approximately 40% of persons aged older than 65, is hypertension (Soldo and Manton 1985). Patients may have either "classic" hypertension (diastolic blood pressure greater than 90 mmHg) or isolated systolic hypertension (systolic blood pressure greater than 160 mmHg and diastolic blood pressure less than 90 mmHg). One precaution to keep in mind is the falsely elevated cuff blood pressure that may be seen in some older patients ("pseudohypertension"). It is probably due to calcification of the brachial artery, and it may be accompanied by a positive "Osler's sign" (a palpable, pulseless, brachial or radial artery after blood pressure cuff occlusion) (Messerli et al. 1985). Secondary causes of hypertension are considered in patients with onset of hypertension after age 55 or accelerated hypertension after age 65. However, an extensive workup is generally recommended in older patients only when hypertension cannot be controlled medically.

Some authorities suggest that older patients with a blood pressure of 160/95 mmHg or greater on several readings should be treated (Byyng 1986). However, older patients are prone to complications of anti-hypertensive therapy, and guidelines for treatment are unclear. Aggressive treatment in patients 80 years of age or older is probably not warranted (Amery et al. 1986).

Nonpharmacologic treatments for hypertension are important, such as salt restriction, weight loss in the obese, smoking cessation, decreasing excessive caffeine use, and a careful exercise plan. In general, pharmacologic agents should be started at a lower dose than in younger patients. One should use simple dosing schedules and slow dosage changes, watch for side effects and drug interactions, and consider whether the patient can afford the financial outlay for the medication chosen. Care should be taken when choosing psychiatric medications in patients who are taking anti-hypertensives with CNS or orthostatic side effects. It may, at times, be desirable to discuss with the primary care physician a change in antihypertensive medication.

Thiazide diuretics are often used in older patients, but they are generally started at lower doses than for younger patients (e.g., 25 mg of hydrochlorothiazide per day). Limiting side effects of diuretics include frequent urination, orthostasis, and dehydration, as well as sodium and potassium depletion. Hyperglycemia, hyperuricemia, and increased lipid levels may also occur. In general, psychiatric symptoms due to diuretic therapy are seen only in patients who develop metabolic derangements.

Beta-blockers can be used in older patients, but with careful attention to the appearance of bradycardia, heart block, bronchospasm, congestive heart failure, and glucose intolerance. Advantages of beta-blockers include antianginal effects, possible cardioprotective effects, and low incidence of orthostatic hypotension. Disadvantages include the major risk of depression and the less serious but significant side effect of somnolence. Calcium-channel blockers may be used, but they carry a risk of heart block in susceptible patients and can decrease cardiac contractility. These agents generally do not cause significant orthostatic hypotension or CNS side effects. Angiotensin-converting enzyme inhibitors are generally well tolerated, but hyperkalemia is a potential complication. CNS side effects are generally not a problem. Centrally acting agents such as clonidine, guanethidine, and methyldopa can produce sedation and depression. Reserpine has also been associated with depression (Applegate 1989; Tuck 1988).

Diabetes Mellitus.   Glucose intolerance increases with age; approximately one-third of patients older than 65 have an abnormal glucose tolerance test. However, whether all these patients require therapy is unclear. An abnormal fasting blood sugar is less common, occurring in only 10% of older patients, and is probably the preferable method of diagnosing diabetes in this population. The majority of older patients with diabetes have type II or non-insulin-dependent diabetes mellitus, although some of these patients may require insulin therapy. Patients are typically overweight and had onset of diabetes after age 40. The required treatment varies considerably and may include diet, weight loss, oral hypoglycemic agents, or insulin; some patients will require a combination. Doses of oral agents or insulin are started low and increased slowly to avoid hypoglycemia, which is a significant risk in older patients. Hypoglycemia may present with psychiatric symptoms ranging from subtle dullness to coma.

Complications of chronic diabetes involve multiorgan disease, and generally reflect microvascular and macrovascular disease or neurologic involvement. Good blood sugar control may decrease the risk of these complications, although this point is not well established, particularly in older patients. Nonspecific complaints such as fatigue may be due to chronic hyperglycemia and may improve with good blood sugar control. Attempts at tight control must be balanced with the risks of hypoglycemia.

Acute hyperglycemia in older diabetics generally presents not as diabetic ketoacidosis, but as hyperglycemic hyperosmolar nonketotic coma (HHNKC). These patients may present with mental status changes in addition to weakness, polyuria, and polydipsia. Mortality is as high as 25% to 50%. Acute hyperglycemia without HHNKC can also cause psychiatric symptoms ranging from subtle personality changes to delirium. The mental status changes of hyperglycemia with or without HHNKC may resolve slowly, particularly in those patients with underlying CNS disease (Cooppan 1987; Riesenberg 1989).

Constipation.   Most healthy older outpatients have a bowel frequency within the same range as their younger counterparts (three times per day to three times per week), but older patients more often complain of constipation and more often use laxatives (Connell et al. 1965; Donald et al. 1985). Factors that may contribute to constipation in older patients include decreased fluid and dietary fiber intake, decreased activity, intrinsic bowel lesions, endocrine and metabolic disorders, and constipating drugs. Constipation can be a significant problem in psychiatric patients, particularly those on medications with anticholinergic effects. Common causes of constipation in older patients are listed in Table 9-4.

The older patient with constipation should have a rectal examination to rule out fecal impaction and anorectal disease such as hemorrhoids or rectal fissure. Those who present with new or worsened constipation without obvious etiology should have some study to visualize their colon. Older patients with weight loss and hemoccult-positive stools should have colonoscopy. Screening blood tests, particularly a complete blood count and thyroid function tests (TFTs), may aid diagnosis.

The first step in treating constipation is to discontinue unnecessary constipating drugs and treat any contributing diseases. Next, patients should be encouraged to increase physical activity, fluid intake, and dietary fiber. Bulk-forming agents such as methylcellulose or psyllium can be added. Patients with hard stools may benefit from a stool softener such as docusate preparations. Other agents to consider are lactulose, enemas, and suppositories.

Table 9-4. Common causes of constipation in the older patient

Intrinsic bowel lesions	Endocrine and metabolic
Colorectal carcinoma	Hypothyroidism
Anorectal disease (e.g., hemorrhoids, fissures)	Adrenal and pituitary hypofunction
Diverticular disease	Hypokalemia
Inflammatory bowel disease	Hypercalcemia
Ischemic bowel disease	Uremia
Irritable bowel disease	
Hypomotility disorders (e.g., idiopathic slow transit, idiopathic megacolon)	**Drugs**
	Analgesics
	Antacids (e.g., calcium carbonate, aluminum hydroxide)
Neurologic	Anticholinergics (e.g., antihistamines, tricyclic antidepressants, antiparkinsonian agents, neuroleptics)
Dementia	
Stroke	
Autonomic neuropathy (e.g., diabetes, pernicious anemia)	
	Antihypertensives, diuretics
Psychiatric	Laxative abuse
Depression	Other (e.g., iron, phenytoin, barium, bismuth)
Chronic psychosis	

Lactulose can be given at a starting dose of 15 to 30 cc at bedtime and increased if necessary. Prepackaged enemas are simple and usually safe. Bisacodyl suppositories are usually more effective than glycerin suppositories.

Some agents require special precautions in older patients. Oral mineral oil is not recommended because of the risks of impaired absorption of fat-soluble vitamins and of aspiration with consequent lipoid pneumonia. Stimulant laxatives are recommended only for short-term use because of cramping and fluid and electrolyte loss. Chronic uses of stimulant laxatives can cause colonic smooth muscle changes resulting in severe, resistant constipation (cathartic colon). Saline laxatives such as magnesium salts carry a risk of fluid loss with chronic use but can be used for short-term therapy. Soapsuds or hydrogen peroxide enemas should not be used because of mucosal irritation.

Fecal impaction should be suspected and a rectal examination performed in patients with severe or chronic constipation, or in patients who develop fecal incontinence or paradoxical diarrhea (i.e., diarrhea in the presence of a fecal impaction). High fecal impaction beyond the range of digital rectal examination may be visualized on plain X rays of the abdomen. If enemas are not successful, careful manual disimpaction with a single well-lubricated finger is required when a fecal impaction is present. A fecal impaction must be removed prior to therapy with stimulant laxatives, because of risk of causing severe cramping or obstruction (Alessi and Henderson 1988).

Weight Loss and Malnutrition. Weight loss is a common symptom in older patients with psychiatric or medical illness. Unintentional weight loss of 5% in 6 months or 10% in 1 year is significant and should be evaluated for an organic cause. In about one-third of patients with weight loss, no physical cause is found. The most common physical causes found are malignancy and gastrointestinal disease. The extent of laboratory testing in the older patient with psychiatric symptoms and weight loss depends on clinical clues of an underlying physical illness, degree of weight loss, and overall status of the patient. Typical screening tests include complete blood count, electrolytes, blood urea nitrogen, creatinine, liver enzyme tests, glucose, serum protein and albumin, calcium, TFTs, erythrocyte sedimentation rate, stools for occult blood, urinalysis, and chest X ray. Further testing is guided by the history, physical examination, and results of screening laboratory tests (Marton et al. 1981; Morley et al. 1986).

The prevalence of malnutrition in older patients varies with the population studied. Malnutrition is reported in less than 5% of ambulatory outpatients but occurs in up to two-thirds of hospitalized and institutionalized older persons. Patients can present with weight loss, weakness, skin problems, and changes in mental status. Laboratory tests to identify malnutrition include serum albumin (a value less than 3 to 3.5 g/dl is significant), total lymphocyte count (values less than 1,500/cm^3 are significant), and the presence of anergy on skin testing. However, in older patients, albumin may not be reliable and anergy may occur without medication. Anthropometric measures can also be used, such as age-adjusted weight and height, skinfold, and arm muscle circumference. Calorie counts can determine if the patient's energy intake is adequate. Treatment of malnutrition includes making food accessible, treating underlying causes, and using nutritional supplements and tube feedings when appropriate (Morley 1986; Morley et al. 1986).

Anemia. Healthy older people maintain a normal hemoglobin value. Those who do not should be evaluated. The classic signs of anemia are pallor, weakness, and fatigue. The older anemic patient, however, may present with behavioral changes or confusion. If the anemia is recognized and treated, the symptoms can respond dramatically to relatively small improvements in hemoglobin. Evaluation of the anemic patient should be approached systematically. A coexisting low platelet count and low white blood cell count suggest pancytopenia. An elevated reticulocyte count suggests that the patient's bone marrow is responding appropriately to some insult, such as hemolysis, blood loss, toxin, or vitamin deficiency. A normal or low reticulocyte count in the face of anemia suggests that the bone marrow is not responding appropriately. Further identification of the anemia (based on the red blood cell size) as microcytic, macrocytic, or normocytic can be made by reviewing the peripheral smear. It should be borne in mind that multiple causes of anemia can coexist in the older patient.

    The patient with a microcytic anemia should have serum iron studies and stool examination for occult blood. A low serum ferritin is diagnostic of iron deficiency, but ferritin can be falsely raised into the normal range by liver disease or inflammatory disorders. Low serum iron and raised total iron-binding capacity can also be seen in iron deficiency anemia, but these tests may not be reliable in older patients because the presence of a chronic disease can lead to a normal or low total iron-binding capacity, even in the presence of an iron deficiency anemia. In some cases, bone marrow aspiration is needed to assess iron stores. Stool examination for occult blood is important; however, negative stool exams should not preclude bowel studies when an iron deficiency anemia is present. Many geriatricians avoid barium studies and evaluate the iron-deficient patient with colonoscopy as the initial test, in order to increase diagnostic accuracy and avoid subjecting the older patient to two bowel preparation procedures.

Anemia of chronic disease is a diagnosis of exclusion made only in patients who have a documented chronic disease and otherwise normal hematologic evaluation. Iron studies typically show both decreased iron and total iron-binding capacity.

Macrocytic anemia from megaloblastic red blood cell changes in older patients can be due to deficiency of folate or vitamin B_{12}. Red cell folate levels are more reliable than serum folate levels but are not available in all laboratories. If there is no malabsorption, folate deficiency can be corrected with folic acid (1 mg orally per day).

The most frequent cause of vitamin B_{12} deficiency in the older patient is pernicious anemia. The normal lower limit of serum vitamin B_{12} level is uncertain in the older patient, and the necessity for a Schilling test to document pernicious anemia in every older patient with a low B_{12} level has been debated. The Schilling test may be useful in patients with borderline B_{12} levels, because vitamin B_{12} deficiency has been associated with a variety of neurologic symptoms including paresthesias, dysesthesias, abnormal proprioception, and dementia. Psychiatric symptoms have also been described, including delirium, hallucinations, personality changes, delusions, depression, acute psychosis, and mania. Neurologic changes of B_{12} deficiency can occur prior to hematologic changes. Patients with vitamin B_{12} deficiency generally require lifelong monthly intramuscular B_{12} injections. Whether folate deficiency alone can cause neurologic symptoms has been debated. Correction of folate deficiency in the face of undiagnosed vitamin B_{12} deficiency can precipitate progression of neurologic symptoms.

Normocytic anemia should be evaluated with stool examination for occult blood, a reticulocyte count, and examination of the peripheral smear for evidence of hemolysis. Testing for iron deficiency anemia and folate and B_{12} deficiency are often recommended in the older anemic patient because of the possibility of early or mixed disease (Cohen and Crawford 1986; Freedman 1985).

Thyroid Disease. The presentation of thyroid disease in the older patient may be subtle or atypical. Symptoms that are attributed by some to "old age"—such as fatigue, constipation, and functional decline—may be seen with thyroid disease. Screening for thyroid disease in older patients with psychiatric symptoms is recommended because thyroid disease in older patients is common and the symptoms can mimic or exacerbate psychiatric illness.

There is disagreement in the literature on which thyroid functions tests (TFTs) to order for screening purposes. The commonly ordered TFTs include thyroxine (T_4), T_3 resin uptake (T_3RU), and thyroid-stimulating hormone (TSH) levels. The free thyroxine index (FTI) is a calculated measure that corrects for protein binding (FTI = $T_4 \times T_3RU$). More recently, new immunoradiometric methods of TSH assay (the so-called supersensitive TSH measures) allow the distinction between normal (euthyroid) and low (hyperthyroid) levels of TSH. These new TSH assays may be useful as single screening tests of thyroid function (Caldwell 1985; Feit 1988).

Older patients with hyperthyroidism may present with the classic signs and symptoms such as heat intolerance, weight loss, tremor, and palpitations. However, older patients may also present with single-organ-system symptoms (such as atrial fibrillation) or with "apathetic hyperthyroidism" (characterized by anorexia, fatigue, weight loss, and general decline) without the hypermetabolic symptoms of hyperthyroidism. Laboratory testing in hyperthyroidism reveals a high serum T_4, high FTI, and a low, generally undetectable TSH. "T_3 thyrotoxicosis" is a hyperthyroid state with elevated serum T_3 but normal serum T_4.

Initial therapy of hyperthyroidism in the older patient generally involves a beta-blocker such as propranolol and an antithyroid medication such as propylthiouracil. Definitive treatment in older patients is usually with radioactive iodine therapy, after which up to one-third of patients become hypothyroid.

The major symptoms of hypothyroidism in older patients are lassitude, constipation, cold intolerance, fatigue, and decreased mentation. Symptoms may develop slowly and be attributed to "aging," depression, or dementia. Patients with myxedema have the features of hypothyroidism along with soft tissue accumulation of mucopolysaccharides. Laboratory testing in hypothyroidism reveals low serum T_4 and FTI with elevated levels of TSH. In frail older patients or those with cardiac disease, thyroid hormone replacement starts at low doses, such as .025 mg of L-thyroxine per day, and is gradually increased by .025 mg at monthly intervals, with monitoring for side effects and normalization of serum TSH levels. Myxedema coma is a life-threatening presentation of hypothyroidism that occurs almost exclusively in patients older than 50. It generally occurs in patients with chronic myxedema who suffer some additional insult such as sedating medications or an acute illness. Myxedema coma is a medical emergency that requires intravenous L-thyroxine therapy (Robuschi 1987).

Three additional patterns of TFT abnormality are euthyroid hyperthyroxinemia, euthyroid sick syndrome, and subclinical hypothyroidism. Euthyroid hyperthyroxinemia is characterized by an elevated T_4 with normal TSH. These patients are clinically euthyroid, and the elevated serum T_4 level generally resolves spontaneously. Euthyroid sick syndrome, which is recognized by low serum T_4 with normal serum TSH, has been described in hospitalized patients with serious systemic illness of various etiologies. Subclinical (compensated) hypothyroidism is a very common pattern of abnormal TFTs in older patients characterized by elevated TSH with normal T_4 and FTI. It may progress to overt hypothyroidism, particularly in patients with TSH values greater than 20 microunits/mL or high-titer positive thyroid microsomal antibodies (Rosenthal et al. 1987).

A significant percentage of newly admitted psychiatric patients who are clinically euthyroid have some abnormality in initial TFTs, particularly an elevated T_4 or FTI, which reverts to normal after approximately 2 weeks. In patients with an acute psychiatric illness, without signs or symptoms of thyroid disease and with mild or nonspecific abnormalities on initial TFTs, it is reasonable simply to observe the patients and repeat the TFTs after approximately 2 weeks (Feit 1988).

Geriatric Syndromes

Certain medical problems are common in older patients yet may go untreated if not specifically addressed. They are singled out here to alert the psychiatrist to recognize these "geriatric syndromes" and refer patients for evaluation when appropriate.

Hearing and Visual Impairment. Hearing impairment occurs in 25% to 45% of persons older than 65, and 90% of those older than 80. The hearing loss is usually in the high-frequency range, which is important in conversation. Hearing impairment can lead to social isolation, depression, and confusion. However, fewer than 20% of those impaired receive any form of hearing aid. When there is a question of hearing impairment, the first step is to examine the ear for cerumen occluding the external ear canal. If the ear is clear of cerumen, patients can be screened with a hand-held audioscope or referred to audiology. A questionnaire for significance of hearing impairment in older persons is also available (American Speech Language and Hearing Association 1989; Lichtenstein et al. 1988; Mader 1984).

Visual impairment is present in almost 15% of persons aged 65 and older, and almost 30% of those over age 85. The most frequent causes of blindness in older patients are cataracts and macular degeneration. Other important causes are glaucoma and diabetic retinopathy. Patients can be screened by testing visual acuity, performing an ophthalmoscopic examination, and checking intraocular pressure (Straatsma et al. 1985).

Urinary Incontinence.   Urinary incontinence is a problem in up to one-third of community-dwelling older patients and in even higher numbers of those acutely hospitalized. The majority of patients with incontinence have some relief of symptoms if the incontinence is recognized by the clinician, properly evaluated, and treated. However, the patient may not mention it unless specifically asked. Incontinence can be an acute or chronic problem. Common causes of acute incontinence are urinary tract infection, restricted mobility, altered mental status, drugs (particularly those with anticholinergic or sedating properties, and diuretics), polyuria, and fecal impaction. Patients who suddenly develop urinary incontinence should have some procedure (straight catheterization or bladder ultrasound) to rule out urinary retention with overflow incontinence. A postvoid residual of more than 100 ml is considered significant (Ouslander 1986).

There are various classifications of chronic urinary incontinence. One commonly used system classifies chronic incontinence as stress, urge, overflow, or functional incontinence. Symptoms of stress incontinence include loss of small amounts of urine with increases in intra-abdominal pressure such as a cough or laugh. Urge incontinence usually presents with an uncontrollable urge to void, with loss of large amounts of urine. Overflow incontinence is the loss of small amounts of urine associated with an overdistended bladder. Functional incontinence is loss of urine associated with an inability to get to the toilet because of immobility or other functional problems. A patient may have multiple causes of incontinence. Chronic urinary incontinence should be evaluated by an experienced clinician. It is not clear if treating asymptomatic bacteriuria in the patient with chronic incontinence is of any benefit; however, most authors recommend a course of antibiotic in this situation (Ouslander 1986).

Falls.   Falls occur to one-third of community-dwelling persons older than 65, and more than one-half of nursing home residents each year. Five percent of falls result in a fracture, and up to 10% of falls result in other serious injury. There is a wide range of etiologies for falls in older persons, including neurologic disorders (such as Parkinson's disease) with gait and postural abnormalities; environmental hazards (such as loose rugs or electric cords); drugs that cause orthostatic hypotension; and mental status changes. In most cases, falls have multiple causes. The psychiatrist should question the older person about falls, particularly when medications are added or dosage changes are made (Tinetti et al. 1988).

Immobility.   Immobility can have serious consequences in older patients, such as contractures (which can develop in days to weeks), deep venous thrombosis and embolization, osteopenia, orthostasis, atelectasis and pneumonia, constipation, urinary retention, and pressure sores. Common conditions that lead to immobility in older patients are arthritis, hip fracture, stroke, generalized weakness, and pain. Patients confined to bed should be mobilized as quickly as possible. While bedridden, patients should have range-of-motion exercises to prevent contractures and subcutaneous heparin therapy to prevent thrombosis, and they should be turned frequently to avoid skin breakdown (Harper and Lyles 1988).

Pressure Sores.   The majority of pressure sores occur in older patients, with a prevalence of up to 30% in older hospitalized patients. More than 90% of pressure sores occur over one of the following sites: sacrum, ischial tuberosity, greater trochanter, calcaneus, and lateral malleolus. Factors that can lead to pressure sores include pressure to one area for more than 2 hours, shearing forces, friction on the skin surface, and moisture (Allman 1989). Methods of preventing pressure sores include mobilizing patients, relieving pressure in bedridden patients (by repositioning the body at a 30-degree angle every 2 hours), keeping skin clean and dry, and maintaining adequate nutrition. Pressure sores that are limited to the dermis (grade I) or subcutaneous fat (grade II) are kept clean and dry. Pressure sores that involve the deep fascia (grade III) or are extensive in depth (grade IV) need debridement followed by saline dressing changes. The clinician should be wary of closed pressure sores, which are extensive deep fascia wounds that appear benign on the surface (Shea 1975).

Nonspecific Decline.   Older patients may present with nonspecific complaints, such as general fatigue or malaise, declining functional status, or a "failure to thrive." These symptoms may be longstanding in patients who have attributed them to "old age." Nonspecific decline can be due to a host of psychiatric and medical illnesses. The evaluation of these symptoms should be guided by coexistent problems such as weight loss, malnutrition, fever, localizing symptoms, cognitive deficits, or mood disturbances. Any new or changed medications, including over-the-counter drugs, should be suspect.

Hypochondriasis.   Older patients have an increased prevalence of disease, and therefore the clinician should be careful when attributing somatic complaints to hypochondriasis. Studies of community-dwelling older patients do not demonstrate the notion that hypochondriasis is common among older patients. In fact, illness and symptoms are generally underreported and attributed to "old age" by older patients.

Patients who do have hypochondriasis present with an unrealistic interpretation of physical signs or sensations, which leads them to believe that they have a serious disease. Therefore, symptoms that might signify underlying disease should be investigated. Moreover, hypochondriacs also get sick. It is important to distinguish hypochondriasis from other psychiatric disorders, particularly depression. Regularly scheduled, frequent, short visits (even when the patients are feeling well) are generally helpful. Sometimes the frequency of visits can be decreased as the patient-physician relationship develops.

Patients with somatization express psychiatric disease or psychological stress with somatic complaints. Somatization can occur with somatoform disorders, affective disorders, anxiety and panic disorders, personality disorders, psychoses, transient emotional stress, and malingering. Coexistent psychiatric disorders should be treated. A helpful patient-physician relationship grows as the physician respectfully but conservatively evaluates somatic symptoms as they occur (Kaplan et al. 1988).

Common Laboratory Abnormalities

As previously discussed, various screening laboratory tests are often obtained in older patients who present with psychiatric symptoms (see Table 10-3). The psychiatrist should be familiar with the initial approach to abnormalities in these tests and obtain referral when appropriate. The approach to anemia, glucose abnormalities, abnormal thyroid function tests, and vitamin B_{12} and folate deficiency have already been addressed.

Serum Electrolytes. Serum sodium level reflects body water balance. Hypernatremia usually is the result of fluid loss (e.g., from diarrhea, osmotic diuresis, sensible losses, diabetes insipidus from lithium therapy), so that these patients (who have increased plasma osmolality) should develop thirst, but older patients have been shown to have a decrease in thirst sensation (hypodipsia) and are at risk for dehydration. Patients with hypernatremia can present with confusion. Treatment of hypernatremia requires clinical assessment of volume status. This assessment is critical because patients with volume excess and edema and those with the syndrome of inappropriate antidiuretic hormone secretion are treated with water restriction, whereas those with decreased volume status are treated with saline (Narins et al. 1982).

Hyponatremia can result from a variety of etiologies. Symptoms depend on the severity of hyponatremia and how rapidly the change in sodium level has occurred. CNS symptoms such as confusion, lethargy, coma, and seizures are associated with sodium levels below 120 to 125 meq/L. The reader is referred to texts of internal medicine for further discussion of serum electrolyte abnormalities.

Blood Urea Nitrogen and Creatinine. Glomerular filtration rate declines with age, placing older patients at increased risk for developing acute renal failure when exposed to insults such as nephrotoxic drugs and dyes or episodes of low renal perfusion. Blood urea nitrogen and creatinine may overestimate renal function in older patients because of decreased protein intake and decreased muscle mass. Thus, serum levels of blood urea nitrogen and creatinine may be within normal limits despite decreased renal function, and minor elevations of these tests may represent significant renal impairment. Therefore, medications with renal excretion (e.g., penicillin and some other antibiotics, aspirin, bronchodilators) should be prescribed initially in low doses in older patients, and drug levels should be monitored if possible.

Liver Function Tests.   In normal older patients, liver function remains adequate throughout life. However, there is evidence that hepatic metabolism of some drugs decreases with age, and caution should be taken with these agents (see Chapter 22).

Commonly ordered screening tests that reflect liver disease include bilirubin, transaminases (Serum Glutamic-Oxalacetic Transaminase, Aspartate and Serum Glutamic-Pyruvic Transaminase, Alanine Trans), and alkaline phosphatase. A full discussion is beyond the scope of this chapter. Patients with abnormalities should be referred. These tests may be abnormal in a variety of disorders such as viral hepatitis, drug-induced hepatitis, cirrhosis, biliary tract obstruction, malignancy, hemolysis, and prolonged fasting. Some psychiatric medications may cause hepatitis. Drug-induced hepatitis can present with a cholestatic, a hepatitic, or a mixed pattern. Phenothiazines can cause a cholestatic-type drug-induced hepatitis with marked bilirubin elevation (primarily direct bilirubin), marked alkaline phosphatase elevation, and only mild to moderate transaminase elevations. Monoamine oxidase inhibitors can cause a predominantly hepatitic picture with marked transaminase elevation and lesser increase in alkaline phosphatase.

Syphilis Serology.   There are two basic types of serologic tests for syphilis. The first is nonspecific reagin antibody testing (e.g., Venereal Disease Research Laboratories, Rapid Plasma Reagin). The second is specific antitreponemal antibody testing (e.g., Fluorescent Treponemal Antibory-Absorption Test for Syphilis, Microhemagglutinations-Treponenia Pallidum). The VDRL and RPR have a high false positive rate, and so positive results should be followed by an FTA-ABS or MHA-TP. A false negative VDRL can occur in patients with primary syphilis who have not yet developed reactivity, and in one-third of patients with latent or tertiary syphilis the VDRL titer can spontaneously decline over time.

Asymptomatic neurosyphilis develops in approximately one-third of patients after 1 year or more of untreated syphilis. Symptomatic neurosyphilis can be meningovascular, parenchymal, or mixed disease. Meningovascular neurosyphilis presents as subacute or chronic meningitis. Parenchymal neurosyphilis may present as general paresis or tabes dorsalis. General paresis is characterized by progressive dementia, alterations in speech, and generalized weakness with hyperreflexia. Irritability, grandiose delusions, and hallucinations may occur. Tabes dorsalis is characterized by progressive ataxia, paresthesias, sharp pains, and sensory dysfunction. The Argyll-Robertson pupil (reacts to accommodation but not to light) may be seen in both general paresis and tabes dorsalis.

The diagnosis of neurosyphilis is based on cerebrospinal fluid findings of an elevated protein level and/or mononuclear pleocytosis. A positive cerebrospinal fluid VDRL is diagnostic but not present in all cases. Older patients with positive serology and neurologic symptoms should have a lumbar puncture.

Penicillin is the treatment of choice for all stages of syphilis. Primary, secondary, and latent syphilis of less than 1 year's duration should be treated with 2.4 million units of benzathine penicillin intramuscularly as a single dose. Neurosyphilis is treated with a 10-day course of intravenous penicillin, followed by three weekly doses of benzathine penicillin.

After therapy for syphilis, the VDRL should be followed for evidence of decline in titer or conversion to seronegative status (which may take months). The FTA-ABS remains positive with or without therapy. Lumbar puncture should be repeated in patients with neurosyphilis to determine adequacy of treatment (Ward and Szebenyi 1986).

Urinalysis.   Urinary tract infection is the most common cause of gram-negative sepsis in older patients. Symptoms of urinary tract infection in older patients can include changes in mental status, functional decline, abdominal pain, or nausea and vomiting in addition to, or instead of, dysuria and urinary frequency. Older patients with serious infection may lack a febrile response. Urinalysis usually reveals bacteriuria, commonly enteric rods. Some older patients may not have significant pyuria. Diagnosis of urinary tract infection is made based on urine culture and sensitivity. Mild symptomatic urinary tract infection in older patients should be treated with a 7- to 10-day course of oral antibiotic rather than the single-dose therapy recommended for younger patients. Intravenous antibiotic is recommended for serious infection. Men with urinary tract infections (not related to recent catheterization) and women with recurrent urinary tract infections should have a urologic referral (Zweig 1987).

Asymptomatic bacteriuria is common in older patients, particularly women, and increases in frequency with age as well as hospitalization and institutionalization. Its significance is unclear.

Treatment of asymptomatic bacteriuria has not been shown to affect subsequent morbidity or mortality and probably should not be undertaken (Nordenstam et al. 1986). However, patients with incontinence and asymptomatic bacteriuria probably deserve a trial of antibiotic therapy. Essentially all patients with chronic indwelling urinary catheters will have bacteriuria and pyuria. These patients should not be treated with antibiotics if asymptomatic (Ouslander 1986).

Medical Clearance for Electroconvulsive Therapy

Pretreatment evaluation of the older patient prior to electroconvulsive therapy (ECT) should focus on neurologic and cardiovascular status. A contraindication to ECT is the presence of increased intracranial pressure. ECT can be safely given in stroke patients after neurologic status has stabilized, or even in patients with brain tumors who are carefully monitored during treatment.

Cardiac events are the major cause of mortality reported from ECT. All older patients should have cardiac monitoring during the ECT treatments. ECT causes a diffuse autonomic discharge, which can lead to severe bradycardia or even asystole, if patients are not given atropine for cholinergic blockade. In patients who are given atropine, however, heart rate, blood pressure, and plasma catecholamines increase immediately after ECT. Pretreatment evaluation of cardiac status should focus on the presence of hypertension, angina, heart failure, and arrhythmias. If these problems are controlled, the patient may have ECT. Patients with hypertension who develop extreme blood pressure rise after ECT may need to have a prophylactic beta-blocker. Beta-blockade may also be necessary in patients with angina. Intravenous lidocaine may be used in patients with a history of ventricular arrhythmia. Pacemaker patients can receive ECT after pacer function has been documented. Demand pacemakers should be converted to fixed mode with an external magnet immediately prior to ECT, and the patient should be appropriately grounded. ECT has been done in the immediate postmyocardial infarction period in severe cases of depression, generally with a resuscitation team present. However, if possible, it is recommended to wait at least 6 weeks after myocardial infarction, to allow cardiac status to stabilize.

Patients with respiratory diseases may be at increased risk from ECT, particularly those with ventilatory compromise and/or carbon dioxide retaining patients with compromised hypoxic drive who may not tolerate the brief period of apnea with ECT. Prolonged apnea has been reported in patients taking the drug echothiopate (even in eyedrop form) to prevent glaucoma. This drug should be discontinued before ECT therapy is instituted.

Many of the potential risks of ECT therapy can be prevented with careful technique. In selected patients, pretreatment oxygen therapy may decrease the risk of memory deficits and cardiac arrhythmias. Succinylcholine is given for muscle relaxation to decrease cardiovascular strain and decrease the risk of fractures; it is particularly important in patients with osteoporosis. Cardiac monitoring is required as previously noted. Atropine can prevent the risk of bradycardia and asystole, but should be decreased in dosage or avoided in patients with pacemakers, arrhythmias, or hypertension. Patients with glaucoma should have adequate topical treatment prior to pretreatment atropine (Elliot et al. 1982; Salzman 1982; Woodcock 1983).

Medical Aspects of Antidepressant Therapy

The major adverse side effects of the tricyclic and tetracyclic antidepressant medications include sedation, anticholinergic, adrenergic, and cardiovascular effects.

The sedative effects of some antidepressants can pose a major problem in older patients. Nighttime dosing of sedating antidepressants (such as tertiary amines) or use of less-sedating drugs (such as secondary amines) can help prevent this problem. Anticholinergic effects can occur with nearly all tricyclic and tetracyclic antidepressants. Newer heterocyclic compounds (e.g., trazodone, fluoxetine) avoid anticholinergic effects. Typical anticholinergic effects include delirium, dry mouth, constipation, tachycardia, blurred vision, and urinary retention. An increase in heart rate may not be tolerated in patients with unstable angina, and patients with chronic atrial fibrillation should be carefully observed. Patients should be questioned about the foregoing symptoms as well as about signs of adrenergic hyperactivity such as tremulousness and sweating.

Clinically significant orthostatic hypotension is common with antidepressant therapy in older patients and is presumably due to antagonism of peripheral alpha-1 adrenergic receptors. The best predictor of postural hypotension with antidepressant therapy is preexisting orthostatic hypotension. Careful monitoring of ortho-static blood pressure and symptoms of hypotension is required be-fore and during treatment. The occurrence of orthostatic hypoten-sion may be reduced with low doses, divided doses, and slowly increasing doses. Paradoxically, pretreatment orthostatic hypoten-sion was shown in a study to predict favorable treatment response (Jarvik et al. 1983).

A quinidinelike effect has been demonstrated by a reduced fre-quency of premature ventricular contractions in patients receiving imipramine, nortriptyline, or maprotiline. In addition, these agents may prolong intracardiac conduction. Caution is recom-mended in patients with preexisting conduction disturbances and those receiving class IA antiarrhythmic drugs such as quinidine. The antiarrhythmic agent may need to be reduced or discontinued while the patient is receiving an antidepressant. In vitro studies have demonstrated that these drugs do not lower cardiac output even in patients with impaired ventricular function.

An electrocardiogram should be taken prior to instituting anti-depressant therapy in older patients. It has been suggested that if bifascicular block, second-degree heart block, or QT prolongation is present, tricyclic antidepressants should not be started unless the patient is under careful observation in a hospital setting. Simple first-degree AV block and bundle branch block do increase the risk of complications to a small degree. A repeat electrocardi-ogram after treatment has begun is necessary in all patients with heart disease to monitor prolongation of the PR, QT, and QRS du-ration (which most patients develop), worsening of AV block, and ventricular arrhythmias (Thompson et al. 1983; Veith 1982). In general, ECT is preferred in patients with significant heart disease and severe depression. If there are no contraindications, some other antidepressants may be useful (e.g., monoamine oxidase in-hibitor).

Conclusion

Careful medical management is an important aspect in the care of older psychiatric patients. These patients frequently have causa-tive or coexistent medical illness that can significantly affect their psychiatric care. The psychiatrist should be able to recognize med-ical problems, initiate treatment if available, and refer to other cli-nicians when appropriate.

References

Abramowicz M: Drugs that can cause psychiatric symptoms. Med Lett Drugs Ther 28:81–86, 1986

Alessi CA, Henderson CT: Constipation and fecal impaction in the long-term care patient. Clin Geriatr Med 4:571–588, 1988

Alexopoulos GS, Young RC, Meyers BS, et al: Late-onset depression. Psychiatr Clin North Am 11:101–112, 1988

Allman RM: Pressure ulcers among the elderly. N Engl J Med 320:850–853, 1989

American Speech, Language, and Hearing Association: Guidelines for the identification of hearing impairment/handicap in adult/elderly persons. American Speech, Language, Hearing Association Journal August:59–63, 1989

Amery A, Brixko R, Clement D, et al: Efficacy of antihypertensive drug treatment according to age, sex, blood pressure, and previous cardiovascular disease in patients over the age of 60. Lancet 2:589–592, 1986

Applegate WB: Hypertension in elderly patients. Ann Intern Med 110:901–915, 1989

Byyng RL: Hypertension in the elderly. Am J Med 81:1055–1058, 1986

Caldwell G, Gow SM, Sweeting VM, et al: A new strategy for thyroid function testing. Lancet 1:1117–1119, 1985

Calkins E, Davis PT, Ford AB (eds): The Practice of Geriatrics. Philadelphia, PA, WB Saunders, 1986

Cassel CK, Walsh JR, Shepard M: Clinical Evaluation of the Patient in: Cassel CK, Reisenberg D, Sorenson LB, et al (eds): Geriatric Medicine, 2nd Edition. New York, Springer-Verlag, 1989, pp 102–110

Cohen HJ, Crawford J: Hematologic problems, in The Practice of Geriatrics. Edited by Calkins E, Davis PJ, Ford AB. Philadelphia, PA, WB Saunders, 1986, pp 519–531

Connell AM, Hilton C, Irvine G, et al: Variation of bowel habits in two population samples. Br Med J 2:1095–1099, 1965

Consensus Conference: Differential diagnosis of dementing diseases. JAMA 258:3411–3416, 1987

Cooppan R: Determining the most appropriate treatment for patients with non-insulin dependent diabetes mellitus. Metabolism 365:17–21, 1987

Cummings JL: Acute confusional states, in Clinical Neuropsychiatry. New York, Grune & Stratton, 1985, pp 68–74

Cummings JL, Benson DF: Dementia: A Clinical Approach. Boston, MA, Butterworths, 1984

Donald IP, Smith RG, Cruikshank JG, et al: A study of constipation in the elderly living at home. Gerontology 31:112, 1985

Elliot DL, Linz DH, Kane JA: Electroconvulsive therapy: pretreatment medical evaluation. Arch Intern Med 142:979–981, 1982

Feit H: Thyroid function in the elderly. Clin Geriatr Med 4:151–161, 1988

Freedman ML (ed): Hematologic disorders, in Clinics in Geriatric Medicine, Vol 4. No 1. Philadelphia, PA, WB Saunders, 1985

Harper CM, Lyles YM: Physiology and complications of bedrest. J Am Geriatr Soc 36:1047–1054, 1988

Jarvik LF, Read SL, Mintz J, et al: Pretreatment orthostatic hypotension in geriatric depression: predictor of response to imipramine and doxepine. J Clin Psychopharmacology 3:368–372, 1983

Kane RL, Ouslander JB, Abrass IB: Essentials of Clinical Geriatrics, 2nd Edition. New York, McGraw-Hill, 1989

Kaplan C, Lipkin M, Gordon GH: Somatization in primary care. J Gen Intern Med 3:177–190, 1988

Kolman PBR: The value of laboratory investigation of elderly psychiatric patients. J Clin Psychiatry 45:112–116, 1984

Lichenstein MJ, Bess FH, Logan SA: Validation of screening tools for identifying hearing-impaired elderly in primary care. JAMA 259:2875–2878, 1988

Lipowski ZJ: Delirium in the elderly patient. N Engl J Med 320:578–581, 1989

Mader S: Hearing impairment in elderly persons. J Am Geriatr Soc 32:548–553, 1984

Marton KI, Sox HC Jr, Krupp JR: Involuntary weight loss: diagnostic and prognostic significance. Ann Intern Med 95:568–574, 1981

Messerli FH, Ventura HO, Amodea C: Osler's maneuver and pseudohypertension. N Engl J Med 312:1548–1551, 1985

Morley JE: Nutritional status of the elderly. Am J Med 81:679–695, 1986

Morley JE, Silver AJ, Fiatarone M, et al: Geriatric grand rounds: nutrition and the elderly. J Am Geriatr Soc 34:823–832, 1986

Moskowitz RW: Primary osteoarthritis: epidemiology, clinical aspects, and general management. Am J Med 83:5–10, 1987

Narins RG, Jones ER, Stom MC, et al: Diagnostic strategies in disorders of fluid, electrolyte, and acid-base homeostasis. Am J Med 72:496–520, 1982

Nordenstam GR, Brandenberg CA, Oden AS, et al: Bacteriuria and mortality in an elderly population. N Engl J Med 314:1152–1156, 1986

Ouslander JG: Illness and psychopathology in the elderly. Psychiatr Clin North Am 5:145–157, 1982

Ouslander JG (ed): Urinary incontinence, in Clinics in Geriatric Medicine, Vol 2. No 4. Philadelphia, PA, WB Saunders, 1986

Riesenberg D: Diabetes mellitus, in Geriatric Medicine, 2nd Edition. Edited by Cassel CK, Reisenberg D, Sorenson LB, et al. New York, Springer-Verlag, 1989, pp 228–238

Robuschi G, Safran M, Braverman LE, et al: Hypothyroidism in the elderly. Endocr Rev 8:142–153, 1987

Rosenthal MJ, Hunt WC, Garry PJ, et al: Thyroid failure in the elderly: microsomal antibodies as discriminant for therapy. JAMA 258:209–213, 1987

Rossman I (ed): Clinical Geriatrics, 3rd Edition. Philadelphia, PA, JB Lippincott, 1986

Rowe JW, Besdine RW (eds): Geriatric Medicine, 2nd Edition. Boston, MA, Little, Brown, 1988

Salzman C: Electroconvulsive therapy in the elderly patient. Psychiatr Clin North Am 5:191–197, 1982

Shea JD: Pressure sores: classification and management. Clin Orthop 112:89–100, 1975

Soldo BJ, Manton KG: Health status and service needs of the oldest old: current patterns and future trends. Milbank Memorial Fund Quarterly, Health and Society 63:286–319, 1985

Sorenson LB: Rheumatology, in Geriatric Medicine, 2nd Edition. Edited by Cassel CK, Reisenberg D, Sorenson LB, et al. New York, Springer-Verlag, 1989, pp 184–211

Straatsma BR, Foos RY, Horwitz J, et al: Aging-related cataract: laboratory investigation and clinical management. Ann Intern Med 102:82–92, 1985

Thompson TL, Moran MG, Nies AS: Psychotropic drug use in the elderly. N Engl J Med 308:194–199, 1983

Tinetti ME, Speechley M, Ginter SF: Risk factors for falls among elderly persons living in the community. N Engl J Med 319:1701–1707, 1988

Tuck ML, Griffiths RF, Johnson LE, et al: Hypertension in the elderly. J Am Geriatr Soc 36:630–643, 1988

U'Ren RC: Anxiety, paranoia, and personality disorders, in Geriatric Medicine, 2nd Edition. Edited by Cassel CK, Reisenberg D, Sorenson LB, et al. New York, Springer-Verlag, 1989, pp 491–500

Veith RC: Depression in the elderly: pharmacologic considerations in treatment. J Am Geriatr Soc 30:581–586, 1982

Vickers R: Medical aspects of aging, in Essentials of Geriatric Psychiatry. Edited by Lazarus LW, Jarvik LF, Foster JR, et al (eds). New York, Springer, 1988

Ward TT, Szebenyi SE: Sexually transmitted diseases: syphilis, in A Practical Guide to Infectious Diseases, 2nd Edition. Edited by Reese RE, Douglas RG. Toronto, Little, Brown, 1986

Woodcock J: Pyschiatry, in Medical Consultation: Role of the Internist on Surgical, Obstetric, and Psychiatric Services. Edited by Kammerer WS, Gross RJ. Baltimore, MD, Williams & Wilkins, 1983

Zweith S: Urinary tract infections in the elderly. Am Fam Physician 35:123–130, 1987

CHAPTER 10

Jeffrey I. Victoroff, M.D.

Neurological Evaluation

The primary goal of the neurological evaluation in geriatric psychiatry is to identify evidence of nervous system dysfunction that may relate to psychiatric status. Traditionally, this evaluation is viewed as the opportunity to discover "organic" causes of psychiatric disturbance. However, our expanding knowledge of the biology of behavior compels us to reconsider this traditional view. Because we accept that all behavior is based on brain function, the distinction between "organic" and "nonorganic or functional" disturbances represents a false dichotomy. We are now endeavoring to understand how neurobiological factors interact with environmental and psychological factors to produce behavior. Therefore, our true goals are to evaluate the role of the geriatric nervous system in mediating both the homeostasis of the internal biopsychological milieu and the patient's responsiveness to his or her environment, and to attempt to identify changes in this nervous system–environment interaction that ultimately may be expressed as changes in behavior. In practical terms, we use the neurological evaluation—in concert with the history, mental status examination, medical examination, and selected laboratory tests—as one component of the integrated neurobehavioral approach to the geriatric psychiatric patient.

There are two kinds of changes in the geriatric nervous system

This work is supported by National Institute on Aging grant T32 AG001172-02, and by the French Foundation for Alzheimer's Research grant L890608. The author thanks Drs. D. Frank Benson and Jeffrey L. Cummings for valuable editorial review and comment.

that may be reflected as changes in behavior: first, there are the changes related to normal aging; second, there are pathological changes—many of which increase in incidence and prevalence among the elderly. I begin this chapter with a brief review of the neurology of normal aging. In the main body of the chapter I address the components of the complete neurological assessment, including the neurological history and examination, with special emphasis on the psychiatric significance of neurological symptoms and signs. I conclude with discussion of the role of the neurological evaluation in the comprehensive assessment of disorders of behavior in geriatric patients.

The Neurology of Normal Aging

Changes attributed to aging of the nervous system are usually regarded as negative and inevitable. However, three factors bear consideration. First, it is often difficult to distinguish normal aging from pathological change. Some investigators argue that the role of aging per se has been overemphasized and that many age-associated decrements in function can actually be accounted for by a wide array of environmental factors (Rowe and Kahn 1987). Second, although there are measurable decrements in some functions, we cannot presume that all of these changes are maladaptive. Third, there is considerable individual variation; some individuals exhibit substantial preservation of function. Nonetheless, the average aging nervous system undergoes several important changes that may have an impact on behavior, both by directly affecting function and by changing the way in which the patient perceives the environment.

Both the peripheral nervous system and the muscular system—the pathway of communication from the central nervous system to the motor system and the final motor effectors themselves—exhibit a progressive and measurable decrement in function with advancing age. In many cases this decrement represents a combination of age-related factors, diseases of the nervous system, and systemic diseases, including endocrine, nutritional, and vascular causes (Baker 1989). Primary sensory receptors change in structure and decline in number with age, and neurons exhibit 1) demyelination and remyelination, 2) greater distal than proximal axonal degeneration, 3) loss of fast-conducting peripheral axons, and 4) lipofuscin accumulation (Spencer and Ochoa 1981). There are age-related declines in the number of anterior horn cells and motor cranial nerve nuclei as well as demyelination and remyelination of motor roots. The result is a progressive decrease in the number of functioning motor units after age 60. Muscle fiber atrophy is common, particularly among the type II fibers, and total muscle mass may decrease by 25% to 43%; remaining fibers exhibit signs of denervation, with the presence of target cells as well as ragged red fibers, ring fibers, lipofuscin accumulation, and increased interstitial connective tissue and fat (Hubbard and Squier 1989; Munsat 1984). Electrophysiology shows decreased amplitude of sensory action potentials, decline in both sensory and motor nerve conduction velocities, increased duration of motor units, and reduced somatosensory evoked potentials with age (Smith 1989).

Most pertinent to the neuropsychiatric evaluation are the age-related changes in the brain. There have been estimates of loss of cortical neurons with aging as high as 30% to 60%, corresponding to roughly 1% loss per annum above age 60, with the greatest losses among large neurons (Anderson et al. 1983; Henderson et al. 1980). Questions have been raised about the techniques used to make these estimates, but the bulk of evidence favors decreases in number of cortical neurons, in neuronal density, and in dendritic arborizations as well as a relative increase in glial cells (Coleman and Flood 1987). There are comparable losses of subcortical and brain stem neurons, especially in the putamen, nucleus basalis of Meynert, substantia nigra, and locus coeruleus (Riederer and Krusik 1987).

Biochemical changes include neurotransmitter and biosynthetic enzyme changes: an age-related increase in monoamine oxidase (MAO) leads to increased catabolism of the catecholamines; dopamine content decreases in striatum, and both synthetic enzymes tyrosine hydroxylase and dopa decarboxylase decrease; acetylcholine levels appear stable despite fall in the rate-limiting synthetic step of choline uptake; synthesis of norepinephrine declines, although results are inconsistent regarding brain content; serotonin appears to remain stable despite increases in MAO (Rogers and Bloom 1985; Selkoe and Kosik 1984). There are age-related decreases in cerebral blood flow, independent of cerebral vascular disease (Takeda et al. 1988). It is less clear whether there is also a decline in cerebral metabolic rate; some investigators find clear age-related declines, particularly in frontal cortex (e.g., Chawluk et al. 1985) and others find no decline with age (e.g., Rapoport 1986). This variability of findings may relate to selection bias in different studies, or to the existence of regional (vs. global) declines in cerebral metabolism with age.

There are age-related changes in function that may relate to the foregoing physiological changes that should be taken into account in the neurological examination of the elderly patient. Both special and general sensory systems suffer a decline in function. Motor performance exhibits an overall decline, more for maximal performance tasks than for habitual tasks (Stones and Kozma 1985). Strength, balance, postural reflexes, and hand steadiness all decline with age (Stelmach et al. 1989; Teravainen and Calne 1983). There is a drop-off in reaction time after the twenties, more marked after age 50 (Welford 1988). Aging may also have an impact on cognition, although it is difficult to determine whether such declines represent normal aging or reflect the earliest signs of progressive dementing processes. These cognitive declines appear in aspects of attention, memory, language, and spatial performance (Binks 1989; Kirasic and Allen 1985; Plude and Hoyer 1985).

In summary, there is age-related decline in the structure and the function of the aging nervous system both centrally and peripherally. There may also be cognitive decline independent of the pathology of recognized dementing diseases. A familiarity with these changes may offer perspective to the neurological evaluation of the elderly psychiatric patient, both by helping distinguish normal from pathological processes and by orienting the examination toward vulnerable systems that may affect behavior.

Neurological Assessment and Potential Relation to Psychopathology

There are a number of ways to regard the relationship between neurological abnormalities and behavioral changes:

- The neurologic condition might be considered the proximate biological cause of the psychiatric condition, such as dementia due to neurosyphilis.
- The neurologic condition and psychiatric condition may be two manifestations of a shared neurobiological change, such as right hemiparesis and depression due to left frontal lobe infarction (Robinson et al. 1984).
- The neurologic condition may represent a psychological stressor that lowers the threshold for appearance of the psychiatric condition, such as an adjustment reaction with depressed mood related to lumbar spondylosis (Love 1987).
- A psychiatric condition may serve as a stress under which a previously covert neurological impairment becomes apparent, for

example, the emergence of an underlying dementia during an episode of depression (Kral 1983).

- The treatment for the neurological condition may produce or exacerbate psychopathology, such as psychosis related to L-dopa therapy in Parkinson's disease (Klawans 1982).
- Treatment of a psychiatric condition may produce or exacerbate a neurological problem, e.g., the wide range of neuroleptic-induced extrapyramidal disorders (Marsden and Jenner 1980).
- A somatoform psychiatric disorder may mimic or embellish a neurologic disorder, as in hysterical paralysis (Strub and Black 1988).
- A psychological factor may lead to elaboration of an underlying neurological disorder; an example would be the co-occurrence of seizures and pseudoseizures.
- The psychological factor and the underlying neurological disorder may be independent but coincident in time.

To determine the causal relationship between co-occurring neurologic and psychiatric conditions is valuable, although in many cases current knowledge does not permit precise determination of causality in behavioral dysfunction. Therefore, in the discussion that follows, the emphasis is on practical strategies to integrate the neurological assessment into the neuropsychiatric evaluation.

The Neurological History

Neurological disorders, including dementias, may be the most common cause of geriatric disability, outpacing respiratory, cardiovascular, orthopedic, and rheumatological disorders (Broe and Creasey 1989; Drachman and Long 1983). With the aging of the population and the advancement of medical treatment for non-neurological conditions, this disproportionate prevalence of neurological disorders will probably increase in the coming decades. Given the behavioral significance of neurologic disease, the geriatric psychiatric evaluation must always include a careful neurological history. In addition, because of the possibilities of denial, somatization, and failing memory, it is important to seek independent confirmation of neurologic complaints or experiences, usually from a spouse or other close relative. Further, because even remote or seemingly unrelated neurological events may be important in the genesis of a behavioral problem (e.g., the minor "bump on the head" that leads to an undetected subdural hemorrhage and gradual personality change), it is important to press for any neurological experiences or symptoms of possible relevance. The focus and depth of this exploration depend on individual circumstances; however, a good general neurologic review should consider the following points.

Cognitive Change

A neurological disorder may produce both cognitive and noncognitive dysfunction (e.g., dementia and paranoia in Alzheimer's disease). Therefore, the interview should include a careful review of subtle new intellectual deficits such as forgetfulness, verbal symptoms such as word-finding difficulty, and visuospatial symptoms such as difficulty navigating through town.

Head Trauma

Two hundred to three hundred people per 100,000 of the population are admitted to hospitals for head trauma each year, and there are probably many more nonhospitalized cases (Jennett and Teasdale 1981). Although the likelihood of behavioral sequelae may increase in cases with loss of consciousness or scalp laceration, even minor head trauma deserves consideration as a possible precipitant of postconcussion syndrome, subdural hemorrhage, and posttraumatic epilepsy. Moreover, injuries without direct trauma to the occiput—such as whiplash—can produce cognitive and affective changes (Yarnell and Rossie 1988). The recovery from head trauma is likely to be slower and less complete in older patients (Wrightson 1989).

Acute Decline in Function

Any acute change in function raises the question of stroke or transient ischemic attack. Small strokes may escape recognition or medical evaluation until the secondary behavioral problems emerge—such as dementia or affective change—because they fail to produce overt focal symptoms or signs. It is also possible for a slowly progressive process to reach a critical stage and then present with acute symptoms suggestive of stroke (e.g., an expanding tumor mass that finally produces observable dysfunction). On the other hand, it is possible for a nonacute process to present in a "pseudo-acute" way when other factors lower the patient's reserve; an example is the appearance of the first signs of primary degenerative dementia during a stressful time such as a move, a loss, or a medical problem.

Transient or Paroxysmal Neurological Symptoms

Syncopal episodes often suggest a cardiac arrhythmia with increased stroke risk (and possible association with anxiety disorders). However, transient ischemic attacks or partial seizures may go unrecognized because of a vague or atypical history. Inquiring about any faints or "funny turns" may elicit this history.

Dizziness

Peripheral vestibulopathy is common in the elderly and may produce both subjective symptoms and gait unsteadiness. In the patient complaining of "dizziness," it is important to distinguish light-headedness (a near-fainting sensation that can be due to postural hypotension, vasovagal responses, or presyncopal symptoms of cardiac arrhythmia) from vertigo (a sense of movement with respect to the surroundings, which may be produced by a wide range of central or peripheral vestibular pathology including behaviorally relevant conditions such as migraine, vertebrobasilar insufficiency, or posterior fossa mass lesions) (Baloh 1984).

Progressive Focal Motor or Sensory Dysfunction

Weakness, numbness, or discoordination of any part of the body requires further neurological evaluation. Although symptoms confined to a single extremity may initially suggest a peripheral process without relevance to behavior, many disorders with potential behavioral associations (e.g., multi-infarct dementia, idiopathic Parkinson's disease, amyotrophic lateral sclerosis) may present with asymmetric or focal symptoms.

Alteration in Special Senses

Changes in hearing or vision, in particular, may relate to psychiatric dysfunction in three ways: 1) primary sensory disorders may produce sensory deprivation that is associated with hallucinations in the affected sensory modality (Benson 1989; Cummings 1985); 2) sensory disorders may create misperceptions of the environment that potentially lead to such problems as the paranoia of the hearing impaired (Cooper and Curry 1976); 3) sensory disorders may be symptomatic of a central dysfunction (e.g., stroke, tumor, demyelinating disease), which itself may alter behavior.

New Headache

Although a lifetime history of vascular or muscle-tension headaches is probably not relevant to a new behavioral disorder, the recent onset of headaches in an elderly patient or a significant change in previous headache symptoms suggests the possibility of intracranial mass lesion or increased intracranial pressure, chronic meningitis, or temporal arteritis (in addition to more common problems such as hypertension, cervical spondylosis, sinusitis, and glaucoma).

Gait Disturbance

Gait disorders have been reported to produce disability in 13% of the aged, even excluding those gait disturbances caused by specific medical disease (Larish et al. 1988). Although geriatric gait disorders are often multifactorial, complaints of new dysfunction can be suggestive of behaviorally relevant disorders (e.g., multi-infarct dementia, increased intracranial pressure, normal pressure hydrocephalus, or Parkinson's disease).

Sleep Disturbance

Aging is associated with decreased slow-wave sleep and increased nocturnal wakefulness. One-third of the elderly experience frequent sleep interruptions because of apnea or hypopnea, even in the absence of complaints about sleep. Snoring, which is increasingly common with age, usually indicates some degree of upper airway obstruction and is associated with hypertension and cardiovascular disease (Dement et al. 1985). Therefore, nocturnal respiratory status may be compromised not only in patients with sleep complaints such as daytime sleepiness, choking attacks, or morning headache, but also in those who simply snore. A history of snoring or other sleep disturbance may be relevant to the presenting psychiatric problem, because there is evidence that sleep apnea may be associated with psychopathology or cognitive deficits (Kales et al. 1985; Telakivi et al. 1988).

Exposure to Centrally Acting Substances

Substance use or abuse can result in neurologic and psychiatric symptoms, sometimes combined. A history of alcohol abuse, even if remote, must be taken into account as a possible cause of cognitive decline. Occupational exposure to toxins such as solvents or heavy metals should be queried. Because the elderly are both exposed to more prescription medications and possibly more sensitive to behavioral side effects than younger patients, it is important to document recent drug use.

The Neurological Examination

The neurological examination requires experience, practice, and sophistication in neuroanatomy to yield the most fruitful results; for this reason, non-neurologists sometimes hesitate to perform a complete examination. However, the elderly psychiatric patient often presents with combined medical, neurologic, and psychiatric symptomatology. Proficiency and confidence in the techniques of the neurological examination put the geriatric psychiatrist in a position to offer a unique synthesis of biological and behavioral knowledge in the assessment of the patient, making the development of these examination skills an extremely valuable asset. Excellent general reviews of the neurological examination are available in standard neurology texts such as that of Adams and Victor (1989) or in specialized references (e.g., Brazis et al. 1985; De Jong 1979). However, the examination of the aged patient requires special knowledge of the neurology of aging. The following discussion focuses on both the distinctive features of the geriatric neurological examination and the behavioral significance of neurological signs.

In this examination, there are three goals: 1) to objectively assess physical signs, and to distinguish the signs of normal aging from pathological abnormalities; 2) to assess the neurological significance of abnormal signs, both by determining the anatomy of the responsible lesion and generating testable hypotheses regarding the differential diagnosis of the abnormality; and 3) to assess the potential behavioral significance of abnormal signs. In performing the examination, the geriatric psychiatrist may be faced with a frightened, confused, distracted, uncooperative, or even frankly combative patient. Establishing rapport and maintaining flexibility can mitigate these factors; however, even the most challenging patients can be assessed in some detail by careful observation of their spontaneous activity and responses to events in the environment.

Observation

The neurological examination begins at the first moment the examiner catches sight of the patient. Throughout the historical interview, important information can be gathered regarding the posture, gait, coordination, and excesses or deficiencies of movement; the symmetry of facial, truncal, and appendicular activity; attention to or neglect of extrapersonal space; eye movements; and the response to visual, auditory, and somatosensory stimuli in the environment. By the time the formal examination begins, the examiner will have formulated questions about apparent dysfunction that can be tested in depth.

Mental Status Examination

The mental status examination is described in Chapter 8. The performance of the patient during the course of both the psychiatric interview and the mental status examination provides clues to focus the detailed neurologic examination. For example, mental slowness may be a sign of subcortical pathology, particularly of the basal ganglia, and therefore mandates a careful search for abnormalities of tone, posture, gait, and the presence of resting tremor. Idiosyncratic speech or paraphasias may be signs of left hemisphere dysfunction and require investigation for evidence of right corticospinal or sensory system pathology.

Cranial Nerves

Both taste and olfaction show age-related decline in sensitivity, especially pronounced after the age of 50, with females exhibiting superiority in olfactory abilities throughout the life span. Sixty percent of those aged 65 to 80 show olfactory impairment; nearly a quarter are anosmic (Doty et al. 1984; Verillo and Verillo 1985). Deficiency of the first cranial nerve is most likely to be behaviorally significant when it is unilateral, suggesting possible basal frontal or mesial temporal pathology on the affected side.

Elderly patients lose visual acuity because of presbyopia and are increasingly vulnerable to ophthalmological disorders—which may be apparent on fundoscopy—including cataracts, glaucoma, age-related muscular degeneration, anterior ischemic optic neuropathy, and retinal vascular disease (Chisholm 1989; Kasper 1989). Visual acuity can be tested with a hand-held Snellen eye chart at 14 inches with and without corrective lenses, but presbyopia may make vision at distance the better measure. Visual fields can be tested by confrontation, testing each eye separately, and overcoming the patient's urge to look directly toward the stimulus by means of brief, unilateral finger movements or rapid simultaneous presentation of fingers to count in opposite fields. Pupils become smaller with aging (senile miosis) and the pupillary light reflex is often diminished or even absent (Chisolm 1989; Loewenfield 1979), although asymmetry of response represents an afferent pupillary defect. The presence of papilledema is an important sign of increased intracranial pressure; however, the absence of papilledema cannot be taken as evidence of normalcy, because even massive hemispheric tumors may not produce this sign, and papilledema does not usually occur in space-occupying intracranial lesions in the elderly (Caird 1982; Fetell and Stein 1989).

Eye movements change with age; there are increased saccadic latencies (the speed of shifting gaze to fixate on a target) and breakdown of smooth pursuit movements; such disruptions of normal movement may themselves impair vision (Hutton and Morris 1989). Normal aging is also associated with limitation of upward gaze, and less so of downward gaze (Chamberlain 1971). This normal restriction must be distinguished from two patterns of eye movements with potential relevance to behavioral disorders: 1) the Parinaud syndrome (upgaze paralysis, retraction nystagmus, and pupillary light-near dissociation), which may be associated with pineal region masses; and 2) marked restriction of vertical gaze with preservation of oculocephalic reflexes, which suggests progressive supranuclear palsy—a degenerative disease with gaze palsy, parkinsonian motor signs, and dementia. Any other paresis of eye movement, nonconjugate movement, or nystagmus requires further investigation of brain stem, cerebellar, and vestibular function.

Facial asymmetry can be a normal variant or a sign of unilateral facial weakness. Because residual weakness from an old Bell's palsy may be misleading, the examiner should inquire about this past condition and examine the patient's driver's license to determine whether an asymmetry is new. Excessive bucco-oral facial movements are sometimes attributable to ill-fitting dentures or gum chewing; these confounding variables should be ruled out by examining patients with their mouths empty. Dyskinetic lingual-facial-buccal movements are fairly common in elderly patients with no history of neuroleptic exposure (Weiner and Klawans 1973), and, in particular, the edentulous state may predispose to oral dyskinesias (Koller 1983), although neuroleptic-induced tardive dyskinesia must be strongly suspected in aged psychiatric patients.

Hearing declines with age, primarily because of presbyacusis, a multifactorial condition that can involve 1) sensorineural hearing loss due to a declining population of cochlear ganglion cells, 2) conductive loss, and 3) possible changes in the central auditory pathway (Mackenzie 1989). The accumulated effect of noise injury—as well as possible effects of toxins, infections, Meniere's disease, and (rarely) neoplasia—can contribute to hearing impairment. The vestibular system declines in function, with up to 40% loss of myelinated fibers in the aged vestibule (Yoder 1989). Although the most important behavioral test of the eighth nerve is frequently the patient's threshold for speech discrimination in ordinary conversation, this test will not reveal subtle or unilateral deficits that may be signs of tumor, stroke, infection, or other labyrinthine disease. Standard eighth-nerve examination should include hearing tests (e.g., rubbing the fingertips near the patient's ear or whispering into one ear with the other occluded) supplemented by the Weber and Rinne tests to distinguish conductive from sensorineural deficits. Given the potential for hearing defects to produce emotional distress in the elderly, particularly paranoia, a significant defect prompts a referral for audiometric evaluation.

Speech may roughen slightly with age, and dysarthria may occur from causes as benign as loose dentures, but progressive hoarseness or nasality may signal more serious problems such as laryngeal neoplasia, myasthenia, or motor neuron disease. Soft, hypophonic speech can be a sign of pathology in subcortical regions, and patients with Parkinson's disease with dementia typically have softer speech with impaired melody than do patients with Alzheimer's disease (Cummings et al. 1988). Excessive movement of the tongue may be a sensitive indicator of tardive dyskinesia, particularly if the patient fails to keep the tongue extended on command. However, fasciculations (a marker of motor neuron disease) can best be observed with the tongue relaxed in the floor of the mouth.

Motor Examination

The initial observation of the patient is a rich source of information about the function of the motor system. Particular emphasis should be placed on the degree and character of spontaneous movement. Movement disorders in the geriatric psychiatry patient constitute a special diagnostic challenge, because they may represent 1) normal aging effects; 2) idiopathic movement disorders, which increase in prevalence among the aged; 3) medication side effects, especially those of neuroleptics; or 4) the consequences of the psychiatric illness. Further, because movement disorders have been associated with depression and dementia (Girotti et al. 1988; Mayeux 1984), the co-occurrence of movement disorder and psychiatric disturbances raises the question of the degree of interdependence of these diagnoses. In order to distinguish psychogenic alterations in movement from neurological movement disorders, it is important to supplement observation with examination of resting tone, muscle bulk, power, and deep tendon reflexes.

Resting tone increases with age, both for limbs and axial muscles, with paratonia or gegenhalten (the tendency to increase tone in response to rapid displacements of the limb by the examiner) occurring in 10% to 12% of those aged 70 to 79, and in 21% of persons aged older than 80. It remains unclear whether paratonia represents a normal finding or a sign of diffuse cerebral dysfunction (George 1989; Jenkyn et al. 1985). However, marked rigidity reflects pathology, particularly when accompanied by either a spastic catch (suggesting upper motor neuron disease) or cogwheeling (suggestive of basal ganglia disease). Reduction of movement or hypokinesis may represent psychomotor retardation, which can signal depression; but it also carries the name "bradykinesia" and is seen in metabolic disorders such as hypothyroidism, and basal ganglia disorders including parkinsonism. The combination of bradykinesia, resting tremor, cogwheel rigidity, and loss of postural reflexes, often combined with masklike face and stooped, small-stepped gait, should be familiar as the syndrome of parkinsonism, which can occur either as the result of degenerative nervous system disease such as Parkinson's disease, striatonigral degeneration, and progressive supranuclear palsy, or as an extrapyramidal side effect of psychotropic medications, most frequently neuroleptics (Adams and Victor 1989; Klawans and Tanner 1984). Parkinson's disease has a rapid age-related increase in prevalence, affecting roughly 1% of persons older than 65 (Jankovic and Caine 1987), and behavior change in patients with Parkinson's disease may affect up to 77% (Mortimer 1988). Thus Parkinson's disease may be an important cause of psychiatric disability among the elderly. Identification of even subtle signs of Parkinson's disease on examination is important because there may be a long subclinical prodrome (Ward 1987) during which the patient may be at risk for behavioral complications such as depression and dementia while showing little overt evidence of the disease. Although it has been proposed that a related pathophysiology underlies all forms of psychomotor retardation (Benson 1990), certain clinical features may help to distinguish Parkinson's disease from the motor slowing of depression and from neuroleptic effects: the bradykinesia of Parkinson's disease, unlike that of depression, is usually associated with rigidity. Neuroleptic-induced parkinsonism may present with cogwheel rigidity, but it is associated with resting tremor less often than is idiopathic Parkinson's disease.

Excessive movements or hyperkinesias may be normal in form (e.g., the hyperactivity of the agitated, manic, stimulant-affected, or akathetic patient) or abnormal in form (as seen in the neuroleptic-induced dyskinesias, or with tremors, tics, and choreoathetosis). Hyperactivity with abnormal form is usually due to basal ganglia pathology; hyperactivity with normal form possibly relates to dysfunction of a limbic-mesencephalic psychomotor activity circuit (Victoroff 1989). In the presence of generalized hyperactivity with normal form, or motor restlessness, clinical features may help to distinguish psychogenic hyperactivity from neuroleptic-induced akathisia: subjective restlessness occurs in both, but akathetic patients may show more inability to remain still and more shifting from foot to foot, and they may exhibit a coarse tremor (Braude et al. 1983).

Truncal and appendicular choreic, athetotic, and otherwise dyskinetic movements may be reduced when the patient is seated, and so they are better examined with the patient standing at rest, walking, and during activating procedures such as touching the thumb with each finger or standing with arms outstretched and eyes closed (Simpson and Singh 1988). Such dyskinetic movements have a differential diagnosis which includes Huntington's disease, Wilson's disease, acquired hepatocerebral degeneration, senile chorea, and tardive dyskinesia (Klawans and Tanner 1984). Because the degenerative causes of dyskinesia are rare (for instance, Huntington's disease affects only four to eight persons per 100,000 (Mayeux 1984)), and because the incidence of tardive dyskinesia is 5% per year, or even greater among the elderly exposed to neuroleptics (Baldessarini 1988), it is probable that neuroleptic-induced tardive dyskinesia is overwhelmingly the most common pathological cause of dyskinesia in geriatric psychiatric patients. However, as many as 32% of non-neuroleptic-exposed elderly may exhibit spontaneous dyskinesias (Blowers et al. 1981), suggesting that the aged nervous system is susceptible to producing these movements and perhaps explaining the age-associated increased vulnerability to neuroleptic effects.

Muscle bulk declines with age. On examination, atrophy of the interosseous muscles of the hands may be particularly evident, and the most common cause of such focal atrophy is probably arthritic joint disease (Baker 1989). However, focal wasting can also occur with limb disuse, from altered activity, trauma, or a cortical insult such as stroke. Neurologically, wasting is important as a sign of lower motor neuron dysfunction—which can be focal (as in spondylosis or spinal mass lesions) or diffuse (as in motor neuron disease). Observation of the resting muscle may reveal fasciculations, which are pathognomonic of lower motor neuron dysfunction. Measurement of homologous parts on opposite sides of the body aid in confirming an impression of asymmetry. Diffuse wasting may also signal the anorexia of depression or medical problems including metabolic, infectious, and neoplastic disorders. Currently, the wasting syndrome of human immunodeficiency virus is emerging as another possible diagnosis.

Examination of strength in each major muscle group requires consideration of the patient's willingness to generate a maximal effort. Elderly patients may—for good reason—fear excessive exertion, and even their best efforts cannot be compared with those of younger patients. Instead, it is better to use each muscle as the control for the contralateral muscle. Diffuse weakness is difficult to interpret; it may represent psychogenic enervation or a wide range of medical conditions, including the neuropathic and myopathic disorders. Unilateral weakness prompts the search for other localizing signs to discriminate upper from lower motor neuron dysfunction and to delineate the extent of the focal lesion.

Hand tremor has been observed in 2% to 43% of normal aged (Hobson and Pemberton 1955; Prakash and Stern 1973); it is usually a fine rapid distal tremor, present on maintaining an antigravity posture, and it should be distinguished from the 5- to 7-Hz resting tremor of parkinsonism. "Essential" tremor is a heredofamilial postural tremor of 6 to 11 Hz, which sometimes first appears in old age (Koller 1984). A rapid distal tremor can also occur either as the effect of medication (including stimulants, antidepressants, or lithium) or drug withdrawal syndromes. Asymmetric or unilateral tremor may be due to asymmetric nervous system dysfunction; however, tremors often appear asymmetrically in parkinsonism, essential tremor, and normal aging.

Coordination

Coordination testing does not assess a single system in isolation, but instead evaluates the orchestration of motor activities due to the harmonious interaction of the pyramidal system, basal ganglia, and cerebellum. Observing fine finger movements such as rapid, successive opposition of the thumb and other digits may elicit defects of corticospinal tract function. The finger-to-nose test may exhibit abnormalities with dysfunction of different systems: corticospinal tract pathology may produce smooth but weak or ineffectual reaching; basal ganglia pathology may produce bradykinesia and tremor that does not increase with arm extension; cerebellar pathology may produce overshooting, lateral dysmetria, or tremor that increases with arm extension. This classic "intention tremor," or dysmetric performance on the finger-to-nose test, appears in 20% of normal aged persons (Howell 1949). Cerebellar dysfunction may also produce disorganized or erratic rapid-alternating movements (dysdiadochokinesis, which is often tested by instructing the patient to alternately slap a surface with the pronated or supinated hand), awkward heel-to-shin performance, and failure to check recoil when the examiner suddenly releases the flexed arm.

Disorders that produce these appendicular signs of cerebellar dysfunction may include lesions intrinsic to or compressing the cerebellum, but they can also occur with lesions of cerebellar connections (e.g., in the vestibular system, red nucleus, inferior olive, ventral lateral thalamus, or even frontal lobe). Causes of this cerebellar type of appendicular incoordination include posterior fossa neoplasm, cerebrovascular disease, demyelinating disease, or, less often, one of several degenerative conditions including olivopontocerebellar atrophy, dentatorubral degeneration, and Azorean disease (a familial condition of cerebellar dysfunction and parkinsonian features in patients of Portuguese-Azorean descent). Olivopontocerebellar atrophy has recently been shown to be associated with cognitive deficits (Kish et al. 1988) and may be one cause of subcortical dementia. Alcoholic cerebellar degeneration may also produce these appendicular cerebellar signs, but more often it produces truncal ataxia due to midline cerebellar degeneration, with relative preservation of appendicular function.

Reflexes

Deep tendon reflexes are reduced with age, most often at the ankle but also, in some studies, at the biceps, triceps, and patella (Howell 1949; Prakash and Stern 1973). Because reflexes may be reduced and anxiety may make relaxation difficult for the elderly patient, reinforcing maneuvers are sometimes required to elicit the reflexes, such as asking the patient to clench his or her teeth while testing the upper extremities, or using the Jendrassik maneuver (tapping the patellae while patients hook their hands in front of the chest and pull in opposite directions).

Diffuse hyporeflexia disproportionate to age may commonly be a sign of peripheral neuropathy, less commonly of myopathy. In hypothyroidism the reflexes may be slow both to respond and to relax.

Unilateral or focal loss of a reflex may represent peripheral or lower motor neuron damage, commonly as the result of cervical or lumbar spondylosis, less commonly as the result of tabes dorsalis, syringomyelia, or spinal tumor.

Diffuse hyperreflexia occurs in bilateral lesions of the pyramidal system above the mid-cervical level, in states of neuromuscular irritability such as tetany, and in hyperthyroidism.

Focally increased reflexes, particularly when combined with pathological signs such as the Babinski or Hoffman, alert the examiner to unilateral pathology affecting the descending pyramidal system; however, it is possible for pathology in cortical regions outside the motor cortex to produce unilateral hyperreflexia (e.g., prefrontal or temporal lesions), possibly by remote effects on the motor strip.

Two patterns of special relevance to behavior are 1) the combination of absent reflexes and positive Babinski signs seen in subacute combined degeneration due to vitamin B_{12} deficiency, which is a cause of reversible dementia; and 2) the combination of hyperreflexia and atrophy with fasciculations seen in amyotrophic lateral sclerosis, which may be associated with both depression and dementia (Davis 1987; Montgomery and Erickson 1987).

A group of reflexes has been referred to as "frontal release signs" or primitive reflexes. They represent the exaggeration of normal reflexes or reappearance of reflexes seen in infancy, thereby indicating an impairment of nervous system function. However, it is important to consider the presence of such reflexes in light of their prevalence among the normal aged. The palmomental reflex (contraction of the mentalis muscle of the face when the palm is stroked) has been found in 41% to 60% of the healthy aged, with increasing frequency for each decade from the sixth through the ninth (Jacobs and Gossman 1980). The snout reflex (puckering or pursing of the lips in response to light pressure above the upper lip) has been found in 26% to 33% of the healthy aged (Jacobs and Gossman 1980; Jenkyn et al. 1985). The glabellar tap response (inability to inhibit blinking during a series of finger taps to the glabellar region) has been found in 37% of healthy aged (Jenkyn et al. 1985). In addition, Jensen et al. (1983) found no difference in the prevalence of the palmomental or glabellar reflexes between normals and patients with cerebral disease, with the exception that patients with basal ganglia disorders more frequently had a positive glabellar tap. Jenkyn and associates (1985) found that 95% of subjects older than 70 had five to seven "abnormal" signs on examination. Further, patients may have substantial frontal lobe damage yet have no grasp, snout, suck, rooting, hyperactive jaw jerk, or palmomental reflexes (Benson et al. 1981). Hence, the presence of these reflexes may reveal evidence of nervous system degeneration, but it cannot be taken as proof of behaviorally significant frontal lobe pathology; nor can the absence of these reflexes be used to rule out such pathology.

Sensation

There is a well-known decline in vibratory sensation beginning by age 50 to 60, and there are lesser declines in thermal, touch, and pain discrimination (Olney 1989; Pearson 1928). These changes probably relate to combined functional declines of sensory receptors, peripheral nerves, roots, and tracts (Baker 1989). Although decreased detection of vibratory stimuli may be due to normal aging, marked vibratory insensitivity combined with poor proprioception and/or a positive Romberg sign (swaying in the standing position, which markedly increases when the eyes are closed), alert the examiner to peripheral neuropathy or posterior column dysfunction as in subacute combined degeneration. There has also been observed an age-related decline in discrimination of competing tactile stimuli presented to different locations (Kokmen et al. 1977; Levin and Benton 1973). This insensitivity to double simultaneous stimulation may complicate diagnosis of sensory neglect unless there is a notable asymmetry.

Gait

Critchley and others have noted that the gait of the normal elderly shares many of the features of Parkinson's disease, with short steps, rigidity, and flexion posture (Coffey 1989; Critchley 1931). Stoplight photography of walking, healthy, elderly men reveals shortened steps, diminished arm swing, and anteroflexion of the upper torso (Murray et al. 1969). However, these findings are confounded by the fact that elderly patients may walk slowly for a variety of reasons, and a decrease in freely chosen walking rate naturally produces a decreased length of stride (Larish et al. 1988). Thus, in the aged patient with gait disturbance, it is often difficult to distinguish pathology from normal aging and to sort out the contribution of multiple potential contributory factors, including 1) decreased proprioception, 2) decreased vision, 3) impaired postural reflexes, 4) weakness, 5) rigidity, 6) extrapyramidal dysfunction, 7) vestibulopathy, 8) cerebellar ataxia, 9) diffuse frontal lobe pathology, 10) cervical or lumbar spondylosis, 11) joint restriction, 12) pain, 13) postural hypotension, 14) medication effect, 15) fear of falling based on prior mishaps, as well as a wide range of focal and diffuse central disorders including stroke, tumor, and hydrocephalus (Adams 1984; Manchester et al. 1989; Stelmach et al. 1989; Tinetti 1989).

To best observe gait impairment, the clinician should examine the patient standing in place, walking, walking on heels and toes, and walking tandem (one foot behind the other). Examining the patient's response to displacement (pushing the standing patient in different directions) tests postural reflexes. Several patterns of gait may have special relevance to geriatric psychiatry: parkinsonian gait, normal pressure hydrocephalus, broad-based gait, and frontal gait "apraxia." Probably the most frequent of these is parkinsonian gait, which may be a sign of neuroleptic exposure or basal ganglia dysfunction as in idiopathic Parkinson's disease, progressive supranuclear palsy, or striatal infarction. Parkinsonian gait is distinguished from normal aging by the degree of the slowing, rigidity, and shortening of steps, by the presence of festination (acceleration as if chasing the center of gravity), and by the association with resting tremor. Again, depression may produce bradykinesia but should not produce rigidity or tremor. Normal pressure hydrocephalus can produce the triad of altered gait, incontinence, and dementia; this gait disturbance includes the short, stiff step of parkinsonism, but there is less slowing, more of a broad base, and no tremor (Adams 1984). Broad-based gait occurs with either cerebellar dysfunction (as in chronic alcoholism) or with loss of proprioception (as in subacute combined degeneration). Frontal gait "apraxia" with poor initiation, halting steps, and an impression of magnetic attachment to the floor can be associated with bilateral frontal lobe dysfunction.

The Integrated Neurobehavioral Evaluation

Significant changes occur with age in the structure and function of both the central and peripheral nervous systems. In addition, the incidence and prevalence of many neurological disorders increase with age. The neurological evaluation should be considered as one component of an integrated neurobehavioral assessment that includes the psychiatric interview and examination, cognitive testing, neurological examination, and laboratory testing. Because there is an increased probability of "organicity" with age, there should be a low threshold for supplementing the neurological examination with laboratory tests. Although this principle is particularly true when the examination suggests a specific central nervous system disorder, we should be modest about the limits of physical diagnosis: even when no focal or localizing signs are identified, laboratory testing may reveal a specific factor that plays a significant role in the genesis of the behavioral disturbance. Although it is often difficult to render a cost-benefit analysis of such testing, the opportunity to discover potentially treatable causes of behavioral disorder is a compelling mandate. As our sophistication in neurobiology grows, so will these opportunities.

The aging of the population will confront the medical community with a large increase in the number of elderly patients who have both psychiatric disturbances and neurologic problems. At the same time, the disciplines of neurology and psychiatry are evolving in concert toward an integrated understanding of the neuropsychiatry of behavioral disturbance. The geriatric psychiatrist is in a unique position, drawing on a broad base of knowledge in gerontology, neurology, and psychiatry, to offer a synthesis of disciplinary approaches in the evaluation and treatment of behavioral distress among the elderly.

References

Adams RD: Aging and human locomotion, in Clinical Neurology of Aging. Edited by Albert ML. New York, Oxford University Press, 1984, pp 381–386

Adams RD, Victor M: Principles of Neurology, 4th Edition. New York, McGraw-Hill, 1989

Anderson JM, Hubbard BM, Coghill GR, et al: The effect of advanced old age on the neuron content of the cerebral cortex. J Neurol Sci 58:235–244, 1983

Baker PCH: The aging neuromuscular system. Seminars in Neurology 9:50–59, 1989

Baldessarini RJ: A summary of current knowledge of tardive dyskinesia. Encephale 14:263–268, 1988

Baloh RW: Dizziness, Hearing Loss and Tinnitus: The Essentials of Neurology. Philadelphia, PA, F.A. Davis, 1984

Benson DF: Disorders of visual gnosis, in Neuropsychology of Visual Perception. Edited by Brown JW. Hillsdale, NJ, Lawrence Erlbaum, 1989, pp 59–78

Benson DF: Psychomotor retardation. Neuropsychiatry, Neuropsychology, and Behavioral Neurology 3:36–47, 1990

Benson DF, Stuss DT, Naeser MA, et al: The long-term effects of prefrontal leukotomy. Arch Neurol 38:165–189, 1981

Binks M: Changes in mental functioning associated with normal aging, in The Clinical Neurology of Old Age. Edited by Tallis R. Chichester, John Wiley, 1989, pp 27–39

Blowers AJ, Borison RL, Blowers CM, et al: Abnormal involuntary movements in the elderly (letter). Br J Psychiatry 139:363–364, 1981

Brazis PW, Masdea JC, Biller J: Localization in Clinical Neurology. Boston, MA, Little, Brown, 1985

Braude WM, Barnes TRE, Gore SM: Clinical characteristics of akathisia, a systematic investigation of acute psychiatric inpatient admissions. Br J Psychiatry 143:139–150, 1983

Broe GA, Creasey H: The neuroepidemiology of old age, in The Clinical Neurology of Old Age. Edited by Tallis R. Chichester, John Wiley, 1989, pp 51–65

Caird FI: Examination of the nervous system, in Neurological Disorders in the Elderly. Edited by Caird FI. Bristol, Wright PSG, 1982, pp 44–51

Chamberlain W: Restriction in upward gaze with advancing age. Am J Ophthalmol 71:341–346, 1971

Chawluk J, Alavi A, Hurtig H, et al: Altered pattern of cerebral glucose metabolism in aging and dementia. J Cerebral Blood Metab 5:(supp 1) s 121–122, 1985

Chisolm I: Visual failure, in The Clinical Neurology of Old Age. Edited by Tallis R. Chichester, John Wiley, 1989, pp 335–346

Coffey DJ: Disorders of movement in aging. Seminars in Neurology 9:46–49, 1989

Coleman PD, Flood DG: Neuron numbers and dendritic extent in normal aging and Alzheimer's disease. Neurobiol Aging 8:521–545, 1987

Cooper AF, Curry AR: The pathology of deafness in the paranoid and affective psychoses of later life. J Psychosom Res 20:97–105, 1976

Critchley M: The neurology of old age. Lancet 1:1221–1230, 1931

Cummings JL: Clinical Neuropsychiatry. New York, Grune & Stratton, 1985, pp 221–233

Cummings JL, Darkins A, Mendez M, et al: Alzheimer's disease and Parkinson's disease: comparison of speech and language alterations. Neurology 38:680–684, 1988

Davis AS: Neuropsychological measures in patients with amyotrophic lateral sclerosis (letter). Acta Neurol Scand 75:284, 1987

DeJong RN: The Neurologic Examination. Hagerstown, MD, Harper & Row, 1979

Dement W, Richardson G, Prinz P, et al: Changes of sleep and wakefulness with age, in Handbook of the Biology of Aging, 2nd Edition. Edited by Finch CE, Schneider EL. New York, Van Nostrand Reinhold, 1985, pp 692–717

Doty RL, Shaman P, Applebaum SL, et al: Smell identification ability: changes with age. Science 226:1441–1443, 1984

Drachman DA, Long RR: Neurological evaluation of the elderly patient, in Clinical Neurology of Aging. Edited by Albert ML. New York, Oxford University Press, 1984, pp 97–113

Fetell MR, Stein BM: General considerations, Chapter V: Tumors, in Merrit's Textbook of Neurology. Edited by Rowland LP. Philadelphia, PA, Lea & Febiger, 1989, pp 275–285

George J: The neurological examination of the elderly patient, in The Clinical Neurology of Old Age. Edited by Tallis R. Chichester, John Wiley, 1989, pp 67–75

Girotti F, Soliveri P, Carella F, et al: Dementia and cognitive impairment in Parkinson's disease. J Neurol Neurosurg Psychiatry 51:1498–1502, 1988

Henderson G, Tomlinson BE, Gibson PH: Cell counts in human cerebral cortex in normal adults throughout life using an image analyzing computer. J Neurol Sci 46:113–136, 1980

Hobson W, Pemberton J: The Health of the Elderly at Home. London, Butterworth, 1955

Howell TH: Senile deterioration of the central nervous system. Br Med J 1:56–58, 1949

Hubbard BM, Squier MV: The physical aging of the neuromuscular system, in The Clinical Neurology of Old Age. Edited by Tallis R. Chichester, John Wiley, 1989, pp 3–26

Hutton JT, Morris JL: Looking and seeing with age related neurologic illness and normal aging. Seminars in Neurology 9:31–38, 1989

Jacobs L, Gossman MD: Three primitive reflexes in normal adults. Neurology 30:184–188, 1980

Jankovic J, Caine DB: Parkinson's disease: etiology and treatment. Current Neurology 7:193–234, 1987

Jenkyn LR, Reeves AG, Warren T, et al: Neurologic signs in senescence. Arch Neurol 42:1154–1157, 1985

Jennett B, Teasdale G: Prognosis after severe head injury, in Management of Head Injuries. Edited by Jennett B, Teasdale G. Philadelphia, PA, F.A. Davis, 1981, pp 317–332

Jensen JPA, Gron U, Pakkenberg H: Comparison of three primitive reflexes in neurological patients and in normal individuals. J Neurol Neurosurg Psychiatry 46:162–167, 1983

Kales A, Caldwell AB, Cadieux RJ, et al: Severe obstructive sleep apnea, II: associated psychopathology and psychosocial consequences. J Chronic Dis 38:427–434, 1985

Kasper RL: Eye problems of the aged, in Clinical Aspects of Aging. Edited by Reichel W. Baltimore, MD, Williams & Wilkins, 1989, pp 445–453

Kirasic KC, Allen GL: Aging, spatial performance, and spatial competence, in Aging and Human Performance. Edited by Charness N. Chichester, John Wiley, 1985, pp 191–224

Kish SJ, el-Awar M, Schut L, et al: Cognitive deficits in olivopontocerebellar atrophy: implications for the cholinergic hypothesis of Alzheimer's dementia. Ann Neurol 24:200–206, 1988

Klawans H: Behavioral alterations and the therapy of Parkinsonism. Clin Neuropharmacol 5(suppl 1):S29–S37, 1982

Klawans H, Tanner CM: Movement disorders in the elderly, in Clinical Neurology of Aging. Edited by Albert ML. New York, Oxford University Press, 1984, pp 387–403

Kokmen E, Bossemeyer RW, Barney J, et al: Neurological manifestations of aging. J Gerontol 32:411–419, 1977

Koller WC: Edentulous orodyskinesia. Ann Neurol 13:97–99, 1983

Koller WC: Diagnosis and treatment of tremors. Neurol Clin 2:499–514, 1984

Kral VA: The relationship between senile dementia (Alzheimer type) and depression. Can J Psychiatry 28:304–306, 1983

Larish DD, Martin PE, Mungiole M: Characteristic patterns of gait in the healthy old. Ann NY Acad Sci 515:18–32, 1988

Levin HS, Benton AL: Age and susceptibility to tactile masking effects. Gerontologia Clinic 15:1–9, 1973

Loewenfield IE: Pupillary changes related to age, in Topics in Neuroopthalmology. Edited by Thompson HS. Baltimore, MD, Williams & Wilkins, 1979, pp 124–150

Love AW: Depression in chronic low back pain patients: diagnostic efficiency of three self-report questionnaires. J Clin Psychol 43:84–89, 1987

Mackenzie I: Disturbances of Hearing and Balance, in The Clinical Neurology of Old Age. Edited by Tallis R. Chichester, John Wiley, 1989, pp 363–375

Manchester D, Woollacott M, Zederbauer-Hylton N, et al: Visual, vestibular and somatosensory contributions to balance control in the older adult. J Gerontol 44:M118–M127, 1989

Marsden CD, Jenner P: The pathophysiology of extrapyramidal side-effects of neuroloptic drugs. Psychol Med 10:55–72, 1980

Mayeux R: Behavioral manifestations of movement disorders. Neurol Clin 2:527–540, 1984

Montgomery GK, Erickson LM: Neuropsychological perspectives in amyotrophic lateral sclerosis. Neurol Clin 5:61–81, 1987

Mortimer JA: The dementia of Parkinson's disease. Clin Geriatr Med 4:785–797, 1988

Munsat TL: Aging of the neuromuscular system, in Clinical Neurology of Aging. Edited by Albert ML. New York, Oxford University Press, 1984, pp 404–423

Murray MP, Kory RC, Clarkson BH: Walking patterns in healthy old men. J Gerontol 24:169–178, 1969

Olney RK: Diseases of peripheral nerves, in The Clinical Neurology of Old Age. Edited by Tallis R. Chichester, John Wiley, 1989, pp 171–189.

Pearson GHJ: Effect of age on vibratory sensibility. Archives of Neurology and Psychiatry 20:482–496, 1928

Plude DJ, Hoyer WJ: Attention and performance: identifying and localizing age deficits, in Aging and Human Performance. Edited by Charness N. Chichester, John Wiley, 1985, pp 47–99

Prakash C, Stern G: Neurological signs in the elderly. Age Ageing 2:24–27, 1973

Rapoport SI: Positron emission tomography in normal aging and Alzheimer's disease. Gerontology 32(suppl 1):6–13, 1986

Riederer P, Krusik P: Biochemical and morphological changes in the aging brain, in The London Symposia (EEG Suppl 39). Edited by Ellingson RJ, Murray NMF, Halliday AM. Elsevier Science, 1987, pp 389–395

Robinson RG, Kubos KL, Starr LB, et al: Mood disorders in stroke patients: importance of location of lesion. Brain 107:81–93, 1984

Rogers J, Bloom FE: Neurotransmitter metabolism and function in the aging central nervous system, in Handbook of the Biology of Aging, 2nd Edition. Edited by Finch CE, Schneider EL. New York, Van Nostrand Reinhold, 1985, pp 645–691

Rowe JW, Kahn RL: Human aging: usual and successful. Science 237:143–149, 1987

Selkoe D, Kosik K: Neurochemical changes with aging, in Clinical Neurology of Aging. Edited by Albert ML. New York, Oxford University Press, 1984, pp 53–75

Simpson GM, Singh H: Tardive dyskinesia rating scales. Encephale 14:175–182, 1988

Smith J: Clinical neurophysiology in the elderly, in The Clinical Neurology of Old Age. Edited by Tallis R. Chichester, John Wiley, 1989, pp 89–97

Spencer PS, Ochoa J: The mammalian peripheral nervous system in old age, in Aging and Cell Structure. Edited by Johnson J. New York, Plenum, 1981, pp 35–103

Stelmach GE, Phillips J, DiFabio RP, et al: Age, functional postural reflexes, and voluntary sway. J Gerontol 44:B100–B106, 1989

Stones MJ, Kozma A: Physical performance, in Aging and Human Performance. Edited by Charness N. Chichester, John Wiley, 1985, pp 261–292

Strub RL, Black FW: Neurobehavioral Disorders: A Clinical Approach. Philadelphia, PA, F.A. Davis, 1988, pp 451–475

Takeda S, Matsuzawa T, Matsui H: Age-related changes in cerebral blood flow and brain volume in healthy subjects. J Am Geriatr Soc 36:293–297, 1988

Telakivi T, Kajaste S, Partinen M, et al: Cognitive function in middle age snorers and controls: role of excessive daytime somnolence and sleep-related hypoxic events. Sleep 10:454–462, 1988

Teravainen H, Calne DB: Motor system in normal aging and Parkinson's disease, in The Neurology of Aging. Edited by Katzman R, Terry R. Philadelphia, PA, F.A. Davis, 1983, pp 85–109

Tinetti ME: Instability and falling in elderly patients. Seminars in Neurology 9:39–45, 1989

Verillo RT, Verillo V: Sensory and perceptual performance, in Aging and Human Performance. Edited by Charness N. Chichester, John Wiley, 1985, pp 1–46

Victoroff JI: Hyperactivity syndrome of Alzheimer's disease. Bull Clin Neurosci 54:34–42, 1989

Ward C: The genetics and epidemiology of Parkinson's disease, in Degenerative Neurological Disease in The Elderly. Edited by Griffiths RA, McCarthy ST. Bristol, Wright, 1987, pp 20–28

Weiner WJ, Klawans HL: Lingual-facial-buccal movements in the elderly, II: pathogenesis and relationship to senile chorea. J Am Geriatr Soc 21:318–320, 1973

Welford AT: Reaction time, speed of performance, and age. Ann NY Acad Sci 515:1–17, 1988

Wrightson P: Management of disability and rehabilitation services after minor head injury, in Mild Head Injury. Edited by Levin HS, Eisenberg HM, Benton AL. New York, Oxford University Press, 1989

Yarnell PR, Rossie GV: Minor whiplash head injury with major debilitation. Brain Injury 2:255–258, 1988

Yoder MG: Geriatric ear, nose, and throat problems, in Clinical Aspects of Aging. Edited by Reichel W. Baltimore, MD, Williams & Wilkins, 1989, pp 454–463

CHAPTER 11

Marilyn S. Albert, PH.D.

Neuropsychological Testing

A variety of cognitive disorders occurs with increasing frequency as people age, including progressive dementing disorders and cognitive disorders secondary to psychiatric syndromes. These cognitive disorders produce considerable morbidity and mortality, and although only some of them can be completely reversed with treatment, appropriate management can substantially improve quality of life and reduce the development of secondary disorders. Thus, it is in the best interest of the patient for health professionals to become increasingly attuned to the possible presence of cognitive dysfunction in older patients, and familiar with appropriate procedures for evaluation and referral. In this chapter I will focus on the role of neuropsychological testing in the assessment of cognitive dysfunction in the elderly, because there is much that a physician, especially a psychiatrist, can do to identify the presence of cognitive dysfunction and to ensure that it is properly assessed.

Neuropsychological Test Batteries

There are at least two basic approaches to the selection of a neuropsychological test protocol. Some individuals use a predetermined test battery, such as the Halstead-Reitan Neuropsychological Test Battery (Reitan 1979) or the Luria-Nebraska Battery (Goldin 1981). Others select from several tests that seem particularly relevant to the diagnostic question. However, even in the latter case, certain core tests tend to be relied on more heavily than others.

If the neuropsychologist is not using the same standard battery

223

in every testing situation, the selection is determined by a number of factors among which the diagnostic issue at hand is of primary importance. If, for example, language abnormalities are prominent and one is trying to determine whether they are the result of strokes or a primary progressive dementia such as Alzheimer's disease (AD), the neuropsychologist may examine reading, writing, comprehension, repetition, naming, and spontaneous speech in some detail, using a standardized aphasia battery such as the Boston Diagnostic Exam (Goodglass and Kaplan 1980) or the Western Aphasia Battery (Kertesz 1980). If language abnormalities are minimal but memory deficits are prominent, and the differential diagnosis is among several primary progressive dementias, then one might choose to limit the language assessment to an evaluation of naming, using a task such as the Boston Naming Test (Kaplan et al. 1982), and examine memory from a variety of perspectives, including immediate and delayed recall and recognition in both the verbal and nonverbal domains.

In selecting tests it is, of course, also important to take the patient's level of impairment into account. If very difficult tests are chosen, moderately and severely impaired patients are likely to become extremely fatigued, feel overwhelmed, and either fail to perform at their best or refuse to continue with the evaluation. Thus, reduced versions of lengthier tests—for example, the reduced Wechsler Adult Intelligence Scale-Revised (WAIS-R; Wechsler 1981)—or tests designed for impaired patients—for example, the Mattis Dementia Rating Scale (Mattis 1976)—would be wise choices rather than a lengthy and complex battery of tests such as the entire WAIS-R or the Halstead-Reitan battery.

Regardless of one's approach, it is useful to organize the neuropsychological report into broad areas of function such as attention, language, memory, visuospatial ability, conceptualization, and general intelligence. In this way, the physician's understanding of the test result is enhanced.

Attention

Attention is important to consider because simple attentional abilities must be preserved for any other task to be performed adequately. If the patient has difficulty keeping his or her mind on the task for 1 to 3 minutes at a time, it will not be possible to assess other areas of function. For this reason, attention is often assessed before other cognitive domains have been evaluated. Auditory and visual attention can be assessed easily by means of digit span and letter cancellation. Several continuous-performance tasks are also available for this purpose. Many of these have been adapted for computer administration so that both accuracy and latency can be recorded.

Aphasia

Language testing for aphasia should, of course, include an evaluation of comprehension, repetition, reading, writing, and naming. Several standardized batteries are available for this purpose (Goodglass and Kaplan 1972; Kertesz 1980). Some include brief aphasia screening tests that are useful for identifying the existence of a problem without giving a detailed analysis (Halstead and Wepman 1949). If aphasia has been ruled out or is not suspected, confrontation naming (Kaplan et al. 1983) should almost always be part of the assessment of an older individual, because decreases in naming ability occur with age and are also a prominent symptom of a number of disorders common among the elderly (e.g., AD).

Memory

A detailed evaluation of memory is essential in the assessment of the elderly patient. Memory dysfunction occurs in almost all of the cognitive disorders common in the elderly, and the nature and severity of the memory impairment can serve as one of the major guidelines to the diagnosis. The assessment of memory is complicated by the fact that changes in memory capacity occur as people age. Therefore, careful testing is often necessary to differentiate normal from pathological memory performance. Fortunately, there are many memory tests from which one can choose. The ones used commonly today are: Wechsler Memory Scale-Revised (WMS-R) (Wechsler 1987); Rey Auditory Verbal Learning Test (Rey 1964); Selective Reminding Test (Buschke and Fuld 1974); Delayed Recognition Span Test (Moss et al. 1986); California Verbal Learning Test (Delis et al. 1986); Randt Memory Test (Randt et al. 1980); and Fuld Object Memory Test (Fuld 1980). Although some of these tests were specifically developed for use with the elderly, most were originally designed for younger populations and are now being applied to older individuals.

Visuospatial Ability

The assessment of visuospatial ability is more difficult in the elderly than in the young because of the prevalence of visual sensory deficits in this age range. In all of the cognitive domains previously discussed, function can be evaluated either orally or visually. However, it is not so for visuospatial ability, and alternate means of administration are more difficult to develop. It is, for example, difficult to enlarge test stimuli such as blocks or sticks. Therefore, figure copying is the method of assessment that is most likely to be successful. Figures can be chosen to span a great range of difficulty and, as mentioned earlier, can be adapted (by using photographic enlargement or a felt-tipped pen) for individuals with moderate sensory impairments. Even then it may be necessary to allow for a greater margin of error.

Perceptual Capacity

In addition to constructional ability one should assess perceptual capacity. Figure-matching tasks are a good analogue for figure copying. They have the added advantage that they can be administered to patients with severe cognitive deficits—patients in whom it is otherwise difficult to assess spatial function.

Conceptualization

Tasks that examine conceptualization include tests of concept formation, abstraction, set shifting, and set maintenance. A partial list of available tests includes the similarities subtest of WAIS-R (Wechsler 1981); Proverbs Test (Gorham 1956); Trail Making Test (Reitan 1958); Modified Card Sorting Test (Nelson 1976); and Visual-Verbal Test (Feldman and Drasgow 1951).

Many of these tests are lengthy, and shortened versions are better for clinical assessment; for example, the Modified Card Sorting Test (Nelson 1976) is the shortened version of the Wisconsin Card Sorting Test (Heaton 1981). The advantage of tasks from the WAIS-R such as proverb interpretation or similarities is that they are generally arranged in order of difficulty. Thus, the harder items can be omitted if the individual fails on easier items. There are, in addition, tasks that have been designed to assess abstraction in patients with moderate to severe cognitive impairments, who fail the standard tests (Mattis 1976).

General Intelligence

In addition, it is also helpful to assess general intelligence. This assessment will allow one to determine whether the individual has access to previously acquired knowledge. The vocabulary subtest of the WAIS-R is well known as the best quick estimate of IQ. However, in order to interpret the results, one must have a general sense of the individual's premorbid level of ability. Because tests that are purported to assess premorbid ability, such as the vocabulary subtest of the WAIS-R and the Nelson Adult Reading Test (Nelson and O'Connell 1978), often show declines even in mildly impaired patients, information regarding education and occupation is important in assessing premorbid cognitive status. There are recent data to suggest that elderly persons with a poor educational background (i.e., 0–8 years) perform worse on a broad range of cognitive tasks than elderly persons with a good educational background (i.e., 10–16 years) (Anthony et al. 1982). Therefore one must be extremely cautious in interpreting the test results of an elderly individual with limited formal education.

Overall Cognitive Function

Physicians often need a screening test to get a quick notion of their patient's overall level of cognitive function. These tests include the Mini-Mental State Exam (Folstein et al. 1975); Short Portable Mental Status Questionnaire (Pfeiffer 1975); Mental Status Questionnaire (Kahn et al, 1960); Blessed Dementia Index (Blessed et al. 1968); and East Boston Memory Test (Scherr et al. 1988).

Limitations of Tests

Although administering such tests is an excellent idea, it is important to know that they are particularly prone to the confounding effects of education. Individuals with high premorbid ability can score in the unimpaired range despite having experienced a substantial amount of cognitive decline. Conversely, individuals with low educational achievement may be misidentified as impaired. In addition, the cutoff points on many of the existing screening tests are generally designed to identify moderately to severely impaired individuals, in order to minimize false positives. Thus, individuals in the early stages of a dementing disorder such as AD may still perform in the unimpaired range on a short screening test. It is also important to note that such tests, by their very nature, were not designed to measure subtle aspects of behavior. Thus, they may show little or no decline over time in a patient who can be shown by other measures to have declined substantially.

Administration of Cognitive Tests

The manner in which the neuropsychological assessment of an older person is conducted can contribute greatly to its success. As in any cognitive evaluation, the testing environment should be quiet and well lit. If there is a window in the room, it should be at the patient's back, because glare can be a particular problem for an older person. Although standard testing stimuli should be used whenever possible, versions that have been especially adapted for the elderly with sensory or other impairments should be available. Visual stimuli can often be enlarged on a photocopy machine if the lines on the original are too thin. Otherwise, it may be necessary to redraw the stimuli with a felt-tipped pen to increase their visibility. If one is planning to present visual stimuli on a computer screen, it is particularly important for the stimuli to be pretested so that they are not only large enough but also presented with sufficient light-dark contrast for the elderly person to view them with ease. It should be possible to adjust the volume on a tape machine for most older people to hear. Despite these adjustments, the presence of sensory limitations should always be noted and factored into the evaluation.

With the elderly probably more than with any other group, it is extremely important to establish a friendly and nonthreatening environment. As a group, the elderly have less education than the young and are more intimidated by the testing situation. If they are experiencing cognitive deficits, they may be aware of them and be embarrassed, afraid, or anxious.

The order in which tests are given can also serve to reduce tension in the test situation. One should begin with tasks that are unlikely to be stressful so that there is time for the patient to become acclimated to the test situation, and for the tester to establish rapport with the patient. Tasks that are stressful should be followed, whenever possible, with tasks that are not. It is important to remember that success on a task need not be equated with an absence of stressfulness. Timed tasks or tasks in which items are repeated over and over again (as in word-list learning) are often stressful, even if the patient ultimately performs with some degree of accuracy.

Older individuals tend to take more time and fatigue more easily than younger persons. There is also the danger of artificially lower scores on later tasks because of fatigue. One must, therefore, be especially attentive to a patient's tiring and be prepared to stop a test session to continue on another day.

The Differential Diagnosis of Common Dementing Disorders

Dementia is the most common syndrome of cognitive decline seen in the elderly. "Dementia" is a general term used to describe a chronic and substantial decline in two or more areas of cognitive function. It is unlike amnesia, which causes a severe and striking deficit in only one area of cognitive function (i.e., memory). Some dementias are nonprogressive (e.g., alcoholic dementia), but most are progressive. Although all dementias are accompanied by a memory impairment, the nature of the impairment differs substantially among patients. For example, AD patients demonstrate a very rapid rate of forgetting during brief delays (Hart et al. 1988, Moss et al. 1986), whereas Pick's patients do not (Moss and Albert 1988); patients with Huntington's disease (HD) show relative preservation of verbal recognition memory versus nonverbal recognition memory (Butters et al. 1983). The other cognitive deficits that accompany memory impairments also vary widely among patient groups.

The nature of the onset and progression of the cognitive deficits also differs greatly among the major dementing disorders. A carefully collected cognitive history is, therefore, an essential adjunct to a dementia workup and often makes the difference between an accurate diagnosis and an inaccurate one. Most of the dementias have an insidious onset and develop slowly and gradually. These include AD, Pick's disease, Parkinson's dementia, and progressive supranuclear palsy (PSP). The most virulent dementing disorder, Creutzfeldt-Jakob disease, develops insidiously too, but it is known for its rapid rate of progression from onset to death (often within 1 year). Personality change or psychiatric syndromes, such as depression, are also seen in dementing disorders, and whether they precede or follow the onset of cognitive decline is critical for an accurate diagnosis. The initial symptoms of a multi-infarct dementia develop acutely, but because multiple large or small cerebral infarcts are the cause of the cognitive decline, the ultimate clinical picture can take many years to develop, albeit in a stepwise and stuttering fashion.

Thus, each dementing disorder has a unique cognitive history and a unique pattern of spared and impaired function that can help the clinician identify it. The most common dementing disorders seen in the elderly as well as the cognitive profile associated with depression are discussed in the following paragraphs.

Alzheimer's Disease

The first and most noticeable symptom generally observed in patients with AD is a severe anterograde memory deficit. Early in the course of disease, it is confined mainly to an impairment of secondary memory, but as the disease progresses, primary memory deficits develop. The striking aspect of this difficulty in acquiring new information is the rapid rate at which information is forgotten in secondary memory. Comparisons of dementias of differing etiologies suggest that AD patients lose more information over a brief delay than patients with HD (Moss et al. 1986), Pick's disease (Moss and Albert 1988), or PSP (Milberg and Albert, in press). It was recently demonstrated by the use of a continuous recognition paradigm that this rapid rate of forgetting is evident chiefly during the initial 10 minutes following exposure to new material (Hart et al. 1988). Therefore, retention intervals falling within this time period are diagnostically the most useful. Recall paradigms with relatively brief intervals between exposure to information and its immediate and delayed recall (e.g., 15 seconds vs. 2 minutes, respectively) are thus best in accentuating differences among patients. Many standard memory tests can be readily adapted to these constraints.

It is likely that the rapid rate of forgetting in AD is the result of the striking damage to the hippocampal complex seen in this disorder. There is a high density of neurofibrillary tangles and neuritic plaques in the medial temporal lobe, particularly the afferent neurons of the entorhinal cortex and the efferent neurons of the subiculum (Hyman et al. 1976). This condition appears to functionally disconnect the hippocampal formation from the rest of the cerebral cortex. The large declines in choline acetyltransferase seen in AD (Davies and Maloney 1976) probably contribute to this memory impairment of AD patients. However, because the alteration in acetylcholine levels is thought to result from neuronal loss in the basal forebrain (Whitehouse et al. 1981) and basal forebrain damage is seen in other dementing disorders with less-severe memory impairment early in the course of disease (Tagliavini and Pilleri 1983), it is unlikely that the cholinergic deficit alone is responsible for the AD patient's particularly severe pattern of memory impairment.

Recent data suggest that, in addition to a memory impairment, the other cognitive deficit most commonly seen in the early stages of AD is difficulty with sequencing, monitoring, and shifting behavior (Grady et al. 1989; Morris and Fulling 1983). Such disabilities have typically been attributed to frontal system dysfunction (Damasio 1985; Milner 1964; Stuss and Benson 1986), but it has been suggested that in AD patients, problems with complex attentional mechanisms secondary to parietal lobe abnormalities may be responsible for the impairments (Grady et al. 1989).

In the most typical presentation of AD, language deficits (e.g., difficulty with confrontation naming) and spatial deficits (e.g., difficulty with figure copying) develop after the onset of memory dysfunction (Bayles and Kaszniak 1987; Rosen 1983). These deficits have been attributed to neurofibrillary tangle and neuritic plaque formation in multimodal association cortices (Kemper 1984; Pearson et al. 1985).

The initial symptoms of a patient with AD typically provide very subtle evidence of memory difficulty. Patients may begin by repeating themselves, forgetting names, or forgetting appointments. Patients are often aware of these difficulties but tend to minimize them. On neuropsychological testing, patients early in the course of AD often have IQs in the normal range (i.e., 110) but have substantial difficulty with memory, set shifting, and conceptualization, and slight difficulty with naming. For example, a patient with an IQ of 110 may have a memory quotient (based on the WMS-R) of 90—a 20-point discrepancy (a person's memory quotient should be approximately equal to the IQ).

Delayed-recall performance on a memory test such as the Delayed Recognition Span Test would also be impaired. Although verbal recognition span may be 8, which is in the low normal range, after 15 seconds a typical patient recalls only two words, and after 2 minutes only one word. Impairments in set shifting and abstraction are often revealed by performance on the Trail Making Test. This task requires an individual to first connect a series of numbers in order, and then connect alternating numbers and letters in order (i.e., 1-A, 2-B, etc.). Mildly impaired AD patients are generally slow on both tasks and make errors on the second. Impairments on the similarities subtest of the WAIS-R are also common. Responses are likely to be concrete (e.g., an apple and an orange are alike because they both have peels). Performance on the Mattis Dementia Rating Scale also reflects these difficulties. A mildly impaired AD patient may score 121 of a possible 144 on the Delayed Recognition Span Test (with losses primarily on the memory and conceptualization subtests). Difficulty in naming may also be apparent on the 10 items from the Boston Naming Test often appended to the Delayed Recognition Span Test (this task consists of a series of line drawings that patients are asked to name). Patients may fail to spontaneously name some of the drawings, giving either category descriptions or semantic associates of the target word (e.g., "ladle" for "funnel," "musical instrument" for "accordion," and "not plier" for "tongs"). Despite these obvious difficulties, performance on the Mini-Mental State Exam may be good in a well-educated, mildly impaired patient (e.g., 28 of 30). In such a patient, errors invariably occur on the recall portion of the test.

Dementia of the Frontal Lobe Type

Several pathologic entities have been associated with a progressive dementing process that involves the frontal lobes. Recently these disorders have been called dementia of the frontal lobe type (DFT) (Neary et al. 1988) to differentiate them from dementia of the Alzheimer's type. To date, three different pathologic entities have been described. These include Pick's disease (Pick 1892), progressive subcortical gliosis (Neuman and Cohn 1967), and frontal lobe degeneration (Brun 1987; Gustafson 1987). Progressive subcortical gliosis has also been called type II Pick's disease (Constantinidis et al. 1974). All of these disorders begin with changes in personality (Neary et al. 1988) such as lack of impulse control, stereotyped behavior, and inappropriate affect. Speech that is either hypophonic or excessively loud has also been noted. Alterations in pain sensitivity may occur.

Although memory function is abnormal early in the course of disease, it is less severely affected than in AD. DFT patients remember less than normals immediately after being exposed to the material, but they do not forget as rapidly as they did initially, thereafter (Moss and Albert 1988). It is, therefore, of considerable interest that the hippocampus has been reported as spared in some DFT patients (Constantinidis et al. 1974), although not invariably (Seitelberger et al. 1983). Spatial ability is typically reported as relatively intact, even in advanced disease (Neary et al. 1988), congruent with the relative absence of pathological changes in the parietal cortex. It is also noteworthy that the electroencephalogram remains normal until late in the course of frontal lobe syndromes (Neary et al. 1988).

The accurate identification of this group of syndromes is particularly important for good patient management. Early in the course of disease, DFT patients give the appearance of having well-preserved abilities because of their relatively mild memory deficit. However, their inappropriate behavior makes them severe management problems, and unprepared families can become distraught (Gustafson 1987). DFT patients profit from being treated like psychiatric patients, with whom they are sometimes confused (Neary et al. 1988). Enabling families to understand that the cause of the disorder is a brain disease generally helps them to adapt to the cognitive and personality changes as well as extremes of behavior DFT patients display. The initial episodes that raise concern generally relate to inappropriate behavior that is uncharacteristic of the patient (e.g., leaving the scene of an accident, making sexually explicit statements in public, developing obsessions with food, compulsively carrying out certain routines). Some patients become emotionally labile and irritable.

On neuropsychological testing early in the course of disease, the DFT patient may appear normal in many respects (e.g., reveal an estimated verbal IQ of 104, a memory quotient of 118, and a score of 29 on the Mini-Mental State Exam). Despite the apparent normality of the scores, however, patients typically have clear cognitive deficits in domains associated with frontal lobe function. They have difficulty with proverb interpretation. For example, when asked to explain the proverb "Barking dogs seldom bite," they may say, "They try to act fiercer to cover up the fact that they're really gentle." Set-shifting abilities are also compromised. They are generally slow on the Trail Making Test and, more important, they make errors. Naming may be impaired; the patient may score 49 out of 60 on the Boston Naming Test. Errors consist primarily of semantic associates of the target word (e.g., "fancy fish" for "seahorse" or "harmonica" for "accordion"). Although the score on the WMS-R may be within the normal range, memory is typically quite variable. For example, on the Delayed Recognition Span Test, verbal recognition span may be 11 (which is normal), but after both the 15-second and the 2-minute delay, the patient may recall only four words (considerably less than one would have predicted given a good recognition span). The items missed on the Mini-Mental State Exam may also be related to recall. Variability, both within and across test sessions, suggests that the patients' memory deficit may be at least partially the result of declines in concentration.

To complicate the foregoing emphasis on personality changes in DFT, patients with a gradually progressive language deficit have also been found to have autopsy-confirmed Pick's disease (Cole et al. 1979; Wechsler et al. 1982) or progressive subcortical gliosis (Moss et al. submitted). Therefore, a gradually progressive language deficit is not restricted to the pathologic diagnosis of AD. Because the early symptoms of DFT mimic a gradually progressive aphasia, these patients benefit from nonverbal communication strategies rather than the mnemonic aids often recommended for AD patients.

Parkinson's Dementia

A significant number of patients with Parkinson's disease (PD) develop a dementia syndrome. Prevalence rates vary from 25% to 40% (Brown and Marsden 1984), but they appear to be higher than would be explained by the co-occurrence of AD and PD. Indeed, some demented PD patients have neuritic plaques and neurofibrillary tangles on autopsy (the pathological hallmarks of AD), although others do not (Jellinger 1987).

Given this complex pathological picture, it is not surprising that the neuropsychological deficits associated with demented PD patients are varied and heterogeneous. Most have the cognitive deficits associated with PD itself, namely, visuospatial dysfunction and difficulty with concept formation and set shifting (Boller et al. 1984; Hovestadt et al. 1987; Taylor et al. 1986). These deficits have been most commonly ascribed to cell loss in the basal ganglia (with projections to the prefrontal cortex), and to the declines in dopamine, which accompany the neuronal loss (Divac 1972).

When dementia develops in PD patients, it generally includes substantial difficulty with memory (El-Awar et al. 1987) and occasionally with linguistic skills such as confrontation naming. Recently, implicit memory problems, both in motor-skill learning (i.e., pursuit rotor) and in verbal priming have been reported in demented PD patients (Heindel et al. 1989). Because AD patients have preserved motor-skill learning but impaired verbal priming (Heindel et al. 1989), it may be that a subgroup of demented PD patients with preserved motor-skill learning and impaired verbal priming identifies the subgroup of demented PD patients with coexistent AD.

Progressive Supranuclear Palsy

Although PSP is an extremely rare disorder, it is being studied with increasing frequency, largely because it is a dementia in which damage is restricted almost entirely to subcortical areas (Steele et al. 1964). Patients with HD ultimately develop neocortical damage (Bruyn et al. 1979), as do demented patients with PD (Divac 1972), leaving PSP as the classic subcortical dementia. Pathologic damage in PSP appears to be limited to the basal ganglia, brain stem, and cerebellar nuclei. It is therefore striking that memory function in the early stages of PSP is near normal levels, even when tasks requiring initiation and sequencing, such as verbal fluency, are devastated (Milberg and Albert, in press). PSP patients also have difficulty with so-called frontal tasks such as card sorting, which is thought to result from a disconnection of the frontal lobes from subcortical structures (Pillon et al. 1986). This hypothesis has received some recent support from single photon emission computed tomography data showing frontal metabolic declines in PSP patients (Goffinet et al. 1988). Although the matter has not been examined, it may be that memory remains relatively intact in PSP patients until late in the course of disease if it is assessed in a manner that minimizes the profound initiation and conceptualization deficit of PSP patients.

The neurologic deficits of PSP (e.g., ophthalmoplegia, gait disturbance) are generally diagnostic of the disorder so that memory testing may not be needed for establishing the diagnosis. However, a demonstration of relatively preserved memory in the face of profound initiation and conceptualization deficits will greatly assist caregivers in patient management.

In a typical PSP patient, the neurologic examination is strikingly abnormal. There is often a masked face, reduced spontaneous blinking, a positive snout and glabellar reflex, hypokinesia, and bradykinesia, as well as an abnormal gait and markedly abnormal eye movements. Lack of vertical eye movements and limited horizontal eye movement are common.

Neuropsychological testing often shows marked impairments in abstraction, response initiation, and motoric set-shifting tasks. Naming and memory may also be deficient but less so. Estimated IQ may be reduced (e.g., Henry and Weingartner 1973), primarily because of difficulty with the similarities and vocabulary subtests of the WAIS-R. For example, a mildly impaired PSP patient may be unable to say how "north" and "west" are alike but know that the distance from New York to Paris is about 3,000 miles. Proverb interpretation is also generally concrete. Difficulty with response initiation is often most dramatic on verbal tasks. Spontaneous speech shows immense latencies. During critical points in a narrative, usually over substantive words or action verbs, a patient may stop for as long as 2 minutes before continuing. This greatly reduced initiation is reflected in a markedly impaired performance on word list generation. For example, when asked to name all the words beginning with the letter S, a mildly impaired PSP patient may produce only three in 1 minute, which is in the 0 percentile of performance. On the other hand, on verbal tasks—in which the stimulus for the response is provided, such as on confrontation naming—a patient may be much less impaired. Thus, a patient who is in the 0 percentile in word list generation may score 67 out of 85 on the Boston Naming Test. Memory may be abnormal but irregularly so. For example, a patient may fail to recall all three of the words on the Mini-Mental State Exam but recall both sentences on the Mattis Dementia Rating Scale. The score on the WMS-R may be clearly impaired (Silbermann et al. 1983), but delayed recall of the stories and figures on the WMS-R may not be substantially worse than immediate recall, suggesting that PSP patients do not have a particularly rapid rate of forgetting.

Huntington's Disease

HD is another dementing disorder that is generally diagnosed by the presence of a characteristic neurologic abnormality (i.e., chorea) (Caine 1986). A history of HD in other family members is, of course, also sought, because HD is a genetic disorder (Weingartner et al. 1981). However, occasionally there is no family history of HD (perhaps because of illegitimacy, broken family, or unknown adoption) and the choreic movements are atypical. In these instances neuropsychologic testing can be very helpful.

HD patients have poor verbal and nonverbal recall and poor nonverbal recognition. However, as mentioned earlier, verbal recognition is relatively well preserved early in the course of disease (Butters et al. 1983; Moss et al. 1986), and so is verbal priming compared to motor-skill learning, as mentioned earlier (Heindel et al. 1989). Early HD patients also have good confrontation-naming ability and relative preservation of many of the verbal tasks on the WAIS-R, such as information, vocabulary, and similarities (Josiassen et al. 1982), while showing impairment in many of the WAIS-R subtests that deal with spatial and arithmetic ability, such as arithmetic, digit span, picture arrangement, and digit-symbol (Butters et al. 1978; Josiassen et al. 1982). A combination of this pattern of preserved and impaired function should be diagnostic. HD patients typically present with a history of motor and cognitive dysfunction. Patients may report "hand spasms" and increasing problems with tripping, even on smooth surfaces, along with mild difficulty with memory that is less evident to others than it is to the patients themselves. The neurologic examination, of course, reveals the characteristic choreic movements of HD.

Neuropsychological testing in a mildly impaired patient may

yield an estimated verbal IQ of 99 (100 being the average for the population), with a memory quotient (WMS-R) of 90, the 9-point differential between the two being suggestive of memory difficulties. However, verbal recognition span tends to be selectively preserved in a mildly impaired patient (e.g., Wechsler 1981), compared to recognition span for faces or spatial positions (e.g., Buschke and Fuld 1974; Rey 1964, respectively). Tasks that require speed, sequential planning, and set formation are also generally deficient. The digit symbol substitution test, a task that requires matching a series of symbols that go with a set of numbers, may be impaired. The Trail Making Test may also be performed poorly, for example, in the 10th percentile on the first portion (Trails A) and the 25th percentile on the second (Trails B). Verbal fluency is also typically impaired (e.g., 27th percentile). Spatial tasks such as figure copying are generally accurate but demonstrate slight difficulty with planning. Naming is often within normal limits.

Multi-infarct Dementia

Cerebrovascular disease most commonly presents clinically as the "stroke syndrome" (Mohr et al. 1980). Although not all forms of vascular disease in the central nervous system involve stroke (e.g., cardiac arrest, prolonged hypotension), the disorders that produce dementia are generally the result of multiple strokes over time. These have been labeled multi-infarct dementia (Hachinski et al. 1974) to emphasize the fact that the deficits result from actual infarcts and not from diffuse narrowing of blood vessels.

These dementias are characterized by at least two clinical pictures. When large-vessel disease produces multiple cerebral emboli, large discrete cerebral infarcts typically occur. The focal cognitive deficits that result include aphasia, apraxia, agnosia, and amnesia, depending on the anatomic distribution of the lesion. Repeated strokes lead to a stepwise development of multiple cognitive deficits.

Medium- or small-vessel disease, secondary to atherosclerosis of the small vessels that penetrate subcortical white matter, produces more incomplete, diffuse infarction of brain tissue. Defined in this manner, the latter encompasses the syndromes known as *état lacunaire*, or lacunar state (Marie 1901) and Binswanger's disease (Fisher 1982). These disorders produce a more insidious decline and are harder to differentiate from progressive primary dementias such as AD than those produced by large-vessel disease. Because the cognitive deficits depend on the location and size of the tissue damage, it has been difficult to identify a consistent cognitive profile (Cummings et al. 1987; Perez et al. 1975). Neuroimaging procedures, such as magnetic resonance imaging, can also be inconclusive because multiple regions of high signal intensity do not always reflect infarction (Johnson et al. 1987) and are often seen in cognitively high-functioning individuals as well as in those with dementia (Brand-Zawadski et al. 1985). At present, the most useful information in the diagnosis of lacunar disease and other associated disorders tends to be provided by a very careful cognitive history and neurologic examination, in combination with neuroimaging procedures.

Neuropsychological testing in a mildly impaired patient with a lacunar disease (i.e., a patient with a score of 19 on the Mini-Mental State Exam) may show cognitive deficits reflective of aphasia. For example, patients may be unable to write single words (e.g., write "squar" for "square" and "scoss" for "cross"). The sentence on the Mini-Mental State Exam may show a similar linguistic impairment (e.g., "I came your by automobile"). There may also be difficulty reading simple sentences and misnaming of letters of the alphabet. Repetition may be impaired. Naming may be below normal but less impaired than reading, writing, and repetition. Consistent with these deficits would be a severe impairment in word list generation. When asked to name in 1 minute all the things one can buy in a supermarket, a mildly impaired patient may produce only three items. Such patients may also show difficulty with even simple alternating movements (e.g., they may not be able to perform even alternate taps with the index finger of each hand). Drawings that involve alternation may also be impaired. Only the simplest verbal and visual abstractions are performed correctly by such patients. Memory impairment may, however, be variable. Orientation may be only mildly impaired; patients may know the month, the year, and the names of the president, the governor, the hospital, and the city. They may recall a simple sentence after 10 minutes, but they may not recall any of the three words on the Mini-Mental State Exam.

Depression

Some depressed patients show a variety of cognitive deficits. The differential diagnosis between depression and the primary progressive dementias such as AD and Pick's disease is, therefore, often difficult. The best method for differentiating these two populations is, unfortunately, still unknown. Patients with depression have been reported to show deficits in vigilance (Byrne 1977; Frith et al. 1983), memory (Breslow et al. 1980; Caine 1986; Cronholm and Ottosson 1961; Henry et al. 1973; Neville and Folstein 1979; Raskin et al. 1982; Silbermann et al. 1983; Sternberg and Jarvik 1976), and conceptualization (Caine 1986; Raskin et al. 1982), all abilities that are impaired in AD and that in some studies were said not to differentiate patients with depression from those with primary progressive dementia. Contradictions in the results of various studies can probably be attributed to the fact that the age of the subjects varied widely as did the severity and type of depression. For example, tests that differentiate 55-year-old depressed and demented patients may not discriminate 70-year-old patients from one another because of the added alterations in test performance introduced by age-related changes in cognition. Seventy-five-year-old patients with multiple treated episodes of depression throughout their lives are likely to be systematically different from 75-year-old patients with a first depressive episode. Patients with atypical depressions and cognitive deficits may differ from patients with a more typical depressive profile. Differences among patient populations along these dimensions are likely to be the cause of some of the differences between published reports.

Nevertheless, some general statements can be made. First, it is essential to clarify the order in which the cognitive deficits occurred relative to the depression. Further, because the order of events must be reconstituted retrospectively, one must attempt to determine whether the patient was truly depressed at the relevant point in time. This determination can often be very difficult because many dementing disorders, particularly AD, produce an apathy and withdrawal from activities that families often interpret as depression. And, in an elderly individual, there are likely to be many real-life events that can reasonably be considered causally related to a depression (e.g., retirement, the death of a close friend or spouse). Therefore, considerable skill is needed to reconstruct these past events from an interview with the patient and the family.

Second, one should attempt to give several different tests within the same cognitive domain to examine intertest variability. Depressed patients often show large differences in performance among tests of a similar nature (e.g., tests of delayed recall), whereas demented patients do not. These fluctuations by the depressed patient are thought to be secondary to changes in attention, motivation, and mood.

Finally, the existing literature indicates that some aspects of cognition are unimpaired in depression. These include recognition of high-imagery words (Silbermann et al. 1983), recall of related words that have previously been sorted (Weingartner et al. 1981), paired associate learning (Breslow et al. 1980), and rate of forgetting over time (Cronholm and Ottosson 1961). Naming and arithmetic ability are also reported to be unimpaired in comparison to normals (Caine 1986).

References

Anthony JC, LeResche L, Niaz U, et al: Limits of the Mini-Mental State as a screening test for dementia and delirium among hospital patients. Psychol Med 12:397–408, 1982

Bayles KA, Kaszniak AW: Communication and Cognition in Normal Aging and Dementia. Boston, MA, Little, Brown, 1987

Blessed G, Tomlinson BE, Roth M: The association between quantitative measures of dementia and of senile changes in the cerebral gray matter of elderly subjects. Br J Psychiatry 114:797–811, 1968

Boller F, Passafiume D, Keefe N, et al: Visual impairment in Parkinson's disease. Arch Neurol 41:485–490, 1984

Brand-Zawadski M, Fein G, Van Dyke C, et al: Magnetic resonance imaging of the aging brain: patchy white matter lesions and dementia. AJNR 6:675–682, 1985

Breslow R, Kocsis J, Belkin B: Memory deficits in depression: evidence utilizing the Wechsler Memory Scale. Percept Mot Skills 51:541–542, 1980

Brown RG, Marsden CD: How common is dementia in Parkinson's disease? Lancet 2:1262–1265, 1984

Brun A: Frontal lobe degeneration of non-Alzheimer type, 1: neuropathology. Arch Gerontol Geriatr 6:193–208, 1987

Bruyn GW, Bots G, Dom R: Huntington's chorea: current neuropathological status, in Advances in Neurology, Vol. 23: Huntington's Disease. Edited by Chase T, Wexter N, Barbeau A. New York, Raven, 1979, pp 83–94

Buschke H, Fuld PA: Evaluating storage, retention, and retrieval in disordered memory and learning. Neurology 11:1019–1025, 1974

Butters N, Sax D, Tarlow S: Comparison of the neuropsychological deficits associated with early and advanced Huntington's disease. Arch Neurol 35:585–589, 1978

Butters N, Albert MS, Sax DS, et al: The effect of verbal mediators on the pictorial memory of brain-damaged patients. Neuropsychologia 21:307–323, 1983

Byrne DC: Affect and vigilance performance in depressive illness. J Psychiatr Res 13:185–191, 1977

Caine E: The neuropsychology of depression: the pseudodementia syndrome, in Neuropsychological Assessment of Neuropsychiatric Disorders. Edited by Grant I, Adams KM. New York, Oxford University Press, 1986

Cole M, Wright D, Banker BQ: Familial aphasia due to Pick's disease. Ann Neurol 6:158, 1979

Constantinidis J, Richard J, Tissot R: Pick's disease: histological and clinical correlation. European Neurology 11:208–217, 1974

Cronholm B, Ottosson J: Memory functions in endogenous depression. Arch Gen Psychiatry 5:193–197, 1961

Cummings JL, Miller B, Hill MA: Neuropsychiatric aspects of multi-infarct dementia and dementia of the Alzheimer type. Arch Neurol 44:389–393, 1987

Damasio A: The frontal lobes, in Clinical Neuropsychology. Edited by Heilman K, Valenstein E. New York, New York University Press, 1985, pp 339–375

Davies P, Malony AJR: Selective loss of central cholinergic neurons in Alzheimer's disease. Lancet 2:1403, 1976

Delis D, Kramer J, Fridlund A, et al: California Verbal Learning Test. San Antonio, TX, Psychological Corporation, 1986

Divac I: Neostriatum and functions of the prefrontal cortex. Acta Neurobiol Exp 32:461–477, 1972

El-Awar M, Becker JT, Hammond KM, et al: Learning deficit in Parkinson's disease: comparison with Alzheimer's disease and normal aging. Arch Neurol 44:180–184, 1987

Feldman MJ, Dragsow JA: A visual-verbal test for schizophrenia. Psychiatr Q Suppl 25:55–64, 1951

Fisher CM: Lacunar strokes and infarcts: a review. Neurology 32:871–876, 1982

Folstein MF, Folstein SE, McHugh PR: Mini-Mental State: a practical method for grading the cognitive state of patients for the clinician. J. Psychiatr Res 12:189–198, 1975

Frith CD, Stevens M, Johnstone EC, et al: Effects of ECT and depression on various aspects of memory. Br J Psychiatry 142:610–617, 1983

Fuld PA: Guaranteed stimulus-processing in the evaluation of memory and learning. Cortex 16:255–272, 1980

Goffinet AM, DeVolder AG, Gillain C, et al: Positron tomography demonstrates frontal lobe hypometabolism in progressive supranuclear palsy. Ann Neurol 25:131–139, 1988

Goldin CJ: A standardized version of Luria Nebraska neuropsychological tests, in Handbook of Clinical Neuropsychology. Edited by Filskov S, Voll TJ. New York, Wiley-Interscience, 1981

Goodglass H, Kaplan E: The Assessment of Aphasia and Related Disorders. Philadelphia, PA, Lea & Febiger, 1972

Gorham DR: A proverbs test for clinical and experimental use. Psychol Rep 1:1–12, 1956

Grady GL, Haxby JV, Horwitz B, et al: Longitudinal study of the early neuropsychological changes in dementia of the Alzheimer type. J Clin Exp Neuropsychol 10:576–596, 1989

Gustafson L: Frontal lobe degeneration of non-Alzheimer type, II: clinical picture and differential diagnosis. Arch Gerontol Geriatr 6:209–223, 1987

Hachinski VC, Lassen NA, Marshall J: Multi-infarct dementia: a cause of mental deterioration in the elderly. Lancet 2:207–209, 1974

Halstead WC, Wepman JM. The Halstead-Wepman aphasia screening test. J Speech Hear Disord 14:9–15, 1949

Hart RP, Kwentus JA, Harkins SW, et al: Rate of forgetting in mild Alzheimer's type dementia. Brain Cogn 7:31–38, 1988

Heaton R: University of Colorado School of Medicine. Psychological Assessment Resource, 1981

Heindel WC, Salmon DP, Shults CW, et al: Neuropsychological evidence for multiple implicit memory systems: a comparison of Alzheimer's, Huntington's, and Parkinson's disease patients. J Neurosci 9:582–587, 1989

Henry GM, Weingartner H, Murphy DL: Influence of affective states and psychoactive drugs on verbal learning and memory. Am J Psychiatry 130:966–971, 1973

Hovestadt A, deJong GJ, Meerwaldt JD: Spatial disorientation as an early symptom of Parkinson's disease. Neurology 37:485–487, 1987

Hyman BT, Van Hoesen GW, Damasio AR, et al: Alzheimer's disease: cell specific pathology isolates the hippocampal formation. Science 225:1168–1170, 1984

Jellinger K: Neuropathological substrates of Alzheimer's disease and Parkinson's disease. J Neural Transm 24 (suppl): 109–129, 1987

Johnson KA, Davis KR, Buonanno FS, et al: Comparison of magnetic resonance and roentgen ray computed tomography in dementia. Arch Neurol 44:1075–1080, 1987

Josiassen RC, Curry L, Roemer RA, et al: Patterns of intellectual deficit in Huntington's disease. J Clin Neuropsychol 4:173–183, 1982

Kahn RL, Goldfarb AL, Pollack M, et al: Brief objective measures for the determination of mental status in the aged. Am J Psychiatry 111:326–328, 1960

Kaplan E, Goodglass H, Weintraub S: Boston Naming Test. Philadelphia, PA, Lea & Febiger, 1983

Kemper T: Neuroanatomical and neuropathological changes in normal aging and dementia, in Clinical Neurology of Aging. Edited by Albert ML. New York, Oxford University Press, 1984, pp 9–52

Kertesz A: Western Aphasia Battery. London, Ontario, University of Western Ontario, 1980

Marie P: Des foyers lacunaires de desintegration et de differents autres etats cavetaures du cerveau. Rev Med 21:281–298, 1901

Mattis S: Dementia Rating Scale, in Geriatric Psychiatry. Edited by Bellack R, Karasu B. New York, Grune & Stratton, 1976

Milberg W, Albert M: Cognitive differences between patients with progressive supranuclear palsy and Alzheimer's disease. J Clin Exp Neuropsychol (in press)

Milner B: Some effects of frontal lobectomy in man, in The Frontal Granular Cortex and Behavior. Edited by Warren JM, Akert K. New York, McGraw-Hill, 1964, pp 313–334

Mohr JP, Fisher CM, Adams RD: Cerebrovascular diseases, in Harrison's Principles of Internal Medicine. Edited by Isselbacher K, Adams RD. New York, McGraw-Hill, 1980, pp 1911–1941

Morris JC, Fulling K: Early Alzheimer's disease: diagnostic considerations. Arch Neurol 45:345–356, 1983

Moss MB, Albert MS: Alzheimer's disease and other dementing disorders, in Geriatric Neuropsychology. Edited by Albert MS, Moss MB. New York, Guilford Press, 1988, pp 145–178

Moss M, Albert M, Butters N, et al: Differential patterns of memory loss among patients with Alzheimer's disease, Huntington's disease, and alcoholic Korsakoff's syndrome. Arch Neurol 43:239–246, 1986

Moss MB, Albert MS, Kemper T: The dementia of progressive subcortical gliosis: a case study. Submitted.

Neary D, Snowden JS, Northen B, et al: Dementia of frontal lobe type. J Neurol Neurosurg Psychiatry 51:353–361, 1988

Nelson HE: A modified card sorting test sensitive to frontal lobe defects. Cortex 12:313–324, 1976

Nelson HE, O'Connell A: Dementia: the estimation of premorbid intelligence levels using the new adult reading test. Cortex 14:234–244, 1978

Neumann M, Cohn R: Progressive subcortical dementia. Brain 90:405–418, 1967

Neville HJ, Folstein MF: Performance on three cognitive tasks by patients with dementia, depression, or Korsakoff's syndrome. Gerontology 25:285–290, 1979

Pearson RCA, Esiri MM, Hiorns RW, et al: Anatomical correlate of the distribution of the pathologic changes in the neocortex in Alzheimer's disease. Proc Natl Acad Sci USA 82:4531–4534, 1985

Perez FI, Rivera VM, Meyer JS: Analysis of intellectual and cognitive performance in patients with multi-infarct dementia, vertebrobasillar insufficiency with dementia, and Alzheimer's disease. J Neurol Neurosurg Psychiatry 38:533–540, 1975

Pfeiffer E: SPMSQ: Short Portable Mental Status Questionnaire. J Am Geriatr Soc 23:433–441, 1975

Pick A: On the relation between aphasia and senile atrophy of the brain, in Classics in Modern Translation. Edited by Rottenberg DA, Hochberg FH. New York, Hasner Press, pp 35–40

Pillon B, Dubois B, Lhermitte F, et al: Heterogeneity of cognitive impairment in progressive supranuclear palsy, Parkinson's disease, and Alzheimer's disease. Neurology 36:1179–1185, 1986

Randt CT, Brown ER, Osborne DJ: A memory test for longitudinal measurement of mild to moderate deficits. Clin Neuropsychol 2:184–194, 1980

Raskin A, Friedman AS, DiMascio A: Cognitive and performance deficits in depression. Psychopharmacol Bull 18:196–202, 1982

Reitan RM: Validity of the Trail Making Test as an indication of organic brain damage. Percept Mot Skills 8:271–276, 1958

Reitan RM: Halstead-Reitan Neuropsychological Test Battery. Tucson, AZ, Neuropsychology Laboratory, University of Arizona, 1979

Rey A: L'examen clinique en psychologie. Paris, Presses Universitaires de France, 1964

Rosen WG: Neuropsychological investigation of memory, visuoconstructional, visuoperceptual, and language abilities in senile dementia of the Alzheimer type, in The Dementias. Edited by Mayeux R, Rosen WG. New York, Raven, 1983, pp 66–74

Scherr PA, Albert MS, Funkenstein HH, et al: The correlates of cognitive function in an elderly population. Am J Epidemiol 28:1084–1101, 1988

Seitelberger F, Gross H, Pilz P: Pick's disease: a neurological study, in Neuropsychiatric Disorders in the Elderly. Edited by Hirano A, Miyashi K. New York, Igaku-Shoin Medical Publishers, 1983, pp 87–117

Silbermann EK, Weingartner H, Laraia, M, et al: Processing of emotional properties of stimuli by depressed and normal subjects. J Nerv Ment Dis 171:10–14, 1983

Steele JC, Richardson JC, Olszewiski J: Progressive supranuclear palsy. Arch Neurol 10:333–359, 1964

Sternberg DE, Jarvik ME: Memory functions in depression. Arch Gen Psychiatry 33:219–224, 1976

Stuss DT, Benson DF: The Frontal Lobes. New York, Raven, 1986

Tagliavini F, Pilleri I: Basal nucleus of Meynert: a neuropathological study in Alzheimer's disease, simple senile dementia, Pick's disease, Huntington's chorea. J Neurol Sci 62:243–260, 1983

Taylor AE, Saint-Cyr JA, Lang AE: Frontal lobe dysfunction in Parkinson's disease. Brain 109:845–883, 1986

Wechsler D: Wechsler Adult Intelligence Scale–Revised. San Antonio, TX, Psychological Corporation, 1981

Wechsler D: Wechsler Memory Scale–Revised. San Antonio, TX, Psychological Corporation, 1987

Wechsler AF, Verity MA, Rosenschein S, et al: Pick's disease: a clinical, computed tomographic, and histologic study with golgi impregnation observations. Arch Neurol 39:287–290, 1982

Weingartner H, Gold P, Ballenger JD, et al: Effects of vasopressin on human memory function. Science 211:601–603, 1981

Whitehouse PJ, Clark DL, Coyle AW, et al: Alzheimer's disease: evidence for selective loss of cholinergic neurons in the nucleus basalis. Ann Neurol 10:122–126, 1981

CHAPTER 12

Richard Margolin, M.D.

Neuroimaging

Introduction

Psychiatric diagnosis in the aged is often difficult. Traditionally, the process has involved interview, general physical and neurological examinations, and laboratory tests. In recent years, these methods have been increasingly complemented by a set of procedures known as *neuroimaging*. This term denotes several methods for creating images of various facets of brain structure or function. Although some neuroimaging techniques were introduced decades ago, the field has become much more sophisticated with the introduction during the past 15 years of powerful computerized methods. The more important and widely utilized of these newer methods include X-ray computed tomography (CT), magnetic resonance imaging (MRI), positron emission tomography (PET), single photon emission computed tomography (SPECT), and computerized electroencephalography. The aim of this chapter is to present an overview of these techniques, including methodology and appropriate use in the geriatric mental disorders. Because it is impossible to discuss the individual techniques comprehensively in this chapter, the reader desiring more information is referred to detailed reviews on CT (Hounsfield 1980), MRI (Partain et al. 1988), PET (Phelps and Mazziotta 1985), and SPECT (Proceedings 1987, 1988). A comprehensive review of the major modalities with particular reference to geriatric psychiatry has also been published (Margolin and Daniel 1990).

Methodology

Although there are many ways to consider the imaging methods, several key concepts deserve special attention. Perhaps the most important is the distinction between structural and functional imaging. *Structural imaging* techniques delineate facets of cerebral anatomy such as the size, location, and shape of brain regions. *Functional imaging* techniques reveal elements of cerebral physiology such as blood flow, metabolism, and parameters of neurotransmission. CT and MRI are structural imaging modalities, whereas PET and SPECT are functional imaging methods.

Another important concept is the spatial nature of the data produced. Earlier brain imaging techniques such as pneumoencephalography were—and so are some techniques still being used (e.g., multiprobe cerebral blood flow [CBF] systems)—essentially planar, collapsing the inherently three-dimensional shape of the brain into two dimensions. The newer methods, by contrast, are all tomographic. A tomogram literally means a picture of a slice. These modalities all produce several parallel, thin, slicelike images of the brain, called tomograms. Tomographic methods are a major advance over planar techniques because they provide markedly increased detail (information density).

A final concept common to all the tomographic techniques is the manner in which their data are collected and displayed. Several standard orientations for data acquisition exist. These are called the transverse, sagittal, and coronal planes. The transverse orientation, although not universally defined in exactly the same way, generally refers to a plane that passes through the orbits and the internal auditory meati. The sagittal plane is roughly perpendicular to the transverse plane and cleaves the midline, through the interhemispheric fissure. The coronal plane is vertically oriented and perpendicular to the sagittal plane.

With regard to data display, sets of images are usually presented using a shades-of-gray scale. The particular meaning of the scale varies with each modality. Color display scales are also employed, but in such schemes individual colors have no special meaning in themselves. Images can be recorded on film or displayed on computer monitors. Currently images are interpreted by a trained radiologist, usually a neuroradiologist, or for some modalities a nuclear medicine specialist. Advances in computer technology and image analysis methods portend semiautomatic interpretation of images in the future.

Computed Tomography

Developed in the 1970s, CT quickly became widely used in neuro-psychiatry. The ability to obtain tomographic images of brain structure noninvasively was perceived by clinicians as a tremendous development. In CT images, gray- and white-matter zones as well as the cerebrospinal fluid (CSF) compartment can be individually visualized. Both normal anatomy and pathological structural alterations can be appreciated. The method uses a thin X-ray beam, which is passed through the head; intervening tissues absorb the beam according to their relative densities. The residual beam is recorded by a detector apparatus. Each image is produced sequentially by slightly advancing the bed on which the patient lies and repeating the data acquisition process. Separately, a computer converts the absorption patterns into images in a procedure called reconstruction. CT can readily distinguish tissues of quite different density but cannot do as well with tissues of marginally different density, such as gray and white matter.

CT is relatively easy for patients to tolerate. Although head-dedicated CT scanners exist, the procedure is generally performed on a device able to admit the torso. Thus, the aperture of the scanner is not confining and a standard examination requires less than an hour. A practical consideration for CT and all the other techniques is that stabilization and immobilization of the patient's head and body during the data acquisition period are essential for high-quality images. Usually, about 15 to 20 slices are obtained in a clinical study; their customary orientation is transverse. In the usual gray-scale display scheme, images are presented with white representing structures of highest density and black those of least density.

CT can be performed with or without "contrast media." This term denotes substances, usually containing iodine, which absorb X rays well. It has been recognized for almost a decade that intracranial blood vessels can be outlined by performing CT after intravenous delivery of contrast media. CT so performed is called a contrast-enhanced scan. Unfortunately, although some pathology is definitely better seen with contrast, a small but significant percentage of patients are allergic to contrast media. Patients at risk cannot always be identified before the procedure is performed. Recently, however, nonionic contrast media with low allergy potential have become available.

Magnetic Resonance Imaging

MRI has become widely used in clinical practice only within the last 5 years. During that time its growth has been phenomenal. In contrast to CT, which measures only tissue density, MRI is actually a set of distinct procedures that as a whole reveals details about various facets of the physicochemical composition of the brain. Magnetic resonance denotes the property of nuclei of certain elements to spin about an axis when exposed to a magnetic field. The most common element possessing this property is hydrogen, and consequently hydrogen (or proton) imaging is the basis of almost all current MRI systems. A magnetic resonance scanner is a device that applies a steady magnetic field together with pulses of radio frequency energy to an area of a patient's body. The scanner also incorporates a receiver that records the response to the applied energy of nuclei in the cells of the body region being scanned.

Two key parameters have been described in MRI that reflect distinct tissue responses to magnetic perturbation. These parameters are called the T1 and T2 relaxation times. Images reflecting either T1 or T2 may be created by varying details of the data acquisition process. The T1-weighted image is somewhat similar to a non-contrast-enhanced CT image of the brain in that it generally represents anatomy and faithfully depicts spatial relationships among structures in the brain. It provides excellent, even extraordinary, visualization of contrast between gray and white matter. T1 MRI is distinctly superior to CT in this regard. The T2-weighted image, on the other hand, is markedly influenced by tissue water content and it does not closely correspond to anatomical detail. It is proving very useful, however, in revealing localized pathology that is not evident on images obtained with other techniques.

A clinical magnetic resonance scan typically includes 15 to 20 images per acquisition. There are quite a number of data acquisition schemes, called *pulse sequences*, currently being explored in cranial MRI, and there is no consensus as to which is the most efficient or useful in neuropsychiatric indications. Probably the most commonly used scheme, however, is the spin echo sequence. In this approach, a proton density and a T2-weighted image are produced essentially simultaneously at each scanning plane. A proton density image is intermediate in appearance between T1- and T2-weighted images. The process is repeated multiple times in order to image the entire brain.

As in CT, a gray-scale image display scheme is customary; however, the term *signal intensity* is used instead of density, reflecting the heterogeneity of the MRI modality. In this scheme, white represents areas of highest signal intensity, and black, the areas of lowest signal intensity. It is important to realize that a given brain structure can appear very different on proton density, T1-weighted, and T2-weighted images; for example, the lateral ventricles are generally seen as black on T1-weighted images and white on T2-weighted images.

In contrast to CT, the patient is not moved between image acquisitions. MRI is somewhat more challenging for patients than CT because the scanner aperture is smaller; thus there is often a feeling of confinement. An MRI examination can sometimes take more than an hour. A significant advantage of MRI is its ability to produce images in any plane, not just the transverse plane. In routine clinical practice, several saggital views and a complete set of transverse images are obtained. However, more extensive saggital or coronal views are very helpful in certain clinical situations. For example, sagittal views image the pituitary gland very well. Contrast media have also been under development for MRI; the first such product, a gadolinium salt, has been approved for clinical use.

Positron Emission Tomography

PET is the most advanced functional neuroimaging modality developed to date. It is a nuclear medicine technique that depends on certain properties of positrons (subatomic particles belonging to the class called antimatter). They have the mass and charge of electrons and are thus also known as antielectrons. Positron-emitting elements for PET do not occur naturally in any quantity but can be produced artificially with a medical cyclotron. Such radioactive elements are then chemically bonded to a molecule of interest in a process known as radiochemistry. Molecules so produced are called radiotracers. In PET, a radiotracer is injected intravenously or inhaled while a patient lies with a part of the body inside the PET scanner's aperture. The PET scanner detects the radiation produced when positrons undergo radioactive decay. Positron radioactive decay is unique in that it produces two gamma rays traveling in essentially opposite directions. The PET scanner uses this property to localize the source of the decay, thus reconstructing images of the distribution of tracer presence.

Many feel that PET has considerable potential in psychiatry. The basis for this viewpoint is twofold. First, positron-emitting isotopes of the key component elements of biologically important molecules exist, including oxygen, carbon, and nitrogen. As a result, among the PET radiotracers that have been created are some very interesting molecules for the study of psychiatric disorders. Second, PET is in principle a quantitative method. Upon introduction to the body, the fate of the PET radiotracer depends on the way the various cellular systems and organs it encounters "see" it. For example, some tracers are extensively metabolized, whereas others are not; some are trapped by the brain, but others remain in the vascular compartment. Although the PET scanner detects only total radioactivity in an organ, a mathematical model can be applied to such uptake data. Such a procedure, called tracer kinetic modeling, enables creation of images that precisely reflect a physiological process.

Although PET brain research began in the 1970s, its applications in psychiatry, and certainly in geriatric psychiatry, are still emerging. With PET several important physiological processes can be imaged, of which regional CBF, regional cerebral glucose metabolism (CMR_{glu}), and regional cerebral oxygen metabolism (CMR_{O_2}) have been the most thoroughly studied so far. However, work with neurotransmission (e.g., dopamine, acetylcholine, and serotonin systems) and protein synthesis is also promising.

Like CT and MRI, PET also generates tomographic images, the exact number being dependent on the particular scanner type. The most current PET scanners produce between 7 and 15 parallel slices simultaneously. For some applications this number suffices; if additional detail is desired, the acquisition can be repeated after moving the patient slightly. From the patient's perspective, PET's endurability is in between that of CT and MRI. Although with some scanners obtaining a single set of slices can take very little time, a complete brain survey (multiple sets of slices) might last from 10 to 30 minutes. At least an intravenous line is almost always necessary, and some types of PET study require arterial catheterization. No contrast media for PET have yet been developed.

Single Photon Emission Computed Tomography

SPECT is a derivation of PET that uses relatively standard nuclear medicine cameras instead of specially developed scanners. The SPECT tracers that have been synthesized until now for neuropsychiatric applications have incorporated isotopes of technetium, iodine, or xenon. Only tracers of CBF have been developed to the level of clinical utility at this time. Two such tracers are now commercially available: ^{123}I-iofetamine (Spectamine, Medi-Physics) and ^{99m}Tc-Hexamethylpropylamine oxime (HMPAO) (Ceretec, Amersham). Although there are complex differences in behavior between these two tracers, the evidence does not suggest the superiority of one or the other in psychiatric applications, and both portray CBF realistically. HMPAO is easier for nuclear medicine departments to use because its radionuclide, technetium, is more available. Although SPECT CBF measurements are approved for clinical use only in stroke so far, research results imply that they are valuable in a variety of neuropsychiatric conditions. New SPECT tracers measuring CBF and other neurochemical processes (e.g., receptor function) are under active development and will likely be available within a few years. Satisfactory quantitative models for SPECT imaging of CBF have not yet been developed for any tracer.

SPECT also produces tomograms, usually about 60. It is quite tolerable for patients. In the most widely implemented system the patient lies on an open bed while a large flat gamma camera orbits the head. No contrast agents for SPECT exist yet.

Practical Considerations in the Use of Neuroimaging in Geriatric Psychiatry

From the perspectives of geriatric psychiatrist, radiologist, and patient, there are many practical distinctions between these methods. Some, such as the length of time for data acquisition and the extent of discomfort, confinement, and invasiveness, are especially important considerations for frail elderly patients and have been discussed. Other factors important in understanding the neuroimaging methods include resolution, hazards, accessibility, and cost. Resolution refers to the detail that can be visualized in an image. Technically it is defined by the smallest objects that can be discriminated within an image. Data concerning these parameters are summarized in Table 12-1.

It is fair to say that each technique has its strengths and weaknesses. In terms of resolution, CT and MRI are clearly superior, but PET has made considerable progress in this respect in recent years; it is approaching a theoretical maximum resolution of approximately 3 mm. The resolution achieved so far with SPECT is quite inferior to that of PET and definitely limits its clinical value; it is still unclear if technological advances will significantly improve SPECT's resolution.

CT, PET, and SPECT all require the use of ionizing radiation,

Table 12-1. Practical considerations in the use of neuroimaging techniques in geriatric psychiatry

Technique	Resolution (mm)	Radiation	Accessibility	Cost per study[a] (dollars)
CT	1–2	Yes	Wide	500
MRI	1–2	No	Fairly wide	750–1,000
PET	5	Yes	Limited	1,200–2,500
SPECT	15	Yes	Increasing	750

[a]Prices do not reflect regional variations unless a range is given and are representative of an average U.S. city market in early 1990. These prices are typical of a "routine" study. Some studies have higher costs if additional optional components are performed.

which is well recognized to carry certain risks. The doses, however, are generally modest and compare favorably with those of traditional radiologic procedures. MRI is alone in not involving radiation exposure. In fact, with the exception of patients with certain types of cardiac pacemaker or surgical clips, its known risks are not significant. As with any new medical procedure or drug, it is possible that long-term risks will become apparent with experience.

Use of Neuroimaging Methods in Geriatric Psychiatry

While neuroimaging has already become useful clinically in some mental disorders of late life (notably the organic dementias), a larger number of conditions have been investigated in research studies. These include organic nondementing syndromes, as well as the psychoses, affective disorders, and anxiety disorders. Only in dementia and normal aging have elderly populations been the specific focus of neuroimaging research programs; in the other disorders, patients and controls of young, middle-aged, and elderly groups have been mixed together. This mixing clearly limits the conclusions that can be drawn at this time about the ultimate value of the imaging techniques in geriatric psychiatry.

In turning to the use of the various imaging methods in geriatric psychiatry, it is reasonable to ask in turn, what is the primary value of the structural and the functional imaging techniques? Anatomic abnormalities in the brain, at the level resolvable with current imaging methods, are "macroscopic." CT and MRI can detect pathology such as atrophy, edema, infarction, and tumor. These disturbances regularly occur in major neuropsychiatric disorders such as dementia, delirium, and poststroke depression. In these conditions the disturbances affect brain structures subserving key psychological processes, for example, cognition, language, mood, and affect. Knowledge of the brain regions affected by such tissue-disruptive processes can enhance the geriatric psychiatrist's understanding of symptomatology.

Potentially much more valuable in appreciating brain-behavior relationships in psychiatric disease are the functional imaging techniques. Details of several neurophysiological processes have now been demonstrated with imaging techniques, including CBF, metabolism, and parameters of neurotransmitter function. It is reasonable to suppose that abnormalities in these physiologic processes may occur in psychiatric disease before their anatomic correlates can be identified. Furthermore, in most psychiatric diseases, anatomic abnormalities are not known. Thus, the functional imaging techniques are regarded by many as promising more sensitive and specific data about neural disturbance in mental disorders than the structural imaging methods can provide.

Aging

Before reviewing neuroimaging findings in individual disorders, it is important to consider briefly some information that has emerged from studies of normal aging. Knowledge of age-specific changes in human neuroanatomy and physiology is developing rapidly. It is already clear that definite structural and physiological changes occur with aging in many brain regions and systems (Veith and Raskind 1988; Waller and London 1987). Some familiarity with the major findings in the neurobiology of aging is crucial because aging-related processes and disease-related processes interact in subtle ways in geriatric psychiatric syndromes. Certain disorders, most notably the dementias, are strongly age associated. Imaging studies inevitably reflect a mixture of age- and disease-related phenomena.

The primary macroscopic morphological change known to occur with aging is brain atrophy, noted as an increase in the volume of the CSF space and a decrease in brain volume (Schwartz et al. 1985). The CSF space in humans is composed of the third, fourth, and lateral ventricles and the subarachnoid space. The ventricles are easily identified on CT or MRI scans in the depths of the brain, whereas the subarachnoid space is visualized as the sulci adjacent to cortical gyri. Besides atrophy, both gray- and white-matter density have also been reported to fall. Finally, white-matter abnormalities of uncertain significance are seen occasionally with CT and regularly with MRI in otherwise normal elderly persons; these abnormalities are discussed in this chapter.

Age-related changes have also been identified in functional measures. CMR_{glu} and CMR_{O_2} seem stable, at least in studies of very healthy individuals, but CBF declines (Duara et al. 1983; Pantano et al. 1984). The regional pattern of these metabolic parameters may change with aging. Ingvar (1979) proposed the term *hyperfrontality* to refer to the normal pattern of frontal CBF being greater than parietal CBF. This pattern is lost with aging. Neurotransmitter physiology changes with age have also been found with PET. For example, Wong and associates (1984) found age-related decrements in dopamine D_2 receptor binding in various cortical regions and the basal ganglia.

Some of the same structural and functional abnormalities that occur in aging have been revealed by neuroimaging methods in various psychiatric diseases in young and middle-aged persons; for example, both ventricular and sulcal enlargement as well as hypofrontality have been found in subpopulations of schizophrenic patients. When patients with such diseases are studied for the first time with imaging procedures in late life, it may be impossible to separate the effects of age and disease. The possibility of dual contributions to imaging findings must, therefore, be borne in mind.

Dementia

Among geriatric psychiatric disorders, dementia is the most common setting for the application of neuroimaging techniques. Two factors have led to this development. The first is the valuable data about cerebral morphology and function, which the techniques now provide. The second is the lack to date of a reliable, biologically based nonimaging method for positive diagnosis of the major dementing disorders. Nevertheless, although the technological advances these techniques have enjoyed in the past two decades have been spectacular, and the likelihood of further progress is substantial, neuroradiological tools have still not replaced the traditional clinical evaluation used in diagnosing dementia and the complementary techniques (e.g., lumbar puncture, electroencephalography, and analysis of blood chemistries) that help identify specific etiologies.

Numerous structural and functional imaging studies of Alzheimer's disease (AD), multi-infarct dementia (MID), and other types of dementia have now been published. In this work CT, MRI,

PET, and SPECT have all been used. A number of well-conducted studies have either focused on individual types of dementia or compared controls with demented patients who had mixed diagnoses. In this section, I first describe the key findings in the several major etiologies, then comment on the clinician's use of the techniques in differential diagnosis.

Alzheimer's Disease

Although presenile-onset and senile-onset dementia of the Alzheimer type have in past times been considered by some to be separate diseases, they are considered in this chapter as one condition called AD. Because AD is the major cause of dementia in developed countries, it is not surprising that this condition has been the dementing disorder most studied by neuroimaging. McGeer (1986) comprehensively reviewed the major neuroimaging studies performed in AD.

Modern structural imaging in AD began with the use of CT. Huckman and colleagues (1975) first found ventriculomegaly with CT in the mid-1970s in virtually all members of a group of elderly dementia victims. Although the severity of brain atrophy has varied, many studies subsequently confirmed the finding in both young (Brinkman et al. 1981) and old (Gado et al. 1982) AD patients.

Because macroscopic cerebral atrophy is generalized in advanced AD, the most common pattern on CT or MRI is matched sulcal and ventricular enlargement. Sulcal enlargement has been less consistently seen than ventriculomegaly, at least in CT studies (Albert et al. 1984a). In addition to global atrophy, various patterns of regional atrophy have also been reported, and the absence of atrophy is commonly encountered, especially in early AD. Thus, AD patients are separable from controls on the basis of CT or MRI findings only statistically in group analyses, not individually.

Besides atrophy, decrements in tissue density (especially in the white matter) have also been reported (Albert et al. 1984b; Bondareff et al. 1981; Naeser et al. 1980). These decrements can be either diffuse and detectable only with quantitative analysis, or focal and identifiable by visual inspection of scans.

Serious efforts have been made to translate findings of atrophy or hypodensity into clinically useful tools for diagnosing AD. Unfortunately, primarily because of the great overlap with findings in normal elderly, it has not been possible to develop either manual or automated schemes for this purpose.

The advent of MRI has occasioned several studies of AD in recent years (Besson et. al. 1983, 1985; Brant-Zawadzki et al. 1985; Erkinjuntti et al. 1984; Fazekas et al. 1987). In an early study, McGeer (1986) confirmed that brain atrophy could be identified with MRI. Besson and associates (1983) found increased T1 values in gray and white matter of many cortical regions; this group (1985) also found increased white-matter proton density values. MRI has produced some intriguing findings, not previously seen clearly with CT, with respect to the status of the white matter in AD. These data are discussed in detail in this chapter.

It is not surprising that AD has been one of the disorders most actively explored by PET investigators. CBF, CMR_{O_2}, and CMR_{glu} changes have all been investigated. Frackowiak (1987) reviewed these studies comprehensively. Two key findings have emerged from this work. The first is that all three parameters of brain metabolism are significantly decreased in advanced AD, on the order of 20% to 30% (Frackowiak et al. 1981). Despite the reductions in blood flow, evidence has been developed that suggests that occult hypoperfusion is not directly involved in the pathogenesis of AD.

Second, a pattern seemingly unique to AD has been noted in imaging of CMR_{glu}; this pattern has been replicated by several groups (Benson et al. 1983; Chase et al. 1984; Duara et al. 1986; Ferris et al. 1983; Friedland et al. 1983). The pattern consists of a localized metabolic deficiency in the posterior parietal and temporal lobes, bilaterally (Chase et al. 1983). With advancing disease the frontal lobes are also affected and the severity of the metabolic dysfunction increases, particularly in the parietal lobes (Jagust et al. 1987). Chase's group (Foster et al. 1983) also demonstrated that the site of focal hypometabolism in AD sometimes parallels predominant features of the clinical presentation. For example, some AD patients with prominent aphasia had focal defects in the left temporal cortex, whereas patients with marked visuospatial incoordination had such abnormalities in the superior right parietal lobe. It is not yet apparent how often these nonparietal or unilateral parietal focal deficits occur.

Two focal points of recent PET work in AD are noteworthy. The first concerns the manifestations of AD early in its course. Haxby and associates (1985) have identified parietal lobe metabolic defects even in minimally demented patients who could not be distinguished from controls in neuropsychological tests thought to be mediated by parietal systems. Another theme of recent research is the comparison of patients with early-onset versus late-onset AD. Small and colleagues (1987) have shown that early-onset patients show parietal hypometabolic defects more significantly than late-onset patients.

A number of SPECT studies of AD have also now been conducted; the results confirm the PET finding of biparietal hypoperfusion (Holman 1986; Testa et al. 1988).

Multi-infarct Dementia

The classic CT signature of MID is the presence of multiple non-enhancing infarcts, which can be of variable size and can be located in the cortex, white matter, or subcortical nuclei. There are several variants of MID, and the terminology needs improvement. One variant of MID, subcortical arteriosclerotic encephalopathy (SAE)—Binswanger's disease—appears on CT as multiple infarcts in the periventricular white matter (Roman 1987). Infarcts caused by occlusion of perforating arteries in the subcortical nuclei and white matter are called *lacunes*. Thus, another variant of MID, in which multiple lacunes exist, is known as the lacunar state. Lacunes are usually less than 1 cm in size, and may be round or slit-like. They account for up to 20% of strokes (Mohr 1983). Unfortunately, the absence of visible strokes on CT scans of patients with dementia does not entirely rule out MID, because some strokes are isodense with surrounding parenchyma (Harsch et al. 1988) and because some may be very small (Cummings 1987; Knopman and Rubens 1986; Kohlmeyer 1979). CT more commonly misses brain stem strokes, but in practice its sensitivity in chronic supratentorial stroke is very high (Aichner and Gerstenbrand 1989).

The MRI features of stroke and MID have been the subject of several careful reviews (Ford et al. 1989; Kessler 1988). Characteristic findings exist for both early and completed stroke. The geriatric psychiatrist generally does not evaluate patients with MID in close proximity to acute strokes; thus the pattern in completed stroke is the more relevant. The majority of strokes are thrombotic in origin; a minority are hemorrhagic. Completed thrombotic infarctions typically demonstrate a pattern of decreased signal intensity on T1-weighted images and increased signal on T2-weighted images. Chronic hemorrhagic infarctions display a core of hyperintense signal on T1- and T2-weighted images surrounded by a rim of hypointense signal, especially on T2-weighted images (Ford et al. 1989). Although the resolution is similar in MRI and CT, MRI is superior in detecting small infarctions, especially lacunes (Brown et al. 1988), and also brain stem strokes.

An important and still imperfectly clarified issue in the application of neuroimaging in dementia is the significance of the white-matter lesions (WMLs) revealed by MRI. Not long after the introduction of MRI into general clinical use, WMLs, particularly in T2-weighted images, were reported in scans of both normal elderly patients and patients with dementia (Bradley et al. 1984; Brant-Zawadzki et al. 1985). A number of groups have now investigated this subject in detail (Fazekas et al. 1987; George et al. 1986) and have identified several distinct patterns, including periventricular lesions, ventricular pole lesions, and focal (punctate) or diffuse (confluent) abnormalities in the deep white matter.

The several patterns previously described have varying significance. Frontal horn capping is not necessarily pathological (Zimmerman et al. 1988). It may represent an age-accentuated pattern of CSF transudation from the interstitial space into the ventricles. Uniform periventricular hyperintensity is of similarly uncertain diagnostic significance, occurring commonly in both normal elderly and demented individuals (Fazekas et al. 1987). Discrete, deep WMLs may have a variety of causes, ranging from frank infarction to chronic vascular insufficiency (Braffman et al. 1988). Vasculitis and multiple sclerosis, known causes in younger persons, must also be considered if the clinical data so indicate.

Considerable variation exists in the frequency of WMLs reported (Erkinjuntti et al. 1984; George et al. 1986), but a rate of about 30% in unselected elderly patients is credible (Braffman et al. 1988). Although these lesions are clearly found in some normal individuals (Fazekas 1989), they are more frequently encountered in dementia than in normal aging (Fazekas et al. 1987). They occur in both AD and MID at a rate higher than that seen in normals; a rate approaching 100% is reported in MID. Suggestive of a vascular etiology, their frequency increases with cardiovascular risk factors, including hypertension and diabetes mellitus (Gerard and Weisberg 1986). However, even in patients with such risk factors, extrapolation from the finding of WMLs to a diagnosis of SAE is a temptation not supported by present knowledge. Many more demented patients have WMLs than meet strict criteria for SAE (Caplan and Schoene 1978). Furthermore, not even prominent WMLs rule out AD.

PET findings in MID are based on the results of stroke research performed with this technique. Several studies have noted the metabolic and blood flow patterns in acute and completed strokes. The examination of CBF, CMR_{glu}, CMR_{O_2}, and the oxygen extraction fraction (OEF) in stroke is useful. Normally these parameters are tightly coupled and blood supply is not limiting. OEF is an indicator of the reserve capacity of blood flow. Although the changes in these parameters during the evolution of a stroke are complex, a completed stroke classically produces a region of matched hypometabolism and decreased blood flow (Frackowiak 1987). OEF is not increased. The zone of hypometabolism is often substantially larger than would be predicted from examining CT or MRI scans. Abnormalities in distant sites are seen which reflect the impact of a stroke on neural connectivity. The larger functional than structural zone of impairment indicates that tissue surrounding the infarct may be damaged but still alive and reflects biochemical processes initiated by the stroke in surrounding tissue. MID presents on PET scans as focal areas of decreased metabolism and blood flow in the areas of known infarcts (Frackowiak 1985). There is no specific regional pattern in MID as there is in AD. Only very incomplete comparison studies of the diagnostic value of PET and CT/MRI in stroke have been executed; the work done so far supports the idea that they could have complementary roles. SPECT studies of MID are yet fragmentary also, but as with AD, they generally confirm the PET findings.

Other Dementias

A multitude of etiologic entities besides AD and MID can cause dementia. These include neurodegenerative dementias such as Pick's disease, progressive supranuclear palsy, Huntington's disease (HD), and the dementia associated with Parkinson's disease (PD); normal pressure hydrocephalus (NPH)-induced dementia; Creutzfeldt-Jakob disease and other infectious disorders; posttraumatic dementia; dementia induced by hypoxia; alcoholic and other metabolic dementias; and endocrine-related dementias. Recently added to this list is dementia due to human immunodeficiency virus (HIV) infection. The neuroimaging findings in all of these dementias cannot be individually reviewed here, but a few comments may be helpful.

Some of these dementias have specific associated neuroimaging findings. In Pick's disease, for example, the diagnosis is supported by the finding of focal frontotemporal atrophy and reductions in CBF and CMR. In progressive supranuclear palsy, retention of a rim of cortical metabolism/flow surrounding a generalized frontal reduction has been claimed. In NPH, ventriculomegaly out of proportion to sulcal atrophy may be seen with either CT or MRI. Periventricular hyperintensity may also be seen on MRI in this condition. Dementia due to HIV infection is frequently associated with the finding of focal areas of white-matter hypodensity on CT or similar zones of increased T2 signal on MRI.

Other Organic Mental Disorders

PD and HD have also been studied by neuroimaging. CT and MRI are not often abnormal in PD, but PET shows some promise in assisting diagnosis of this condition in that CMR_{glu} is reduced by approximately 20% (Kuhl et al. 1984). Imaging of dopamine receptors in the basal ganglia is being investigated and might even more directly facilitate assessment of the condition in the future. Psychiatric complications of PD, including dementia, and L-dopa–induced psychosis are common, but studies of subgroups of PD patients with and without these complications have not yet been undertaken.

HD is commonly associated with psychiatric symptoms. In advanced disease, caudate head atrophy can be seen with structural imaging. Earlier in the course of the disease a characteristic metabolic signature has been demonstrated with PET (Phelps et al. 1982), namely, a marked reduction in basal ganglia CMR_{glu}. The concept has been advanced that this phenomenon may be detectable even preclinically (Mazziotta et al. 1987).

Psychoses

Considerable neuroimaging research has been conducted in schizophrenia. Shelton and Weinberger (1986) and Coffman and Nasrallah (1986) summarized the structural studies using CT and MRI, respectively. As these reviews indicate, many studies using CT and several using MRI have replicated the original finding of ventriculomegaly in schizophrenia (Johnstone et al. 1978) or found sulcal enlargement. Nasrallah and associates (Coffman and Nasrallah 1986) have suggested that these phenomena may be related to fetal or peripartum events with prolonged or delayed neurodevelopmental expression. Because increase of CSF space is also associated with aging, prudence is advised in the interpretation of scans from elderly schizophrenics.

Several groups have studied schizophrenia with PET. The major finding in these studies has been hypofrontality of CBF and CMR (Buchsbaum et al. 1984; Wolkin et al. 1988). A correlation with chronicity and negative symptoms has been suggested. Few of these studies included many elderly patients. It is also worth noting that no study has yet been published concerning the very important geriatric psychiatric syndrome of late-onset psychosis or paraphrenia. The appropriate clinical use of neuroimaging in elderly schizophrenics is currently limited to the setting of a change in psychopathologic symptoms, suggestive of the onset of another condition, particularly an organic brain disorder.

Affective Disorders

The relatively few structural imaging studies in affective disorders have rarely focused on elderly patients. Jaskiw and colleagues (1987) and Schlegel and Kretzschmar (1987a, 1987b) reviewed the majority of studies performed. In adult patients of diverse ages, several investigators noted relative ventricular enlargement as well as associations between ventriculomegaly and the presence of various indices of severity, including delusions, chronicity, and number of hospitalizations. The results, overall, did not reveal consistent anatomic abnormalities in such conditions as major depression, bipolar disorder, or dysthymia.

In view of the essential absence of known anatomic correlates of affective disorders, and because of their cyclic nature, the functional neuroimaging techniques are best fitted for investigating them. The first such studies of affective disorders actually used a nonimaging technique, namely, the multiple probe ^{133}Xe techniques (both intraarterial and inhalational) of regional CBF. These studies had predictably complex results (reviewed by Margolin and Daniel 1990) with both the presence of differences (Mathew et al. 1980) and the absence of differences (Gur et al. 1983; Silfverskiold and Risberg 1989) being reported between unipolar depressed, bipolar depressed, and bipolar manic patients and controls studied at rest. Treatment response was also investigated.

Although the Xenon probe techniques are still being used, methodological complexities and limitation of the data produced to cortical structures are factors favoring the replacement of these methods by PET and SPECT. Again, few if any studies specifically focusing on elderly patients have been reported. PET studies have explored CMR_{glu} differences between various mood disorder groups and controls. In two early studies (Baxter el al. 1985; Buchsbaum et al. 1984), no difference in whole brain metabolism was found between unipolar depressives and controls. The Baxter study found relatively reduced values in a bipolar depressed subgroup, however, and the Buchsbaum study reported hypofrontality, again especially in the bipolar depressed subgroup. A more recent study by Baxter and associates (1989) reported a localized deficiency in left anterolateral prefrontal cortex in both unipolar and bipolar depressives, versus normals or bipolar manics. With medication and especially response to medication, this abnormality normalized. It is interesting that the location of this abnormality is the same as the predominant location of cortical damage in stroke patients who become depressed (Robinson et al. 1984). Unfortunately, the sample size in all these studies was small, limiting permissible conclusions.

Neuroimaging and Differential Diagnosis

From the geriatric psychiatrist's perspective, perhaps the most important use of neuroimaging is in differential diagnosis, because a variety of distinct neurological and psychiatric disorders present in late life with a common set of psychopathological features. The primary differential diagnostic use of neuroimaging in geriatric psychiatry so far has been in the evaluation of dementia. Not only can various neurological and systemic conditions cause dementia, but functional psychiatric conditions, usually severe depression, can imitate it (depressive pseudodementia) (Wells 1979).

Both structural and functional neuroimaging methods have potential roles in the differential diagnosis of dementia. CT and MRI are useful in the exclusion of a number of structural brain diseases that can cause dementia. CT's value as a screening tool in this process is indisputable; its relatively limited cost is a particular asset.

Using pulse sequences producing both T1- and T2-weighted images, MRI is superior to CT for detecting cerebral atrophy and structural abnormalities. Virtually all the disorders that can be detected by CT can be appreciated at least as well by MRI. Whether MRI will replace CT as the primary neuroimaging screening tool depends primarily on economic factors (MRI is still moderately

Table 12-2. Common geriatric psychiatric disorders that can be evaluated by structural neuroimaging

Alzheimer's disease
Stroke and multi-infarct dementia
Tumors (both benign and malignant)
Hydrocephalus, including normal pressure hydrocephalus
Brain trauma and hemorrhage
Subdural hematoma
Abscess
Encephalitis, HIV-induced neuropathology

Source. Adapted from Margolin and Daniel 1990, Table 4.

more expensive) and other practical factors. Table 12-2 shows a number of disorders that entail associated cognitive, affective, or personality changes, the diagnosis of which can be facilitated by CT or MRI. Figure 12-1 shows images typical of some of these conditions.

In addition to positively identifying specific dementing etiologies, structural imaging can be used for true differential diagnosis by subgrouping patients on the basis of their imaging findings. For example, Naeser and colleagues (1980), using CT attenuation values as an indicator of brain density, were able to differentiate patients with presenile dementia from patients with pseudodementia.

Because cerebral dysfunction is likely to occur earlier than structural pathology in most geriatric psychiatric disorders, PET and SPECT should enable advances in differential diagnostic capabilities. Their use for this purpose has been documented in dementia. Kuhl (1984) demonstrated that PET can distinguish dementia of the Alzheimer type (DAT), MID, and depressive pseudodementia (Figure 12-2). It should be remembered that, in the absence of postmortem histopathological examination, no "gold standard" exists against which imaging findings must be compared.

Serial scans can be helpful in distinguishing etiologies, and occasionally specialized neuroimaging modalities are appropriate. An example of a specialized procedure is radionuclide cisternography, which can help to distinguish NPH dementia from AD. Sluggish CSF dynamics, as demonstrated by prolonged lateral ventricle retention of a radiotracer injected into the lumbar CSF space, correlates with NPH dementia. Similarly, angiography may be helpful in suspected cerebral vasculitis.

Future Prospects

Structural neuroimaging will remain essential for detecting several key neurological disorders of late life associated with significant mental symptoms, at least until definitive biological tests become available for specific disorders. CT's long-term future in this area is uncertain because MRI is likely to assume an increasingly routine role. In MRI, postmortem correlations are urgently needed to clarify the issue of the significance of white-matter pathology that is found so frequently (Braffman et al. 1988).

Although structural imaging tools will remain valuable, the ar-

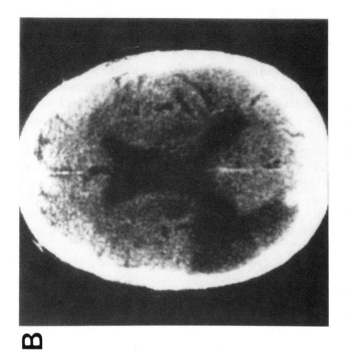

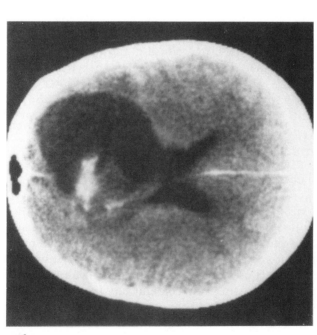

Figure 12-1. A: CT image of a low-grade astrocytoma presenting clinically as insidiously progressive dementia without localizing signs. B: CT image of a right parietal lobe (nondominant hemisphere) stroke, presenting with behavior change out of proportion to focal neurological findings. C: MRI image of extensive white-matter abnormalities in an elderly patient with clinically mixed dementia, Alzheimer type, and multi-infarct dementia. D: MRI image of an arachnoid cyst; chemical characteristics of the cyst fluid distinguished it from subdural hematoma, obviating a diagnostic trephination.

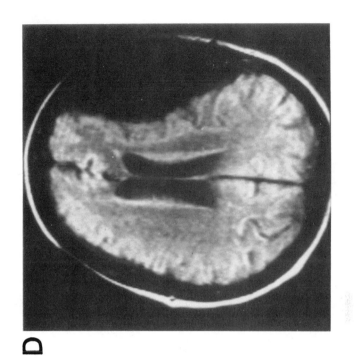

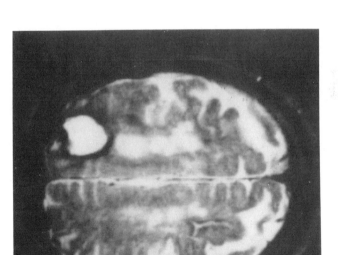

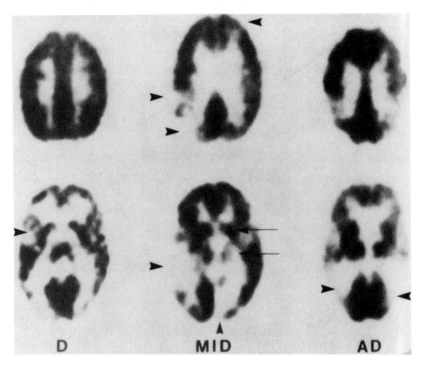

Figure 12-2. From Kuhl (1984) and reproduced by permission. Three clinical entities (*left, right,* and *middle* image sets) studied by PET. For each case the *upper* image represents a higher slice and the *lower* image represents a lower brain slice. The *left* image set demonstrates the left anterior prefrontal lobe metabolic deficit noted in depression. The *center* image set displays irregular zones of reduced metabolism compatible with areas of infarction seen on CT and with anatomical defects seen later on postmortem examination. This pattern is seen in multi-infarct dementia. The *right* image set demonstrates the bilateral parietal defect characteristic of AD.

rival of functional neuroimaging techniques (PET and SPECT) may genuinely alter the diagnostic strategy in geriatric psychiatry. The change will come about if the promise of these techniques in such areas as the imaging of neurotransmitter physiology and the brain correlates of mental or emotional activity can be realized and made practical in clinical situations. For example, it is possible that studies of cholinergic systems in AD (Coyle et al. 1983), norepinephrine and serotonin in mood disorders, and dopamine in schizophrenia and late-onset psychosis will become regular components of future diagnostic evaluations. Such studies might be performed at baseline and after administration of a potentially effective course of pharmacotherapy. Alternatively, future metabolic or blood flow investigations in depression or dementia might employ cognitive tasks during imaging, to differentially activate specific brain regions. For PET to fulfill its potential, cost and access obstacles must fall; for SPECT to achieve recognized clinical status, quantitative models for the physiological processes being imaged must be developed. Whatever the details, however, reasoned speculation suggests that neuroimaging has a substantial future in geropsychiatry.

References

Aichner F, Gerstenbrand F: Computed tomography in cerebrovascular disease, in Handbook of Clinical Neurology, vol 10. Vascular diseases series, part II. Edited by Toole JF. Amsterdam, Elsevier Science, 1989

Albert M, Naeser MA, Levine HL, et al: Ventricular size in patients with presenile dementia of the Alzheimer's type. Arch Neurol 41:1258–1263, 1984a

Albert M, Naeser MA, Levine HL, et al: CT density numbers in patients with senile dementia of the Alzheimer's type. Arch Neurol 41:1264–1269, 1984b.

Baxter LR, Phelps ME, Mazziotta JC, et al: Cerebral metabolic rates for glucose in mood disorders. Arch Gen Psychiatry 42:441–447, 1985

Baxter LR, Schwartz JM, Phelps ME, et al: Reduction of prefrontal cortex glucose metabolism common to three types of depression. Arch Gen Psychiatry 46:243–250, 1989

Benson DF, Kuhl DE, Hawkins RA, et al: The fluorodeoxyglucose 18F scan in Alzheimer's disease and multi-infarct dementia. Arch Neurol 40:711–714, 1983

Besson JA, Corrigan FM, Foreman EI, et al: Differentiating senile dementia of Alzheimer type and multi-infarct dementia by proton NMR imaging. Lancet 2:789, 1983

Besson JA, Corrigan FM, Foreman EI, et al: Nuclear magnetic resonance (NMR), 2: imaging in dementia. Br J Psychiatry 146:31–35, 1985

Bondareff W, Baldy R, Levy R: Quantitative computed tomography in senile dementia. Arch Gen Psychiatry 38:1365–1368, 1981

Bradley WG, Waluch V, Brant-Zawadzki M, et al: Patchy periventricular white matter lesions in the elderly; a common observation during NMR imaging. Noninvasive Medical Imaging 1:35–41, 1984

Braffman BH, Zimmerman RA, Trojanowski JQ, et al: Brain MR: pathologic correlation with gross and histopathology, 2: hyperintense white-matter foci in the elderly. AJR 151:559–566, 1988

Brant-Zawadski M, Fein G, Van Dyke C, et al: MR imaging of the aging brain: patchy white-matter lesions and dementia. AJNR 6:675–682, 1985

Brinkman SD, Sarwar M, Levin HS, et al: Quantitative indexes of computed tomography in dementia and normal aging. Radiology 138:89–92, 1981

Brown JJ, Hesselink JR, Rothrock JF: MR and CT of lacunar infarcts. AJR 151:367–372, 1988

Buchsbaum MS, DeLisi LE, Holcomb HH, et al: Anteroposterior gradients in cerebral glucose use in schizophrenia and affective disorders. Arch Gen Psychiatry 41:1159–1166, 1984

Caplan LR, Schoene WC: Clinical features of subcortical arteriosclerotic encephalopathy (Binswanger disease). Neurology 28:1206–1215, 1978

Chase TN, Foster NL, Mansi L: Alzheimer's disease and the parietal lobe. Lancet 2:225, 1983

Chase TN, Foster NL, Fedio P, et al: Regional cortical dysfunction in Alzheimer's disease as determined by positron emission tomography. Ann Neurol 15(suppl):S170–S174, 1984

Coffman JA, Nasrallah HA: Magnetic resonance imaging in schizophrenia, in The Neurology of Schizophrenia. Edited by Nasrallah HA, Weinberger DR. Amsterdam, Elsevier, 1986

Coyle JT, Price DL, DeLong MR: Alzheimer's disease: a disorder of cortical cholinergic innervation. Science 219:1184–1190, 1983

Cummings JL: Multi-infarct dementia: diagnosis and management. Psychosomatics 28:117–125, 1987

Duara R, Margolin RA, Robertson-Tchabo EA, et al: Resting cerebral glucose utilisation as measured with positron emission tomography in 21 healthy men between the ages of 21 and 83 years. Brain 106:761–775, 1983

Duara R, Grady C, Haxby J, et al: Positron emission tomography in Alzheimer's disease. Neurology 36:879–887, 1986

Erkinjuntti T, Sipponen JT, Iivanainen M, et al: Cerebral NMR and CT imaging in dementia. J Comput Assist Tomogr 8:614–618, 1984

Fazekas F: Magnetic resonance signal abnormalities in asymptomatic individuals: their incidence and functional correlates. Eur Neurol 29:164–168, 1989

Fazekas F, Chawluk JB, Alavi A, et al: MR signal abnormalities at 1.5 T in Alzheimer's dementia and normal aging. AJR 149:351–356, 1987

Ferris SH, de Leon MJ, Wolf AP, et al: Positron emission tomography in dementia, in The Dementias. Edited by Mayeux R, Rosen WG. New York, Raven, 1983, pp 123–129

Ford CS, Buonanno FS, Kistler PJ: Magnetic resonance imaging in cerebrovascular disease, in Handbook of Clinical Neurology, vol 10. Vascular diseases series, Part II. Edited by Toole JF. Amsterdam, Elsevier Science Publishers, 1989

Foster NL, Chase TN, Fedio P, et al: Alzheimer's disease: focal cortical changes shown by positron emission tomography. Neurology 33:961–965, 1983

Frackowiak RS: The pathophysiology of human cerebral ischaemia: a new perspective obtained with positron tomography. Q J Med 57:713–727, 1985

Frackowiak RS: Energy metabolism and neurotransmitter function in ageing and the dementias, in Clinical Efficacy of Positron Emission Tomography. Edited by Heiss W-D, Pawlik G, Herholz K, et al. Amsterdam, Martinus Nijhoff, 1987

Frackowiak RS, Pozzilli C, Legg NJ: Regional cerebral oxygen supply and utilisation in dementia: a clinical and physiological study with oxygen-15 and positron tomography. Brain 104:753–778, 1981

Friedland RP, Budinger TF, Ganz E: Regional cerebral metabolic alterations in dementia of the Alzheimer type: positron emission tomography with (18-F)-2-fluorodeoxyglucose. J Comput Assist Tomogr 7:590–598, 1983

Gado M, Hughes CP, Danziger W, et al: Volumetric measurements of the cerebrospinal fluid spaces in demented subjects and controls. Radiology 144:535–538, 1982

George AE, de Leon MJ, Kalnin A, et al: Leukoencephalopathy in normal and pathologic aging, 2: MRI of brain lucencies. AJNR 7:567–570, 1986

Gerard G, Weisberg LA: MRI periventricular lesions in adults. Neurology 36:998–1001, 1986

Gur RE, Skolnick BE, Gur RC: Brain function in psychiatric disorders, II: regional cerebral blood flow in medicated unipolar depressives. Arch Gen Psychiatry 41:695–699, 1983

Harsch HH, Tikofsky RS, Collier BD: Single photon emission computed tomography imaging in vascular stroke. Arch Neurol 45:375–376, 1988

Haxby JV, Duara R, Grady CL, et al: Relations between neurophysiological and cerebral metabolic asymmetries in early Alzheimer's disease. J Cereb Blood Flow Metab 5:193–200, 1985

Holman LB: Perfusion and receptor SPECT in the dementias—George Taplin memorial lecture. J Nucl Med 27:855–860, 1986

Hounsfield GN: Computed medical imaging. J Comput Assist Tomogr 4:665–674, 1980

Huckman MS, Fox JH, Topel JL: The validity of criteria for the evaluation of cerebral atrophy by computerized tomography. Radiology 116:85–92, 1975

Ingvar D: Hyperfrontal distribution of the cerebral grey matter flow in resting wakefulness: on the functional anatomy of the conscious state. Acta Neurol Scand 60:12–25, 1979

Jagust WJ, Budinger TF, Reed BR: The diagnosis of dementia with single photon emission computed tomography. Arch Neurol 44:258–262, 1987

Jaskiw GE, Andreasen NC, Weinberger DR: X-ray computed tomography and magnetic resonance imaging in psychiatry, in Psychiatry Update: American Psychiatric Association Annual Review, Vol 6. Edited by Hales RE, Frances AJ. Washington DC, American Psychiatric Press, 1987, pp 260–299

Johnstone EC, Crow TJ, Frith CD: The dementia of dementia praecox. Acta Psychiatr Scand 57:305–324, 1978

Kessler RM: NMR imaging of ischemic cerebrovascular disease, in Magnetic Resonance Imaging, 2nd Edition. Edited by Partain CL, Price RR, Patton JA, et al. Philadelphia, PA, WB Saunders, 1988

Knopman DS, Rubens AB: The validity of computed tomographic scan findings for the localization of cerebral functions: the relationship between computed tomography and hemiparesis. Arch Neurol 43:328–332, 1986

Kohlmeyer K: A comparison of cerebral angiography and computer tomography in patients with stroke. Fortschr Geb Roentgenstr Nuklearmed 131:361–368, 1979

Kuhl DE: Imaging local brain function with emission computed tomography. Radiology 150:625–631, 1984

Kuhl DE, Metter EJ, Riege WH: Patterns of cerebral glucose utilization in Parkinson's disease and Huntington's disease. Ann Neurol 15(suppl):S170, 1984, pp 119–125

Margolin RA, Daniel DG: Neuroimaging in geropsychiatry, in Clinical and Scientific Psychogeriatrics, Vol 2. Edited by Bergener M, Finkel SI. New York, Springer, 1990, pp 162–186

Mathew RJ, Meyer JS, Francis DJ: Cerebral blood flow in depression. Am J Psychiatry 137:1449–1450, 1980

Mazziotta JC, Phelps ME, Pahl JJ, et al: Reduced cerebral glucose metabolism in asymptomatic subjects at risk for Huntington's disease. N Engl J Med 316:357–362, 1987

McGeer PL: Brain imaging in Alzheimer's disease. Br Med Bull 42:24–28, 1986

Mohr JP: Lacunes. Neurol Clin 1:201–221, 1983

Naeser MA, Gebhardt C, Levine HL: Decreased computerized tomography numbers in patients with presenile dementia. Arch Neurol 37:401–409, 1980

Pantano P, Baron JC, Lebrun-Grandie P: Regional cerebral blood flow and oxygen consumption in human ageing. Stroke 15:635–641, 1984

Partain CL, Price RR, Patton JA, et al (eds): Magnetic Resonance Imaging, 2nd Edition. Philadelphia, PA, WB Saunders, 1988

Phelps ME, Mazziotta JC: Positron emission tomography: human brain function and biochemistry. Science 228:799–809, 1985

Phelps ME, Mazziotta JC, Huang S-C: Study of cerebral function with positron computed tomography. J Cereb Blood Flow Metab 2:113–162, 1982

Proceedings of the clinical SPECT symposium. Am J Physiol Imaging 2:127–166, 1987

Proceedings of the hexamethyl-propylene amine oxime (HM-PAO) symposium. J Cereb Blood Flow Metab 8(suppl):S95-S123, 1988

Robinson RG, Kubos KL, Starr LB, et al: Mood disorders in stroke patients: importance of location of lesion. Brain 107:81–93, 1984

Roman GC: Senile dementia of the Binswanger type: a vascular form of dementia in the elderly. JAMA 258:1782–1788, 1987

Schlegel S, Kretzschmar K: Computed tomography in affective disorders,

Part I: ventricular and sulcal measurements. Biol Psychiatry 22:4–14, 1987a

Schlegel S, Kretzschmar K. Computed tomography in affective disorders, Part II: brain density. Biol Psychiatry 22:15–23, 1987b

Schwartz M, Creasey H, Grady CL, et al: Computed tomographic analysis of brain morphometrics in 30 healthy men, aged 21 to 81 years. Ann Neurol 17:146–157, 1985

Shelton RC, Weinberger DR: X-ray computed tomography studies in schizophrenia: a review and synthesis, in Handbook of Schizophrenia, Vol 1. Edited by Nasrallah HA, Weinberger DR. Amsterdam, Elsevier, 1986

Silfverskiold P, Risberg J: Regional cerebral blood flow in depression and mania. Arch Gen Psychiatry 46:253–259, 1989

Small GW, Kuhl DE, Riege WH, et al: Cerebral glucose metabolic patterns in Alzheimer's disease: effect of gender and age at dementia onset. Arch Gen Psychiatry 46:527–532, 1989

Testa HJ, Snowden JS, Neary D, et al: The use of [99mTc]-HM-PAO in the diagnosis of primary degenerative dementia. J Cereb Blood Flow Metab 8(suppl):S123–S126, 1988

Veith RC, Raskind MA: The neurobiology of aging: does it predispose to depression? Neurobiol Aging 9:101–117, 1988

Waller SB, London ED: Noninvasive diagnostic techniques to study age-related cerebral disorders, in Psychogeriatrics: An International Handbook. Edited by Bergener M. New York, Springer, 1987

Wells CE: Pseudodementia. Am J Psychiatry 136:895–900, 1979

Wolkin A, Angrist B, Wolf A, et al: Low frontal glucose utilization in chronic schizophrenia: a replication study. Am J Psychiatry 145:251–253, 1988

Wong DF, Wagner HN, Dannals RF, et al: Effects of age on dopamine and serotonin receptors measured by positron tomography in the living human brain. Science 226:1393–1396, 1984

Zimmerman RD, Fleming CA, Lee BC, et al: Periventricular hyperintensity as seen by magnetic resonance: prevalence and significance. AJNR 7:13–20, 1988

CHAPTER 13

Andrew Leuchter, M.D.

Electroencephalography

Introduction

The electroencephalogram (EEG) was developed as a clinical test in the 1930s by a psychiatrist, Dr. Hans Berger. Ironically, in the more than five decades since its introduction into clinical practice, it has become a technique most commonly performed under the supervision of, and interpreted by, neurologists. Neurologists have in fact made the greatest use of this test, using it to help corroborate the diagnosis of seizure disorders.

Since its introduction, however, it has been clear that the EEG has a special role in the assessment of older adults. Berger (1937) himself reported that the EEG changes with aging and is abnormal in a high proportion of individuals with dementia. To date, the EEG remains the single most cost-effective physiologic test to indicate the presence of an encephalopathy. It therefore is incumbent on the geriatric psychiatrist to understand the fundamentals of EEG interpretation.

Despite the frequency with which the test is ordered, the specific indications for the test as well as the guidelines for interpreting the results remain unclear. This chapter reviews the major clinical uses of the EEG, its role in evaluating common clinical syndromes, and the usefulness of EEG results.

Indications for Electroencephalography

There are two primary reasons to perform an EEG in geriatric psychiatry: 1) to evaluate a possible organic mental disorder, and 2) to evaluate a possible seizure disorder. Although the test is commonly ordered to "rule out" one of these conditions, normal EEG results cannot rule out brain disease; they simply establish that the presence of such disease is less likely.

An EEG is not indicated whenever brain disease is known or suspected to exist. Rather, the test is useful primarily in four situations: 1) the presence of brain disease is suspected, but there is no clear etiology or the presentation is unusual; 2) the presence of brain disease is possible, but it is difficult to differentiate from some other psychiatric illness (e.g., depression); 3) the course of a psychiatric illness is unusual or the illness is refractory to treatment; and 4) a structural imaging study would be advisable but is unavailable.

Electroencephalogram Findings of Normal Aging

Any discussion of the application of electroencephalography must consider that the normal EEG in the elderly may differ significantly from that seen in young adults. The EEG cannot fully exclude a diagnosis of brain disease in the elderly, because many of the findings of "normal" aging may mimic brain disease.

Although there is considerable variation in the normal EEG at any age, a typical EEG in a young adult (aged 20–60) who is resting and awake with eyes closed shows a pattern of moderate-amplitude, sinusoidlike electrical activity in the back of the head at a frequency of 8 Hz to 12 Hz (the so-called posterior dominant or "alpha" rhythm), with a mean frequency for young adults of 10 Hz. Visual inspection of the EEG shows negligible slow-wave activity in the 0- to 4-Hz range ("delta") and little detectable in the 4- to 8-Hz range ("theta"), except when the patient is drowsy. Low-amplitude fast activity (greater than 12 Hz, or "beta" rhythms) predominates in the anterior and central head regions.

In adults aged over 60, increased "slowing" is said to occur as a normal finding. This slowing may be of two types. First, there commonly is slowing of the posterior dominant rhythm. This rhythm remains in the alpha range, but the mean for a group of elderly subjects reportedly slows to 9 Hz by age 90. Some normal elderly subjects have been reported to have alpha rhythms as slow as 8 Hz, but a posterior dominant rhythm below the alpha range in the waking and alert state always is considered pathologic (Obrist 1976; Obrist et al. 1966).

The second type of normal slowing is intermittent theta slowing seen over the temporal regions. This slow activity, which is intermixed with the normal background rhythms, commonly occurs at a frequency of 6 Hz to 8 Hz and may occur in brief runs. It has been reported to occur in up to 40% of normal volunteers (Busse et al. 1954; Torres et al. 1983). Some investigators believe that this pattern of mild, intermixed slowing is indicative of subclinical cerebrovascular disease, and they have shown that in carefully screened controls the true prevalence drops tenfold. For current clinical standards, however, this finding is still considered within normal limits (Niedermeyer 1987a).

Slowing may be accentuated by drowsiness in either young or old, but it is particularly likely to emerge early in drowsiness among elderly subjects. This slowing is most often seen in the frontal regions, where trains of semirhythmic delta activity may be seen. This delta slowing may occasionally be mistaken for frontal intermittent rhythmic delta activity (FIRDA), a pathologic rhythm often associated with metabolic encephalopathy and sometimes deep midline lesions (Zurek et al. 1985). The elderly may be more likely to become drowsy during EEG recordings because of sensory losses, so it is vital that they be alerted often during the procedure and that their state of arousal is noted in the report.

Other EEG changes also are commonly seen with aging. Amplitude of the signal generally decreases, as does the response to photic stimulation (Niedermeyer 1987a). In some individuals, there is an increase in the amount of sharp-wave activity seen in the temporal regions intermixed with slowing, but this activity should be readily distinguishable from true epileptiform activity. The changes in beta activity with aging are unclear, with equal numbers of studies finding either increases or decreases in fast activity (Niedermeyer 1987a; Spehlmann 1981).

Electroencephalogram in the Evaluation of Specific Disorders

Many of the various clinical situations that may prompt the geriatric psychiatrist to order an EEG are discussed in the following sections.

Primary Degenerative Dementia of the Alzheimer's Type

The finding that first generated clinical interest in the EEG was that institutionalized demented patients demonstrated excessive, diffuse slowing of background rhythms, as well as slowing of the posterior dominant rhythm. This finding proved to be nonspecific, seen primarily in more advanced cases of dementia as well as in a variety of organic conditions.

Five decades of clinical experience, however, have demonstrated that the EEG has clear uses in patients with possible or definite organic mental disorders. The most common use is in the initial evaluation of possible Alzheimer's disease (AD). Experts differ as to the indications for an EEG in the initial evaluation: some believe that it should be ordered in all cases; a National Institutes of Health consensus conference concluded that the test should be ordered when the etiology of the dementia is unclear or the presentation is unusual (Group for the Advancement of Psychiatry 1988). Because the etiology of dementia is usually unclear and presentations frequently are unusual, an EEG is ordered in most cases in clinical practice.

The EEG frequently is not ordered in the initial evaluation of a patient with possible AD because it is generally believed that the EEG is normal in cases of mild dementia (Cummings and Benson 1983). A recent study found, however, that among 104 patients whose testing had shown normal or equivocal mental status and were to be evaluated for possible dementia, the EEG was abnormal in more than 40% of cases (Daly and Leuchter 1990). These findings suggest that the standard EEG is highly sensitive to the presence of even mild encephalopathy. Replication of these results is necessary before the EEG is made an integral part of the initial evaluation of all subjects.

When a baseline tracing from the patient's premorbid state is available, the EEG may be particularly helpful in the evaluation of subsequent dementia. A patient's EEG may remain within normal limits for all, but it may eventually show slowing that is excessive for that individual. Baseline tracings, however, are seldom available.

Other Causes of Dementia

The EEG does have some utility in the differential diagnosis of dementia, and it may help to distinguish AD from other dementing illnesses.

Multi-infarct dementia commonly shows focal or lateralizing abnormalities, in contrast to the diffuse and symmetric pattern of slowing seen in AD. Focal abnormalities frequently are absent in cases of multi-infarct dementia, however; cases of diffuse deep white-matter ischemic disease (i.e., Binswanger's disease) where there are no cortical infarcts or lesions "undercutting" the cortex may show a pattern indistinguishable from that of AD. Structural imaging studies of the brain (computed tomography, magnetic resonance imaging) clearly are most useful in corroborating the diagnosis of multi-infarct dementia.

In Creutzfeldt-Jakob disease, an uncommon cause of dementia in the elderly, the EEG reveals frontally predominant triphasic waves, paroxysmal lateralizing epileptiform discharges, or some other pseudoperiodic sharp-wave complex, within 12 weeks of onset of clinical symptoms in more than 90% of cases (Spehlmann 1981). As the disease progresses, these sharp-wave complexes attenuate and disappear into a background of slow-wave activity. Although it is not pathognomonic of the illness, the presence of a pseudoperiodic discharge in the presence of a rapidly progressive dementia is highly suggestive of the diagnosis. The absence of these periodic discharges after 10 weeks of clinical symptoms makes the diagnosis suspect (Chiappa and Young 1978).

Huntington's chorea frequently presents with a progressive loss of amplitude of the EEG, with or without slowing. The dementia accompanying thyroid disease may present with dramatic attenuation of EEG amplitude. Other forms of dementia, such as Pick's disease, or the dementia accompanying Parkinson's disease or progressive supranuclear palsy, do not have characteristic EEG presentations that help distinguish them from AD (Niedermeyer 1987b; Spehlmann 1981).

Even in the forms of dementia that do have particular EEG presentations, the EEG usually is primarily a tool for confirming the diagnosis; clinical history and physical examination are likely to be more useful in establishing the diagnosis.

Depression

The EEG is particularly useful in cases in which there is a suspicion that cognitive impairment is caused by depression. Neuropsychologic tests, commonly used in such cases, are liable to be adversely affected by motivational or attention problems. The EEG, however, is a clinically available measure of brain function that can help distinguish between these two illnesses. Abnormal EEG results are not seen in uncomplicated depression (Small 1987). Normal EEG results may be seen early in the course of a dementia, however, so that follow-up testing may be necessary to detect an encephalopathy.

Toxic and Metabolic Conditions

The EEG is useful in detecting excess morbidity due to reversible toxic or metabolic conditions, because it is a sensitive (albeit nonspecific) screen for encephalopathic conditions. For example, a patient with mild cognitive impairment but severe slowing on EEG may have another disease process instead of, or in addition to, AD (Cummings and Benson 1983).

A common finding in the elderly is that one or more medications that a patient is receiving are causing a toxic encephalopathy. Such an encephalopathic process would be expected to present electrographically with increased slow-wave activity as well as slowing of the posterior dominant rhythm. It may be difficult to determine when medications are causing or contributing to an encephalopathy, because, even in therapeutic dosages, many psychoactive and nonpsychoactive drugs may cause EEG changes. Antidepressants or neuroleptics commonly cause slowing of the posterior dominant rhythm and an increased amount of slow-wave activity (Fink 1968). Lithium similarly may cause increased slowing, and at toxic levels it may cause focal abnormalities or spike discharges (Law 1979). Benzodiazepines and other sedative-hypnotics usually cause increased beta activity in therapeutic doses (Fink 1968), most commonly a pattern of frontocentrally predominant, 20- to 25-Hz, beta activity. In high doses, these drugs may cause increased slowing as well.

One of the most common causes of drug-induced cognitive dysfunction in the elderly is drugs with anticholinergic effects. These drugs routinely cause increased amounts of slowing in the EEG (Pfefferbaum et al. 1979). If increased slowing is detected in the EEG of a patient taking a drug known to cause cognitive dysfunction, it may be prudent to discontinue or replace the drug with a nonoffending agent.

The EEG may help to detect unsuspected metabolic derangements, because blood chemistry panels cannot screen for all possible endocrinopathies, electrolyte imbalances, and toxic substances. Apart from increased slowing, other patterns that may be seen in metabolic encephalopathy include FIRDA, triphasic waves, and sharp waves. Depending on the distribution and the frequency of occurrence of these waveforms, they may suggest a specific etiology of metabolic encephalopathy. For example, the most common cause of 2- to 3-per-second frontally predominant triphasic waves is hepatic encephalopathy. Such waveforms also may be seen, however, in patients with chronic renal failure (Hughes 1982). The clinical history and other laboratory tests clearly are necessary to interpret these nonspecific findings.

Delirium and Changes in Mental Status

Although the EEG is most often ordered in the elderly for evaluating possible dementia, the most justifiable use is in the evaluation of delirium. It was first established in the 1940s that the degree of slowing in the EEG among delirious patients is directly related to the level of confusion, and that improvements in the EEG reflect improvements in mental status (Engel and Romano 1944; Romano and Engel 1944). The EEG, therefore, is an important confirmatory tool, and it is difficult to make the diagnosis of delirium in the absence of EEG slowing (Lipowski 1987). The EEG may also be useful in evaluating the course of delirium. Interventions to improve the patient's condition should diminish EEG slowing, and persistent severe slowing suggests either that the cause of the delirium has not been corrected or that another illness (i.e., dementia) exists. It is unclear how long EEG slowing may persist after the resolution of a delirium.

When a patient's mental status has declined acutely and a cerebrovascular accident is suspected, the EEG will demonstrate focal slowing to document a cerebrovascular accident, whereas the CT scan may not show any changes for 5 days (Niedermeyer 1987c). In situations in which a structural imaging study of the brain is desirable but unavailable, the EEG may be used. It is important to note that there may be a significant mass lesion, particularly in the deep white matter, without any EEG changes.

Finally, the EEG may be useful in following the course of a dementing illness. As a patient's mental status declines, the EEG is marked by concomitant increased slowing, loss of the posterior dominant rhythm, and, occasionally, the emergence of spike foci. If the patient has had a baseline EEG and later suffers an abrupt decline in function, a repeat tracing may be useful in determining the cause of the loss in functional status. For example, a significant decline in function with no change in EEG patterns would be unusual and might suggest the development of superimposed depression.

Seizure Disorders

Most patients who develop seizure disorders do so before age 65. The most common causes of seizures with onset late in life are stroke, trauma, and mass lesions. Among these individuals, the EEG is useful to confirm the diagnosis, to help establish the type of seizure, and to define the area of origin of the epileptic discharge. The geriatric psychiatrist generally does not establish the diagnosis of epilepsy or initiate treatment of seizures; these tasks usually are performed by a consulting neurologist. In this section I therefore focus primarily on clinical guidelines for the ordering and interpretation of EEG in patients with possible seizures.

Seizures in the elderly most commonly present with periodic alterations in level of consciousness or behavior. In most cases the diagnosis is straightforward, with frank lapses of consciousness that may be associated with loss of motor tone or abnormal movements, incontinence, and postictal confusion. In such cases, the EEG provides confirmatory evidence and may help guide treatment.

In some cases—such as patients with possible loss of consciousness, episodic confusion, waxing and waning mental status, refractory depression, or panic attacks—a seizure disorder enters the differential diagnosis. The discovery of a seizure focus in these patients may be clinically significant, because there are reports in the literature of individuals with seizure foci whose refractory depressions or panic disorders are responsive to anticonvulsants. The index of suspicion for seizures usually is not high in such cases, and the EEG typically is ordered for "atypical" cases, such as a patient with panic attacks who is briefly unresponsive; it is not routinely recommended for evaluation of patients with panic disorder. The test usually is requested to "rule out seizures." The EEG, however, cannot rule out a seizure disorder; it has been estimated that 15% to 30% of patients with seizure disorders have normal EEGs (Niedermeyer 1987d).

To perform an adequate electrographic screen for a seizure disorder, a recording at least 30 minutes long should be performed; using several different electrode montages. Furthermore, if the patient's physical health and mental state permit, activation procedures such as hyperventilation, photic stimulation, stage II sleep, and sleep deprivation may be useful to activate an underlying seizure focus.

In cases in which epileptiform abnormalities (i.e., spikes or spike-and-wave complexes) are detected, a diagnosis of a seizure disorder is not certain. Depending on the location and nature of the abnormality, epileptiform abnormalities predict the existence of a clinical seizure disorder with certain degrees of reliability: frequent spike-and-wave complexes in the anterior temporal region are correlated with clinical seizures in more than 90% of otherwise healthy adults; isolated occipital spikes have less than a 40% correlation with seizures (Niedermeyer 1987d). The surest method to establish a link between an observed epileptiform abnormality and a possible seizure disorder is to perform prolonged (possibly ambulatory) EEG recording and to observe changes in the state or behavior of the patient that are linked to electrographic changes.

In interpreting the significance of epileptiform abnormalities, the clinical history and condition of the patient must be considered. Some chronic illnesses (such as renal failure) or degenerative diseases of the brain (such as AD) may lead to the development of generalized sharp waves or spike foci that have a low association with clinical seizures. In the final analysis, seizures are diagnosed on the basis of clinical presentation (Pinkus and Tucker 1985).

Conclusion

The EEG plays a prominent role in the evaluation of brain disease among geriatric psychiatry patients, and it is generally quite sensitive to the presence of encephalopathic conditions as well as seizure disorders. The EEG tracing generally does not yield results that are diagnostic for any illness; rather its findings are either consistent with (e.g., slowing in AD), supportive of (e.g., triphasic waves in Creutzfeldt-Jakob disease), or highly suggestive of the presence of a particular illness (e.g., anterior temporal spike-and-wave foci in a seizure disorder).

The most common use of the EEG, for the evaluation of possible encephalopathy, is limited somewhat by difficulties in quantitating "normal" amounts of slowing in the elderly. This limitation may soon be eased by the use of brain mapping (i.e., quantitative electroencephalography), which can both quantitate the amount of slowing in an individual's EEG and compare it to age- and gender-based norms. Computer-based techniques have been shown to enhance the sensitivity of conventional EEG in the detection of abnormal brain electrical activity in dementia (Brenner et al. 1988). Brain mapping is not yet in clinical use, and it probably will never supplant the EEG in certain clinical situations such as detection of seizure foci. The more widespread application of computer-based techniques in the near future probably will significantly expand the usefulness of electroencephalography in geriatric patients.

References

Berger H: On the electroencephalogram of man: twelfth report. Archiv für Psychiatric und Nervenkrankheiten 106:165–187, 1937

Brenner RP, Reynolds CF, Ulrich RF: Diagnostic efficacy of computerized spectral versus visual EEG analysis in elderly normal, demented, and depressed subjects. Electroencephalogr Clin Neurophysiol 69:110–117, 1988

Busse EW, Barnes RH, Silverman AJ, et al: Studies of the process of aging: factors that influence the psyche of elderly persons. Am J Psychiatry 110:897–903, 1954

Chiappa K, Young R: The EEG as a definitive diagnostic tool early in the course of Creutzfeldt-Jacob disease. Electroencephalogr Clin Neurophysiol 45:26p 1978

Cummings J, Benson D: Dementia: A Clinical Approach. Boston, MA, Butterworths, 1983

Daly K, Leuchter A: The diagnostic usefulness of the electroencephalogram early in the course of a dementing illness. Proceedings of the Combined Southern California Regional Meeting of the Society of General Internal Medicine and the American Geriatrics Society, Los Angeles, March 1990

Engel G, Romano J: Delirium, II: reversibility of the electroencephalogram with experimental procedures. Archives of Neurology and Psychiatry 51:378–392, 1944

Fink M: EEG classification of psychoactive compounds in man: a review and theory of behavioral associations, in Psychopharmacology: A Review of Progress 1957–1967. Edited by Effron DH. Washington, DC, U.S. Government Printing Office, 1968, pp 497–507

Group for the Advancement of Psychiatry: The Psychiatric Treatment of Alzheimer's Disease. New York, Brunner/Mazel, 1988

Hughes JR: EEG in Clinical Practice. Boston, MA, Butterworths, 1982

Law MD: Evaluation of psychiatric disorders and the effects of psychotherapeutic and psychomimetic agents, in Current Practice of Clinical Electroencephalography. Edited by Klass DW, Daly DD. New York, Raven, 1979, pp 395–419

Lipowski Z: Delirium (acute confusional states). JAMA 258:1789–1792, 1987

Niedermeyer E: EEG and old age, in Electroencephalography: Basic Principles, Clinical Applications, and Related Fields, 2nd Edition. Edited by Niedermeyer E, Lopes da Silva F. Baltimore, MD, Urban and Schwarzenberg, 1987a, pp 301–308

Niedermeyer E: EEG and dementia, in Electroencephalography: Basic Principles, Clinical Applications, and Related Fields, 2nd Edition. Edited by Niedermeyer E, Lopes da Silva F. Baltimore, MD, Urban and Schwarzenberg, 1987b, pp 309–315

Niedermeyer E: Cerebrovascular disorders and EEG, in Electroencephalography: Basic Principles, Clinical Applications, and Related Fields,

2nd Edition. Edited by Niedermeyer E, Lopes da Silva F. Baltimore, MD, Urban and Schwarzenberg, 1987c, pp 275–299

Niedermeyer E: Epileptic seizure disorders, in Electroencephalography: Basic Principles, Clinical Applications, and Related Fields, 2nd Edition. Edited by Niedermeyer E, Lopes da Silva F. Baltimore, MD, Urban and Schwarzenberg, 1987d, pp 405–510

Obrist WD: Problems of aging, in Handbook of Electroencephalography and Clinical Neurophysiology, Vol 6A. Edited by Remond A. Amsterdam, Elsevier, 1976, pp 207–229

Obrist WD, Henry CE, Justiss WA: Longitudinal changes in the senescent EEG: a 15-year study. Proceedings of the Seventh International Congress of Gerontology. Vienna, International Association of Gerontology, 1966

Pfefferbaum A, David KL, Coulter CL, et al: EEG effects of physostigmine and choline chloride in humans. Psychopharmacology 62:225–233, 1979

Pinkus J, Tucker G: Behavioral Neurology. New York, Oxford University Press, 1985

Romano J, Engel G: Delirium, I: electroencephalographic data. Archives of Neurology and Psychiatry 51:356–377, 1944

Small J: Psychiatric disorders and EEG, in Electroencephalography: Basic Principles, Clinical Applications, and Related Fields, 2nd Edition. Edited by Niedermeyer E, Lopes da Silva F. Baltimore, MD, Urban and Schwarzenberg, 1987, pp 523–539

Spehlmann R: EEG Primer. Amsterdam, Elsevier, 1981

Torres F, Faoro A, Loewenson R, et al: The electroencephalogram of elderly subjects revisited. Electroencephalogr Clin Neurophysiol 56:391–398, 1983

Zurek R, Schiemann Delgado J, Froescher W, et al: Frontal intermittent rhythmic delta activity and anterior bradyrhythmia. Clin Electroencephalogr 16:1–10, 1985

SECTION 3

Psychiatric Disorders

CHAPTER 14

Stephen Read, M.D.

The Dementias

Cognitive disorders are frequent concerns for the geriatric psychiatrist. Acquired cognitive impairment can be caused by at least 70 known disorders, including primary brain diseases as well as diseases of other organ systems causing secondary brain dysfunction (Cummings and Benson 1983). Chronic mental impairment due to brain disease is an epidemic problem in developed countries. It was estimated in 1987 (U.S. Congress Office of Technology Assessment 1987) that approximately 1.5 million Americans now suffer severe dementia and an additional 1 million to 5 million have mild to moderate dementia. The startlingly high frequency reported from a community survey in Boston (Evans et al. 1989)—especially the 46% for people older than 85 years—lacks neuroimaging as well as pathologic confirmation but is in line with frequencies reported for dementia as a whole. Because dementia is more common among the elderly than among other age groups, the number of severely demented will increase by 60% by the year 2000 and by 400%—to 7.4 million—by 2040 if current trends continue. In the absence of effective treatments for the most common of these illnesses, the burden is expected to fall heavily on community resources and institutions providing long-term care.

The recognition little more than a decade ago that dementia is a major and growing public health problem (Plum 1979) has resulted in increasing research efforts and a flow of new information. Clinical, pathological, and neurobiological definitions of these illnesses are evolving rapidly and so the synopses in this chapter are necessarily brief. Most attention is properly directed to Alzheimer's disease (AD), the most common cause of dementia; other dementias are often discussed in compendia concerning AD (e.g., Cummings and Benson 1983; Reisberg 1983).

Diagnosis and Symptomatology

"Dementia" designates an organic mental syndrome defined by the presence of cognitive deficits, most particularly memory impairment. A variety of psychological and behavioral disturbances may be present, but they do not contribute directly to the diagnostic criteria. Clinical diagnosis is supported by finding a specific organic factor causing brain dysfunction (e.g., hypothyroidism) or by recognizing a characteristic clinical syndrome, such as AD, which cannot yet be confirmed by laboratory testing; evidence for these "specific etiological factors" are discussed more fully in this chapter and in Chapter 9. Evaluation for dementia may be requested by the patient or—because the illness may blunt the patient's insight—by family members or a community agency; or another physician may refer the patient because of suspected impairment in thinking, change in personality, or disturbance in mood or behavior.

DSM-III-R (American Psychiatric Association 1987) requires five criteria for the diagnosis of dementia (see Table 14-1). Memory impairment is the cardinal symptom. Suspicion of a memory disorder also makes suspect the patient's anamnesis; history should be elicited from collateral sources in addition to the patient whenever possible. Both short- and long-term memory processes are impaired in dementia, although the former may be more prominent and appear earlier. Isolated short-term memory deficit (anterograde amnesia) is characteristic of amnestic disorder (see Chapter 15).

In addition to memory impairment, there must be at least one

Table 14-1. DSM-III-R diagnostic criteria for dementia

A. Impairment of short- and long-term memory
B. One of the following:
  (1) Impaired abstract thinking
  (2) Impaired judgment
  (3) Aphasia, apraxia, agnosia, constructional difficulty
  (4) Personality change
C. Disturbance of work and/or social relationships or activities
D. Not occurring exclusively during the course of delirium
E. Evidence for, or reasonable presumption of, an organic etiologic factor

Source. From American Psychiatric Association 1987. Reprinted with permission.

additional deficit to diagnose dementia; usually several coexist. Problem solving is hampered by deterioration of abstract thinking. Various degrees of language disturbance (aphasia), inability to carry out verbal commands (apraxia), or impaired capacity to understand perceptions (agnosia) are common. Mood and personality frequently change. Patients commonly have poor insight into their decreased capacities, and their judgments may be impulsive and imprudent.

"Significant interference" with daily functioning may be subtle or obvious, but it requires exploration of the difficulties actually present and allows for rating the degree of dementia as mild, moderate, or severe. A functional evaluation based on activities of daily living provides a useful framework for review. Self-care activities include dressing, grooming, eating, moving about, sleeping, and toileting. So-called "instrumental" activities include skills such as shopping, driving, handling money, using the telephone, and using tools. A review of these activities of daily living also provides an opportunity to define the onset, progression, duration, and persistence of symptoms and to explore situational and physical factors. Standard scales for activities of daily living are available, but they are not always sufficient; some emphasize "physical functioning," and others have proved more useful measures of caregiver perception and stress than of actual patient capacities (Kane and Kane 1981).

Confusion or "clouded sensorium" is the typical presentation in metabolic encephalopathy, referred to as the syndrome of delirium in DSM-III-R. Although patients with dementia may suffer from superimposed delirium, one must always be on the lookout for the encephalopathy masquerading as dementia. Disturbance of attention is one of the most prominent features of delirium and is commonly tested by repetition (digits forward or repeating sentences of increasing difficulty), but it may be revealed only by failure at a more stringent task requiring sustained attention (cf. Chapter 11). A diffusely abnormal electroencephalogram is common in delirium but unusual in early dementia. The laboratory may be helpful in the differential diagnosis.

Differential Diagnosis and Evaluation

Disorders to be considered in the differential diagnosis of dementia (see Table 14-2) may be grouped as follows: 1) syndromes other than dementia; 2) identifiable disorders causing a secondary de-

Table 14-2.   Differential diagnosis of dementia

Nondementias
  "Normal" aging
  Mental retardation
  Focal brain syndromes (e.g., amnesia, aphasia)
  Delirium

Illnesses with a secondary dementia
  Psychiatric
    Mood disorders, especially depression
    Factitious/conversion disorder
    Schizophrenia
  Medical
    Major organ system impairment
    Endocrine
    Infectious
    Other
  Neurologic
    Movement disorders
      Huntington's disease (chorea)
      Parkinson's disease
      Progressive supranuclear palsy
    Hydrocephalus
    Mass lesions
  Vascular (multi-infarct dementia)

Primary dementias
  Alzheimer's disease
  Pick's disease
  Creutzfeldt-Jakob disease

mentia; and 3) primary dementias or illnesses of brain in which the dementia is the major manifestation (Cummings and Benson 1983; U.S. Congress Office of Technology Assessment 1987). For the most part, this differential diagnosis involves clinical recognition of disparate syndromes; laboratory evaluation will play an important and (it is hoped) growing role in the future.

Dementia is acquired; mental retardation is congenital. Confusion may arise for clinicians who encounter an anonymous patient (who wanders, for example, into an emergency room) or who are deciding whether a mentally retarded patient suffers decline from a previously attained capacity (in which case dementia is properly diagnosed). Amnestic syndrome is the only focal brain syndrome specifically recognized by DSM-III-R, but a Wernicke's aphasia, a frontal lobe personality syndrome due to tumor, or a right parietal syndrome due to middle cerebral artery stroke can mimic dementia. Diagnostic studies, especially neuroimaging, may or may not reveal such lesions, and careful clinical evaluation and mental status testing are critical skills for detecting them. Neuropsychological testing is an important tool to document the pattern of cognitive deficits and provide a baseline against which future progression can be measured. Psychometric tests are also the current "gold standard" for determining efficacy in experimental drug testing; these topics are discussed in Chapter 11.

Improvement in patients mistakenly diagnosed as suffering from the progressive dementia of a degenerative brain disorder is frequently due to the failure to recognize psychiatric disorders (Nott and Fleminger 1975; Ron et al. 1979). Such patients are often said to suffer from "pseudodementia," although functional and cognitive impairment clearly accompany the episode. The term *pseudodementia* has fallen out of favor and is being replaced, for example, by "dementia syndrome of depression" (Folstein et al. 1975; Reifler 1982). Mania, psychosis, anxiety, personality, and conversion disorders have been reported, but depression remains by far the most frequent psychiatric disorder mimicking and/or associated with dementia, especially in older patients (Caine 1981; Wells 1979). The reader is referred to the specific chapters in this book for descriptions of these conditions.

Although medical disorders constitute a minority of cases in reported series, failure to identify a treatable illness is a grave injustice to the patient. Fiscal policies that discourage full evaluation are also shortsighted. The clinical workup should be guided by the findings in each case, but at a minimum should include complete blood count, blood chemistries, thyroid function studies, electrocardiogram, and neuroimaging before the diagnosis of a progressive degenerative brain disorder such as AD is made.

Treatment for specific causes of dementia are addressed in this chapter. The concept of controlling risk factors for dementia has emerged, but at this time it cannot be extended much beyond indications for controlling risk factors for cardiovascular disease and general health. Definition of nutritional, environmental, and metabolic factors that are associated with dementia may lead to more helpful recommendations in the future.

Management Considerations

In addition to the diagnostic considerations outlined in the previous section, a comprehensive evaluation requires characterization of behavior patterns, definition of degree of progression, and assessment of the strengths and weaknesses of the patient's support network. Dementia is a chronic disorder, and a long-term perspective should be adopted from the outset, with the interaction of medical, behavioral, family, and community factors (Cummings and Miller 1990; Jarvik and Winograd 1988). Periodic evaluation, with determination of functional level, supports reevaluation of whether a new symptom—agitation, incontinence, weight loss—represents the appearance of a new disorder or is explicable in terms of the dementia.

Psychiatric and behavioral disorders are serious concerns for many dementia caregivers (Rabins et al. 1982). Understanding that many of these abnormalities are an outgrowth of the primary dementing illness may be comforting to the family. Environmental manipulation is sufficient to manage some situations. For example, installing a second lock that must be opened simultaneously with the more familiar first one may be enough to prevent a patient from wandering away from home. For others, the problem may be more severe or refractory to a behavioral approach and may require medical intervention. Dangerous, acutely developing behaviors and refractory symptoms may be managed best in an inpatient psychiatry unit.

Psychotropic medicines, reviewed by Satlin and Cole (1988), are frequently prescribed for dementia patients. Sometimes the indication is a fully developed psychiatric syndrome such as paranoia or major depression, but the psychotropics are often prescribed for a more vaguely defined complex such as "agitation." There are few studies to support this practice; most reports are anecdotal, and even attempts at controlled studies often have heterogeneous patient populations and poorly defined outcome measures. In this state of ignorance, it is especially appropriate to emphasize caution because of the multiple potential side effects of these agents. Review of clinical experience, however, suggests that judicious use may sustain the patient in a given supportive network, facilitate needed care activities, reduce potentially dangerous behaviors, and delay the need for institutionalizing some patients.

Several types of agents can be considered. Neuroleptics appear to have replaced minor tranquilizers as the most frequently used agents to "calm" patients, although a recent review of their use (Gottlieb and Piotrowski 1990) confirmed an absence of compelling efficacy studies. No agent is clearly better than another, although side-effect profiles may dictate a choice. When neuroleptics are prescribed, low doses are recommended. Patients are monitored closely for gait and postural instability due to secondary parkinsonism, orthostatic hypotension, lethargy, and oversedation. Akathisia can make patients more agitated. Periodic observation for the development of dyskinesia is prudent. After stabilization, periodic dose reductions are necessary to enable an assessment of continued utility.

It is not surprising to find few clear guidelines for the use of antidepressants, given the controversy and problems with the evaluation of depression in dementia patients (discussed more fully in the "Alzheimer's Disease" section). Alleviation of severe depression, however, can produce an impressive improvement in function. There are case reports to support the use of most types of antidepressant treatment in the dementia patient, including tricyclics, monoamine oxidase inhibitors, stimulants, and electroconvulsive therapy (Gierz et al. 1990). The use of these agents is reviewed elsewhere, but recommendations again include initiating treatment with low doses, small dose increments, and close monitoring to minimize morbidity from side effects such as confusion, sedation, excitement, urinary retention, and orthostatic hypotension.

Community resources should be evaluated for their availability and applicability to the patient's situation (Read 1990). Safety and security of the home, availability of space to walk when the patient is no longer oriented, and the safety of the neighborhood are factors in deciding place of residence. Transportation may become a major difficulty, especially if the patient used to be the principal driver in the household. If the current situation is appropriate, stability tends to favor the cognitively impaired patient's ability to live in the community by maximizing the use of residual habits and memory.

The severity of dementia provides a rough guide to the degree of support required and the optimal treatment setting. The patient with mild impairments has difficulty with abstract tasks and instrumental activities but can generally stay at home and possibly even continue to work at a reduced level of responsibility. A moderate degree of dementia signals the need for assistance with personal care. Structured social activity in community-based day care or in-home support by family members or hired assistants provides a stable and stimulating but nonthreatening program for the patient and a rest for the caregiver. Availability and reimbursement for these services vary widely; precise indications and benefits remain poorly defined (Vogel and Palmer 1982). In severe dementia, the demands for care are heavy, requiring full-time nursing care either at home or in an institutional setting.

Careful review of financial resources and legal status is warranted, preferably early in the patient's course. The patient's realization that the illness will lead to loss of independence can produce anxiety, fears of abandonment, loss of self-esteem, and guilt. Although it may be potentially threatening, discussing plans for the future and concrete actions to clarify his or her affairs and ensure security can be very comforting to the dementia patient. More concrete benefits may derive from arrangements for retirement, health plans, consideration of long-term care insurance, and disposition of assets. Clear expressions of preferences with regard to surrogate decisionmakers and desired intensity of medical intervention help ensure that future care will be guided by the patient's values.

In eliciting symptoms and defining their context, the psychiatrist also learns about the caregivers' capacities and the resources available or needed in each case; the demands on caregivers often seem to constitute a "36-hour day" (Mace and Rabins 1982). Care can be physically difficult and may involve emotional relearning and redefinition of interpersonal roles (Jarvik and Small 1988). The patient's physician must be aware of the caregiver's needs and resources because the patient's well-being is inextricably dependent on the continued attention of the caregiver. Breakdowns in this system may lead to neglect or even physical abuse.

Regular meetings with other dementia caregivers provide emotional and practical sustenance important for the endurance of many caregivers; referrals to existing support groups may be made through local resources or by contacting the national office of The Alzheimer's Association. Depression appears in caregivers more commonly than in control populations (Brody 1989). Appropriate attention to caregiver dysfunction and health may be the most beneficial action possible for a given family system.

Decisions about institutional placement are particularly difficult for the caregiver. The disability leading to the need for full-time nursing care generally develops insidiously, but it may become evident with a sudden deterioration in the patient's condition or external situation. Caregivers must weigh their needs and perceptions as well as those of the patient. Reality testing concerning both the patient's current condition and the available resources can help to resolve the caregiver's feelings. Perhaps the most common problem is guilt or denial on the part of the caregiver, which may motivate an attempt to keep the patient at home longer than is prudent. Other families may seek institutional care before the patient's condition warrants. When available, short-term admissions that provide respite to the support system can delay the need for permanent placement and may accustom both patient and caregiver to the separation process.

Alzheimer's Disease

Etiology

The cause of AD is not yet known. Several hypotheses have been summarized in the second edition of *Dementia: Guidelines for Diagnosis and Treatment* (U.S. Department of Veterans Affairs 1989).

Acetylcholine Hypothesis. Disruption of cholinergic mechanisms damages memory in animals and humans. Acetylcholine (ACh) is consistently reduced in AD and may play a specific role in brain dysfunction, especially memory impairment (Bartus et al., 1982). Although ACh receptor density is relatively unchanged in AD, choline acetyltransferase activity is reduced, especially in the temporal lobes. In addition, decreases in ACh markers correlate with the degree of cognitive impairment in AD. Cortical cholinergic innervation appears to arise from small groups of cells anteroinferior to the putamen; these basal nuclei (sometimes called "of Meynert") are selectively devastated in AD. These observations form the basis of a cholinergic hypothesis of AD and provide the rationale for cholinergic augmentation (Coyle et al. 1983).

Genetic Hypothesis. Genetic factors are suspected as etiologically significant in at least some patients with AD. Approximately 10% of AD patients report other affected family members, and a recent review tallied 88 reported families in whom 48.6% of adults overall developed AD (St. George-Hyslop et al. 1989). These patients with positive family histories often have early onset of their disease, and the pattern is most consistent with autosomal dominant transmission. Some (e.g., Breitner et al. 1988) have suggested that in apparently sporadic cases a genetic factor is disguised by mortality from other causes before AD appears, but this contention remains controversial. Molecular genetic investigations, following Davies (1986), have also produced conflicting results: a marker on chromosome 21, explored because of the high frequency of AD pathology in aging Down's syndrome patients, has been claimed and challenged, another locus has been reported but unconfirmed, and the likelihood of heterogeneity has been raised again; see the commentaries following George-Hyslop and colleagues' review (1989).

Microtubule Hypothesis. This hypothesis proposes that a defect in microtubules (which form the spindle that spatially orients chromosomes, control directed cell migration, and facilitate transport of neurotransmitters in neurons) represents a common pathologic mechanism for AD and Down's syndrome. The hypothesized microtubular defect in AD is consonant with other findings, including 1) the observation of an impaired philothermal response in Alzheimer's patients, 2) increased numerical chromosome abnormalities found in Alzheimer's patients, 3) the association between Down's syndrome and AD, 4) delayed reappearance of microtubule network following colchicine treatment of skin fibroblasts from Alzheimer's patients compared to controls, and 5) defective microtubule assembly in Alzheimer brain (Matsuyama and Jarvik 1989).

Aluminum Hypothesis. Aluminum remains the most popular candidate for an environmental factor in the etiology of AD. Essentially absent in normal brain, it is not only present in AD, but appears to be particularly associated with senile plaques (SPs) and neurofibrillary tangles (NFTs). What type of exposure to this ubiquitous element would lead to AD, however, remains undiscovered.

Glutamatergic Hypothesis. Degeneration of glutamatergic nerve terminals has been reported to occur in brain specimens from patients with histopathologically confirmed AD. L-Glutamate is an excitatory amino acid neurotransmitter that is thought to be used by the pyramidal cell in the cerebral cortex. Pyramidal cell neurons contribute significantly to major neocortical efferent and intracortical associational pathways. These neurons degenerate in AD. Also, the content of L-glutamate in the terminal projections of the perforant pathway is markedly reduced in AD. L-Glutamate is a principal neurotransmitter of this efferent projection from the entorhinal cortex to the hippocampus. The existence of glutamatergic abnormalities in AD should stimulate novel experimental approaches to pharmacologic intervention.

Philothermal Hypothesis. This hypothesis is based on the observation that the migration of white blood cells toward warmer temperatures is impaired in some Alzheimer's patients. It proposes that individuals with impaired philothermal response also have reduced ability to respond to infectious, toxic, and other noxious influences throughout the body as well as in the brain, and it is consistent with the hypothesis of a microtubular defect in patients with AD.

Abnormal Protein/Autoimmune Hypothesis. AD has been associated with abnormal proteins (e.g., amyloid, MAP tau, and the antigen that binds Alz 50). New technologies are being used to study those proteins as well as decreased protein synthesis, reduced amounts of total protein in the brain, and low levels of the protein that slows degeneration of ribonucleic acid. Numerous questions are being asked, including whether the proteins themselves or just their accumulation is abnormal, and—if the proteins are abnormal—whether they are encoded by defective genes or reflect modifications at later steps of their production.

Infectious Agent Hypothesis. "Slow viruses" have been implicated in several degenerative neurological diseases, including three that cause dementia in humans: Creutzfeldt-Jakob disease (CJD), Gertsmann-Straussler syndrome, and kuru. Viruslike particles have been found in the brains of these patients, and both CJD and kuru can be transmitted to animals by injecting extracts of deceased patients' brains. At present, there is no confirmed infectious agent for AD, despite numerous attempts to identify one.

Head-Injury Hypothesis. Patients with dementia of the Alzheimer type have been shown to have had a history of head injury with loss of consciousness at some time in the past, compared with matched hospital controls. Others have also suggested a role for head injury in AD based on dementia pugilistica, the dementia seen in prizefighters who sustain repeated blows to the head. Although the mechanism is not known, one possibility is that trauma damages the blood-brain barrier.

Blood-Flow Hypothesis. Advanced scanning devices such as single photon emission computed tomography (SPECT) and positron emission tomography (PET) have been used to document decreased blood flow, decreased oxygen consumption, and increased glucose uptake in the brains of living Alzheimer's patients. Research has not yet demonstrated whether the changes are a cause or an effect of brain disease.

Other Hypotheses. In addition to aluminum, other minerals, heavy metals, environmental toxins (pesticides and other chemicals), neurotoxic plants, nutritional deficiencies, alcohol, and drugs have all come under consideration as potential causes of AD.

There is no certainty that all cases of AD have the same etiology. It is possible that a combination of mechanisms may be operative, or that different mechanisms in different people may be responsible for their dementia. AD may represent a common final pathway for divergent causes, it may have a single underlying cause with multiple manifestations that eventually converge, it may require a threshold of vulnerability to be reached before one or a combination of several factors produce the disorder, or it may follow some yet unsuspected model.

Diagnosis and Symptomatology

From the first clinicopathological description in 1907 until recent years, AD was diagnosed only when dementia appeared prior to age 65; patients with dementia of later onset were diagnosed with "senile dementia" (Amaducci et al. 1986). The term *Alzheimer's disease* is now proper at all ages, however, because similar pathology appears in patients regardless of age at onset (Tomlinson et al. 1970).

Certain diagnosis of AD still requires confirmation based on histological examination of brain tissue. The clinical problem still is how to recognize it accurately in life: using highly detailed criteria based on typical cases entails the risk of excluding the diagnosis when AD is present; when less-restrictive criteria are used, the risk is that other illnesses may be overlooked. DSM-III-R criteria for "primary degenerative dementia of the Alzheimer type" include insidious onset and steady progression of dementia (see Table 14-1) in the absence of other clear disorder, but they do not add further specification of the clinical picture to distinguish AD from other dementias.

These issues were addressed by a 1984 task force with members from the National Institute of Neurological and Communicative Disorders and Stroke and the Alzheimer's Disease and Related Disorders Association (McKhann et al. 1984). These guidelines are more descriptive of the dementia syndrome expectable with AD. The issue of heterogeneity is raised, and subtyping of AD is encouraged. Recognizing the necessary ambiguity of clinical diagnosis, the task force recommended the terms "possible Alzheimer's disease" and "probable Alzheimer's disease" for degrees of uncertainty in clinical diagnosis, and "definite Alzheimer's disease" only following histological confirmation. Carefully used, the specificity of these criteria may approach 90% as evaluated by autopsy. Accuracy and sensitivity in a heterogeneous community sample, however, is a more difficult question not fully addressed at this time.

Pathology

The brain appears grossly normal in the early phases of AD, but it undergoes widespread atrophy as the disease advances. Histopathological examination of brain tissue with special silver stains is required to display the SPs and NFTs that are considered the most characteristic features of AD, although other abnormalities such as granulovacuolar degeneration and Hirano bodies can also be identified. It should be emphasized that none of these findings alone is pathognomonic of AD, but the density, conjunction, and distribution of SPs and NFTs in relation to the patient's age are critical (Khachaturian 1985). SPs occur in the neuropil and consist of a core of proteinaceous material deposited in a configuration known as amyloid; there is a halo of adjacent degenerating nerve processes. NFTs are intraneuronal, consisting of abnormal protein and endogenous neurofilaments condensed into a paired helical configuration. These lesions are always found in the hippocampus and amygdala and, when present in the cortex, are found preferentially in inferior temporal, postcentral parietal, posterior cingulate, and prefrontal cortex. Primary motor and sensory cortex, cerebellum, and spinal cord are usually spared.

Laboratory Findings

Hematological, metabolic, and endocrine parameters are normal in AD, and the absence of a confirmatory laboratory test continues to be frustrating. Characterization of the abnormal proteins that make up SPs and NFTs, particularly the amyloid and its precursors, is an area of active research (Selkoe 1989): it seems that amyloid deposits appear in brain tissue prior to cellular response; precursors to the amyloid may originate outside the brain. Neuronal and glial responses imply a role for endogenous neurotrophic factors in the pathogenesis of AD.

Although loss of brain tissue is seen by both X-ray computed tomography (CT) and magnetic resonance imaging (MRI), structural brain imaging techniques have not shown changes specific to AD. Techniques that examine brain activity may be more promising, although problems continue with accessibility and standardization of criteria. PET with oxygen utilization or glucose uptake reveals hypoactivity bilaterally in the posterior temporoparietal lobes in patients with AD; the affected areas correspond to association cortex known to have high counts of SPs and NFTs. Blood flow by SPECT shows similar patterns and may prove to be more available. The routine electroencephalogram appears normal in early AD and shows nonspecific slowing later, but computer-assisted Fourier analysis and evoked potential techniques may improve specificity.

Course and Prognosis

At this time the prognosis for AD is relentless progression of disability due to dementia. Variations in the rate of progression are common, and some patients appear to have extended periods with little or no increase in their functional impairment, whereas others worsen noticeably between visits. Currently, there are no clear predictors for the course of any given individual.

Psychiatric and behavioral disorders are common in AD (Wragg and Jeste 1989). Disturbances of thought and mood occur in 30% to 40% of AD patients, with diagnosable psychotic or mood disorders in approximately one-third of these. General management issues have been discussed, but it should be noted that although formal, insight-oriented psychotherapy with AD patients would be ambitious, there is increasing support in the literature for the use of supportive individual and group therapies (Sadavoy and Robinson 1989); these topics are covered more fully in Chapters 24 and 26.

Delusions are usually simple and derive from the core cognitive syndrome (e.g., the mislaid keys have been "stolen"), but they can be more elaborately paranoid (e.g., "My daughter stole them because she wants to sell my car for the money"). Other delusions may be based on agnosia or misrecognition, for example, the patient who believes there are strangers living in the house because she does not recognize herself in the mirror.

Incidence of depression in AD patients is controversial, with reported frequencies varying from 0% to 88%, although most studies place the incidence between 10% and 25% (Wragg and Jeste 1989). Referral bias may explain some of the wide discrepancies in these figures, but it is likely that more fundamental factors are involved, including the identification of depression in AD patients. Stability and expression of depressive symptoms are affected by the dementia. Sadness, loss of self-worth, and anxiety are commonly reported by patients, but mood is more often labile and reactive than pervasive. Guilt is uncommon, but poor appetite, restless pacing, sleep disturbance, and anhedonia are seen without primary mood change in many AD patients.

Other behavioral abnormalities are not well classified by DSM-III-R categories. It is common for the moderately demented AD patient to pace aimlessly. Some are at high risk for wandering away from a home they may no longer recognize. Patients with AD often become apathetic and disengaged. A significant percentage develop egocentricity, lability, and impulsivity. Irritability can lead to verbal or physical altercation. Overt disinhibition with financial or sexual impropriety may also occur.

Treatment

Treatment for AD remains experimental, and no clearly beneficial agent has emerged (Dysken 1987). Piracetam is a "nootropic" agent postulated to provide nonspecific stimulation of neuronal metabolism. The use of dihydroergotamine mesylate is supported by several studies showing positive, albeit small, effects. Removal of amyloid protein or aluminum salts remains experimental.

Responses to cholinergic agents continue to encourage therapeutic trials, although no agent has yet received marketing approval. Nutritional enrichment with choline precursors alone (lecithin) has little short-term benefit. Physostigmine and tetrahydroaminoacridine inhibit the enzyme acetylcholinesterase, thus prolonging the activity of ACh at the synapse; some patients may respond to these agents, at least temporarily, but dose windows, duration of effect, and toxicity are not fully determined. Direct cholinergic agonists and agents to stimulate the regrowth of cholinergic neurons remain in development, as does treatment with NGF.

Multi-infarct Dementia

Diagnosis, Symptoms, and Pathology

Although arteriosclerosis has been discredited as the major cause of senile memory impairment, cerebrovascular disease (CVD) remains the second most common cause of dementia. Whereas approximately 50% of autopsies in dementia have AD pathology, 20% show CVD and another 12% have evidence of both (Tomlinson et al. 1970). Furthermore, many ischemic brain lesions recognized at autopsy have been clinically silent, but the demonstration of CVD does not in itself demonstrate a vascular cause of a patient's dementia. DSM-III-R criteria for multi-infarct dementia (MID) include dementia (see Table 14-1) with the addition of sudden onset or irregular course and a history of stroke, lateralizing neurologic signs, and uneven or "patchy" mental status deficits. All the following types of insults are now included in the definition of MID (Glatt and Katzman 1984):

- Large-vessel occlusion, which is recognizable by the predominance of a conventional stroke syndrome such as fluent or nonfluent aphasia.
- Lacunae, which are small pockets of fluid of less than 2 cm diameter that appear to be residua of small-vessel occlusion, especially in the cerebral white matter. Hypertension is the most commonly associated condition, and lesions are particularly frequent in the basal ganglia and pons.
- Small-vessel occlusions in the cortex, which can result from repeated microemboli (e.g., from atrial fibrillation), from inflammatory arteritis, or rarely from idiopathic thrombosis (so-called Torvik's disease). These lesions may not be revealed by structural neuroimaging, and if they accrue over time, they can mimic idiopathic degenerative disease.
- Cerebral white-matter pathology, in which the primary lesion is probably sclerosis of the recurrent arteries penetrating subcortical white matter from the cortex, most commonly due to chronic hypertension. Ischemia from intermittent hypotensive hypoperfusion is also a favored mechanism. Perhaps best defined by the pattern referred to as "leukoaraiosis" on magnetic resonance imaging, it may be referred to as subcortical arteriosclerotic encephalopathy or as Binswanger's disease.
- Border-zone infarction, which is a diffuse injury resulting from episodes of ischemia and/or hypotension rather than focal-vessel occlusion and stroke. Association cortex tends to be affected, and memory impairment is also common, probably because the hippocampus is especially sensitive to hypoxia.

Laboratory Evaluation

Electrocardiogram is recommended in the workup of all dementia patients because of the high incidence of ischemic lesions and rhythm abnormalities, which may be related to previously unsuspected CVD; other vascular studies may be indicated in selected cases. Blood work may suggest other disorders contributing to CVD, including hyperlipidemia, abnormalities of platelets or other formed blood elements, or inflammatory markers in vasculitis.

Neuroimaging techniques play an important role. MRI appears to be more sensitive to vascular lesions than CT scanning, especially for lesions of the cerebral white matter and brain stem. Functional imaging may also be useful: Hachinski and associates (1975) found that dementia patients with high scores on an ischemic scale had multiple scattered areas of hypoperfusion as defined by Xenon blood flow studies, whereas patients with probable AD had low scores and normal blood flow distribution. PET and SPECT studies may distinguish these same patterns (see Chapter 12).

Course, Prognosis, and Treatment

As may be expected, the course of MID is variable, depending mostly on the type and course of vascular disease present. There is no direct treatment for the cognitive dysfunction at this time, but recognition and treatment of accompanying disorders may be beneficial.

Controlling risk factors for vascular disease—cessation of smoking, control of hypertension and arrhythmia, diet, and exercise—may improve prognosis and even short-term clinical functioning. The MID patient also may benefit from treatment of accompanying psychiatric disorder. Although data are scanty on MID, poststroke depression is common and treatments are often effective. Treatment of paranoia, delusions, and anxiety may also be beneficial in selected cases. Principles have been discussed; the interaction of psychopharmacological agents with cardiovascular medications must be followed closely in MID (Signer and Read 1989).

Pick's Disease

This uncommon disorder involves relatively focal degeneration of the frontal and anterior lobes, which may be suggested by CT or MRI scan. Affected cortex reveals Pick bodies: distinctive ballooning of nerve cells with inclusions stained by silver compounds. Gustafson (1987) has also described frontal lobe degeneration with dementia, but without this histological appearance. Although less common than AD in every age bracket, Pick's and other frontal lobe disorders may be relatively more frequent in dementia of middle than of late life (Heston et al. 1987). There are no standard diagnostic criteria, but patients typically develop personality change with apathy and sometimes disinhibition prior to frank cognitive impairments. Motor function, as in AD, is normal until the disease is far advanced. Memory per se is not severely affected early in the disease, decreased speech output precedes formal aphasia, and some cognitive tasks such as arithmetic and the ability to copy drawings may be preserved until the overall dysfunction is far advanced. There is no known treatment, and the disease progresses relentlessly to complete disability and death.

Parkinson's Disease

Contrary to Parkinson's early assertions, cognitive impairment is now recognized as a frequent concomitant of Parkinson's disease (PD). Forgetfulness, slowed thinking, or apathy and depression may develop in early PD prior to the identification of the more characteristic movement disorder. Dementia occurs in 25% to 40%, depending on criteria and source, and it may be more common in those patients without prominent tremor, suggesting subtypes of PD (Chui 1989). Whether PD causes dementia without concomitant other disorder, especially AD, is disputed by some experts.

PD is diagnosed clinically by the presence of tremor, rigidity, and bradykinesia. There is destruction of dopaminergic cells originating from the substantia nigra in the midbrain and projecting to the basal ganglia. Although the etiology is unknown, the precipitation of PD by exposure to a specific environmental toxin (a contaminant of synthetic opiates) has opened new possibilities for understanding the pathogenesis of PD and other degenerative neuropsychiatric disorders.

Improved cognition is seen in many patients upon treatment of PD. The most common agent has been l-dopa, a dopamine precursor usually combined with the peripheral dopa decarboxylase inhibitor carbidopa to reduce peripheral side effects. Other agents include the receptor agonists amantadine and bromocryptine. Deprenyl, a selective monoamine oxidase inhibitor, may slow the progression of PD, possibly by delaying the metabolism of an endogenous MPTP-like substance (Tetrud and Langston 1989).

Psychiatric syndromes are common in PD. Delusions can be difficult to manage because the blockade of dopamine receptors by neuroleptics tends to aggravate the core PD symptoms. Standard treatments are often effective for the depression commonly seen in PD, but these patients may be more sensitive to side effects, especially hypotension, bowel inactivity, and confusion.

Huntington's Disease

The patient with Huntington's disease (HD) suffers the clinical triad of dementia, psychosis, and choreiform movements, any of which may dominate the initial presentation. Onset is insidious, usually around age 40. Late-onset HD may not display prominent chorea and tends to progress more slowly. Both sexes are affected equally, and the family history usually reveals affected individuals in multiple generations.

The dementia syndrome is marked by changes in personality and judgment along with memory loss, but with relative preservation of other higher cortical functions. This pattern, which has some features in common with the cognitive impairments found in PD and other movement disorders, is sometimes referred to as "subcortical dementia" (McHugh and Folstein 1975).

Degeneration of the caudate nucleus is demonstrated by CT or MRI scanning in established HD, and hypometabolism has been demonstrated much earlier with PET. HD is like a genetic disorder with autosomal dominant transmission and high penetrance. The HD gene has been localized to chromosome 4, and premorbid ascertainment of risk is available (Hayden et al. 1988; Meissen et al. 1988).

Neuroleptics can improve function by alleviating the choreiform movements and psychosis and by tempering the sometimes outrageous behavior of the disinhibited HD patients. Psychiatric morbidity is high. Depression is six times more common in patients with early HD than in age-matched controls. Suicide causes significant mortality in these patients. Tricyclic antidepressants are the most commonly used agents for depression. Other patients may develop schizophreniform psychoses and require neuroleptic treatment. Psychiatrists may also be important in assisting with the management of secondary disturbances (e.g., guilt, stress, and depression) in patients and family members.

Creutzfeldt-Jakob Disease

CJD is an uncommon cause of dementia, with an incidence significantly less than 1 person per 100,000. It is the human representative of an intriguing group of disorders, including scrapie in sheep, which are transmitted under the (fortunately) unusual condition of the direct inoculation of infected brain tissue into a donor. Most remarkably, this transmission can be accomplished by an inoculate containing protein, but no nucleic acid; the term "prion" has been proposed for this novel proteinaceous infectious material (Prusiner 1982). Normal contact appears to carry no risk for infection, but passage has been verified in recipients of human growth hormone (which is harvested from cadavers) and, rarely, by corneal transplant from a donor whose CJD went unrecognized. A minority of cases occur in restricted pedigrees and may be genetically transmitted, but the origin of most cases is idiopathic (Manuelidis and Manuelidis 1989; Prusiner 1989).

Most often the disease evolves over weeks or months; sometimes in retrospect there is an acute but nonspecific phase to the illness. The patient has a global dementia, often with a quality of confusion or befuddlement. Generalized myoclonus is also usually present, which is exacerbated or elicited when the patient is startled. Characteristic periodic discharges are seen in the electroencephalogram of a majority of fully developed cases. Pathologically, the disorder is referred to as a spongiform encephalopathy because of the multiple extracellular vacuoles seen microscopically in brain tissue. There is accumulation of protein in an amyloid configuration, although its relationship to the amyloid in AD is unclear. The distribution of pathology is irregular among cortex, deep nuclei, and cerebellum (Roos et al. 1973).

References

Amaducci LA, Rocca WA, Schoenberg BS: Origin of the distinction between Alzheimer's disease and senile dementia: how history can clarify nosology. Neurology 36:1497–1499, 1986

American Psychiatric Association: Diagnostic and Statistical Manual of Mental Disorders, 3rd Edition, Revised. Washington, DC, American Psychiatric Association, 1987

Bartus RT, Dean RL, Beer B, et al: The cholinergic hypothesis of geriatric memory dysfunction. Science 217:408–417, 1982

Breitner JCS, Murphy EA, Silverman JM, et al: Age-dependent expression of familial risk in Alzheimer's disease. Am J Epidemiol 128:536–548, 1988

Brody EM, Family at risk. Alzheimer's Disease, Treatment and Family Stress. Edited by Light E, Lebowitz B. (DHHS Publication No. (ADM) 89-1569) Alcohol, Drug Abuse, and Mental Health Administration, National Institute of Mental Health, 1989

Caine ED: Pseudodementia: current concepts and future directions. Arch Gen Psychiatry 38:1359–1364, 1981

Chui HC: Dementia: a review emphasizing clinico-pathologic correlation and brain-behavior relationships. Arch Neurol 46:806–814, 1989

Coyle JT, Price DL, DeLong MR: Alzheimer's disease: a disorder of cortical cholinergic innervation. Science 219:1184–1190, 1983

Cummings JL, Benson DF: Dementia: A Clinical Approach. Boston, MA, Butterworths, 1983

Cummings JL, Miller BL (eds): Alzheimer's Disease: Treatment and Long-term Management. New York, Marcel Dekker, 1990

Davies P: Genetics of Alzheimer's disease: a review and a discussion of the implications. Neurobiol Aging 7:459–466 1986

Dysken M: A review of recent clinical trials in the treatment of Alzheimer's dementia. Psychiatr Annals 17:178–191, 1987

Evans DA, Funkenstein H, Albert MS, et al: Prevalence of Alzheimer's disease in a community population of older persons: Higher than previously reported. J Am Med Assoc 262:8:2551–2556, 1989

Folstein MF, Folstein SE, McHugh PR: Mini-Mental State. J Psychiatr Res 12:189, 1975

Gierz M, Zweifach M, Jeste DV: Antidepressant agents, in Alzheimer's Disease: Treatment and Long-term Management. Edited by Cummings JL, Miller BL. New York, Marcel Dekker, 1990

Glatt S, Katzman R: Multi-Infarct Dementia, in Annual Review of Gerontology and Geriatrics. Edited by Eisdorfer C. New York, Springer, 1984, pp 61–86

Gottlieb GL, Piotrowski LS: Neuroleptic treatment, in Alzheimer's Disease: Treatment and Long-term Management. Edited by Cummings JL, Miller BL. New York, Marcel Dekker, 1990

Gustafson L: Frontal lobe degeneration of non-Alzheimer type, II: clinical picture and differential diagnosis. Arch Gerontol Geriatr 6:209–223, 1987

Hachinski VC, Iliff LD, Zilka E, et al: Cerebral blood flow in dementia. Arch Neurol 32:632–637, 1975

Hayden MR, Robbins C, Allard D, et al: Improved predictive testing for Huntington disease by using three linked DNA markers. Am J Hum Genet 43:689–694, 1988

Heston LL, White JA, Mastri AR: Pick's disease: clinical genetics and natural history. Arch Gen Psychiatry 44:409–411, 1987

Jarvik L, Small G: Parentcare: A Commonsense Guide for Adult Children. New York, Crown, 1988

Jarvik LF, Winograd CH (eds): Treatments for the Alzheimer Patient. New York, Springer, 1988

Kane RA, Kane RL: Assessing the Elderly. Toronto, DC Heath, 1981

Khachaturian ZS: Diagnosis of Alzheimer's disease. Arch Neurol 42:1097–1105, 1985

Mace NL, Rabins PV: The 36-Hour Day: A Family Guide to Caring for Persons with Alzheimer's Disease, Related Dementing Illness, and Memory Loss in Later Life. Baltimore, MD, Johns Hopkins University Press, 1982

Manuelidis EE, Manuelidis L: Suggested links between different types of dementias: Creutzfeldt-Jakob disease, Alzheimer disease, and retroviral

CNS infections. Alzheimer Disease and Associated Disorders 3:100–109, 1989

Matsuyama SS, Jarvik LF: Hypothesis: microtubules, a key to Alzheimer disease. Proceedings Natl Academy of Science, Neurobiology 86:8152–8156, 1989

McHugh P, Folstein MF: Psychiatric syndromes of Huntington's chorea: a clinical and phenomenologic study, in Psychiatric Aspects of Neurologic Disease. Edited by Benson DF, Blumer D. New York, Grune & Stratton, 1975, pp 267–285

McKhann G, Drachman D, Folstein M, et al: Clinical diagnosis of Alzheimer's disease: report for the NINCDS-ADRDA work group under the auspices of Department of Health and Human Services Task Force on Alzheimer's Disease. Neurology 34:939–944, 1984

Meissen GJ, Myers RH, Mastromauro CA, et al: Predictive Testing for Huntington's Disease with Use of a Linked DNA Marker. March 3, 1988

Nott PN, Fleminger JJ: Presenile dementia: the difficulties of early diagnosis. Acta Psychiatr Scand 51:210–217, 1975

Plum F: Dementia: an approaching epidemic. Nature 279:372–374, 1979

Prusiner SP: Novel proteinaceous infectious particles cause scrapie. Science 216:136–144, 1982

Prusiner SB: Creutzfeldt-Jakob disease and scrapie prions. Alzheimer Disease and Associated Disorders 3:54–76, 1989

Rabins PV, Mace NL, Lucas MJ: The impact of dementia on the family. JAMA 248:333–335, 1982

Read S: Community resources, in Alzheimer's Disease: Treatment and Long-term Management. Edited by Cummings JL, Miller BL. New York, Marcel Dekker, 1990

Reifler BV: Arguments for abandoning the term pseudodementia. J Am Geriatr Soc 30:665, 1982

Reisberg B (ed): Alzheimer's Disease. New York, Free Press, 1983

Ron MA, Toone BK, Garralda ME, et al. Diagnostic accuracy in presenile dementia. Br J Psychiatry 134:161–168, 1979

Roos R, Gajduseek DC, Gibbs CJ: The clinical characteristics of transmissible Creutzfeldt-Jakob disease. Brain 96:1–20, 1973

Sadavoy J, Robinson A: Psychotherapy and the cognitively impaired elderly, in Psychiatric Consequences of Brain Diseases in the Elderly. Edited by Conn D, Grek JA, Sadavoy J. New York, Plenum, 1989, pp 101–135

Satlin A, Cole JO: Psychopharmacologic interventions, in Treatments for the Alzheimer Patient. Edited by Jarvik LF, Winograd CH. New York, Springer, 1988

Selkoe DJ; Molecular pathology of amyloidogenic proteins and the role of vascular amyloidosis in Alzheimer's disease. Neurobiol Aging 10:387–395, 1989

Signer SF, Read SL: The patient with stroke, in Treatments of Psychiatric Disorders: A Task Force Report of the American Psychiatric Association,

Vol. 2. Washington, DC, American Psychiatric Association, 1989, pp 867–876

St. George-Hyslop PH, Myers RH, Haines JL, et al: Familial Alzheimer's disease: progress and problems. Neurobiol Aging 10:417–425, 1989

Tetrud JW, Langston JW: The effect of deprenyl (Seligiline) on the natural history of Parkinson's disease. Science 245:519–522, 1989

Tomlinson BE, Blessed G, Roth M: Observations on the brains of demented old people. J Neurol Sci 11:205–242, 1970

U.S. Congress Office of Technology Assessment: Losing a Million Minds: Confronting the Tragedy of Alzheimer's Disease and Other Dementias (OTA-BA-323). Washington, DC, U.S. Government Printing Office, 1987

U.S. Department of Veterans Affairs, Office of Geriatrics and Extended Care: Dementia: Guidelines for Diagnosis and Treatment, 2nd Edition. Washington, DC, U.S. Department of Veterans Affairs, 1989

Vogel RJ, Palmer HC (eds.): Long-term Care: Perspectives From Research and Demonstrations. U.S. Department of Health and Human Services, Health Care Financing Administration, 1982

Wells CE: Pseudodementia. Am J Psychiatry 136:895–900, 1979

Wragg RE, Jeste DV: Overview of depression and psychosis in Alzheimer's disease. Am J Psychiatry 146:577–587, 1989

CHAPTER 15

David K. Conn, M.B.B.CH.

Delirium and Other Organic Mental Disorders

In this chapter I will focus on delirium and the other organic mental disorders as defined in DSM-III-R, with special reference to their occurrence in the elderly (American Psychiatric Association 1987). They include amnestic syndrome, organic mood syndrome, organic anxiety syndrome, organic delusional syndrome, organic hallucinosis, and organic personality syndrome. Intoxication and withdrawal of psychoactive substances are described in Chapter 19. The new classification of organic mental disorders in DSM-III represented a radical departure from previous classification systems (American Psychiatric Association 1980). Although it has been generally accepted in North America, it is still the subject of some controversy.

In discussing the approach of DSM-III, Lipowski (1984) noted that the essential feature of the newly described syndromes was no longer cognitive impairment but "the psychological or behavioral abnormality associated with transient or permanent dysfunction of the brain." The concept of organicity was no longer synonymous with the presence of cognitive impairment. The division of organic syndromes into acute and chronic subtypes was abandoned in DSM-III because it forced the clinician to classify the patient's condition as either reversible or not, on the basis of a purely cross-sectional assessment. A number of criticisms have been leveled against the new classification system (Spitzer et al. 1983). It has been accused of being overinclusive and overcomplex, possibly hindering case finding for epidemiologic studies, imposing premature closure on the issue of cause, and in general leaving too much to the clinician's judgment. It is certainly noteworthy that the organic mental syndromes and disorders constitute the only section in DSM-III-R in which the clinician must make an etiologic diagnosis.

In the decade since the introduction of the new diagnostic categories of organic disorders there has been little systematic research—and therefore few data—on the epidemiology of the other organic syndromes. There are a few exceptions, particularly in the category of organic mood syndrome, such as the work relating to poststroke depression and depression in patients with Parkinson's disease (Robinson and Rabins 1989). Much of the literature on the etiology of organic mental syndromes is based on short series or case reports. There have been few controlled trials of treatment.

The clinician using the DSM-III-R diagnostic system may encounter difficulties. Using history, physical examination, or laboratory tests, the clinician must judge whether a specific factor is etiologically relevant to particular psychopathology. When a patient has a past psychiatric history and/or strong family psychiatric history plus significant medical disease, it may be virtually impossible to determine which of these factors is most relevant. Patients often have features of several organic syndromes, and it may therefore be necessary to use the residual category of organic mixed syndrome. Patients with mild symptoms of depression, an organic labile (pseudobulbar) affect, or localized cognitive impairment may not fulfill diagnostic criteria and therefore are difficult to classify. However, in spite of the potential problems, the new system clearly offers advantages.

One particular clinical concern relates to the consequence of establishing a definitive etiology. For example, if a patient's depression is attributed entirely to his or her stroke, then other etiological factors such as early-life experiences, family history of depression, medications, and other recent losses may be overlooked. It is vitally important, therefore, that the clinician, in spite of establishing an etiological factor, continue to search for other contributing factors and thereby consider the full array of potential interventions (Conn 1989).

Delirium

Delirium has been described as one of the most common and important forms of psychopathology in later life (Lipowski 1989). More than 20 other terms have been used to describe this syndrome, including acute confusional state, acute brain syndrome, acute brain failure, acute organic psychosis, acute organic syndrome, metabolic encephalopathy, reversible toxic psychosis, and toxic confusional state (Liston 1982). The elderly are especially susceptible to delirium as a consequence of virtually any physical illness or the toxic effects of a vast number of commonly used drugs, even if used at therapeutic dosages. A number of factors predispose the elderly to delirium, including structural brain disease, reduced capacity for homeostatic regulation, impaired vision and hearing, a high prevalence of chronic disease, reduced resistance to acute stress, and age-related change in the pharmacokinetics and pharmacodynamics of drugs (Lipowski 1989). Other contributing factors include sleep loss, sensory deprivation, sensory overload, and psychosocial stress related to such factors as bereavement or relocation.

From a clinical standpoint it is crucial that delirium be recognized and investigated as soon as possible. Delirium is often the first sign of an underlying medical problem such as an acute infection or myocardial infarction, and failure to recognize delirium may lead to failure to diagnose and treat the underlying medical disorder. There is a high mortality related to delirium (Rabins and Folstein 1982); these patients are at high risk for injury, and their care may be difficult.

Epidemiology

Data concerning the epidemiology of delirium are relatively limited. The incidence of delirium among patients in medical and surgical units of general hospitals is reported to be 10% to 15% (Beresin 1988), although in elderly patients the incidence appears to be at least 30% (Gillick et al. 1982). In contrast, retrospective studies using hospital charts suggest that fewer than 1% of patients actually receive a diagnosis of delirium (Henker 1979), pointing to the fact that delirium is often overlooked. A study of patients aged older than 65 admitted to a university general hospital, revealed that in 76.9% of cases, cognitive deficits were missed by the examining physicians (McCartney and Palmateer 1985). The incidence of delirium increases with age and is therefore most frequent in the most elderly (Warshaw et al. 1982).

Diagnosis and Clinical Features

The diagnostic criteria for delirium are delineated in Table 15-1 (American Psychiatric Association 1987). One of the cardinal fea-

Table 15-1. Diagnostic criteria for delirium

A. Reduced ability to maintain attention to external stimuli (e.g., questions must be repeated because attention wanders) and to appropriately shift attention to new external stimuli (e.g., perseverates answer to a previous question).

B. Disorganized thinking, as indicated by rambling, irrelevant, or incoherent speech.

C. At least two of the following:

   (1) Reduced level of consciousness (e.g., difficulty keeping awake during examination).

   (2) Perceptual disturbances; misinterpretations, illusions, or hallucinations.

   (3) Disturbance of sleep-wake cycle with insomnia or daytime sleepiness.

   (4) Increased or decreased psychomotor activity.

   (5) Disorientation to time, place, or person.

   (6) Memory impairment (e.g., inability to learn new material, such as the names of several unrelated objects after 5 minutes, or to remember past events, such as history of current episode of illness).

D. Clinical features develop over a short period of time (usually hours to days) and tend to fluctuate over the course of a day.

E. Either of the following:

   (1) Evidence from the history, physical examination, or laboratory tests of a specific organic factor (or factors) judged to be etiologically related to the disturbance.

   (2) In the absence of such evidence, an etiologic organic factor can be presumed if the disturbance cannot be accounted for by any nonorganic mental disorder (e.g., manic episode accounting for agitation and sleep disturbance).

Source. Reprinted from DSM-III-R with permission from the American Psychiatric Association. Copyright 1987.

tures of delirium is a reduction in the ability to focus, maintain, and shift attention. In DSM-III-R the term *clouding of consciousness* has been excluded from the first criterion because of disagreement about the precise meaning of this term. Levels of arousal may be either reduced, with decreased wakefulness and alertness (occasionally mutism or catatonia), or increased, with high levels of vigilance and an increased response to external stimuli. Three clinical variants are described: hypoalert-hypoactive, hyperalert-hyperactive, and mixed (Lipowski 1980). Patients may develop involuntary movements such as tremor, asterixis, or myoclonus.

The history is a crucial component of diagnosis. Rapid onset, diurnal fluctuation of symptoms, and a relatively short course of illness are highly suggestive of a diagnosis of delirium. Changes in the emotional state of the patient are frequent, with dramatic mood shifts and high levels of anxiety and fear, particularly in response to hallucinations or paranoid thoughts. Patients often are highly agitated and restless and may try to climb out of bed, pull out intravenous and other lines, and try to leave the unit.

Some authorities subdivide the DSM-III concept of delirium into two separate diagnostic entities. Many neurologists tend to view the hyperactive delirious patient ("acute agitated delirium") as suffering from a different disorder than the patient with reduced alertness and psychomotor activity (Adams and Victor 1985). The latter are referred to as suffering from an "acute confusional state." The former are typified by the patient with "delirium tremens," experiencing vivid hallucinations, delusions, extreme agitation, irritability, and signs of overactivity of the autonomic nervous system.

Etiology

Many articles contain exhaustive and unmemorizable lists of illnesses and drugs that can precipitate delirium. Wise (1987) invented a mnemonic, "I WATCH DEATH," to assist the clinician in recalling the main etiologic categories of delirium (see Table 15-2). This mnemonic, although initially rather startling, serves a second purpose by reminding us that delirium should be treated as a medical emergency with prompt initiation of appropriate investigations and treatment. Levkoff and associates (1988), in a large study of elderly hospitalized patients, noted four factors that distinguished 80% of all cases of delirium: urinary tract infection, admission laboratory findings of low serum albumin, elevated white blood cell count, or proteinuria.

Table 15-3 summarizes some of the commonly used drugs that can cause delirium in the elderly. Estroff and Gold (1986) pointed out that most of the evidence implicating specific reactions to drugs is based on single case reports, that many of these reports originate from nonpsychiatric physicians who may not have been well trained in describing psychiatric and behavioral disorders, and that the literature prior to the development of criteria (e.g., DSM-III and Research Diagnostic Criteria) is of untested reliability. For example, reports that may have described a patient as being psychotic may, in retrospect, have been describing a misdi-

Table 15-2. Causes of delirium (mnemonic: I WATCH DEATH)

Category	Examples
I: Infections	Urinary tract infection, encephalitis, any systemic infection
W: Withdrawal	Alcohol, benzodiazepines
A: Acute metabolic disorder	Acidosis, alkalosis, electrolyte disturbance, hepatic or renal failure, dehydration
T: Trauma	Head injury, postoperative, hyperthermia, hypothermia
C: CNS pathology	Hemorrhage, seizures, stroke, transient ischemic attack, tumors
H: Hypoxia	Anemia, hypotension, pulmonary/cardiac failure, pulmonary embolus
D: Deficiencies	Vitamin B_{12}, thiamine
E: Endocrinopathies	Thyroid dysfunction, adrenal dysfunction, hyperglycemia, hypoglycemia, hyperparathyroidism
A: Acute vascular	Shock, hypertensive encepatholopathy
T: Toxins/drugs	See Table 15-3
H: Heavy metals	Lead, manganese, mercury

Source. Reprinted from Wise 1987 with permission from American Psychiatric Press, Inc. Copyright 1987.

Table 15-3. Some commonly used drugs causing delirium

Group	Examples
Analgesics	Opiates, salicylates
Antiarrhythmics	Lidocaine, procainamide
Antibiotics	Cephalexin, gentamicin, penicillin
Anticonvulsants	Phenytoin
Antihypertensives	Methyldopa
Anti-inflammatory	Indomethacin, steroids
Antineoplastic	5-fluorouracil, methotrexate
Antiparkinsonian	Levodopa, bromocriptine
Gastrointestinal	Cimetidine
Psychotropics	Antidepressants, barbiturates, benzodiazepines, lithium, neuroleptics
Sympathomimetics	Amphetamines, phenylephrine
Miscellaneous	Drug withdrawal (alcohol, barbiturates, benzodiazepines)
	Bromides
	Disulfiram
	Timolol eyedrops
	Theophylline

agnosed delirium. Causality has often been inferred by the clearing of symptoms following discontinuation of a drug. However, the patient is rarely rechallenged with the suspected culprit, and blood levels are often not reported.

Differential Diagnosis

The main differential diagnoses are dementia and psychoses. In the elderly it can be difficult to separate delirium from dementia. Indeed, the two syndromes frequently coexist. One report suggests that approximately 40% of patients with dementia aged 55 or older were suffering from delirium on admission to hospital and that 25% of all delirious patients also suffered from dementia (Erkinjuntti et al. 1986). None of the DSM-III-R criteria for delirium are pathognomonic. The major differentiating features are the history of acute onset, short course, and pronounced diurnal fluctuations. A number of clinical conditions presenting with delirium (e.g., cerebral hypoxia following cardiac arrest, meningitis, or encephalitis) may ultimately progress to chronic cognitive impairment with features of dementia.

Functional psychosis in the elderly individual, especially if also cognitively impaired, may resemble delirium. The term "pseudodelirium" has been proposed for these patients. The patient with a functional psychotic illness is more likely than the delirious patient to have a psychiatric history, systematized versus fleeting delusions, and inconsistent cognitive performance, and to display features of a mood or schizophrenic disorder (Lipowski 1989).

Differential diagnosis also includes the more focal organic syndromes, which are discussed later in this chapter.

Diagnosing Delirium

Because of the importance of getting an accurate history of the onset and development of signs and symptoms, a corroborative history from family members or nursing staff is often vital. Subsequently, it is necessary to examine the mental status and to complete a thorough physical evaluation of the patient. The Mini-Mental State Exam (Folstein et al. 1975) is useful, particularly with regard to documenting change over time. However, it has definite limitations and should not be used as the sole basis for a cognitive mental status evaluation. Most patients with delirium display major abnormalities in their ability to write (Chedru and

Geschwind 1972). It may be useful to test various integrative tasks including visual-spatial ability, and to test praxis and motor fluency.

In the institutional setting a full review of the chart is useful, especially noting changes in the patient's behavior; medications, including changes in dosage or recent additions; and results of current laboratory tests.

Table 15-4 delineates an etiological workup for the patient with delirium. It is not possible to give an absolute formula for which tests should or should not be done. The choice of tests depends very much on the clinical situation and setting. The clinician should consider the indications for possible investigations in each individual case. Some of the tests are necessary for a basic workup, whereas others should be performed only when there is a high suspicion of a specific abnormality (Tobias et al. 1989; Wise 1987).

Electroencephalogram abnormalities virtually always accompany delirium and may be useful in differentiating delirium from dementia (cf. Chapter 13).

Table 15-4. Suggested laboratory workup for delirium

Basic tests
  Blood count with differential
  ESR
  Blood chemistry (electrolytes, BUN, creatinine, glucose, calcium, phosphate, liver function, albumin)
  Urinalysis
  Chest X ray
  Electrocardiogram

Other studies as indicated
  Arterial blood gases
  Toxicological screen of urine/blood
  Serology for syphilis
  Electroencephalogram
  Computed tomography or magnetic resonance imaging scan of head
  Thyroid function
  Vitamin B_{12}, folate
  Magnesium
  Cerebrospinal fluid examination
  Le Prep, ANL
  Heavy metals
  Urine test for porphobilinogen

Note. ESR = Erythrocyte sedimentation rate. Le Prep = Lupus erythematosus prep. ANL = Antinuclear antibody.

Pathophysiology

Our current knowledge of the pathogenesis and pathophysiology of delirium is rather limited. A number of theoretical mechanisms have been proposed and reviewed (Lipowski 1980, 1987). Delirium is probably the manifestation of a final common pathway resulting from acute brain failure. Given the multiple possible causes of delirium, a variety of different alterations in the brain may be responsible for its development. The major theories are that delirium is caused by 1) a general reduction in cerebral oxidative metabolism, which can result from a decrease in the supply, uptake, or utilization of substrates for brain metabolic activity; 2) damage to enzyme systems, the blood-brain barrier, or cell membranes; 3) reduced brain metabolism resulting in decreased acetylcholine synthesis with ensuing cholinergic deficiency; 4) an imbalance of central cholinergic and adrenergic function; 5) raised plasma cortisol in response to acute stress, which has a pathological effect on the anatomical substrates of attention and information processing; and 6) dysfunction of the right hemisphere, which is important for the process of attention.

Management

Diagnosis. The cornerstone of management is correct diagnosis. If an underlying cause is known or suspected, the approach must focus on the treatment or elimination of the disorder or factors responsible, whether requiring active medical or surgical treatment or discontinuation of drugs.

Supportive Care. It is important to ensure that supportive measures are carried out to maintain fluid balance, nutrition, sedation and rest, and general comfort, and that the physical examination and blood work be repeated on a regular basis. Frequently delirium is the harbinger of medical disorder (e.g., urinary tract infection, congestive heart failure), and failure to make an early diagnosis may delay important medical treatment.

Because many patients with delirium are critically ill, good nursing care is vital. The nursing care plan requires close observation of the patient with particular regard to changes in vital signs, behavior, and mental status.

To both patient and family the delirious state is often an understandably frightening situation. It is, therefore, necessary to offer explanation, support, and reassurance. The patient may benefit from family visits and from care in a quiet, well-lit room providing optimal levels of stimulation. It is often useful to have a low-level night light. Frequent reorientation of the patient with the use of clocks, calendars, photos of families, and other personal possessions may be helpful. For some patients the use of a radio or television may be of benefit; however, for the acutely agitated patient it may be too much stimulation. For patients suffering sensory impairment it is important to make sure that eyeglasses and hearing aids are being used properly.

Medication.   Empirical data on pharmacological management of delirium are sparse. The decision to prescribe medication should be related to the presence of specific symptoms (e.g., aggression, agitation, hallucinations) that require treatment, with consideration of likely side effects (particularly anticholinergic effects, hypotension, and respiratory suppression).

For most delirious patients, haloperidol appears to be the drug of choice because of minimal anticholinergic and hypotensive effects. However, it does cause frequent extrapyramidal symptoms. For the elderly person, starting doses are 0.5 mg to 2 mg orally or intramuscularly (the lower dose is preferable). It may be necessary to repeat the dosage every 30 minutes until sedation is achieved. Close follow-up is critical. After the confusion has cleared, the drug dosage should be reduced gradually over a period of 3 to 5 days (Wise 1987). Although it is not universally accepted, and not approved by the Food and Drug Administration, intravenous haloperidol has been used successfully to treat agitated delirious patients (Tesar et al. 1985).

Benzodiazepines with short half-lives, such as oxazepam and lorazepam, are still considered to be the drugs of choice for withdrawal syndromes such as delirium tremens. Particular concerns about benzodiazepines include the risk of increased sedation and disinhibition. A recent study suggested that haloperidol in combination with a benzodiazepine leads to a decreased level of extrapyramidal symptoms as compared to haloperidol alone. No adverse effects were seen in any of the 14 patients receiving the combination (Menza et al. 1988).

In severe anticholinergic delirium, physostigmine has been used in doses of 1 mg to 2 mg intravenously or intramuscularly. However, contraindications are said to include a history of heart disease, asthma, diabetes, peptic ulcer, and bladder or bowel obstruction (Lipowski 1987).

Psychological Care. Richeimer (1987) categorized four types of intervention to help the delirious patient compensate for cognitive impairments: 1) clarification of perceptions, 2) verification and validation of perceptions that are accurate, 3) explanation of events and why they are difficult to understand, and 4) repetition of all important and helpful information. Further interventions to help support the patient's emotional state include 1) acknowledging feelings, 2) providing familiarity, 3) alleviating isolation, 4) fostering a sense of control, and 5) responding to the need of the patient for hope as well as realistic information. Some patients may develop posttraumatic stress disorder following delirium and may require a considerable degree of support following such an episode.

Course and Prognosis

Delirium has a variable course, which, as previously mentioned, fluctuates. The end result is either recovery, incomplete recovery with some residual cognitive impairment, or a downward course that sometimes progresses to stupor, coma, and eventually death. In the hospitalized patient, delirium is likely to increase the length of stay and hence the cost of care (Thomas et al. 1988). Hence it is emphasized that vigorous measures should be taken for the early detection and treatment of delirium. The mortality rate appears to depend on the setting; the rates for the elderly vary from 17% to 75% (Liston 1982; Rabins and Folstein 1982).

In an elderly population, delirium may represent the terminal state prior to death. My clinical impression is that many patients on a palliative care unit for the elderly develop an acute confusional state in the days prior to death. For some patients this change in mental status appears to have an adaptive function. Extremely agitated and anxious patients frequently become quietly confused and disoriented and appear to suffer less during the final hours of their life.

Amnestic Syndrome

The diagnostic criteria for amnestic syndrome include 1) evidence of both short-term memory impairment and long-term memory impairment and 2) no evidence of delirium or dementia (American Psychiatric Association 1987). Clinically, three types of memory are recognized: 1) immediate memory, as measured (for example) by digit span, which is highly dependent on capacity for attention; 2) short-term memory—for example, recall after a short period of distraction (there are differences of opinion as to how long this period should be, but most clinicians use a period of 2 to 5 minutes); and 3) long-term memory, measured (for example) by recall of early-life events or historical figures.

The central feature of the amnestic syndrome is the inability to store, retain, and reproduce new information, leading to antero-grade amnesia (i.e., an impairment in the ability to lay down new memories during the period following the onset of an illness). By contrast, the ability to immediately recall information is pre-served. Although less severe than the loss of short-term memory, defects in long-term memory are usually present. The result is ret-rograde amnesia: impaired ability to recall information that ex-isted prior to the onset of an illness. Neuropsychologists divide the deficits in anterograde amnesia into 1) faulty encoding, 2) faulty consolidation, 3) accelerated forgetting, and 4) faulty retrieval (Kopelman 1987). Confabulation (the production of inaccurate, er-roneous answers to straightforward questions) may occur in the amnestic patient. Patients may provide incorrect answers based on personal or past experiences, in which case the responses are co-herent and reasonable, or they may give impossible, inappropriate, adventurous, or even gruesome responses ("fantastic" confabula-tion).

The most common cause of amnestic syndrome is Wernicke's encephalopathy, which is believed to be caused by thiamine defi-ciency (Adams and Victor 1985). It is most often seen in chronic alcoholics, but it may also occur in the isolated elderly (who may have a primary psychiatric diagnosis such as depression or para-noid disorder producing nutritional deficiencies).

Prompt treatment with parenteral thiamine is critical. The ma-jority of patients subsequently develop Korsakoff's syndrome, which is chronic and characterized by severe anterograde and moderate retrograde amnesia (cf. Chapter 19). Patients with Kor-sakoff's syndrome often have severely compromised insight, and only 25% of patients make a full recovery (Victor et al. 1971).

Disease processes that affect the diencephalic and medial tem-poral structures (i.e., mamillary bodies, fornix, and hippocampus) can cause the amnestic syndrome (see Table 15-5). In patients with thiamine deficiency the symptoms appear to be related to bilateral sclerosis of the mamillary bodies and degenerative changes in the dorsal medial nucleus of the thalamus (Horvath 1988; Stoudemire 1987).

Table 15-5. Causes of amnestic syndrome, with differential diagnosis

Causes	Differential diagnosis
Wernicke's encephalopathy	Transient global-amnesia
Korsakoff's syndrome	Psychogenic amnesia
Head injury	Postictal states
Postanoxia	
Herpes simplex encephalitis	
Hippocampal infarctions	
Neoplasm	

Differential Diagnosis

Transient global amnesia is a syndrome characterized by the development of anterograde amnesia, which may persist for several hours, and a short period of retrograde amnesia. Patients are bewildered but have no other clinical or neurological deficits. The syndrome may be related to decreased blood flow in the posterior hemispheric or inferior temporal regions.

Psychogenic amnesia is characterized by inability to recall vital personal information, for example, one's name. There may be a loss of specific emotionally charged information, for example, memory of a recent loss. Major depression can also be present, and patients may display "la belle indifférence."

Treatment

Medical treatment of the primary etiological factor is the first consideration. Subsequently, rehabilitation may involve specific therapies (both cognitive and behavioral) to maximize the individual's level of functioning. Strategies useful at any age to help patients increase memory function include reorientation therapy; the programmed use of diaries, notebooks, or other aids; and specific memory training programs based on the cognitive psychology of memory.

Organic Mood Syndrome

Organic mood syndrome is characterized by a mood disturbance similar to that of major depression or mania, but it is caused by a specific organic factor. The diagnosis can be made only when there is evidence of a direct link between the organic disorder and depression. The phenomenology is essentially the same as that of the primary mood disorders. In addition, mild cognitive impairment is frequently observed. Psychotic symptoms such as delusions or hallucinations may be present, particularly in the manic form (American Psychiatric Association 1987).

Psychiatrists are frequently consulted to rule out depression in the medically ill, and a number of diagnostic difficulties may emerge. Many physical illnesses and drugs may cause symptoms that are used in physically healthy patients to make a diagnosis of depression (e.g., fatigue, decreased energy, insomnia, weakness, poor concentration, and anorexia). It is at times difficult for the clinician to decide whether or not to attribute these symptoms to depression. The rate of depression in medical populations appears to be between 12% and 32% (Stoudemire 1988). Approximately 20% of nursing home residents and 35% of elderly patients in chronic care hospitals have symptoms suggesting the presence of major depression (Katz et al. 1989; Sadavoy et al. 1990).

Many patients with neurological disease display evidence of aprosdia or organic emotional lability. Prosody is the affective and inflectional coloring of speech, including syllable and word stress, rhythm, cadence, and pitch. Along with gesture and mimicry, prosody provides the emotional element to speech. Prosody can be disturbed by right-hemisphere lesions and also by disorders of the basal ganglia, cerebellum, and brain stem. As a result the patient may present with a flat, rather monotonous voice, which can lead to either underestimation or overestimation of the severity of an emotional disorder such as depression. The flat, emotionless voice may be mistaken for depression or, conversely, genuine feelings of sadness and distress may be unconvincingly presented. Patients with brain disease have organic emotional lability, that is, they cry (or occasionally laugh) frequently and intensely with decreased control, often in response to a question or other interaction that produces emotional change. This behavior may also give the clinician the false impression of depression. However, organic labile affect may be a signal of an underlying depressive illness (Ross and Rush 1981) and may improve with antidepressants (Schiffer et al. 1985).

Many illnesses and drugs are said to cause depression. However, it would be more accurate to state that many of these conditions are associated with depression. Stoudemire (1987) cautioned that the attribution of "medication or disease as the cause of depression should be approached with some degree of caution and skepticism and case reports and lists of such should be approached and evaluated critically." The medical diseases and drugs that are commonly associated with depression are listed in Chapter 9.

In the elderly, both stroke and Parkinson's disease are associated with depression. At least one-fourth of stroke victims appear to develop a major depression, and depressive symptoms may occur in more than one-half of all patients following stroke (Robinson et al. 1984). Follow-up studies report that the high-risk period for poststroke depression lasts for approximately 2 years (Robinson and Price 1982). According to Robinson and colleagues (1983), patients with left-hemisphere strokes are more vulnerable to depressive symptoms, particularly when the lesion is closest to the frontal pole. Other studies, however, have failed to show a consistent association between side of lesion and presence of depression (House 1987). There is evidence that poststroke depression may be related to widespread depletion of norepinephrine following a localized lesion of the cortex.

Studies of the frequency of depression vary considerably but suggest that 30% to 70% of patients with Parkinson's disease suffer from depression. Depressed patients with Parkinson's disease have lower levels of 5-hydroxyindoleacetic acid in their cerebrospinal fluid than do nondepressed patients with Parkinson's disease (Mayeux et al. 1984). The degree of physical disability and the duration of the disease do not seem to correlate with the severity of the depression. Parkinson's disease can present with depression (Kearney 1964) but this relation has not been well studied.

Other disorders that are clearly associated with depression include endocrine disorders, particularly hypothyroidism, Addison's disease, and Cushing's syndrome. Hyperthyroidism too may present with depressive symptoms in the elderly ("apathetic hyperthyroidism"). Other important conditions include occult carcinomas (particularly of the pancreas), viral illnesses, pernicious anemia, and collagen-vascular diseases.

Medications associated with depression include antihypertensives, especially reserpine and methyldopa. The evidence that other antihypertensives (such as propranolol) cause depression is much weaker (Paykel et al. 1982). Some clinicians believe that beta-blockers such as atenolol, which are less likely to cross the blood-brain barrier than others such as propranolol, are consequently less likely to cause depression. Steroids appear to cause depression, although a labile emotional state with features of euphoria and anxiety is also commonly associated with use of steroids.

Factors that alter the major neurotransmitter systems implicated in primary mood disorders (norepinephrine and serotonin) or limbic-hypothalamic functions probably precipitate the development of organic mood disorders (Cummings 1985a).

Mania also appears to be associated with a variety of medical conditions and drugs (Krauthammer and Klerman 1978). In comparison with depressive symptoms, which are very common in the elderly medically ill population, the manic state is rarer. The presentation includes pressure of speech, flight of ideas, hyperactivity, insomnia, distractibility, grandiosity, and poor judgment. A variety of conditions can mimic mania, such as agitated delirium or the disinhibited subtype of frontal lobe syndrome, which might account for some of the conditions that are said to be associated with secondary mania. Table 15-6 lists the more common diseases and drugs associated with secondary mania in the elderly. In elderly patients who develop mania for the first time at age 60 or older, there appears to be a preponderance of cerebral organic disorders, particularly among men (Shulman and Post 1980). Cummings (1985a) suggested that the localized neurological conditions linked to mania appear to include right-hemisphere lesions or lesions close to the third ventricle and hypothalamus.

The treatment of organic mood syndrome essentially parallels the treatment of depression or mania (see Chapter 22). There is evidence that both antidepressants and electroconvulsive therapy can be effective in the treatment of mood disorder accompanying stroke or Parkinson's disease (Harvey 1986; Lipsey et al. 1984; Murray et al. 1986). Treatment of the acute manic state generally requires major tranquilizers. Lithium has been shown effective in

Table 15-6. Important causes of organic mood syndrome (mania) in the elderly

Medical illnesses	Medications
Central nervous system	Corticosteroids
stroke/cerebral neoplasms	Thyroxin
(especially right hemisphere)	Levodopa
Multiple sclerosis	Bromocriptine
Encephalitis	Sympathomimetics
Syphilis	Amphetamines
Post-head injury	Cimetidine
Hyperthyroidism	
Uremia	
Hemodialysis	

treating secondary mania occurring in conjunction with brain disease, although extra care must be taken to avoid toxicity (Rosenbaum and Barry 1975; Young et al. 1977). In the same way that patients with a primary mood disorder may benefit from a combination of psychopharmacological agents and psychotherapy, patients with secondary depression may also benefit greatly from a variety of psychiatric treatments. Individual supportive therapy and group therapy may be of great benefit. The families of elderly patients who are suffering from physical illness and an associated mood disturbance often require a great deal of support.

Organic Anxiety Syndrome

The essential feature of organic anxiety syndrome is recurrent or persisting anxiety and/or panic due to a specific organic factor (American Psychiatric Association 1987). Common symptoms include feelings of apprehension, tension, dread, or panic; and autonomic and visceral symptoms including tachycardia, hyperventilation, increased sweating, dizziness, numbness and tingling, dilatation of the pupils, diarrhea, and urinary frequency. Other symptoms include decreased concentration, tremor, restlessness and occasionally perceptual changes such as derealization, depersonalization, or even hallucinations.

Anxiety may be a learned response, or—in the case of organic anxiety syndrome—it may reflect a neurotransmitter abnormality. Factors predisposing an individual to anxiety (e.g., genetic and psychodynamic factors) probably play a role in the development of organic anxiety syndrome. The most likely etiologies of this disorder include hyperthyroidism, hypercortisolism, hypoglycemia, and some potentially toxic agents such as amphetamines and other psychostimulants, caffeine, and sympathomimetic agents (Cummings 1985a; Stoudemire 1987). Rare etiologies include pheochromocytoma, carcinoid syndrome, brain tumors, and epilepsy, particularly complex partial seizures. Any condition that causes hypoxia is likely to cause anxiety. Alcohol and drug withdrawal syndromes produce an anxiety syndrome but are separately classified (cf. Chapter 19).

Management should focus on identifying and treating the primary cause. While this process is under way, benzodiazepines may be helpful in controlling the symptoms of anxiety. Beta-blockers are also said to have a role in the management of anxiety, especially when these symptoms are primarily of a somatic nature, but their use in this capacity has not been well studied in the elderly. Psychotherapy, relaxation techniques, and hypnosis may also help the patient.

Organic Delusional Syndrome

Organic delusional syndrome is characterized by the occurrence of prominent delusions that can be attributed to an organic factor. Exclusion criteria include dementia and delirium. Hallucinations may be present but are not usually prominent (American Psychiatric Association 1987). The delusions may be simple and persecutory in nature, or they may be complex, systematized beliefs. The delusions may be related to specific neurological deficits such as anosagnosia, denial of blindness (Anton's syndrome), or reduplicative paramnesia (in which a patient claims to be present simultaneously in two locations). Specific delusions such as Capgras syndrome (the delusion that significant people have been replaced by identically appearing imposters), delusional jealousy, delusions of infestation, and De Clerambault's syndrome (erotomania) have all been linked to specific organic causes as discussed in Cummings' (1985b) extensive review of organic delusions.

Cummings documented approximately 70 medical causes, drugs, and toxic agents that have been implicated in producing delusions. However, he noted that many of these appear to occur in the setting of an acute confusional state and others appear to be linked to dementia. These conditions, therefore, would not qualify for a diagnosis of organic delusional syndrome. Because most of the literature in this area predated the diagnostic concept of organic delusional syndrome, it is difficult, in retrospect, to define which of these disorders may specifically cause a delusional state. Table 15-7 lists some of the possible causes of organic delusional syndrome in the elderly (Cummings 1985b; Stoudemire 1987).

Certain conditions and medications have been clearly linked to the development of delusions. These conditions include central nervous system disorders such as Huntington's disease, Parkinson's disease, ideopathic calcification of the basal ganglia, and spinocerebellar degenerations. Disorders affecting the temporal-limbic regions (e.g., epilepsy and herpes encephalitis) and tumors or strokes involving the temporal lobe or subcortical regions are all implicated in the development of delusions. A variety of medi-

Table 15-7. Important causes of organic delusional syndrome in the elderly

Medical illnesses	Drugs and toxins
Central nervous system	Levodopa
Stroke	Bromocriptine
Parkinson's disease	Amantadine
Epilepsy	Isoniazid
Idiopathic basal ganglia	Corticosteroids
calcification	Digitalis
Spinocerebellar degeneration	Amphetamines
Herpes encephalitis	Methylphenidate
Huntington's disease	Lidocaine
Endocrine	Procainamide
Thyroid and adrenal disorders	Ephedrine
Vitamin deficiency	Phenytoin
Vitamin B_{12}	
Folate	
Collagen-vascular disease	
Systemic lupus erythematosus	

cations and toxic agents have been linked to the development of psychosis, but psychosis may in some cases be related to delirium. Prospective studies with a view to determining this relationship to delirium would be useful. Certain medications such as levodopa and corticosteroids appear to be frequent culprits.

Cummings (1985b) suggested that the etiology of organic delusional syndrome arises from the disruption between cortical function and the limbic system. He proposed that limbic or basal ganglia dysfunction predisposes to abnormal emotional experiences, which are subsequently interpreted by the intact cortex and lead to complex intricately structured delusions. Subcortical and limbic lesions may disrupt ascending dopaminergic pathways, which have been implicated in schizophrenia. He noted that predisposing factors include genetic constitution, early-life experiences, personality characteristics, the location and extent of lesions, and the age of onset.

In conjunction with treatment of the primary condition, the use of neuroleptic medications may also be indicated in the treatment of organic delusional syndrome. Cummings' (1985b) prospective study of 20 consecutive patients with organic delusions suggested that the response to treatment was variable. Simple delusions, which are more common in patients with dementia, responded best to neuroleptic treatment, whereas complex delusions were more resistant. It should be noted, of course, that simple delusions tend to have a better prognosis even without treatment. The delusions, particularly complex delusions, can lead to misguided actions, which may be highly disruptive to family or nursing home routines. As a result, staff or families may need a considerable degree of support and education with regard to the management of patients with persisting delusions. Because paranoid thinking may be linked to cognitive impairment and misinterpretation of the environment, the gradual development of a trusting relationship with staff and ongoing reorientation and reassurance may be particularly beneficial. Although the mainstay of treatment is psychopharmacological, other approaches (e.g., behavioral management and psychotherapy) may play an important role (Proulx 1989; Sadavoy and Robinson 1989).

Organic Hallucinosis

The essential feature of organic hallucinosis is the presence of prominent, persistent, or recurrent hallucinations that are due to a specific organic factor. The hallucination must not occur during the course of delirium or dementia (American Psychiatric Association 1987). Hallucinations can occur in any sensory modality (auditory, visual, tactile, olfactory, or gustatory) and can vary from simple and unformed to highly complex and organized. The individual may be aware that the hallucinations are imaginary or may be convinced of their reality.

Sensory deprivation related to loss of vision or hearing is a frequent cause of hallucinations in the elderly. In a study of visual hallucinations in the elderly, 29% of 150 successive referrals to a geriatric psychiatrist reported visual perceptual disturbances. There was a significant correlation between the presence of hallucinations and eye pathology (Berrios and Brook 1984). Visual hallucinations have been subdivided into "release" and "irritable" types (Brust and Behrens 1977). Release hallucinations are usually formed images and tend to occur in the area of a field deficit. They are associated with any focal lesion in the visual pathway. Irritable (ictal) hallucinations are brief, stereotyped visual experiences. With primary eye disease the hallucinations may be simple or complex, for example, following eye surgery (especially if the eyes are patched).

Other causes of hallucinations include alcoholic hallucinosis (auditory), delirium tremens (visual and tactile), complex partial seizures, and lesions, especially of temporal-limbic structures. The differential diagnosis includes schizophrenia, especially when auditory hallucinations occur.

Medications and toxic agents responsible for hallucinations include hallucinogens, amphetamines, antiparkinsonian agents, thyroxin, steroids, antibiotics (especially intravenous penicillin), digoxin, sympathomimetics, cimetidine, narcotics, and heavy metals.

Tactile hallucinations are said to occur most commonly in toxic and metabolic disturbances or drug withdrawal states (Berrios 1982). Olfactory and gustatory hallucinations are most commonly caused by complex partial seizures.

Mechanisms suggested in the pathophysiology of hallucinations include a "perceptual release theory" (i.e., decreased sensory input results in the release of spontaneous central nervous system activity); the intrusion of dreams into the waking state (narcolepsy, hypnogogic hallucinations), serotonin antagonism (hallucinogens), and the role of hemispheric specialization (more commonly right-hemisphere lesions or seizure foci) (Cummings 1985a).

Management includes ensuring maximum sensory input through treatment of underlying disorders or through improved hearing or visual aids. Anticonvulsants such as carbamazepine are indicated for the treatment of seizures. The use of neuroleptics may be helpful, but this possibility has not been well studied. Neuroleptics may help to decrease anxiety or fear associated with the hallucinations.

Organic Personality Syndrome

The cardinal feature of the organic personality syndrome is a marked change in personality due to a specific organic factor. The personality disturbance should be persistent and may be either lifelong or represent a change or accentuation of a previously characteristic trait involving at least one of the following: 1) affective instability (e.g., marked shifts from normal mood to depression, irritability, or anxiety); 2) recurrent outbursts of aggression or rage that are grossly out of proportion to any precipitating psychosocial stressors; 3) markedly impaired social judgment (e.g., sexual indiscretions); 4) marked apathy and indifference; and 5) suspiciousness or paranoid ideation. Exclusion criteria include delirium and dementia. Where outbursts of aggression or rage are the predominant feature, a subtype entitled "explosive type" is used (American Psychiatric Association 1987).

Any disease that damages frontal lobes may lead to a "frontal lobe syndrome." Neoplasms, head trauma, cerebrovascular accidents, multiple sclerosis, and Huntington's disease are all associated with this syndrome. An insidious presentation of personality change may herald the onset of a more global dementia, particularly in patients with Pick's disease, which primarily affects the frontal lobes; the same can also be true of other dementias such as Alzheimer's disease.

Cummings (1985a) has described three separate frontal lobe syndromes, although in practice they tend to overlap. The syndromes described are 1) orbitofrontal syndrome characterized by disinhibition and impulsive behavior ("pseudopsychopathic"); 2) frontal convexity syndrome, in which apathy predominates; and 3) medial-frontal syndrome, which is associated with akinesia. Disinhibited behavior may cause dramatic behavioral change, and there may be totally uncharacteristic behavior incorporating loss of social tact; rude, tasteless, or inappropriate language; and antisocial behavior. The emotions may be labile with episodic euphoria as well as inappropriate jocularity and hyperactivity. There may be inappropriate sexual behavior. Individuals are often highly distractible and lack the ability to monitor and evaluate their own behavior and performance. Insight and judgment are often significantly impaired. On examination patients may display some of these behaviors, or conversely, be quite apathetic. Patients' inability to program new motor tasks (e.g., the fist-cut-slap test) may lead to motor perseveration or impersistence. There may be decreased word fluency, impaired abstraction and categorization skills, and difficulty shifting set (e.g., Wisconsin Card Sorting Test).

Another organic personality syndrome is described in some patients with long-standing seizure disorders, particularly complex partial seizures. The essential features consist of emotional "viscosity" (pedantic and overinclusive thinking), hyperreligiosity, hypergraphia, intense emotional reactions, humorlessness, hypermoralism, and changes in sexual behavior, most frequently hyposexuality (Bear and Fedio 1977). There are no specific data for the elderly.

Frontal lobe syndrome may cause dramatic problems for the patient and the family. Behavior may be frightening to others, and at times the police or outside agencies are called. Because of decreased insight it may be difficult to involve the individual in a treatment program. Patients with disinhibited behavior may require a combined behavioral and pharmacological approach. Various medications have been used in an attempt to control disinhibited and aggressive behavior. The first line of treatment is generally a neuroleptic. Other drugs reported anecdotally to improve this behavior include propranolol, lithium, trazodone, and carbamazepine. Behavior management programs may be of benefit but require the cooperation of families or caregivers living with the patient (Haley 1983; Proulx 1989).

Conclusion

There is clearly a need for further research as we attempt to understand the complex relationships between behavior and neuropsychiatric disorders. Although the emphasis from an etiological standpoint is on organic factors, it is also important to consider factors predisposing to the development of these disorders. These predisposing factors—such as premorbid personality style, previous life experiences, family psychodynamics, and environmental-cultural influences—may be important in developing a formulation and management plan. Optimal care of these patients, whether in the institution or in the community, requires an integrated and multidisciplinary approach. The primary interventions often involve treating the underlying organic factors and using psychopharmacological agents. However, other interventions such as individual and family psychotherapy, behavioral management programs, and environmental manipulations may be important adjuncts in the care of these patients.

References

Adams RD, Victor M: Principles of Neurology, 3rd Edition. New York, McGraw-Hill, 1985

American Psychiatric Association: Diagnostic and Statistical Manual of Mental Disorders, 3rd Edition. Washington, DC, American Psychiatric Association, 1980

American Psychiatric Association: Diagnostic and Statistical Manual of Mental Disorders, 3rd Edition, Revised. Washington, DC, American Psychiatric Association, 1987

Bear DM, Fedio P: Quantitative analysis of interictal behaviour in temporal lobe epilepsy. Arch Neurol 34:454–467, 1977

Beresin EV: Delirium in the elderly. Journal of Geriatric Psychiatry and Neurology 1:127–143, 1988

Berrios GE: Tactile hallucinations: conceptual and historical aspects. J Neurol Neurosurg Psychiatry 45:285–293, 1982

Berrios GE, Brook P: Visual hallucinations and sensory delusions in the elderly. Br J Psychiatry 144:662–664, 1984

Brust JCH, Behrens MM: "Release hallucinations" as the major symptom of posterior cerebral artery occlusion: a report of 2 cases. Ann Neurol 2:432–436, 1977

Chedru F, Geschwind N: Writing disturbances in acute confusional states. Neuropsychologia 10:343–353, 1972

Conn DK: Neuropsychiatric syndromes in the elderly: an overview, in Psychiatric Consequences of Brain Disease in the Elderly—A Focus on Management. Edited by Conn DK, Grek A, Sadavoy J. New York, Plenum, 1989

Cummings JL: Clinical Neuropsychiatry. New York, Grune & Stratton, 1985a

Cummings JL: Organic delusions: phenomenology, anatomical correlations, and review. Br J Psychiatry 146:184–197, 1985b

Drewe EA: The effect of type and area of brain lesion on Wisconsin Card Sorting Tests Performance. Cortex 10:159–170, 1974

Erkinjuntti T, Wikström J, Palo J, et al: Dementia among medical inpatients: evaluation of 2000 consecutive admissions. Arch Intern Med 146:1923–1926, 1986

Estroff TW, Gold MS: Medication-induced and toxin-induced psychiatric disorders, in Medical Mimics of Psychiatric Disorders. Edited by Extein I, Gold MS. Washington, DC, American Psychiatric Press, 1986, pp 163–198

Folstein MF, Folstein SE, McHugh PR: Mini-Mental State: a practical method for grading the cognitive state of patients for the clinician. J Psychiatr Res 12:189–198, 1975

Gillick MR, Serrell NA, Gillick LS: Adverse consequences of hospitalization in the elderly. Social Science and Medicine 16:1033–1038, 1982

Haley WE: A family-behavioural approach to the treatment of the cognitively impaired elderly. Gerontologist 23:18–20, 1983

Harvey NS: Psychiatric disorders in parkinsonism, I: functional illness and personality. Psychosomatics 27:91–103, 1986

Henker FO III: Acute brain syndromes. J Clin Psychiatry 40:117–120, 1979

Horvath TB: Organic brain syndromes, in Psychiatry, Revised Edition. Edited by Michels R, Cooper AM, Guze SB, et al. Philadelphia, PA, JB Lippincott, 1988

House A: Mood disorders after stroke: review of the evidence. International Journal of Geriatric Psychiatry 2:211–221, 1987

Katz IR, Lesher E, Kleban M, et al: Clinical features of depression in the nursing home. International Psychogeriatrics 1:5–15, 1989

Kearney TR: Parkinson's disease presenting as a depressive illness. J Irish Med Assoc 54:117–119, 1964

Kopelman MD: Amnesia: organic and psychogenic. Br J Psychiatry 150:428–442, 1987

Krauthammer C, Klerman GL: Secondary mania: manic syndromes associated with antecedent physical illness and drugs. Arch Gen Psychiatry 35:1333–1339, 1978

Levkoff SE, Safran C, Cleary PD, et al: Identification of factors associated with the diagnosis of delirium in elderly hospitalized patients. J Am Geriatr Soc 36:1099–1104, 1988

Lipowski ZJ: Delirium: Acute Brain Failure in Man. Springfield, IL, Charles C Thomas, 1980

Lipowski ZJ: Organic mental disorders—an American perspective. Br J Psychiatry 144:542–546, 1984

Lipowski ZJ: Delirium (acute confusional states). JAMA 258:1789–1792, 1987

Lipowski ZJ: Delirium in the elderly patient. N Engl J Med 320:578–582, 1989

Lipsey JR, Robinson RG, Pearlson GD, et al: Nortriptyline treatment of post-stroke depression: a double-blind treatment trial. Lancet 1:297–300, 1984

Liston EH: Delirium in the aged. Psychiatr Clin North Am 5:49–66, 1982

Mayeux R, Stern Y, Cote L, et al: Altered serotonin metabolism in depressed patients with Parkinson's disease. Neurology 34:642–646, 1984

McCartney JR, Palmateer LM: Assessment of cognitive deficit in geriatric patients—a study of physician behavior. J Am Geriatr Soc 33:467–471, 1985

Menza MA, Murray GB, Holmes VF, et al: Controlled study of extrapyramidal reactions in the management of delirious medically ill patients: intravenous haloperidol versus intravenous haloperidol plus benzodiazepines. Heart Lung 17:238–241, 1988

Murray GB, Shea VA, Conn DK: Electroconvulsive therapy for post-stroke depression. J Clin Psychiatry 47:258–260, 1986

Paykel ES, Fleminger R, Watson JP: Psychiatric side effects of antihypertensive drugs other than reserpine. J Clin Pharmacol 2:14–39, 1982

Proulx GB: Management of disruptive behaviours in the cognitively impaired elderly: integrating neuropsychological and behavioural approaches, in Psychiatric Consequences of Brain Disease in the Elderly: A Focus on Management. Edited by Conn DK, Grek A, Sadavoy J. New York, Plenum, 1989

Rabins P, Folstein MF: Delirium and dementia: diagnostic criteria and fatality rates. Br J Psychiatry 140:149–153, 1982

Richeimer SH: Psychological intervention in delirium. Postgrad Med 81:173–180, 1987

Robinson RG, Price TR: Post-stroke depressive disorders: a follow-up study of 103 out-patients. Stroke 13:635–641, 1982

Robinson RG, Rabins PV (eds): Aging and Clinical Practice—Depression and Coexisting Disease. New York, Igaku-Shoin, 1989

Robinson RG, Kubos KL, Starr LB, et al: Mood changes in stroke patients: relationship to lesion location. Compr Psychiatry 24:555–566, 1983

Robinson RG, Starr LB, Price TR: A two-year longitudinal study of mood disorders following stroke: prevalence and duration at six months follow-up. Br J Psychiatry 144:256–262, 1984

Rosenbaum AH, Barry MJ Jr: Positive therapeutic response to lithium in hypomania secondary to organic brain syndrome. Am J Psychiatry 132:1072–1073, 1975

Ross ED, Rush J: Diagnosis and neuroanatomical correlates of depression in brain-damaged patients. Arch Gen Psychiatry 38:1344–1354, 1981

Sadavoy J, Robinson A: Psychotherapy and the cognitively impaired elderly, in Psychiatric Consequences of Brain Disease in the Elderly. Edited by Conn DK, Grek A, Sadavoy J. New York, Plenum, 1989

Sadavoy J, Smith I, Conn DK, et al: Depression in geriatric patients with chronic medical illness. International Journal of Geriatric Psychiatry 5:187–192, 1990

Schiffer RB, Herndon RM, Rudick RA: Treatment of pathological laughing and weeping with amitriptyline. N Engl J Med 312:1480–1482, 1985

Shulman K, Post F: Bipolar affective disorder in old age. Br J Psychiatry 136:26–32, 1980

Spitzer RL, Williams JBW, Skodol AE: International Perspectives on DSM-III. Washington, DC, American Psychiatric Press, 1983

Stoudemire A: Depression in the medically ill, in Psychiatry, Revised Edition. Edited by Michels R, Cooper AM, Guze SB, et al. Philadelphia, JB Lippincott, 1988

Stoudemire GA: Selected organic mental disorders, in Textbook of Neuropsychiatry. Edited by Hales RE, Yudofsky SC. Washington, DC, American Psychiatric Press, 1987, pp 125–139

Tesar GE, Murray GB, Cassem NH: Use of high-dose intravenous haloperidol in the treatment of agitated cardiac patients. J Clin Psychopharmacol 5:344–347, 1985

Thomas RI, Cameron DJ, Fahs MC: A prospective study of delirium and prolonged hospital stay. Arch Gen Psychiatry 45:937–940, 1988

Tobias CR, Lippmann S, Tully E, et al: Delirium in the elderly: a commonly misunderstood disorder. Postgrad Med 85:117–130, 1989

Victor M, Adams RD, Collins GH: The Wernicke-Korsakoff Syndrome. Oxford, Blackwell Scientific Publications, 1971

Warshaw GA, Moore JT, Friedman SW, et al: Functional disability in the hospitalized elderly. JAMA 248:847–850, 1982

Wise MG: Delirium, in The American Psychiatric Press Textbook of Neuropsychiatry. Edited by Hales RE, Yudofsky SC. Washington, DC, American Psychiatric Press, 1987, pp 89–103

Young LD, Taylor I, Holmstrom V: Lithium treatment of patients with affective illness associated with organic brain symptoms. Am J Psychiatry 134:1405–1407, 1977

CHAPTER 16

Andre Allen, M.D.
Dan G. Blazer II, M.D., PH.D.

Mood Disorders

Introduction

Among the mood disorders in the elderly aged older than 65, dysthymia, major depression, and mania constitute the prototypes and depressed mood is the most frequent symptom. Clinicians, however, must differentiate between normal variations in mood and clinical depression (Blazer et al. 1987b). A depressive disorder may be diagnosed by DSM-III-R if the depressive symptoms interfere with work, family, or social functioning; if the individual seeks mental health services (or is referred for mental health services); or if the individual has received medication for the disorder (American Psychiatric Association 1987).

Depression as a generic term ncompasses several psychiatric syndromes, which in turn are presentations of a variety of medical and psychiatric disorders. Depressive symptoms are observed and diagnosed at all ages, but they have been reported to differ in the elderly versus the middle-aged, especially in terms of increased frequency of somatic complaints and decreased expression of guilt (Small et al. 1986).

The issue continues to be scrutinized; recent reports have emphasized more similarities than differences, especially when it is taken into account that problems associated with old age—such as cognitive impairment, physical illness, and functional disability—

In this work, Dr. Blazer was supported in part by the National Institute of Mental Health–sponsored Duke Clinical Research Center for the Study of Psychopathology in the Elderly (MH-40159).

rather than age per se, may contribute to differences in presentation (Klerman and Weissman 1989; Myers et al. 1984).

Epidemiology

A historical review of epidemiologic studies of depression in late life reveals many discrepancies, in large part because of problems with definitions and diagnosis in the 1960s and 1970s (Blazer 1989). The current operational diagnoses in DSM-III-R reflect Research Diagnostic Criteria (Spitzer et al. 1978) diagnoses. The sources of data used for studying the epidemiology of depression have been psychiatric case registers, general population surveys, and surveys of acute and long-term care facilities. Prevalence estimates vary across these sites. Recent community surveys fielded in the early 1980s—the Epidemiologic Catchment Area (ECA) projects—show a consistently low prevalence of major depression in persons aged 65 and older (1%–2%) (Blazer et al. 1987a). These results differ sharply from earlier reports of frequencies around 10% (Gurland et al. 1980; Post 1987) in the United States and Europe.

In a community survey that included more than 1,306 adults older than 60, a large proportion of people over 65 (27%) were found to experience depressive symptomatology across a variety of depressive syndromes that do not always fit DSM-III-R categories. These subtypes included mild dysphoria (19%), dysthymia (2%), major depression (0.8%), and mixed depression and anxiety (1.2%). No cases of manic episodes were located among the subjects interviewed (Blazer et al. 1987a). In many community studies, no manic episodes were found (Bremer 1951; Hare and Shaw 1965; Juel-Nielsen 1961; Myers et al. 1984; Sorensen and Stromgren 1961). Bipolar disorder is rare. Interestingly, in one of the few studies of elderly bipolar patients aged older than 65, Shulman and Post (1980) found that the disorder was of late onset in about two-thirds of the cases. Spar (1979) also showed that bipolar disease is a diagnosis that is often missed in hospitalized older patients.

The prevalence of major depression is much greater in institutions providing long-term care (12%), or in hospitals providing acute care (12%), than in the community; significant depressive symptomatology is found among another 31% and 23% retrospectively of those populations (Koenig et al. 1988; Parmelee et al. 1989). As in other age groups, major depression is more prevalent in women than in men (Myers et al. 1984).

The prevalence of depression in the elderly over 65 is not a static figure. It varies over time, for the cohort into which a person is born appears to carry factors that influence the prevalence of depression at a given age. The prevalence of depression does not increase with age longitudinally, as the follow-up Midtown Manhattan study has shown (Srole and Fisher 1980). Currently, major depression is less prevalent in age cohorts over 65 than in younger cohorts (Myers et al. 1984). In the past, depression was regarded as a disorder of middle-aged and elderly persons, in whom the risk of depression increased with age. However, there is increasing evidence that the prevalence of depression does not increase with age when other risk factors are controlled (e.g., physical illness, functional disabilities, and cognitive impairment) (Berkman et al. 1986).

Although suicide (both overall and in white males) is more prevalent in the elderly, the rate of suicide for subjects over 65 had been steadily declining from the 1930s to 1980. However, it has been rising again slowly since 1980. In 1933, the rate was 45.3 per 100,000, which declined to a low of 17.65 per 100,000 in 1980. In 1986, it was up to 21.6 per 100,000 (a 25% increase since 1980). In comparison, the national suicide rate was 12.8 per 100,000 in 1986. A factor considered important in influencing suicide rate is economic status, which had improved greatly since the 1930s, especially with the institution of Medicare and Medicaid (NCHS 1989).

Studies of need for and use of psychiatric treatment demonstrate that the majority of the elderly with major depression do not receive mental health services. The recent ECA studies show a pattern of underuse of mental health services by all age groups, but especially by the population over 65 (Shapiro et al. 1984). The Baltimore ECA data analyzed by German and colleagues (1985) revealed that 4.2% of those aged 65 to 75 and 1.4% of those 75 and older had made a mental health visit to a specialist or a primary care physician.

Etiology

Even though the concept of social stressors contributing to depression in late life is intuitively attractive, it is not well established (George et al. 1989). In major depression, the most frequently associated stressor is an actual or perceived loss. Late-life psychosocial stressors include physical illness, surgery, limited mobility,

sensory deprivation with deafness and blindness, retirement, economic deprivation, poor living conditions, social isolation, loss of
others (especially the spouse), and rejection by children (Ruegg et
al. 1988).

Physical illness and the resulting disabilities are believed to be
the most significant stressors and contribute to the loss of resources necessary for the maintenance of self-esteem. The relationship between stressors and depression is complex. When comparing the number of stressful agents, Murphy (1982) showed a
greater number of depressed patients had experienced at least one
stressful event compared with normal subjects (48% vs. 23%). The
loss of loved ones and retirement are expected life events and may
not result in life crises unless their timing is "off." When events are
anticipated and rehearsed, the grief work can be completed before
the loss occurs and the individual adapts to the loss with effective
coping strategies (Neugarten 1970). Resolution of stressful events
probably depends on a variety of factors including genetic predisposition, prevailing early-life experiences, adequacy of previous
adaptive and coping mechanisms, patterns and profiles of premorbid personality, and presence or absence of support system. These
factors need further study.

Physiologic changes from aging (Finch 1977) have also been hypothesized to produce age-related, biologic vulnerabilities to
depression. In the central nervous system, reduction of biogenic
amines (e.g., acetylcholine, dopamine, and norepinephrine) occurs
with advancing age. The level of the enzyme involved with the destruction of these monoamines—monoamine oxidase (MAO)—increases with age (Robinson et al. 1971). A study of unmedicated,
elderly, depressed subjects demonstrated higher MAO activity
than in sex- and age-comparable controls (Schneider et al. 1986).
Although biologic vulnerabilities to depression secondary to neurotransmitter dysregulation appear intuitively important, a causal
link has not yet been demonstrated.

Neuroendocrine changes are common in late life and depressive
illness (Janowsky and Sulser 1987; Watson et al. 1987). Physical
and psychological stressors stimulate the secretion of cortisol via
the hypothalamic-pituitary-adrenal (HPA) axis. Biogenic amines
regulate hypothalamic function. Abnormalities in the HPA are
found both in normal elderly subjects and in depressed patients
(Rosenbaum et al. 1984). The 24-hour circadian secretion of cortisol has been found to be disrupted, with an increased cortisol level
(Sachar 1975). Desynchronization of circadian rhythms is a rela-

tively new theoretical contributor to the etiology of depressive disorders. The phase advance of the internal circadian rhythm occurring in depressive illness results in disruption of the sleep-wake cycle (Vogel et al. 1980).

An increased frequency of structural changes in subcortical brain tissue in depressed patients over the age of 45 has been found on magnetic resonance imaging (MRI) scan. Leukoencephalopathy (patchy, deep white-matter lesions of abnormal signal intensity on T2-weighted images) resembles that seen in cerebral infarction and far exceeds that seen in the brains of nondepressed, age-matched controls. It is possible that these lesions may be causally related to the occurrence or outcome of depression in the elderly (Krishnan et al. 1988). Familial or genetic contribution to unipolar disorders appears less robust in late life than at earlier stages of the life cycle (Hopkinson 1964; Mendelwicz 1976; Schulz 1951).

A multitude of drugs can cause depression (see Table 16–1). The relationship is complex between medical illnesses and depression (see Chapter 9 for a table listing physical disorders associated with depression in the elderly).

Diagnostic Workup

Depression associated with dementia (cf. Chapter 14) and other organic disorders (cf. Chapters 9, 10, and 15) are discussed elsewhere in this text. As stated earlier, the diagnosis of depression is made on the basis of the clinical presentation, present and past psychiatric history, prior response to medication, family history of affective disorder, and collateral information. Physical workup is important and includes general health history, present health status, and physical and neurological examination. Nonspecific or multiple somatic symptoms should be investigated and should not be attributed to somatization until physical illnesses are excluded. Screening laboratory tests for medical illnesses presenting with depressive symptoms are listed in Chapter 15. Computed tomography (CT) is used in routine diagnostic workup. The MRI scan of the brain provides greater anatomic detail and greater sensitivity to tissue injury than does the CT scan.

The dexamethasone suppression test (DST) is not diagnostic for major depression because of its low sensitivity. A number of physical illnesses (e.g., diabetes mellitus, Cushing's disease, infectious diseases), drugs (e.g., alcohol, barbiturates, meprobamate, pheny-

Table 16-1.   Commonly prescribed or recreational drugs that can cause depression

Alcohol

Analgesics
  Non-narcotic: indomethacin
  Narcotic: morphine, codeine, meperidine, pentazocine,
    propoxyphene

Antihypertensives
  propranolol, alpha methyldopa, reserpine, clonidine, hydralazine,
    guanethidine

Antibacterials

Antiparkinsonian drugs
  levodopa

Cancer chemotherapeutic agents
  tamoxifen, vincristine, vinblastine, hexamethylamine

Cardiovascular medications
  digitalis, lidocaine

Estrogens

Gastrointestinal medications
  cimetidine

Hypoglycemic agents

Progestational agents

Sedatives
  barbiturates, benzodiazepines, meprobamate, chloral hydrate,
    flurazepam

Steroids

Sources. Hall 1980; Levenson et al. 1981.

toin), low body weight, and ongoing weight loss produce false positive test results, and false negatives are common too. However, nonsuppression of cortisol after treatment may be suggestive of a poor prognosis (Hirschfeld et al. 1985).

Another biological marker for depression—platelet tritiated imipramine binding—is still an experimental tool, but it may offer some specificity in the diagnosis of major depression. Patients with major depression exhibit a significant reduction in the number of platelet tritiated imipramine binding sites, with no change in binding affinity, whereas patients with probable Alzheimer's disease show no alteration in platelet tritiated imipramine binding (Nemeroff et al. 1988).

A finding yet to be evaluated for its usefulness in the differential diagnosis of depression and dementia is that patients whose cognitive impairment worsened during nortriptyline therapy exhibited increased platelet membrane fluidity (Zubenko et al. 1988).

Sleep electroencephalography can be a useful tool to identify depression, because alteration in the sleep characteristics of depression include delayed onset of sleep with early morning awakening, decreased rapid eye movement (REM) latency, increased REM density, and increased sleep discontinuity. Similar findings have been found in the young and in the elderly (Kupfer et al. 1978).

Depression rating scales may be useful clinically for diagnostic screening for depressive symptoms or measuring changes in symptomatology. Most have been developed to test adult patients of various ages, although the Geriatric Depression Scale, a self-report questionnaire (Yesavage et al. 1983), is specifically intended for initial screening in the elderly. The Beck Depression Inventory (Beck 1978), also a self-report questionnaire, has been found to be reliable and valid in older adults (Gallagher 1982). Some scales have limited reliability in detecting depression in older patients because they are loaded with somatic items, for example, the Zung Self-Rating Depression Scale (Zung 1965). The Montgomery-Asberg Depression Rating Scale (MADRS) (Montgomery and Asberg 1979), with excellent interrater reliability, high validity for severity, and high sensibility to change, is a useful scale for monitoring progress in treatment.

Clinical Presentation

The depressed elderly may be reluctant to seek psychiatric care; they tend to attribute their symptoms to medical illnesses and usually see their family doctor for the somatic complaints that are common in late-life depression (DeAlarcon 1964). Families may not recognize that the patient suffers from serious illness and may see the symptoms as willful.

Some patients are labeled as suffering "masked" depression because they insist that physical complaints are the problem and deny that they are depressed, yet they present with the classic depressive syndrome except for the denial of depression (Davies 1965; Lesse 1974).

Although the elderly may not complain of feeling depressed, they may acknowledge loss of interest and say that they do not feel like their old selves. They verbalize less guilt than other age groups

(Dovenmuehle et al. 1970). They are often anxious. Although they are no more likely than middle-aged persons to report cognitive problems, they do suffer more cognitive dysfunction during an episode of depression (Caine 1981).

In psychotic depression the elderly manifest ideas of reference, delusional beliefs, and particularly suspiciousness of others, with paranoid ideation often revolving around being perceived as a bad person or being tortured (Roose et al. 1983).

Clinical and Differential Diagnosis

Although the character of late-life depression is in some ways different from that at earlier ages, the DSM-III-R criteria for mood disorders remain useful for the elderly. A major clinical task is to differentiate major depression from other depressive syndromes. The reader is referred to DSM-III-R for the description of the operational criteria for diagnosis of mood disorders.

Adjustment disorder with depressed mood, major depression, dysthymia, and organic mood disorder are the four diagnostic categories of mood disorders. These are syndromes, however, rather than disease entities. Adjustment disorder with depressed mood is the mildest disorder of mood and the most common. By definition, adjustment disorder is self-limited and lasts less than 6 months. There is an identifiable stressor that constitutes a hardship. As a result, the patient suffers significant interpersonal, social, or occupational distress and impairment. The most common stressor is physical illness.

Major depression is the most severe form of depression. In melancholia, five of the following criteria must be present to make the diagnosis: lack of reactivity to stimuli, diurnal variation, early morning awakening, psychomotor agitation or retardation, significant weight loss or anorexia, more than 5 pounds weight loss, no significant personality disturbance prior to the first episode, one or more previous episodes, or previous good response to antidepressants or electroconvulsive therapy (ECT). Although older adults suffering major depression often suffer melancholic symptoms, recent studies show that there are no significant differences between the elderly melancholic and the younger melancholic in terms of symptom profile. Constipation was found more often in the elderly (Blazer et al. 1987b).

Hypochondriacal symptoms are frequent in the depressed elderly. In DeAlarcon's (1964) study of 152 patients, 65% of men and 62% of women reported such symptoms. Hypochondriacal complaints in this sample increased risk of attempted suicide (24.8% with hypochondriacal symptoms vs. 7.3% without). True hypochondriasis generally begins in mid-life and lacks a cyclical quality in contrast to depression (Blazer 1989).

Psychotic (delusional) depression is more prevalent in late life than in other stages of the life cycle and has a worse prognosis and different family history and biological markers than nonpsychotic depression (Myers et al. 1984; Nelson and Bowers 1978). Psychotic depression rarely responds to an antidepressant alone, necessitating the adjunctive use of a neuroleptic, or treatment with ECT.

Dysthymia is a chronic and less severe form of depression and must last at least 2 years to be diagnosed. Dysthymia is more common among the elderly than episodes of major depression and does not vary in prevalence with age (Myers et al. 1984). A major depressive episode may be superimposed in clinical samples, for example, so-called double depression.

Organic mood disorder is discussed in Chapter 15.

"Pseudodementia"—or the "dementia syndrome of depression"—is rare, according to current anecdotal evidence. It is diagnosed when significant cognitive dysfunction subsides with the resolution of depression. The major clinical features that differentiate pseudodementia and dementia are listed in Table 16-2. In about 20% of diagnosed cases of dementia, a major depression coexists (Reifler et al. 1982). In these cases, mood and function may improve when treated with an antidepressant, but the basic cognitive impairment remains.

Table 16-2. Characteristics distinguishing pseudodementia from dementia

Dementia	Pseudodementia
Insidious and indeterminant onset	Rapid onset
Symptoms usually of long duration	Symptoms usually of short duration
Mood and behavior fluctuate	Mood is consistently depressed
"Near miss" answers are typical	"Don't know" answers are typical
Patient conceals disabilities	Patient highlights disabilities
Level of cognitive impairment is relatively stable	Level of cognitive impairment fluctuates

Source. Adapted from Wells 1979.

Disorders presenting with paranoid delusions, such as late on-set schizophrenia and delusional disorders, may be difficult to distinguish from psychotic depression, and response to treatment is sometimes used as a guide to diagnosis. Although late-onset schizophrenia may be responsive to neuroleptics alone, psychotic depressions may improve only when a neuroleptic is combined or ECT is used.

Treatment

Treatment must encompass all diagnosed psychiatric and physical problems. Treatable depression is often overlooked in patients with physical illness, and physical problems too often receive inadequate therapy in patients treated primarily for depression. In an organic mood disorder the underlying medical problem should be addressed first, because its treatment may lead to the resolution of the symptoms of depression; concurrent treatment for depression is often necessary, however.

The modes of treatment for depression, which are similar throughout adulthood, include psychotherapy, somatic treatment with drugs, and/or ECT. Family involvement is often desirable at all stages of treatment because the older patient frequently is dependent on family members for support. Marital and/or family therapy may be indicated.

Psychotherapy alone is of value primarily in dysthymia and nonmelancholic major depression. Short-term cognitive therapy, behavioral therapy, and brief psychodynamic psychotherapy have been found to be effective, without medications, in high-functioning elders suffering from major depression with minimal or no cognitive impairment (Gallagher and Thompson 1982; Thompson et al. 1987). Although empirical studies are not available, cognitive-behavioral therapy may be the treatment of choice in the depressed medically ill. Antidepressant medication in these patients is often not tolerated because of side effects or is not effective (Gallagher and Thompson 1982; Thompson et al. 1987).

Somatic treatment is indicated for major depression with melancholia, although adjunct psychotherapy may improve response to medication and decrease the likelihood of relapses. Some patients suffering major depression without melancholia or a milder form of depression (classified in DSM-III-R as depressive disorder not otherwise specified) may also respond to antidepressants.

Complications

The major complication of major depression is suicide. Elderly white males have the highest suicide rate among different age, sex, and racial groups in the United States. The profile of the person at greatest risk for suicide is a widowed elderly man who lives alone, has few social contacts, suffers a physical illness, has made one or more previous suicide attempts, has had past episodes, and has current delusions. Nevertheless, clinicians are notoriously inadequate in recognizing which person will make a serious attempt or commit suicide, possibly because suicide is usually an impulsive event. Therefore, family contact is important in the prevention of suicide, although many of the old-old (aged 85 and over) do not have living close relatives. Families can decrease the risk by removing the agents of suicide (weapons, medications) and supervising the patient during a crisis. Nonetheless, when suicide risk is significant the patient should be hospitalized.

Outcome

Major depression is characterized by remissions and relapses. In general, recovery from major depression occurs in approximately one-half of patients who are hospitalized. Within 1 year, one-third to one-half of those who recover will suffer a relapse. Evidence has not shown that major depression is more chronic in late life (Keller and Shapiro 1981; Murphy 1983). Ayd (1983) asserts that in patients aged 31 to 50 the natural untreated length of depression is 9 to 18 months. while after age 50 it increases to 3 to 5 years. In recent studies, a concurrent medical illness has been found to be a predictor of poor outcome (Balldwin and Jolley 1986; Murphy 1983) both in terms of remission of symptoms and in survival. (The data on long-term outcome of depression, especially when complicated by other age-related disorders, are sometimes contradictory, and no definitive statement can be made.)

The size of the social network and subjective social support are significant predictors of depressive symptoms at follow-up. Subjective social support is one of the most reliable social support predictors of the outcome of depressive illness (George et al. 1989). Social factors may be less predictive in the elderly, however. Males and patients in poor physical health have lower rates of recovery (Balldwin and Jolley 1986). Chronicity is strongly related to noncompliance and physical disability. Because of the potential poor outcome, long-term follow-up and long-term use of antidepressant medication should be considered. Nevertheless, response to antidepressant medications is generally good (Gerson et al. 1988), and depression remains the most treatable of the psychiatric disorders of late life.

References

Ayd F: Continuation and maintenance antidepressant drug therapy, in Affective Disorders Reassessed. Edited by Ayd F, Taylor I, Taylor B. Baltimore, MD, Ayd Medical Communications, 1983

American Psychiatric Association: Diagnostic and Statistical Manual of Mental Disorders, 3rd Edition, Revised. Washington, DC, American Psychiatric Association, 1987

Balldwin RC, Jolley DJ: The prognosis of depression in old age. Br J Psychiatry 149:574–583, 1986

Beck AT: Depression Inventory. Philadelphia, PA, Philadelphia Center for Cognitive Therapy, 1978

Berkman WF, Berkman CS, Kaol S, et al: Depression symptoms in relation to physical health and functioning in the elderly. Am J Epidemiology 124:372–388, 1986

Blazer D: Depression in the elderly. N Engl J Med 320:164–165, 1989

Blazer D, Hughes DC, George LK: The epidemiology of depression in an elderly community population. Gerontologist 27:281–287, 1987a

Blazer D, Bachar JR, Hughes DC: Major depression with melancholia: a comparison of middle aged and elderly adults. J Am Geriatr Soc 35:927–932, 1987b

Bremer TA: A social psychiatric investigation of a small community in northern Norway. Acta Psychiatrica Scandinavica Suppl 62, 1951

Caine ED: Pseudodementia: current concepts and future directions. Arch Gen Psychiatry 38:1359–1364, 1981

Davies BM: Depressive illness in the elderly patient. Postgrad Med 38:314–320, 1965

DeAlarcon R: Hypochondriasis and depression in the aged. Gerontology Clinic 6:266–277, 1964

Dovenmeuhle RH, Reckless JB, Newman G: Depressive reactions in the elderly, in Normal Aging. Edited by Palmore E. Durham, NC, Duke University Press, 1970

Finch CE: Neuroendocrine and autonomic aspects of aging, in The Handbook of the Biology of Aging. Edited by Finch CE, Hayfick L. New York, Van Nostrand Reinhold, 1977, pp 262–280

Gallagher D: Assessment of Depression by Interviewing Methods. Psychiatric Rating Scales. Handbook for Clinical Adults. Edited by Poon LW, Crook T, Dansk L. Washington, DC, American Psychological Association, 1986, pp 202–213

Gallagher D, Thompson LW: Differential effectiveness of psychotherapies for the treatment of major depressive disorder in older adult patients. Psychotherapy 19:482–490, 1982

George LK, Blazer D, Hughes DC, et al: Social support and the outcome of major depression. Br J Psychiatry 154:478–485, 1989

German PS, Shapiro S, Skinner EA: Mental health of the elderly: use of health and mental health services. J Am Geriatr Soc 33:246–252, 1985

Gerson SC, Plotkin DA, Jarvik LF: Antidepressant drug studies, 1964–1986: empirical evidence for aging patients. J Clin Psychopharmacology 8:311–322, 1988

Gurland B, Dean L, Cross P, et al: The epidemiology of depression and dementia in the elderly: the use of multiple indicators of these conditions, in Psychopathology in the Aged. Edited by Cole JO, Barrett JE. New York, Raven, 1980

Hall RCW (ed): Psychiatric Presentations of Medical Illness–Somatopsychic Disorders. New York, SB Medical and Scientific Books, 1980

Hare EH, Shaw GK: Mental Health on a New Housing Estate. Maudsley Monograph 12. London, Oxford University Press, 1965

Hershfeld RMA, Koslow SA, Kupfer DJ (eds): Clinical Utility of the Dexamethasome Suppression Test (DHHS Pub No. (ADM) 85-1318). Washington, DC, U.S. Department of Health and Human Services, 1985

Hopkinson G: A genetic study of affective illness in patients over 50. Br J Psychiatry 110:244–254, 1964

Janowsky A, Sulser F: Alpha and beta adrenoceptors in brain, in Psychopharmacology: The Third Generation of Progress. Edited by Meltzer HY. New York, Raven, 1987

Juel-Nielsen H: Frequency of depressive states within geographically limited population groups. Acta Psychiatr Scand [Suppl] 162:69–80, 1961

Keller MB, Shapiro RW: Major depressive disorder: initial results from a one-year prospective naturalistic follow-up study. J Nerv Ment Dis 169:761–767, 1981

Klerman GL, Weissman MM: Increasing rates of depression. JAMA 261:2029–2035, 1989

Koenig HG, Meador KG, Cohen HJ, et al: Depression in elderly hospitalized patients with medical illness. JAMA 148:1929–1936, 1988

Krishnan KRR, Goli V, Ellinwood EH, et al: Leukoencephalopathy in patients diagnosed as major depressive. Society of Biological Psychiatry 23:519–522, 1988

Kupfer DJ, Foster FG, Coble P, et al: The application of EEG for the differential diagnosis of affective disorders. Am J Psychiatry 135:69–74, 1978

Lesse S: Masked Depression. New York, Jason Aronson, 1974

Levenson AJ, Hall RCW (eds): Neuropsychiatric Manifestations of Physical Disease in the Elderly. New York, Raven Press, 1981

Mendlewicz J: The age factor in depressive illness: some genetic considerations. J Gerontol 31:300–303, 1976

Montgomery SA, Asberg MA: A new depression scale designed to be sensitive to change. Br J Psychiatry 134:382–389, 1979

Murphy E: Social origins of depression in old age. Br J Psychiatry 141:135–142, 1982

Murphy E: The prognosis of depression in old age. Br J Psychiatry 142:111–119, 1983

Myers BS, Kalayman B, Meital V: Late onset delusional depression: a distinct clinical entity? J Clin Psychiatry 45:347–349, 1984

Myers JK, Weissman MM, Tischler GL, et al: Six month prevalence of psychiatric disorders in three communities. Arch Gen Psychiatry 41:959–967, 1984

National Vital Statistics of the United States (1980–1985) as reported by Nancy Osgood. National Center for Health Statistics (NCHS) at the Boston Geriatric Society meeting, 1989

Nelson JC, Bowers MB: Delusional unipolar depression: description and drug responses. Arch Gen Psychiatry 35:1321–1328, 1978

Nemeroff CB, Knight DL, Krishnan KRR, et al: Marked reduction in the number of platelet-tritiated imipramine binding sites in geriatric depression. Arch Gen Psychiatry 45:919–923, 1988

Neugarten BL: Adaptation and the life cycle. J Geriatr Psychol 4:71–87, 1970

Parmelee PA, Katz IR, Lawton MP: Depression of institutionalized aged: assessment and prevalence. J Gerontol 44:M22–M29, 1989

Post F: Depression, alcoholism, and other functional syndromes, in Psychogeriatrics: An International Handbook. Edited by Bergener M. New York, Springer, 1987, pp 223–250

Reifler B, Larson E, Hanley R: Coexistence of cognitive impairment and depression in geriatric outpatients. Am J Psychiatry 139:623–626, 1982

Robinson DS, Davies JM, Nies A, et al: Relation of sex and aging to monoamine oxidase activity of human plasma and platelets. Arch Gen Psychiatry 24:536–541, 1971

Roose SP, Glassman AH, Walsh BT, et al: Depression, delusions and suicide. Am J Psychiatry 140:1159–1162, 1983

Rosenbaum AH, Schatzberg AF, MacLaughlin MS, et al: The DST in normal control subjects: a comparison of two assays and the effects of age. Am J Psychiatry 141:1550–1555, 1984

Ruegg RG, Zisook S, Swendlow NR: Depression in the aged. Psychiatr Clin North Am 11:1, 83–89, 1988

Sachar EJ: Neuroendocrine abnormalities in depressive illness, in Topics in Psychoendocrinology. Edited by Sachar EJ. New York, Grune & Stratton, 1975

Schneider LS, Severson JA, Pollock V, et al: Platelet monoamine oxidase activity in elderly depressed outpatients. Biol Psychiatry 21:1360–1364, 1986

Schulz B: Auszahlungen in der verwandtshaft von nach erkrankungsalter und geschlechtgrupierten manisch-depressien. Archiv fur Psychiatric un Nerven Krankheiten 186:560–576, 1951

Shapiro S, Skinner EA, Kessler LG, et al: Utilization of health and mental health services—three epidemiologic catchment area sites. Arch Gen Psychiatry 41:1971–1978, 1984

Shulman K, Post F: Bipolar affective disorder in old age. Br J Psychiatry 136:26–32, 1980

Small G, Ramanujam K, Michael BS, et al: The influence of age on guilt expression in major depression. International Journal of Geriatric Psychiatry 1:121–126, 1986

Sorensen A, Stromgren E: Frequency of depressive states within geographically delimited population groups, II: prevalence (the Samso investigation). Acta Psychiatr Scand [Suppl] 162:62, 1961

Spar JE: Bipolar affective disorder in aged patients. J Clin Psychiatry 40:504–507, 1979

Spitzer RL, Endicott J, Robins E: Research Diagnostic Criteria: rationale and reliability. Arch Gen Psychiatry 35:773–782, 1978

Srole L, Fisher AK: The Midtown Manhattan Longitudinal Study versus "The Mental Paradise Lost." Arch Gen Psychiatry 37:209–221, 1980

Thompson LW, Gallagher D, Breckenridge JS: Comparative effectiveness of psychotherapies for depressed elders. J Consult Clin Psychol 55:385–390, 1987

Vogel GW, Vogel F, McAbee RS, et al: Improvement of depression by REM sleep deprivation: new findings and a theory. Arch Gen Psychiatry 37:247–253, 1980

Watson M, Roeske WR, Yamamura HI: Cholinergic receptor heterogeneity, in Psychopharmacology: The Third Generation of Progress. Edited by Meltzer HY. New York, Raven, 1987

Wells CF: Pseudodementia. Am J Psychiatry 136:895–900, 1979

Yesavage J, Brink T, Rose T, et al: Development and validation of a geriatric screening scale: a preliminary report. J Psychiatr Res 17:37–49, 1983

Zubenko GS, Reynolds CF, Perel GM, et al: Platelet membrane fluidity and treatment response in cognitively impaired depressed elderly: initial results. Psychopharmacology 94:347–349, 1988

Zung WWK: A self-rating depression scale. Arch Gen Psychiatry 12: 63–70, 1965

CHAPTER 17

Dilip V. Jeste, M.D.
Michael Manley, M.D.
M. Jackuelyn Harris, M.D.

Psychoses

Psychoses are among the most severe psychiatric disorders in any age group, including the elderly. These disorders are characterized by delusions, hallucinations, thought disorder, bizarre behavior, or other evidence of loss of touch with reality. Almost any type of psychosis that occurs in younger persons can be seen in older patients. There are, however, some important epidemiologic and clinical differences between early-onset and late-onset psychoses. Discussed in this chapter are the more common psychoses such as schizophrenia, delusional disorder, and psychotic features complicating dementia. Psychotic symptoms secondary to other organic mental syndromes, and mood disorders with psychotic features are considered elsewhere in this book.

Late-onset Schizophrenia

Historical Background

Nearly 100 years ago Kraepelin used the term *dementia praecox* to refer to a disorder we now know as schizophrenia. Dementia praecox suggested an onset in youth and a deterioration of function in the "emotional and volitional spheres of mental life" (Kraepelin 1919). Kraepelin himself later came to doubt the appropriateness of his terminology because the "dementia" of dementia praecox

This work was supported in part by National Institute of Mental Health grants 5R37-MH43693, RO1-MH45131, and P50-AG05131-06, and by the Veterans Administration.

was not always accompanied by permanent deterioration; remissions did occur in some cases. In addition, not all of the patients first presented in youth. There were subsets of patients with onset of symptoms well into the fifth, sixth, and seventh decades of life. Kraepelin applied the diagnosis paraphrenia to those patients with a relatively late onset of delusions and hallucinations, characterized by a predominance of paranoid symptoms. Although Kraepelin stressed the disintegration of personality in dementia praecox versus paraphrenia, he described some paraphrenics with a predominantly downhill course, whereas a subset of patients with dementia praecox did not suffer a marked deterioration in social and personal functioning. Indeed, follow-up studies of Kraepelin's paraphrenics by other investigators indicated that some of the patients diagnosed as having paraphrenia had features similar to those of dementia praecox (Mayer 1921).

The earlier versions of the Diagnostic and Statistical Manuals did not have an upper age limit for the diagnosis of schizophrenia. It was not until DSM-III (American Psychiatric Association 1980) that it was first stipulated that onset of symptoms for schizophrenia must begin before age 45. DSM-III-R (American Psychiatric Association 1987), on the other hand, has allowed an onset of schizophrenic symptoms after age 44, and it has used the term *late-onset schizophrenia* for these individuals. DSM-III-R does not include paraphrenia as a diagnostic entity.

Epidemiology

Although there is a body of literature on late-onset schizophrenia dating back to 1913, there are several important problems with its interpretation. First, there has been no general agreement on the definition of late onset. Some studies chose 40 years of age, but others examined patients with onset after 45, 60, or 65 years of age (Harris and Jeste 1988). The criteria used to establish the diagnosis of schizophrenia were not always mentioned in these studies. Also, it is often difficult to objectify the assessment of age at onset of schizophrenia. Elderly patients may not remember and significant others may have died, making corroboration of the patient's history difficult. The presence of premorbid paranoid or schizoid personality traits may further confuse the issue, and older patients with schizophrenic symptoms may be thought to have organic mental syndromes, mood disorders, or simple sensory deficits (Harris et al. 1988).

Harris and Jeste (1988), on analyzing data from the psychiatric literature, estimated that 13% of all hospitalized schizophrenic patients have onset of psychosis in their fifties, 7% have onset in their sixties, and only 3% first present after age 70. Most studies of late-onset schizophrenia show a 2- to 10-times higher proportion of women than men. Several factors, such as greater longevity of women and neuropsychosocial stressors, have been suggested as possible explanations for the higher prevalence of late-onset schizophrenia in women. The precise contribution of these and other factors to the onset of schizophrenia in females in later life is unclear.

Diagnosis

The patient should meet the DSM-III-R criteria for schizophrenia (including duration of at least 6 months), with the additional requirement that onset of symptoms—including the prodrome—must be at or after age 45. The typical clinical picture is that of an elderly, never-married woman who exhibits persecutory delusions and, frequently, auditory hallucinations; has a chronic course and a premorbid schizoid and paranoid personality disorder; and shows some improvement with low-dose neuroleptic therapy.

Symptomatology

Late-onset schizophrenia is often characterized by bizarre delusions that have a predominantly persecutory flavor. Systematized delusions of physical or mental influence are seen in a considerable proportion of patients. Grandiose, erotic, or somatic delusions may occur in some cases. Auditory hallucinations are the second most prominent psychotic symptom. Schneiderian first-rank symptoms, such as thought broadcasting or two voices arguing with each other, are not rare. Symptoms of depression are reported by a number of these patients. In contrast, looseness of association and inappropriateness of affect are less common than in younger schizophrenic patients (Jeste et al. 1988). There is an insidious deterioration of personal and social adjustment. It is important to establish an absence of even prodromal symptoms of schizophrenia up to age 45 to exclude the diagnosis of early-onset schizophrenia. (Prodrome is characterized by a clear deterioration in functioning before the active phase of psychosis; it includes symptoms such as marked social isolation, blunted or inappropriate affect, and marked impairment in personal hygiene.)

Pathogenesis and Etiology

The etiology and pathophysiology of late-onset schizophrenia are not well understood. The following variables have been explored in some detail.

Genetics. Studies that have examined the prevalence of schizophrenia in families of late-onset schizophrenic patients have had methodologic problems. For example, not all family members have been followed into old age to ensure that every case of late-onset schizophrenia is detected. Physical illness and geographic relocation of relatives also make it difficult to conduct such studies. The published studies suggest that the prevalence of schizophrenia (whether early or late in onset) is approximately 7% in siblings and 3% in parents of all probands with late-onset schizophrenia. The overall prevalence of schizophrenia in first-degree relatives of late-onset schizophrenic patients tends to be lower than that in families of early-onset schizophrenic patients, but greater than that in families of normal probands.

Premorbid Personality. Some studies (Herbert and Jacobson 1967; Kay and Roth 1961) have noted that a sizable proportion of late-onset schizophrenic patients had abnormal premorbid personality traits of a paranoid or schizoid nature. Many patients were never married and were considered by neighbors to be eccentric. Nevertheless, when compared to earlier-onset schizophrenics, patients with late-onset schizophrenia are more likely to have been married, held a job, and had children (Jeste et al. 1988).

Sensory Deficits. Several studies have reported an association between hearing impairment and late-onset schizophrenia. Cooper and Porter (1976) noted an increased incidence of cataracts in a population of paranoid patients compared to affective controls. Cooper and Curry (1976) went on to demonstrate an association between bilateral conductive hearing loss and paranoid illness. Because of methodological shortcomings of such studies, however, the relative contribution of sensory deficits to late-onset schizophrenia requires further elucidation.

Differential Diagnosis

Whenever an aged patient presents with psychotic symptoms, organic pathology must first be ruled out of the differential diagnosis. This step is especially important because a number of potentially reversible medical and surgical illnesses (e.g., certain endocrinopathies) can produce a clinical picture similar to schizophrenia (see Table 17-1). A careful neurologic examination accompanied by laboratory tests (including thyroid function), as well as serologic tests for syphilis are usually part of the assessment. Other appropriate laboratory tests may be needed in individual patients. Modern imaging methods (e.g., magnetic resonance imaging) may identify cases where structural abnormalities coexist with late-onset psychosis (Miller et al. 1989).

Table 17-1.   Disorders associated with secondary psychosis in the elderly

Endocrinopathies
  Hyperthyroidism
  Hypothyroidism
  Addison's disease
  Cushing's disease
  Hyperparathyroidism
  Hypoparathyroidism
  Hypoglycemia

Neurological disorders
  Parkinson's disease
  Alzheimer's disease
  Pick's disease
  Multi-infarct dementia
  Seizure disorders
  Hydrocephalus
  Demyelinating diseases (multiple sclerosis)
  Neoplasms
  Encephalopathies (posttraumatic, hepatic, postanoxic, toxic)
  Viral encephalitis
  Spinocerebellar degeneration
  Neurosyphilis

Vitamin deficiencies
  Thiamine
  Vitamin B_{12}
  Niacin
  Folate

Other conditions
  Systemic lupus erythematosus
  Temporal arteritis
  Hyponatremia
  Delirium

Caution is required in using the diagnosis of late-onset schizophrenia strictly on the basis of a first psychiatric hospitalization for psychosis after age 44. It is prudent to obtain a detailed history of the disease from both the patient and his or her family or friends, because some patients may have had the prodromal symptoms for some time prior to the first hospitalization. The prodrome differs from premorbid personality traits in that it requires a clear deterioration in a previous level of functioning. Also, some patients with an apparently late onset of psychosis may have had a more benign illness that never required hospitalization until age 45.

Mood disorders with psychotic features may present for the first time after age 44 and can be confused with late-onset schizophrenia. The predominance of affective symptoms and periodicity of the illness should prompt the clinician to consider a mood disorder.

Delusional disorder may mimic late-onset schizophrenia, but the latter diagnosis is more likely in the presence of bizarre delusions or prominent auditory hallucinations, Schneiderian first-rank symptoms, deteriorated functioning, and flattening of affect. (See the section on "Late-Life Delusional Disorder" for further discussion of this differential diagnosis.)

Treatment

Available studies suggest that a significant number of late-onset schizophrenics improve symptomatically with neuroleptic treatment (Jeste et al. 1988). An important consideration is the higher incidence of side effects seen in the elderly versus younger patients upon administration of a given amount of neuroleptic. Some studies have shown positive correlations between age and serum level of neuroleptic when equivalent doses of neuroleptic were administered (Yesavage et al. 1982). Usually, small doses of neuroleptics are sufficient for improvement in older patients. The clinician needs to monitor the elderly patient closely for sedation, autonomic effects, parkinsonism, and tardive dyskinesia.

In this age group, as well as in the early-onset schizophrenic group, neuroleptic drugs are the mainstay of therapy. The clinician should advise the patient and family of the possibility of adverse effects including sedation, anticholinergic effects, parkinsonian reactions, postural hypotension, neuroleptic malignant syndrome, and tardive dyskinesia. Periodic assessment (at least once in several months) for the emergence of involuntary movements is also recommended. At present, there is no satisfactory evidence to indicate superiority of one or more specific neuroleptic drugs in the treatment of late-onset schizophrenia. In individual patients, specific drugs may be preferred on the basis of their side-effect profiles. For example, low-potency neuroleptics with marked anticholinergic activity (e.g., thioridazine) may be avoided in men with prostatic hypertrophy and urinary retention. On the other hand, high-potency neuroleptics with an increased liability of parkinsonian reactions (e.g., haloperidol) may not be the drugs of choice for patients with preexisting rigidity or tremor.

Course and Prognosis

Studies of the course of late-onset schizophrenia have generally found it to be chronic (Herbert and Jacobson 1967; Kay and Roth 1961). Spontaneous remissions seem to be uncommon, and discontinuation of neuroleptics (frequently because of noncompliance) tends to exacerbate psychosis. With good compliance and supportive psychosocial therapies, the outlook can be better.

Aging of Early-Onset Schizophrenic Patients

Many schizophrenic patients survive into old age, yet comparatively little is known about the long-term course of schizophrenia. A recent review of the literature on the course of schizophrenia suggests that approximately one-third of patients either undergo remission or are left with mild symptoms over the long term (McGlashan 1986). The more positive, dramatic symptoms of schizophrenia seem to lessen in severity with the passage of time. Rates of partial or complete remittance, ranging from 6% to greater than 50%, have been reported in individual studies (Harding et al. 1987; McGlashan 1986). However, heterogeneity of outcome is a constant attribute of these studies. Many attempts have been made to uncover associations between specific factors and outcome in schizophrenia. A number of patient-related and illness-related factors have been associated with outcome in the literature, but most of these are of little value for predicting the course in a particular patient (Prudo and Blum 1987). Differences in the methods by which information was obtained, lack of adequate control groups, and inattention to such details as drug history or specific subtype of schizophrenia make conclusions difficult to draw.

Research is needed to examine the impact of the changes in social structure and other age-related changes on the course and outcome of schizophrenia. Retirement, for example, may markedly alter the pattern of psychosocial stressors and may have a favorable impact (because of removal of work-related stresses) or an unfavorable effect (secondary to a reduction in income as well as a decrease in employment-associated self-esteem) on the outcome of schizophrenia. Biologic factors (e.g., hormonal changes in the climacterium) also may be important. Differences in the pharmacokinetics and pharmacodynamics of neuroleptics, and a tendency for milder symptoms in elderly schizophrenics, may result in the need for lower doses of these drugs.

Late-Life Delusional Disorder

Persecutory delusions in the elderly psychotic patient usually occur in the context of another, underlying neuropsychiatric disorder (e.g., schizophrenia, mood disorder, dementia). Occasionally, however, a primary delusional disorder is implicated. Conceptualization and study of this disorder have been hampered by inconsistencies in nomenclature and diagnostic criteria.

Kraepelin (1919) defined paranoia as an often incurable disorder characterized by the development of a chronic, well-systematized, delusional state with little or no impairment of orientation, memory, or intellect and an absence of hallucinations. Kraepelin's paraphrenia, on the other hand, included both paranoid delusions and systematized hallucinations, and its onset was typically in later life.

DSM-III described "paranoid disorder" as consisting of at least 1 week's occurrence of persistent delusions of persecution or jealousy with emotion appropriate to the content of the delusions, without evidence of schizophrenia or affective disorder and without prominent hallucinations or evidence of organic dysfunction. "Paranoia" was described as a chronic and stable persecutory delusional system of greater than 6 months' duration. In DSM-III-R the term "paranoid disorder" has been replaced by "delusional disorder" and the criteria for the delusional content have been broadened to include erotomanic, grandiose, jealous, persecutory, somatic, and unspecified types; also, the minimum required duration of symptoms has been increased to 1 month.

Prevalence

Studies suggest that between 2% and 8% of the psychiatric population suffers from some type of paranoid symptom (Leuchter and Spar 1985). DSM-III-R estimates the population prevalence of delusional disorder at 0.3%, with a lifetime risk of 0.5% to 0.1%. A recent study of the incidence of paranoid or delusional disorder by Heston (1987) indicated that although only about 2% of patients satisfied DSM-III criteria for paranoid disorder, another 13% had paranoid ideation.

Delusional disorder can occur in young people, but it usually presents first in mid- to late adulthood. The average age of onset is somewhat earlier for men (40–49) than for women (60–69).

Diagnosis and Symptomatology

The patient should meet the DSM-III-R criteria for delusional disorder. The occurrence of nonbizarre delusions—defined by DSM-III-R as delusions involving situations that may occur in real life (e.g., being followed, poisoned, loved at a distance)—is fundamental to this illness. Auditory or visual hallucinations, if present, are not prominent, and affective symptoms, if any, are of brief duration and did not antedate the delusional syndrome. The predominant theme or themes of the delusion may be erotomanic, grandiose, jealous, persecutory, somatic, or of unspecified type.

Pathogenesis and Etiology

Several factors have been postulated to contribute to the development of delusional disorder, although the available evidence in favor of each of these needs verification.

Genetics. Some, but not all, studies have found an increased incidence of schizophrenia in families of patients with delusional disorder (Kendler and Davis 1981; Winokur 1977).

Premorbid Personality. Persons with avoidant, paranoid, or schizoid personality disorders may be more likely to develop delusional disorder (American Psychiatric Association 1987).

Sensory Deficits. Some studies have demonstrated an association between hearing loss and paranoia in the elderly (Cooper and

Curry 1976), whereas other systematic studies have failed to confirm this relationship (Moore 1981).

Socioeconomic Status. There is some evidence that immigration or low socioeconomic status can predispose to delusional disorder (American Psychiatric Association 1987).

Differential Diagnosis

In order to make the diagnosis of late-life delusional disorder, organic causes must first be investigated and excluded. Organic delusional syndromes associated with early dementia can resemble delusional disorder (American Psychiatric Association 1987). The relative absence of cognitive impairment in delusional disorder should help to rule out dementia. The differentiation from late-onset schizophrenia has been discussed previously.

Delusions can accompany mood disorders. Therefore, for a diagnosis of delusional disorder to be made, one must establish that the delusions preceded the onset of mood disorder. Depressive symptoms frequently occur in delusional disorder, but they usually begin subsequent to the development of delusions.

DSM-III-R requires that symptoms have been present for at least 1 month. Otherwise, a diagnosis of "psychotic disorder not otherwise specified (NOS)" should be considered.

Treatment

Antipsychotic drugs are often efficacious, especially in agitated delusional patients, but they need to be administered cautiously in the elderly patient. (Also, some patients may be refractory to neuroleptic therapy.) One common problem in the treatment of patients with delusional disorder is noncompliance. Raskind and colleagues (1979) have suggested that parenteral depot neuroleptics may be preferable to oral, daily medication because of problems with compliance. From the viewpoint of therapeutic efficacy, however, there is little evidence that any one type of neuroleptic is superior to others. Psychotherapy is an important modality of treatment (Verwoerdt 1987). For some delusional patients, a somewhat distant, medical-type approach is more acceptable and less threatening. Antidepressant drugs, electroconvulsive therapy, and psychotherapeutic approaches have all been tried with variable success.

Course and Prognosis

The data on prognosis are limited, making it difficult to draw conclusions. The course may be chronic, especially in those with the persecutory type. Others may have remissions and relapses.

Psychotic Disorders Not Elsewhere Classified

DSM-III-R describes several other less well-defined psychotic disorders. There is a relative paucity of literature on the characterization of these disorders in the elderly. The conditions in this category include the following.

Brief Reactive Psychosis

This disorder is characterized by sudden onset of psychotic symptoms of less than 1 month's duration, precipitated by a stressful situation, with eventual complete return to premorbid level of functioning.

Schizophreniform Disorder

This disorder is similar to schizophrenia except that the duration of symptoms (including the prodromal and residual phases) is less than 6 months.

Schizoaffective Disorder

This diagnosis is applied when patients do not meet criteria for schizophrenia but have presented with schizophrenic symptoms (criterion A of DSM-III-R), a mood disturbance at some time, and psychotic features in the absence of prominent mood symptoms for at least 2 weeks.

Induced Psychotic Disorder

This diagnosis is used when a close relationship with a person (or persons) with an already present delusion results in the new development of a similar delusion in the second person. McNiel and associates (1972) described induced psychotic disorder (also called folie à deux) in two elderly persons with shared persecutory delusions. The authors noted that the disorder in their patients was similar to that in younger persons, except for an unusually strong interdependence in the elderly couple.

Psychotic Disorder Not Otherwise Specified (Atypical Psychosis)

DSM-III-R describes "psychotic disorder NOS" as a disorder with clearly psychotic symptoms that do not meet the criteria for any other "nonorganic" psychotic disorder. In essence, this category is a residual one to be used in those situations in which either the patient's history and symptoms do not fit into any other category, or not enough information is available to make a diagnosis. The diagnosis of "atypical psychosis"—the DSM-III equivalent of psychotic disorder NOS—was often made for patients with onset of a schizophrenialike illness in later life, because DSM-III did not recognize late-onset schizophrenia. With the specification of late-onset schizophrenia in DSM-III-R, it is expected that the number of patients carrying the psychotic disorder NOS diagnosis will decrease.

Psychosis in Patients With Dementia

Alzheimer's disease (AD) is the most common type of dementia in the elderly. Psychotic symptoms and disruptive behaviors are present in a sizable proportion of Alzheimer's patients and can cause considerable stress to family members.

Prevalence

In a review of psychiatric features occurring in patients with AD, Wragg and Jeste (1989) noted that about 30% of patients (range 10%–73%) exhibit delusions, often of a persecutory nature. The delusions are usually concrete and interpersonal and may be stimulated by environment. The more common types of delusions refer to specific persons (e.g., daughter-in-law or neighbor) stealing things or spying on the patient, and someone impersonating the spouse or a significant other. Complex or elaborate systematized delusions that characterize schizophrenia or delusional disorder are rarely seen in Alzheimer's patients. Hallucinations are reported to occur in about 21% to 49% of the patients, with a tendency toward a higher incidence in an inpatient population. Visual hallucinations are slightly more frequent than auditory hallucinations. Women with AD may be slightly more likely than men to develop psychotic symptoms.

Diagnosis and Symptomatology

Psychotic symptoms in the demented patient may present as disordered perception and thought content. Because of cognitive impairment, patients may be unable to verbalize their thoughts or perceptions properly. In such cases, the occurrence of delusions or hallucinations can only be inferred from the patient's behavior (e.g., responding to a visual or auditory hallucination). Isolated psychotic symptoms such as persecutory delusions are more frequent than diagnosable psychotic or mood disorders in patients with AD (Teri et al. 1988; Wragg and Jeste 1989).

Pathogenesis/Etiology

Association of psychotic symptoms with specific neuropsychiatric features has been attempted. For example, Mayeux (1985) noted an increased incidence of psychotic symptoms in Alzheimer's patients with coexistent extrapyramidal disorder. Both visual and auditory deficits have been positively associated with psychotic symptoms in the demented population. There is no consistent association of psychosis with severity or stage of AD. A past history of psychiatric disorder may be positively associated with psychotic symptoms in AD (Berrios and Brook 1985).

Differential Diagnosis

Delirium due to medications or medical disorders may occur in the context of dementia, and it is an important consideration in the differential diagnosis of psychotic symptoms in patients with AD. The onset of dementia of the Alzheimer's type or other dementing illness prior to the development of psychotic symptoms should help differentiate these patients from elderly schizophrenic or delusional disorder patients who have subsequently developed some cognitive impairment.

Treatment

Few well-controlled, systematic studies have examined the effects of treatment of psychotic symptoms in patients with AD or other dementing illnesses. The available data suggest that treatment with neuroleptic medications results in improvement (Spira et al. 1984). The various neuroleptic drugs seem to be equally effective in these patients, but, as stated previously, caution is advised in administering these medications. Particular care is taken to exclude delirium before commencing neuroleptic therapy with drugs possessing substantial anticholinergic effects, for they may worsen the cognitive impairment. Alternative treatment options for the management of the demented patient should be considered (Wragg and Jeste 1988). These options include benzodiazepines, which may be of benefit in reducing anxiety and agitation, but not specific psychotic symptoms. Trazodone, because of its sedative effects, may also have efficacy in this regard. Supportive psychotherapy may be beneficial for patients in the earlier stages of dementia, and behavioral modification may be valuable in various stages of the illness.

Course and Prognosis

Although there have been few systematic studies of the course of psychosis in AD, Cummings and colleagues (1987) suggested that as the severity of the dementia increases, the psychotic symptoms tend to decrease; that is, some level of cognitive integrity is necessary for the expression of psychotic symptoms.

Summary

Psychotic symptoms can develop in the elderly in a variety of different conditions. With increasing research in this area the terminology and classification have improved, although much remains to be learned about the etiopathology of these disorders. Late-onset schizophrenia (i.e., schizophrenia with onset after age 44) is usually characterized by bizarre, persecutory delusions; auditory hallucinations; chronic course; and a variable degree of symptomatic improvement with low-dose neuroleptics. Delusional disorder presents with nonbizarre delusions without prominent hallucinations. It is of utmost importance to exclude neurological, endocrine, and other medical conditions in evaluating an older patient with new-onset psychosis. Patients diagnosed as having AD or other dementias may also develop psychotic symptoms. Other conditions associated with late-life psychosis include mood disorders with psychotic features, recurrence of earlier-onset schizophrenia, and psychoses NOS. An appropriately detailed medical, psychosocial, and laboratory workup and a comprehensive psychobiosocial approach to management, with an emphasis on using relatively low doses of medications, are highly recommended.

References

American Psychiatric Association: Diagnostic and Statistical Manual of Mental Disorders, 3rd Edition. Washington, DC, American Psychiatric Association, 1980

American Psychiatric Association: Diagnostic and Statistical Manual of Mental Disorders, 3rd Edition, Revised. Washington, DC, American Psychiatric Association, 1987

Berrios GE, Brook P: Delusions and the psychopathology of the elderly with dementia. Acta Psychiatr Scand 72:296–301, 1985

Cooper AF, Curry AR: The pathology of deafness in the paranoid and affective psychoses of later life. J Psychosom Res 20:97–105, 1976

Cooper AF, Porter R: Visual acuity and ocular pathology in the paranoid and affective psychoses of later life. J Psychosom Res 20:107–114, 1976

Cummings JL, Miller B, Hill MA, et al: Neuropsychiatric aspects of multi-infarct dementia and dementia of the Alzheimer type. Arch Neurol 44:389–393, 1987

Harding CM, Brooks GW, Ashikaga T, et al: The Vermont longitudinal study of persons with severe mental illness, II: long-term outcome of subjects who retrospectively met DSM-III criteria for schizophrenia. Am J Psychiatry 144:727–735, 1987

Harris MJ, Jeste DV: Late-onset schizophrenia: an overview. Schizophr Bull 14:39–55, 1988

Harris MJ, Cullum CM, Jeste DV: Clinical presentation of late-onset schizophrenia. J Clin Psychiatry 49:356–360, 1988

Herbert ME, Jacobson S: Late paraphrenia. Br J Psychiatry 113:461–469, 1967

Heston LL: The paranoid syndrome after mid life, in Schizophrenia and Aging. Edited by Miller NE, Cohen GD. New York, Guilford Press, 1987

Jeste DV, Harris MJ, Pearlson GD, et al: Late-onset schizophrenia: studying clinical validity. Psychiatr Clin North Am 11:1–14, 1988

Kay DWK, Roth R: Environmental and hereditary factors in the schizophrenias of old age ("late paraphrenia") and their bearing on the general problem of causation in schizophrenia. J Ment Sci 107:649–686, 1961

Kendler S, David KL: The genetics and biochemistry of paranoid schizophrenia and other paranoid psychoses. Schizophr Bull 7:689–709, 1981

Kraepelin E: Dementia praecox and paraphrenia (1919). Translated by Barclay RM. New York, Robert E. Krieger Publishing, 1971, pp 282–329

Leuchter AF, Spar JE: The late-onset psychoses. J Nerv Ment Dis 173:488–494, 1985

Mayer W: On paraphrenic psychoses (in German). Zeitschrift fur Gesamte Neurologie und Psychiatrie 71:187–206, 1921

Mayeux R, Stern Y, Spanton S: Heterogeneity in dementia of the Alzheimer type: evidence of subgroups. Neurology 35:453–461, 1985

McGlashan TH: Predictors of shorter-medium and longer-term outcome in schizophrenia. Am J Psychiatry 143:50–55, 1986

McNiel JN, Verwoerdt A, Peak D: Folie à deux in the aged: review and case report of role reversal. J Am Geriatr Soc 20:316–323, 1972

Miller BL, Lesser IM, Boone K, et al: Brain white-matter lesions and psychosis. Br J Psychiatry 155:73–78, 1989

Moore NC: Is paranoid illness associated with sensory defects in the elderly? J Psychosom Res 25:69–74, 1981

Prudo R, Blum HM: Five-year outcome and prognosis in schizophrenia: a report from the London field research centre of the international pilot study of schizophrenia. Br J Psychiatry 150:345–354, 1987

Raskind M, Alvarez C, Merlin S: Fluphenazine enanthate in outpatient treatment of late paraphrenia. J Am Geriatr Soc 27:459–463, 1979

Spira N, Dysken MW, Lazarus LW, et al: Treatment of agitation and psychosis, in Clinical Geriatric Psychopharmacology. Edited by Salzman C. New York, McGraw-Hill, 1984, pp 49–76

Teri L, Larson EB, Reifler BV: Behavioral disturbance in dementia of the Alzheimer's type. J Am Geriatr Soc 36:1–6, 1988

Verwoerdt A: Psychodynamics of paranoid phenomena in the aged, in Treating the Elderly With Psychotherapy. Edited by Sadavoy J, Leszcz M. Madison, CT, 1987, pp 67–93

Winokur G: Delusional disorder (paranoia). Compr Psychiatry 18:511–521, 1977

Wragg RE, Jeste DV; Neuroleptics and alternative treatments: management of behavioral symptoms and psychosis in Alzheimer's disease and related conditions. Psychiatr Clin North Am 11:195–214, 1988

Wragg R, Jeste DV: An overview of depression and psychosis in Alzheimer's disease. Am J Psychiatry 146:577–587, 1989

Yesavage JA, Becker J, Werner PD, et al: Serum level monitoring of thiothixene in schizophrenia: acute single-dose levels at fixed doses. Am J Psychiatry 139:174–178, 1982

CHAPTER 18

Robert Abrams, M.D.

Anxiety and Personality Disorders

Anxiety Disorders

Epidemiology

Epidemiologic data suggest that anxiety syndromes have their on-set in early life and have lower prevalence in old age (Regier et al. 1988). Most phobic disorders emerge during childhood through the mid-twenties, and the mean age of onset for panic disorder is in the mid-thirties (Weissman 1988). A mixed-age study found a younger age of illness onset among patients with both major depression and anxiety disorders than among patients with major depression alone (Leckman et al. 1983b). By age 65, the prevalence of anxiety disorders declines. Based on 1-month prevalence rates from the National Institute of Mental Health Epidemiologic Catchment Area (ECA) study, the prevalence for anxiety disorders is lower for both men and women in the over-65 group than for younger age groups (Regier et al. 1988).

A sex differentiation has also been found in the recent data on geriatric anxiety disorders. Following the pattern of the younger age groups, older women in the ECA study were more likely than older men to receive an anxiety disorder diagnosis. The rates for older men were 3.6% for all anxiety disorders, 2.9% for phobias, 0% for panic disorder, and 0.7% for obsessive-compulsive disorders, whereas the rates for older women were 6.8% overall, 6.1% for phobias, 0.2% for panic disorder, and 0.9% for obsessive-compulsive disorders (Regier et al. 1988).

The data showing early onset of anxiety disorders and reduced prevalence in old age must be interpreted with caution, however.

For example, it is not clear whether these data represent the natural course of anxiety disorders (i.e., diminution of prevalence and severity with aging), underreporting by elderly subjects in the study, or cohort differences in which prevalence rates reflect circumstances associated with specific generations (Liptzin 1989). There is evidence that older persons with anxiety disorders rarely seek help (Thompson et al. 1988), and it is also possible that elderly patients are more likely to report some anxiety symptoms more frequently than others. For example, panic disorder is the most common anxiety disorder diagnosis among people of all ages seeking treatment, but it may not be so for the older segments of the population. These methodological issues require further study before it can be confidently asserted that phobias, for example, are more likely than obsessional or panic syndromes to persist into old age.

Other factors may also influence the epidemiologic data on anxiety disorders in the elderly. An example is the heterogeneity of geriatric populations. The current cohort aged older than 65 may actually encompass three groups: the "young-old" under 75, the "old-old" over 85, and those in between. These subgroups may prove to have distinct psychosocial and biological characteristics, and different prevalence patterns of illness, which are obscured in the larger cohort. Moreover, current epidemiologic data do not distinguish late-onset anxiety disorders from early-onset anxiety disorders that persist into old age. These conditions may eventually be shown to have different clinical features, outcomes, and predictors of outcomes.

Another problem is that epidemiologic data in this area focus on anxiety disorders per se, or conditions that meet DSM-III-R (American Psychiatric Association 1987) criteria for diagnosis. Signs and symptoms of anxiety not meeting such criteria (subsyndromal anxiety) have not been studied systematically in the geriatric population. Also, there is considerable comorbidity of anxiety and major depression (Alexopoulos 1989) as there is with other medical and psychiatric syndromes in the geriatric population. The implications of comorbidity for evaluation, diagnosis, and treatment of anxiety syndromes are discussed in the following sections. However, the net effect of diagnostic and comorbidity factors may be to reduce the number of individuals meeting full criteria for a DSM-III-R anxiety disorder, with signs and symptoms of anxiety subsumed under other Axis I categories. The relationship between anxiety and depression—syndromal and subsyndromal—is especially important in the geriatric population. Nosological ambiguities, clinical overlap between signs and symptoms of depression and anxiety (Tyrer et al. 1983), evidence for a nonspecific genetic predisposition to anxiety and depression (Kendler et al. 1987), and the relative lack of specificity of antianxiety and antidepressant drugs (Johnstone et al. 1980) may all contribute to diagnostic blurring and limited accuracy of current epidemiologic data.

Evaluation and Diagnosis

Recent factor and cluster analyses of signs and symptoms of anxiety have identified two fundamental categories, often labeled 1) "cognitive" or "psychic" anxiety and 2) "somatic" anxiety because of their predominant characteristics (Cloninger 1986; Sigvardsson et al. 1986). Cognitive anxiety involves muscular tension, apprehensiveness, and hypervigilance in response to actual or potential danger signals; somatic anxiety involves autonomic hyperactivity, a feeling of overall uneasiness, distractibility, and often multiple bodily aches and pains that are not prompted by a signal or precipitant. Aspects of both cognitive and somatic anxiety can be found in all anxiety disorders and can also occur as isolated symptoms outside the context of DSM-III-R anxiety disorders.

In the elderly, however, the problem of evaluation and diagnosis of anxiety symptomatology and disorders lies less in the identification of basic phenomena such as cognitive and somatic anxiety than in their etiologic attribution. For example, signs and symptoms of cognitive and somatic anxiety can occur in the setting of medical illnesses common in the elderly and thus be mistaken for a primary anxiety disorder. This diagnostic confusion is of greater importance in the geriatric population because the elderly are more likely than the young to have significant health problems and functional disability. Anxiety of syndromal severity often accompanies such manifestations of cardiovascular disease as palpitations, dysrhythmias, and angina. Awareness of the potentially fatal consequences of chest pain by a cardiac patient is a realistic source of anxiety, which, in this case, can function as both a precipitant and a consequence of the cardiac manifestations. Similarly, it can be difficult to determine the precise role of symptomatic anxiety in the clinical presentation of chronic obstructive respiratory disease, thyroid disease, Parkinson's disease, and a spectrum of movement disorders. Overall, a conservative approach to diagnosis is probably most reasonable when medical comorbidity is present, reserving the diagnosis of anxiety disorder for patients in whom the signs and symptoms of anxiety not only meet DSM-III-R criteria but also clearly precede the medical condition or present independent from it.

Signs and symptoms of anxiety are also associated with specific pharmacological treatments of medical and psychiatric disorders. Examples include steroids, theophylline, thyroid replacement therapies, neuroleptics, and antidepressant medications, among many others. Anxiolytic and sedative-hypnotic drugs themselves are associated with rebound anxiety and insomnia when discontinued after chronic use (Liptzin and Salzman 1988).

The general phenomena of insomnia and chronic pain pose similar problems in the diagnosis of anxiety disorders, namely, the difficulty in determining whether anxiety is primary or secondary. In the elderly, reduced time spent in both rapid eye movement (REM) and deeper stages of sleep is nearly universal (Miles and Dement 1980); a healthy older person may lie awake for 20% of the night; by age 75, nearly half of all healthy persons will have complained of some form of insomnia. Thus, the clinician should not assume that complaints of sleep problems in older persons are invariably related to anxiety and depression. Chronic pain is not exclusively the consequence of physical conditions, but on closer examination it may represent the clinical expression of underlying anxiety or dysphoria.

Negative life events must be evaluated carefully in older patients before the signs and symptoms of anxiety that accompany them can be attributed to anxiety disorders. Death of a spouse, serious illness in a family member, institutionalization, and victimization by crime are among the life crises that have been shown to occur frequently in geriatric populations (Murphy 1983). Attention is directed to the timing and duration of signs and symptoms of anxiety as well as the patient's premorbid functioning to assess accurately the impact of a traumatic life event. However, just as late-onset alcoholism has been conceptualized as a maladaptive response to age-related events, it is possible that late-onset anxiety disorders may first emerge, or be exacerbated, after age-related precipitants.

Psychiatric comorbidity, however, is probably the greatest source of confusion in the diagnosis of geriatric anxiety symptoms and disorders. The overlap between anxiety and depression syndromes is substantial. In a study of mixed-age outpatients with unipolar or bipolar major depression, 58% of the sample also had an anxiety disorder (Leckman et al. 1983a); of the patients with both anxiety and depression, approximately one-third met criteria for an anxiety disorder even during depression-free intervals. Also, differences in family history distinguished depressed from anxious-depressed patients. First-degree relatives of patients with both major depression and an anxiety disorder were at greater risk to develop either of these conditions than were relatives of individuals with major depression alone (Leckman et al. 1983a), suggesting that anxiety-depression syndromes may differ genetically as well as clinically from "pure" depression. Hyer and associates (1987) showed that hospitalized elderly men tended to have combined symptoms of depression, anxiety, and hypochondriasis during a single episode of illness. Examining the comorbidity of anxiety and depression in 45 geriatric patients consecutively admitted to an outpatient psychiatric clinic, Alexopoulos (1989) found that only 2% had an anxiety disorder alone, but 38% of patients with major depression also met DSM-III-R criteria for an anxiety disorder. This finding suggests that geriatric patients have anxiety-depression comorbidity at a rate only slightly lower than that of younger patients (e.g., 58% in the mixed-age sample of Leckman et al. [1983a]). However, the reluctance of geriatric patients with anxiety disorders to seek help might distort the comorbidity findings. Moreover, the fact that there is a dearth of relevant studies precludes firm conclusions at this time.

Signs and symptoms of anxiety (rarely DSM-III-R anxiety disorders) are also observed in the context of geriatric alcoholism and may be related to the abrupt drop in blood alcohol levels that follows an episode of heavy drinking (Schuckit 1979), to the general central nervous system depressant effects of alcohol, or to an underlying anxiety-depression syndrome. Paniclike experiences, as well as auditory hallucinations and paranoid delusions, are not infrequently reported by older alcoholics (Victor and Hope 1958). Although alcohol does not appear to affect total sleep time, REM and delta sleep are both decreased, resulting in irritability and lethargy (Bienenfeld 1990). Some elderly individuals use alcohol as self-medication for insomnia, especially sleep-onset difficulties. However, there is often a rebound wakefulness later on in the night, which appears to be related to falling blood alcohol levels. Physiologic and pharmacokinetic changes of aging are likely to result in increased vulnerability to these complications of alcoholism. As noted previously, many of these same complications, particularly rebound anxiety phenomena, are also observed in elderly benzodiazepine users. Decreased tolerance of stimulant drugs such as caffeine may produce physiologic manifestations of anxiety in older persons. Certainly, a careful review of the elderly patient's substance abuse history must be undertaken before other Axis I diagnoses are assigned.

There is relatively little information on the nature of anxiety symptoms and disorders in geriatric depression, although Alexopoulos (1989) has reported preliminary data in hospitalized elderly depressives suggesting that 1) severe psychic anxiety is considerably more frequent than intense somatic anxiety in geriatric major depression, and 2) psychic or cognitive anxiety, but not somatic anxiety, appears to vary inversely with the chronicity of depression. There is probably also considerable comorbidity of anxiety signs and symptoms in dementing disorders, particularly those with a component of agitation; there may also be further overlap in the area of personality disorders (Abrams 1990).

In summary, the evaluation of symptomatic anxiety and anxiety disorders in the elderly is made considerably more complex by the multiple overlapping clinical contexts in which they arise. Anxiety disorders may appear de novo in old age, may represent an exacerbation of previous symptomatology that had hitherto failed to meet DSM-III-R criteria for diagnosis, or may be the continuation into old age of a lifetime condition. As often as not, anxiety disorders in the elderly accompany chronic medical illness, the use of multiple medications and alcohol, or other Axis I disorders (see Table 18-1). Of all these conditions, the anxiety disorder may be the least likely to be appropriately evaluated and treated.

Treatment

Treatment of anxiety disorders in the elderly is mainly psychopharmacologic, but the medications are usually prescribed by nonpsychiatrists. Most patients, including the elderly, receive psychotropic medication prescriptions from their primary care practitioners (Beardsley et al. 1988); nonpsychiatric primary care practitioners are most likely to prescribe an antianxiety medication, in contrast to psychiatrists, who most often prescribe antidepressants. These prescribing patterns may partly explain the contradiction of a low prevalence of bona fide anxiety disorders in the over-65 U.S. population and a high use of antianxiety medications by the same group. Although the ECA program placed the overall rate for anxiety disorders in persons 65 years and older at 5.5% (Blazer 1989), a household survey of medication use by persons aged 60 to 74 years—quoted by Atkinson and Schuckit (1983)—

Table 18-1. Summary of conditions associated with anxiety in the elderly

DSM-III-R anxiety disorders (e.g., panic disorders, agoraphobia, social phobias, simple phobia, obsessive-compulsive disorder, posttraumatic stress disorder, generalized anxiety disorder)

Other Axis I syndromes: major depression, senile dementia

Personality disorders

Alcoholism; benzodiazepine abuse and dependence

Chronic pain syndromes

Chronic insomnia

Transient anxiety associated with negative life events

Medical conditions (e.g., cardiovascular disease, chronic respiratory disease, Parkinson's disease, movement disorders, thyroid dysfunction)

Pharmacological treatments (e.g., corticosteroids, theophylline, thyroid replacement therapies, antipsychotic and antidepressant medications)

found that 11% of the men and 25% of the women used anxiolytic drugs. Although comprising only 10% of the U.S. population, patients over 65 accounted for more than 21% of all prescriptions for diazepam (Atkinson and Schuckit 1983).

An analysis of National Ambulatory Medical Care Survey (Beardsley et al. 1988) data also showed that psychiatrists were more likely than primary care physicians to attempt nonpharmacological interventions as first-line treatment for all mental disorders. This finding has important implications for geriatric patients, in whom side effects and adverse drug interactions are of greater frequency and significance than in younger patients. Because many more elderly patients receive care from primary physicians than from psychiatrists, this finding may account for the relative neglect of psychotherapeutic and behavioral approaches in the treatment of anxiety disorders in particular.

Anxiolytic drugs nevertheless comprise the mainstay of treatment for anxiety disorders in the elderly. Since their introduction in the 1960s, benzodiazepines have supplanted meprobamate as the drugs of choice both for treating transient or "reactive" anxiety and for long-term management of chronic anxiety states. In recent years geriatric clinicians have tended to favor benzodiazepines with shorter half-lives (e.g., lorazepam) to avoid potentially toxic accumulations of drug that occur as a result of the slowed pharmacokinetics of the elderly (Liptzin and Salzman 1988). However, some patients with both daytime anxiety and nighttime insomnia require relatively constant 24-hour levels of medication, and other geriatric patients have been maintained for years on longer-acting drugs. According to Liptzin (1989) these two groups of patients may never achieve satisfactory benefit from the shorter-acting benzodiazepines and stand as exceptions to the general principle of geriatric pharmacotherapeutics, which calls for use of the shortest-acting drug. Also, symptoms of withdrawal from benzodiazepines—which can include rebound anxiety and insomnia as well as tachycardia and other physiological signs—may, in the elderly, be more associated with the use of shorter-acting benzodiazepines than longer-acting ones (Woods et al. 1988).

Although the possibility of drug dependence or abuse should be carefully considered in each case and the lowest effective doses used, recent data do not support the idea that elderly patients are likely to become benzodiazepine abusers (Pinsker and Suljaga-Petchel 1984). On the contrary, the typical elderly patient in these studies used the medications with extreme caution, a finding that suggests that some clinicians may be adopting an overconservative approach to benzodiazepines and thereby unnecessarily prolonging their patients' suffering.

Increasing attention has recently been given to the use of serotonin reuptake inhibitors for obsessive compulsive disorder in younger patients (Goodman et al. 1989). Sufficient data will eventually be available to assess these agents' utility for both anxiety disorders and subsyndromal anxiety symptomatology in the geriatric population.

The coexistence of medical illness or concurrent Axis I conditions frequently complicates the treatment of anxiety syndromes in the elderly. Often, however, treatment of the depressive disorder also provides significant relief of anxiety-related symptomatology; the converse occurs as well. Pharmacological approaches to these combined syndromes are frequently determined by the clinician's perception of anxiety as primary or secondary to the signs and symptoms of depression, or dictated by limiting conditions such as cardiovascular disease—which, for example, might reduce the safety of tricyclic antidepressants. Where anxiety is felt to be a significant component of the clinical picture in dementia, it seems prudent to avoid low-potency neuroleptic drugs and such medications as diphenhydramine hydrochloride (Benadryl), which might induce anticholinergic toxicity. The use of alcohol as an anxiolytic for demented patients in nursing homes and hospitals is probably counterproductive because of the likelihood of rebound phenomena.

Personality Disorders

General Considerations

At present there is relatively little cross-sectional information on DSM-III-R personality disorders in the older age groups, and no longitudinal studies of personality disorder patients are available that track their symptoms into senescence. Much of what is known about personality disorders in the elderly is, therefore, culled from the classic literature on geriatric depression, in which personality traits helped to distinguish clinical subgroups (Post 1962, 1972).

Moreover, the underlying issue of personality changes in normal aging is not settled. Although some large-scale cross-sectional studies using the Minnesota Multiphasic Personality Inventory (MMPI) (Hathaway and McKinley 1943) have shown older subjects to obtain higher scores on scales measuring introversion, concern with health, depression, and immaturity, and lower scores on scales measuring impulsivity, sociopathy, and hostility, these findings have not been borne out in longitudinal MMPI studies; the longitudinal studies have instead emphasized stability of personality profiles of the individual over time (Gynther 1979). Similarly, dimensional scores on the Eysenck Personality Inventory psychoticism, extraversion, and neuroticism subscales show substantial persistence over 30-year periods (Eysenck 1985). Sadavoy and Fogel (in press) in their review point out the conflicting data from cross-sectional, longitudinal, and cross-sequential studies, but highlight how little change seems to occur in personality over time.

However, based on cross-sectional regression analysis of the relationships of different personality disorder traits with age, Tyrer (1988) has suggested that personality disorders can be divided into "mature" and "immature" categories. The mature disorders include obsessive-compulsive, schizotypal, schizoid, and paranoid; these personality disorders show more stability and less variation with age than others. The immature, or flamboyant, personality disorders include the borderline, antisocial, narcissistic, histrionic, and passive-aggressive categories; these personality disorders are more evident in younger individuals, may have earlier onset than mature personality disorders, and tend to become less evident with time. Other authors (McGlashan 1986; Stone 1985) have commented, on the basis of follow-up data, that the florid borderline symptomatology seen at index admissions is much attenuated by age 30, or in the second decade of follow-up. However, while instrumental functioning improved in midlife, relationships remained loose and distant. McGlashan's suggestion that these deficits in relationships may "haunt" the aging borderline is borne out in an upturn in symptoms in patients followed for more than 20 years after diagnosis. Tyrer (1988) reviewed data suggesting that patients with personality disorders have a greater mortality by suicide than other psychiatric patients for a period of 5 years from diagnosis; differences in suicide rates between personality disorder and other psychiatric patients become negligible afterward. The mortality data have been interpreted by Tyrer to support a maturation hypothesis, especially for antisocial and the other immature personality disorders, in which impulsiveness and suicide become less likely over time; however, these data do not follow patients into middle and old age. It is also possible that mature personality disorders are more frequent in the geriatric population than immature personality disorders. Again, longitudinal studies are required.

The maturation hypothesis does not address the problem of theoretical and clinical applicability of DSM-III-R personality disorders to geriatric populations. In the introduction to personality disorders in DSM-III-R (American Psychiatric Association 1987), these entities are described as "often recognizable by adolescence or earlier and continue throughout most of adult life, though they often become less obvious in middle or old age." In a study of geriatric depressives and normal elderly subjects, relatively few individuals met full criteria for DSM-III-R personality disorders, despite a wide range of Axis II symptomatology in the sample population (Abrams et al. 1987). It is possible, however, that these impressions reflect an age bias of DSM-III-R as well as the influences of selective mortality or the natural course of personality disorders. The argument for age bias is that DSM-III-R criteria have limited relevance to the experiences of late life and are less likely to result in diagnosis of personality disorders in the elderly. With its emphasis on "social and occupational functioning," for example, Axis II appears to have been designed using a modal young adult expected to be making career and life-partner choices. As discussed in the following section, interpretation of criteria in a geriatric context requires creativity, flexibility, and probably some loss of diagnostic accuracy.

Evaluation and Diagnosis of DSM-III-R Personality Disorders

Coexistence of Personality Dysfunction and Depression. The complex relationship between depressive and personality symptomatology often confounds the psychiatric evaluation of the geriatric patient. Confusion is encountered particularly in the attempt to differentiate personality traits from features of depression. The dependency, helplessness, somatic preoccupations, and negative self-evaluation frequently observed in elderly depressives can be understood to represent either depressive phenomena or pathological personality functioning. Clinical decisions regarding hospitalization, pharmacotherapy, and suitability for psychotherapy may depend on whether symptoms are seen to reflect stable personality traits or acute depression (Abrams 1989). Although efforts are usually made to obtain an impression of the "baseline" personality functioning of depressed geriatric patients, Axis II disorders are generally diagnosed sparingly during an acute depressive episode because of the unavoidable influence of the Axis I illness. Reports (Reich et al. 1986, 1987) indicate that acute anxiety states also distort self-assessment on a battery of personality assessment instruments, although this phenomenon has been studied much less than the depression-personality confound.

Some forms of chronic depression seen in geriatric populations seem especially closely related to personality disorders. Dysthymia, for example, is a low-grade depressive syndrome that appears in as much as 15% of the geriatric population (Blazer and Williams 1980; Moore 1985). Dysthymia could equally well be deemed an affective disorder with prominent character pathology, or a personality disorder with secondary affective symptomatology, although there may actually be subgroups of each, depending on response to antidepressant drugs (Akiskal 1983). Another chronic depressive disorder often seen in the geriatric population, and again associated with significant personality psychopathology, is "double depression." Post (1962, 1972) used the term "depressive invalidism" to describe double depression in the elderly, referring to a group of geriatric patients having severe recurrent depression with incomplete remissions. Finally, the term "masked depression" has been used to describe a depression syndrome, believed to be more common after midlife, in which cognitive or somatic symptoms are more prominent than sadness, tearfulness, or other affective manifestations (Kielholz 1973; Pissot and Hassan 1973). Thus, masked depression not only may present as a mixed personality disorder in geriatric patients, but also has been associated with a number of dysfunctional premorbid personality traits (Jacobowsky 1961; Lesse 1968; Lindberg 1965).

It is fair to conclude from this discussion that in the geriatric population, where chronic or recurrent depression is common and may also be accompanied by cognitive changes, "clean" personality diagnosis may be impossible. In these circumstances, the clinician must rely on collateral sources of information and in some cases may be forced to defer the designation of an Axis II diagnosis until sufficient historical and observational data can be obtained.

The Time Frame Problem.   Another difficulty in examining geriatric patients for the presence of Axis II disorders is the selection of an appropriate time frame for duration of symptoms. This point is important because with elderly patients there is an entire lifetime to review. DSM-III-R stipulates that criteria for personality disorders should reflect current (1 year) and long-term functioning, but it is not clear whether this stipulation requires dysfunctional behavior patterns to be present continuously from adolescence to old age in order to qualify for a personality disorder. Also, DSM-III-R does not specifically acknowledge past personality disorders (those that have been present throughout much of adult life but are attenuated in old age) nor late-onset personality disorders (those first appearing or meeting full criteria in middle age or later). It is hoped that the recent development of standardized instruments for Axis II diagnoses will produce information on the natural course of personality disorders and the prevalence of past and late-onset disorders (Loranger et al. 1987). For the moment, it is left to the geriatric clinician to determine an appropriate time frame for making a personality disorder diagnosis. It is recommended that the presence or absence of Axis II symptomatology in young adulthood be established first, and information then pursued decade by decade through middle age to the present. This approach can help the clinician to appreciate whether current behavior represents long-standing personality functioning or is more closely related to chronic depression, organic brain changes, or a reaction to age-related life events.

Individual Personality Disorders.   When examining the current period of old age for evidence of personality disorder criteria, it is necessary to interpret those criteria in a geriatric context. For example, in the odd-eccentric (Cluster A) personality disorders (including paranoid, schizoid, and schizotypal personality disorders), care must be taken to consider whether suspiciousness of exploitation or harm (in paranoid personality disorder) or social and sexual isolation (in schizoid personality disorder) are not indeed realistic behaviors in the case of an impoverished, infirm, elderly widower living in a crime-ridden neighborhood.

Cluster B, the dramatic-emotional personality disorders (antisocial, borderline, histrionic, and narcissistic) are assigned to geriatric patients especially infrequently, possibly because they are truly "immature" syndromes that prove unstable over long periods of time and also because much latitude is required to fit the criteria to the experiences of older people. As an example, the "borderline" criteria for idealization should include consideration of such behavior when directed toward caregivers in a hospital or nursing home. "Self-damaging impulsiveness" should not be limited to reckless driving or sexual activity, and "frantic efforts to avoid real or imagined abandonment" should not be confused with reactions to age-related losses or institutionalization. Thus, some criteria (e.g., "self-damaging impulsiveness") must be broadened to include the geriatric context, while others (e.g., "frantic efforts to avoid abandonment") should be narrowed to exclude the impact of realistic events.

The same caveat is true for Cluster C personality disorders, also called the anxious-fearful cluster, which include avoidant, dependent, obsessive-compulsive, and passive-aggressive personality disorders. Reactions and attitudes toward caregivers provide an appropriate context for many elderly patients in which to interpret Cluster C criteria, particularly those for passive-aggressive and dependent disorders. However, the effects of chronic illness on dependency can confuse the issue, because the long-standing illness might make the dependent behavior appear more like personality functioning. In all these disorders, it seems most appropriate to err on the side of conservatism or specificity in diagnosis. Obviously, the clinician can be most confident of the assessment when antecedents of criteria are traceable to the past, but there remains an obligation to determine what is and is not pathological in the older person's present reality.

Treatment

General Principles. Although geriatric patients with personality disorder comprise a more heterogeneous group than might first be imagined, it is possible to set forth some general principles of management:

- Postpone treatment efforts directed toward the personality disorder component until treatment of a concurrent Axis I condition, particularly an affective disorder, has been completed or has reached maximum efficacy.

- Establish clearly the patient's state of physical health. Chronic medical illnesses are associated with unfavorable outcome of treatment in geriatric depression and may likewise adversely affect the course of personality disorders.
- Make creative use of family and institutional supports.
- Set limited, realistic goals for psychotherapy and somatic therapies, based on a collaterally informed picture of the patient's long-term functioning.

Psychotherapy. Patients with personality disorders approach old age ill-equipped to cope with its stresses; a lifetime of disturbed interpersonal relationships and distorted self-attitudes has preceded them. Although difficulty adjusting to the stresses and losses of old age is to some extent universal, in patients with personality disorder the difficulty is increased and has real psychosocial consequences. These individuals tend to experience the inevitable losses of aging as narcissistic assaults, and they respond with primitive defenses involving splitting and interpersonal manipulativeness. An underlying intolerance for anxiety and affect is coupled with an incapacity to grieve, both for losses of significant others and for their own eventual death.

Thus, the psychotherapist working with elderly personality disorder patients faces a daunting task. Impaired interpersonal relationships and denial in the face of unpleasant realities do not suggest significant potential for psychotherapeutic change. However, if a basic alliance can be forged with the therapist, the elderly patient may be able to recognize the attitude of genuine concern and accept truths that, from others, might be rejected as intolerable.

The psychotherapist treating older patients in general, and personality disorder patients in particular, most operate within the patient's social system. Family involvement is crucial, as is work with the staff for institutionalized patients. For patients in nursing homes, the therapist alternately protects the patient from the social system, and the social system from the patient. However, issues of confidentiality and psychotherapeutic boundaries require careful thought. A psychiatrist involved in conservatorship proceedings or long-term care placement may not be able to function at the same time as a psychotherapist for that patient.

A major difference between psychotherapy of older and younger patients is the time frame covered. Transference issues continue to be directed from childhood sources and early parental relationships, but they often contain an overlay from experiences later in life (Sadavoy 1987). The initial focus should be on the patient's present reality and the relationship with the therapist as it unfolds;

this approach has been recommended as a compelling strategy to cope with the interpersonal distortions of personality disorder patients (Kernberg 1976), and with elderly persons it similarly provides a point of shared reality that patient and therapist can examine together. Issues from the past then emerge more naturally, in an unforced and relevant fashion. Patients probably do have a need to mourn past losses, but as Sadavoy (1987) pointed out, such mourning is done neither globally nor in a predictable sequence.

A psychotherapy relationship cannot reasonably be expected to resolve the psychological deficits, and the consequences of those deficits, of elderly patients with personality disorders—a lifetime of missed opportunities, failed relationships, and unused talents. Nevertheless, the impetus provided by aging and restricted opportunities for expression of pathological behaviors may render older patients amenable to a process of growth and change.

References

Abrams RC: Personality disorders in the elderly, in Verwoerdt's Clinical Geropsychiatry, 3rd Edition. Edited by Bienenfeld D. Baltimore, MD, Williams & Wilkins, 1990

Abrams RC, Alexopoulos GS, Young RC: Geriatric depression and DSM-III-R personality disorder criteria. J Am Geriatr Soc 35:383–386, 1987

Akiskal HS: Dysthymic disorder: psychopathology of proposed chronic depressive subtypes. Am J Psychiatry 140:11–20, 1983

Alexopoulos GS: Anxiety and depression in the elderly. Paper presented at a Harvard-NIMH Conference on Anxiety in the Elderly, Boston, January 9–10, 1989

American Psychiatric Association: Diagnostic and Statistical Manual of Mental Disorders, 3rd Edition, Revised. Washington, DC, American Psychiatric Association, 1987

Atkinson JH, Schuckit MA: Geriatric alcohol and drug misuse and abuse. Advances in Substance Abuse 3:195–237, 1983

Beardsley RS, Gardocki GJ, Larson DB, et al: Prescribing of psychotropic medication by primary care physicians and psychiatrists. Arch Gen Psychiatry 45:1117–1119, 1988

Bienenfeld D: Substance abuse in the elderly, in Verwoerdt's Clinical Geropsychiatry, 3rd Edition. Edited by Bienenfeld D. Baltimore, MD, Williams & Wilkins, 1990

Blazer D, Williams CD: Epidemiology of dysphoria and depression in an elderly population. Br J Psychiatry 137:439–444, 1980

Blazer D: Epidemiology and Clinical Interface. Paper presented at a Harvard-NIMH Conference on Anxiety in the Elderly. Boston, January 9–10, 1989

Cloninger CR: A unified biosocial theory of personality and its role in the development of anxiety states. Psychiatr Dev 3:167–226, 1986

Eysenck HJ, Eysenck MW: Personality and Individual Differences. New York, Plenum, 1985

Goodman WK, Price LH, Rasmussen SA, et al: Efficacy of fluvoxamine in obsessive-compulsive disorder. Arch Gen Psychiatry 46:36–44, 1989

Gynther MD: Aging and personality, in New Developments in the Use of the MMPI. Edited by Butcher JN. Minneapolis, MN, University of Minnesota Press, 1979

Hathaway SR, McKinley JC: Minnesota Multiphasic Personality Inventory. Minneapolis, MN, University of Minnesota, 1943

Hyer L, Gonveia I, Harrison WR, et al: Depression, anxiety, paranoid reactions, hypochondriasis, and cognitive decline of later-life inpatients. J Gerontol 42:92–94, 1987

Jacobowsky B: Psychosomatic equivalents of endogenous depression. Acta Psychiatr Scand 162:253–260, 1961

Johnstone EC, Cunningham Owens DG, Frith CD, et al: Neurotic illness and its response to anxiolytic and antidepressant treatment. Psychol Med 10:321–328, 1980

Kendler KS, Heath AC, Martin WG, et al: Symptoms of anxiety and symptoms of depression: same genes, different environments? Arch Gen Psychiatry 44:451–457, 1987

Kernberg OF: Borderline Conditions and Pathological Narcissism. New York, Jason Aronson, 1976

Kielholz P: Masked depressions and depressive equivalents, in Masked Depression: An International Symposium. Edited by Kielholz P. Berne, Switzerland, Hans Huber, 1973

Leckman JF, Merikanges KR, Pauls DL, et al: Anxiety disorders and depression: contradictions between family study data and DSM-III conventions. Am J Psychiatry 140:880–882, 1983a

Leckman JF, Weissman MM, Merikanges KR, et al: Panic disorder and major depression. Arch Gen Psychiatry 40:1055–1060, 1983b

Lesse S: The multivariant masks of depression. Am J Psychiatry 124(suppl 1):35–40, 1968

Lindberg BJ: Somatic complaints in the depressive symptomatology. Acta Psychiatr Scand 41:419–427, 1965

Liptzin B: Masked anxiety—alcohol/drug issues. Paper presented at a Harvard-NIMH Conference on Anxiety in the Elderly, Boston, January 9–10, 1989

Liptzin B, Salzman C: Psychiatric aspects of aging, in Geriatric Medicine. Edited by Rowe JW, Besdine RW. Boston, MA, Little, Brown, 1988

Loranger AW, Susman VL, Oldham JM, et al: The Personality Disorder Examination: a preliminary report. Journal of Personality Disorders 1:1–13, 1987

McGlashan TH: The Chestnut Lodge follow-up study, III: long-term outcome of borderline personalities. Arch Gen Psychiatry 43:20–30, 1986

Miles L, Dement W: Sleep and aging. Sleep 3:119–220, 1980

Moore JT: Dysthymia in the elderly. J Affective Disord 1 (suppl):515–521, 1985

Murphy E: The prognosis of depression in old age. Br J Psychiatry 142:111–119, 1983

Pinsker H, Suljaga-Petchel K: Use of benzodiazepines in primary-care geriatric patients. J Am Geriatr Soc 32:595–597, 1984

Pissot P, Hassan S: Masked depression and depressive equivalents, in Masked Depression: An International Symposium. Edited by Kielholz P. Berne, Switzerland, Hans Huber, 1973

Post F: The Significance of Affective Symptoms in Old Age. Maudsley Monographs 10. London, Oxford University Press, 1962

Post F: The management and nature of depressive illness in late life: a follow-through study. Br J Psychiatry 121:393–404, 1972

Regier DA, Boyd JH, Burke JD, et al: One-month prevalence of mental disorders in the United States. Arch Gen Psychiatry 45:977–986, 1988

Reich J, Noyes R, Coryell W, et al: The effect of state anxiety on personality measurement. Am J Psychiatry 143:760–763, 1986

Reich J, Noyes R, Hirschfeld R, et al: State and personality in depressed and panic patients. Am J Psychiatry 144:181–187, 1987

Sadavoy J: Character disorders in the elderly: an overview, in Treating the Elderly With Psychotherapy: The Scope for Change in Later Life. Edited by Sadavoy J, Leszcz M. Madison, CT, International Universities Press, 1987, pp 175–229

Sadavoy J, Fogel B: Personality disorders in late life, in Handbook of Mental Health and Aging. Edited by Birren JE, et al. Orlando, FL, Academic Press (in press)

Schuckit MA: Drug and Alcohol Abuse: A Clinical Guide to Diagnosis and Treatment. New York, Plenum, 1979

Sigvardsson S, Bohman M, von Knorring A-L, et al: Symptom patterns and causes of somatization in men, I: differentiation of two discrete disorders. Genet Epidemiol 3:153–169, 1986

Stone MH: Long-term outcome in borderline adolescents, in Proceedings of IVth Congress on Biological Psychiatry. Edited by Shagass C. New York, Elsevier, 1985

Thompson JW, Burns BJ, Bartko J, et al: The use of ambulatory services by persons with and without phobia. Med Care 26:183–198, 1988

Tyrer P: Personality Disorders: Diagnosis, Management, and Course. London, Wright, 1988

Tyrer P, Casey P, Gall J: Relationship between neurosis and personality disorder. Br J Psychiatry 142:404–408, 1983

Victor M, Hope JM: The phenomenon of auditory hallucinations in chronic alcoholism. J Nerv Ment Dis 126:451–481, 1958

Weissman MM: The epidemiology of panic disorder and agoraphobia, in American Psychiatric Press Review of Psychiatry, Vol 7. Edited by

Frances AJ, Hales RE. Washington, DC, American Psychiatric Press, 1988, pp 54–66

Woods JH, Katz JL, Winger G: Use and abuse of benzodiazepines—issues relevant to prescribing. JAMA 260:3476–3480, 1988

CHAPTER 19

Norman S. Miller, M.D.

Alcohol and Drug Dependence

Epidemiology

The prevalence of alcohol dependence among the elderly has been determined in systematic epidemiologic studies (Robins et al. 1988). The prevalence of drug dependence in the geriatric age group is less clearly documented than the prevalence of alcohol dependence, although there is considerable evidence that it is a significant problem, particularly with prescription and over-the-counter (OTC) medications. The use of illicit drugs by the geriatric population is generally not considered a common problem, although narcotic and other similar drugs are obtained by the elderly through prescriptions (Baum et al. 1985; Beers et al. 1988; Schweizer et al. 1989).

The rates of lifetime and recent prevalence of alcohol and drug dependence have been determined by the national cooperative Epidemiologic Catchment Area (ECA) study in five major U.S. cities: Baltimore, Los Angeles, New Haven, Durham, and St. Louis (Robins et al. 1988). This study was unique because it determined the prevalence of actual diagnoses according to DSM-III-R criteria (American Psychiatric Association 1987), whereas all preceding national studies had been based on estimates of consumption and of social, occupational, and health consequences of alcohol and drug use.

Alcohol Dependence

The findings relevant to age were that the prevalence rates for alcohol dependence are higher for younger than for older ages and for men than for women. For men, lifetime prevalence for alcohol dependence varied from 27% (ages 18–29) to 28% (ages 30–44), 21% (45–64 years), and 14% (65 years and older). Among women, the corresponding prevalence rates were 7%, 6%, 3%, and 1.5%. The remission rates tended to rise consistently with increasing age. Although alcohol dependence is a disorder predominantly of males, there is substantial evidence that the prevalence for women is increasing dramatically, especially at the youngest ages (18–29). Other studies of prevalence report wide variation in prevalence rates at all ages, mostly because of the inherent bias in the methods for ascertaining prevalence (i.e., estimates, not actual diagnostic criteria) (Atkinson and Schuckit 1983; Bienenfeld 1990; Hartford and Samorajski 1982). (See Table 19-1.)

The age of onset of alcohol dependence for the 18- to 29-year-old cohort was 17.8 years in men and 18.4 in women; for the age 30–50 cohort it was 24.2 years in men and 27.3 years in women; and for the age 60 and older cohort, age of onset was 31.0 years in men and 40.6 years in women (Robins et al. 1988). (See Table 19-2.)

There are two major explanations for the distribution of the prevalence and the age of onset of alcohol dependence in the geriatric population. First, alcohol dependence is a progressive disorder that has a peak prevalence in early to mid-adulthood (Robins et al. 1988). Second, alcohol dependence can occur as a later-onset phenomenon in the 60-and-older group, engendered by factors in later life (Atkinson et al. 1985; Vaillant 1983).

Table 19-1.   Rates of lifetime alcohol disorder by age, sex, and race (all sites of ECA study)

Age (years)	Men			Women		
	White	Black	Other	White	Black	Other[a]
18–29	29	13[b]	27	7	4[b]	5
30–59	24	32	29	4	7	5
60 +	13	24	22	2	3	1
All ages	23	24	28	4	6	5

[a] This category is dominated by Los Angeles Hispanics, whose male rates exceed whites, and whose female rates are below whites.
[b] The low rate in young blacks is found in all four sites with substantial black populations.
Source. Robins et al. 1988.

Table 19-2. Onset, remission, and duration of alcohol disorders

Age at interview (years)	Mean age at onset (years)		Mean age at last symptom if none recent (years)		Mean duration (years)	
	Men	Women	Men	Women	Men	Women
18–29	17.8	18.4	21.3	20.8	3.5	2.4
30–59	24.2	27.3	32.6	33.5	8.4	6.2
60 +	31.0	40.6	51.0	55.7	20.0	15.1

Source. Robins et al. 1988.

Drug Dependence

Although prevalence rates for prescription medications are not available in the ECA data published thus far, it has been well established that the elderly are the largest users of legal drugs in the national population, accounting for approximately 30% of all prescriptions (Beardsley et al. 1988; Koch and Knapp 1987; Schweizer et al. 1989; Stephens et al. 1981). The 1985 National Ambulatory Medical Care survey of office physicians revealed that for patients over 65 years of age, at least one drug was prescribed in more than 68% of office visits (Koch and Knapp 1987). The most commonly prescribed drugs are cardiovascular medications, sedatives-hypnotics, tranquilizers, and analgesics. It is estimated that 25% of all individuals of geriatric age (over 55) use psychoactive drugs and are at risk for development of drug abuse and dependence (Beardsley et al. 1988).

The propensity of the elderly to use multiple drugs in addition to the high rate of use of at least one drug, when combined with their enhanced sensitivity to drug toxicity, accentuates the problem of psychoactive drug use in the elderly. It has been reported that as many as 20% of the geriatric patients admitted to a general hospital had a drug-induced disorder (Atkinson and Schuckit 1983). A study of nursing home residents (confirmed by other studies) revealed that 50% of them received psychotropic drugs, particularly benzodiazepines, sedatives-hypnotics, and antipsychotic drugs. Moreover, for elderly persons living independently, analgesics, anxiolytics, and sedative-hypnotic drugs constitute the greatest source for the development of drug dependence and its consequences (Koch and Knapp 1987; Stephens et al. 1981). In a recent survey, as many as 33% of chronic daily benzodiazepine users were elderly (aged over 55) (Mellinger et al. 1984). The use of benzodiazepines by the elderly is disproportionate to their numbers. Other survey data from the National Disease and Therapeutic Index indicate that 26% of benzodiazepine prescriptions for anxiety, and 40% of hypnotics, are given to patients aged 65 and older (Schweizer et al. 1989).

In the vast majority of cases the source of the drugs is the physician (Beardsley et al. 1988; Koch and Knapp 1987). The general practitioner or primary care physician leads the list of physician types, followed by the psychiatrist. Physicians' prescribing practices and attitude toward drug abuse and dependence are critical determinants in the frequency and prevalence of drug abuse and dependence in the geriatric population (Beardsley et al. 1988; Koch and Knapp 1987).

Illicit Drug Use

Use of illicit drugs such as cannabis, cocaine, and phencyclidine is not prevalent. Most information regarding illicit drug use among the elderly, however, is obtained from small series or case reports (Atkinson and Schuckit 1983; Baum et al. 1985; Robins et al. 1988). Among those of all ages who did not meet lifetime criteria for alcohol dependence, 3.5% had a diagnosis of illicit drug dependence, whereas in those with alcohol dependence, that rate was 18%. The lifetime prevalence rates for illicit drug dependence according to age were 17% for 18- to 29-year-olds, 4% for ages 30 to 59, and less than 1% for age 60 and older. Prevalence rates for patient populations are much higher—as high as 60% among adult populations of alcoholics. One should always suspect illicit drug use in the presence of alcohol dependence and/or atypical psychiatric syndromes in the elderly.

Over-the-Counter Medications

OTC medications are frequently a major source of drug toxicity and of abuse and dependence. Of the 69% of persons over the age of 60 who use OTC drugs, 80% use alcohol. It is well known that OTC use increases with advancing age, especially in women, and approximately two-thirds of all persons over the age of 60 consume at least one nonprescription drug daily (Beers et al. 1988; Schuckit 1983). OTC drugs are defined as drugs obtainable without prescription (analgesics, laxatives, antihistamines, antiulcer drugs, vitamins). They may be taken mistakenly by individuals with impaired cognition and judgment (Baum et al. 1985).

Special Populations

The prevalence of alcohol and drug dependence is estimated to be 25% to 50% in general medical populations and 50% to 75% in general psychiatric populations (Curtis et al. 1989; Miller and Gold 1989). The elderly comprise a majority of the general medical populations and a significant proportion of the general psychiatric populations. Furthermore, there is no significant age-related decrease in drinking problems associated with alcohol abuse and dependence in the elderly (Robins et al. 1988). The clinical diagnosis of alcohol and drug dependence in the geriatric population as determined by clinicians is considerably less than the prevalence rates determined in the ECA studies (Koch and Knapp 1987; Stephens et al. 1981; Whitcup and Miller 1987).

Identification and Diagnosis

Dependence Syndrome

The essential features of the dependence syndrome as defined by the DSM-III-R criteria include the behaviors of addiction and pharmacologic tolerance and dependence. The behaviors of addiction are 1) preoccupation with the acquisition of alcohol or drugs, 2) compulsive use, and 3) a pattern of relapse. Preoccupation is manifested by a persistent drive to acquire alcohol or a drug and having alcohol or drug use a high priority; compulsion is continued use in spite of adverse consequences. Relapse to the drug is manifested by an inability to reduce or abstain from the use of the drug in spite of recurrent, adverse consequences (Hartford and Samorajski 1982).

Tolerance is defined as either a loss of an effect at a particular dose or the need to increase the dose to maintain the same effect. Dependence is defined as the onset of stereotypic and predictable signs and symptoms on cessation of a drug. Because six of the criteria for a diagnosis of dependence syndrome do not depend on pharmacological tolerance and dependence, the criteria for the dependence syndrome in DSM-III-R may be met without them. Furthermore, tolerance and dependence are not specific to addiction and may occur in the absence of addiction. Tolerance and dependence are particularly poor indicators of "dependence on alcohol and drugs" in the elderly because they do not develop dramatically. The ability to develop tolerance and dependence actually diminishes with increasing age. Clinically, tolerance and dependence for alcohol, anxiolytics, sedatives-hypnotics, and other drugs develop only to a minimal or moderate extent in all ages, making them marginal clinical markers (Hartford and Samorajski 1982; Miller and Gold 1989b).

Denial is a common accompaniment of addiction. Making a diagnosis of drug or alcohol addiction is usually tenuous if only the patient's account is obtained. The patient's objective behavior regarding preoccupation with, and compulsive use of, alcohol or drugs, and corroborative history from others is the key to making a proper diagnosis. Usually the patient minimizes or rationalizes drug and alcohol use and its consequences. Direct confrontation is sometimes helpful in obtaining more information, but sometimes it may anger the patient. This reaction may be instructive in itself, for most nonaddicted people do not mind a sincere inquiry into possibly harmful effects from alcohol and drugs (Hartford and Samorajski 1982; Miller and Gold 1989).

The DSM-III-R criteria are difficult to apply in the case of the elderly when the diagnostic emphasis is on the consequences of alcohol and drug use (Miller and Gold 1989a; Whitcup and Miller 1987), because the consequences are often considerably different than for younger individuals. For instance, the elderly are frequently unemployed, living alone or apart from family, and not experiencing significant legal problems as a result of their alcohol and drug dependence. Psychiatric and medical problems constitute the major consequences of drug and alcohol dependence for the elderly population.

Common Patterns of Use of Alcohol and Drugs

Many of the signs and symptoms produced by alcohol dependence are also produced by the benzodiazepines and sedative-hypnotic drugs. Anxiety, depression, and insomnia are frequent consequences of chronic alcohol intake of moderate to high doses in many, and of low doses in some. These are symptoms for which benzodiazepines and sedatives-hypnotics are frequently prescribed, and these drugs may be used as substitutes for alcohol when alcohol is not available (Hartford and Samorajski 1982; Miller and Gold 1989b). Unfortunately, although the drugs may transiently relieve these symptoms—as did alcohol at one time— as long as the alcohol dependence continues, the need for the drugs will also continue (as will consequences of the alcohol dependence).

Furthermore, as the benzodiazepines and sedatives-hypnotics are used repetitively, dependence on them develops and sometimes leads to confusion with target symptoms for which the drugs were initially prescribed, namely, anxiety, depression, and insomnia (Hartford and Samorajski 1982; Miller and Gold 1989b).

Psychiatric Complications

The psychiatric complications of alcohol and drug dependence are similar in the aged to those found in any population, with some shift in emphasis. As previously mentioned, anxiety and depression are common consequences of alcohol and drug dependence (Curtis et al. 1989; Schuckit 1983). The depressant drugs such as alcohol, anxiolytics, and sedatives-hypnotics produce depression during intoxication and anxiety during withdrawal. By contrast, stimulant drugs such as caffeine and ephedrine produce anxiety during intoxication and depression during withdrawal. These drugs may also produce psychotic symptoms such as delusions and hallucinations, which are particularly troublesome for elderly individuals with diminished vision and hearing who are already vulnerable to misperceptions. Drug-induced delusions are frequently paranoid and terrifying; the hallucinations are more often visual than auditory.

Impaired cognition is a potential problem when alcohol, anxiolytic, sedative-hypnotic, anticholinergic, and antihistaminic drugs are used on a chronic basis, individually or in combination. Studies of alcohol-induced dementia cite age as the most important risk factor in the severity of the dementia; older alcoholics sustain the more severe decline in intelligence (Parsons et al. 1987). Age is a greater risk factor than frequency, duration, and amount of alcohol consumption in determining the severity of the alcoholic dementia. Computed tomography scans reveal significant cerebral atrophy among alcoholics, particularly older alcoholics. The extent to which the atrophy is reversible in the older alcoholic remains to be established. Early identification of an alcohol-or drug-induced dementia or delirium may prevent costly evaluations for other etiologies (Hartford and Samorajski 1982).

Suicide is a particularly common problem associated with alcohol and drug dependence. Next to advanced age in men, alcohol dependence and drug dependence are among the greatest risk factors for suicide (Atkinson and Schuckit 1983; Curtis et al. 1989; Koch and Knapp 1987).

Medical Complications

The medical complications of alcohol and drugs are numerous and are referable to the cardiovascular, gastrointestinal, metabolic, central nervous, and vascular systems. Alcohol by itself has been reported to cause liver disease, hypertension, myocardial infarction, cardiac arrhythmias, stroke, peptic ulcer disease, immunosuppression, accidents, dehydration, and electrolyte abnormalities, just to name some of the complications (Hartford and Samorajski 1982; Lieber 1982).

Delirium tremens (DT) as part of the alcohol withdrawal syndrome remains a significant source of morbidity and mortality. DT is defined as confusion with hallucinations, tremors, and excessive autonomic discharge. Across all ages, the death rate from DT may be as high as 20% to 40% if appropriate treatment is not instituted in time (Miller et al. 1988). The typical history reflects chronic consumption of alcohol, with a previous history of DT and significant elevation of vital signs in early withdrawal. Hypertension, tachycardia, and hyperthermia in the setting of coarse tremors of the extremities and body, and anxiety and agitation within hours of the last drink, represent an increased risk for the development of DT. Moreover, one-third of the cases of DT are preceded by an alcohol withdrawal seizure (Lieber 1982). DT must be differentiated from intoxication from stimulants.

Usually the withdrawal seizures occur within 12 to 24 hours of cessation of drinking, followed by the onset of the autonomic signs and the onset of terrifying hallucinations, extreme agitation, and delusions within 3 to 4 days. The total course is typically 1 week, followed by a period of prolonged prostration. The best alternative is to prevent DT if possible by adequate suppression of withdrawal with benzodiazepines, hydration, and administration of thiamine and other B-complex vitamins (Adam and Victor 1986). Although this profile is a classic one in adults, there are no age-specific data available for the elderly.

Wernicke Korsakoff (W-K) syndrome consists of a continuum of two disorders that are clinically distinct and related to a common pathogenesis, namely, a thiamine deficiency. Wernicke's syndrome is a confusional state, characterized by a clouded sensorium associated with one or more neurological abnormalities (ataxia, ophthalmoplegia—commonly sixth-nerve paresis—and peripheral neuropathy) may occur in any combination with delirium (Lieber 1982) but must also be distinguished from delirium, especially in the older patient. Because W-K syndrome may last for weeks, followed by a gradual clearing and a residual deficit for recent memory, the differential diagnosis from dementia of other causes must be made. The loss in recent memory is out of proportion to the relative sparing of other cognitive functions in W-K syndrome. Confabulation or a tendency to rationalize the memory loss is a popular sign associated with the Korsakoff's syndrome.

Etiology and Pathogenesis

Genetics of Alcoholism

The specific etiology of alcoholism and drug dependence is not known. What is known from twin, adoption, familial, and high-risk studies is that the genetic background of an individual is an important determinant in the development of alcoholism (Goodwin 1985). Other factors are operative and pertain to the exposure to alcohol and the factors that control the exposure.

Those with a family history of alcoholism tend to have an earlier onset and a more rapid course of alcoholism (Atkinson et al. 1985). Familial alcoholics also appear to have more, and more serious, consequences of alcoholism. When onset occurs later (i.e., in midlife and geriatric age groups), there appears to be less familial alcoholism (Goodwin 1985). The occasional study has shown that a family history of alcohol dependence is present also in persons dependent on cocaine and heroin (Kosten et al. 1987).

Exposure

For the geriatric population, exposure to alcohol is determined by a number of conditions. Data are sparse, but common sense dictates that the availability of alcohol and drugs is the rate-limiting step in exposure. Although it may be under the ultimate control of the individual, availability is influenced by other less controllable factors. For instance, many retirement communities have cocktail hours, which by themselves are apparently harmless sources of congeniality and congregation. For those who have a genetic predisposition, however, repeated exposure to alcohol represents a risk of developing alcoholism.

Aging often brings freedom from children and the rigors of a career, as well as increasing independence in a marital relationship. The sense of fewer responsibilities may ease self-imposed controls and lead to greater use of alcohol and drugs.

Differential Diagnosis

Alcohol and drug dependence are primary disorders according to the dependence syndrome defined in DSM-III-R. The relationship to other disorders is better understood if the alcohol and drug dependence are recognized as capable of producing virtually any psychiatric syndrome, particularly depression, anxiety, and cognitive difficulties in the elderly.

The prevalence rates for depression among alcoholics range from 5% to 59% with the average around 15%; the rates are higher for women—as much as twofold to threefold in some studies. Rates for the elderly are not available, for most of the studies were performed on age-heterogenous populations (Schuckit 1986).

Anxiety symptoms are very common among alcoholics—rates as high as 63% have been reported—but separate rates for the elderly are not available (Small et al. 1984).

Treatment

Effective treatments for alcohol and drug dependence exist and are available to the elderly. As with every aspect of geriatric psychiatry, the attitude that the elderly are unable to benefit from treatment of alcoholism and drug dependence is to be avoided, although the treatment may need to be modified to take into consideration the physical and psychological differences associated with aging.

Reduced Tolerance to Drugs

Age-related changes in the distribution and metabolism of drugs may result in increased sensitivity to, and prolonged effects from, low levels of drugs including alcohol. These age changes include a slowed metabolic breakdown of alcohol and drugs by hepatic enzymes; and a decreased lean body mass with a relative increase in body fat, reducing the intravascular volume. Serum proteins are also reduced and, in combination with the other factors, contribute to an increased free-concentration of alcohol and drugs in the water compartment. Furthermore, the neuroreceptors are more sensitive to alcohol and drugs with advancing age (Atkinson and Schuckit 1983; Whitcup and Miller 1987).

Perhaps less well appreciated is the fact that some drugs accumulate by being taken up in the fat and muscle stores and persist for prolonged periods of time after the drug is discontinued. Because of slow release over time from the stores back into blood, the protracted effect of the drug on cognition, memory, and mood may be experienced for weeks to months, even in the elderly, who have reduced muscle mass and fat deposits (Miller and Gold 1989b).

Tolerance to alcohol and drugs is reduced in the elderly, and the withdrawal syndrome may be more severe and prolonged. Typically, the complete withdrawal from alcohol and drugs may take weeks to months in the elderly versus days or weeks in younger individuals, and it requires reduced doses of drugs for detoxification. Correspondingly, the cognitive improvement, reduction in anxiety and depression, chronic pain, and insomnia originating from alcohol and drug dependence may resolve more gradually. Patience is needed, for rapid evaluations are frequently not possible in the population of elderly patients. Hospitalization may be indicated because of increased medical risks of outpatient detoxification in the elderly. Although the risks from inpatient hospitalization itself must be included in the decision to hospitalize, the added advantage of enhancing abstinence and compliance with detoxification in a structured environment is achieved. For medically stable and motivated persons, outpatient detoxification is possible and may be desirable.

Treatment of Acute Withdrawal

The treatment of acute withdrawal should be modified for the elderly. Because of the enhanced sensitivity to drugs, including the benzodiazepines, doses required to suppress the signs and symptoms of withdrawal are usually one-half to one-third the requirement for middle-aged adults. Benzodiazepines are the drugs of choice, and short- to intermediate-acting forms may be used. Longer-acting preparations may result in an accumulation and undesired prolonged effects from the drugs.

There are many detoxification schemes available, employing various benzodiazepines including lorazepam, diazepam, and chlordiazepoxide. It is suggested that the clinician become familiar with one type of benzodiazepine to maximize efficacy and minimize untoward effects. Chlordiazepoxide may produce a smoother withdrawal and promotes less drug-seeking behavior than many other benzodiazepines.

The elderly patient should also receive 100 mg of thiamine daily (for 3 days intramuscularly and then orally if debilitated) as well as multivitamins daily. The thiamine should be administered before any intravenous dextrose is given, to avoid precipitating a Wernicke's encephalopathy by using up marginal stores of thiamine.

The patient may also need hydration with intravenous fluids if unable to take sufficient fluids orally. It is important to assess daily the need for hydration in the acute withdrawal period, when the water loss in an already dehydrated patient may be high. Also, the patient may be sedated from the medication used to treat the withdrawal and may not take as much fluid as needed. Electrolytes should be checked, for many elderly patients are on drugs that may promote electrolyte loss—as do vomiting and diarrhea from acute and chronic alcohol withdrawal.

The detoxification from dependence on benzodiazepines, barbiturates, and sedatives-hypnotics in the elderly is adjusted to the duration of action of the drug that is being detoxified. Usually 2 weeks are sufficient to withdraw a patient from a shorter-acting preparation such as alprazolam or seconal, and 4 weeks from longer-acting preparations such as diazepam or meprobamate. The initial dose is determined from the estimated daily dose used by the patient, taking into account errors of estimate. The dose equivalency is calculated according to conversion criteria in order to use a selected benzodiazepine, such as chlordiazepoxide (see Table 19-3). The total calculated dose is reduced by 50%, given in three or four divided doses, and tapered gradually over the desired time. Exact daily reductions in dose are not necessary, especially if intermediate-acting preparations are used. It is suggested that the short-acting preparations not be used for withdrawal because of the more intensive withdrawal effects from the steeper slope in the blood level of the drug during elimination.

Treatment of Coexisting Psychiatric Disorders

The treatment of coexisting psychiatric disorders may be necessary after a sufficient period of abstinence from alcohol and drugs has elapsed. In general, medications should be used either when there is no improvement in affective or anxiety symptoms, or when a plateau has been reached after an initial period of improvement. Because those who suffer from addiction (dependence) are prone to use the complaints of anxiety, depression, and chronic pain as justifications for drug-seeking behavior, medicating these symptoms is to be discouraged and avoided whenever possible. Although no specific data are available for the elderly, they may do well in traditional forms of long-term treatment for alcoholism and drug dependence such as Alcoholics Anonymous and Narcotics Anony-

Table 19-3. Dose conversions for sedative-hypnotic drugs equivalent to secobarbital 600 mg and diazepam 60 mg

Drug	Dose (mg)
Benzodiazepines	6
Alprazolam	
Chlordiazepoxide	150
Clonazepam	24
Clorazepate	90
Flurazepam	90
Halazepam	240
Lorazepam	12
Oxazepam	60
Prazepam	60
Temazepam	90
Barbiturates	600
Amobarbital	
Butabarbital	600
Butalbital	600
Pentobarbital	600
Secobarbital	600
Phenobarbital	180
Glycerol	2,400
Meprobamate	
Piperidinedione	1,500
Glutethimide	
Quinazolines	1,800
Methaqualone	

Note. For patients receiving multiple drugs (e.g., flurazepam 30 mg/day, diazepam 30 mg/day, phenobarbital 150 mg/day), each drug should be converted to its diazepam or secobarbital equivalent. In the preceding example the patient is receiving the equivalent dose of diazepam 100 mg/day or secobarbital 1,000 mg/day.
Source. Adapted from Perry and Alexander 1986.

mous. It is important for them to select meetings that are made up of individuals in similar age groups. Family therapy is applicable to the elderly, as it is to other age groups.

Supportive and cognitive psychotherapies are often useful in guiding the elderly alcoholic toward a life without alcohol and as many other drugs as possible.

Prognosis and Outcome

The prognosis for untreated alcoholism and drug dependence in the elderly is poor (Gitlow and Peyser 1988). Alcoholism and drug dependence are chronic, progressive, relapsing disorders that require continuous treatment for permanent remission. Many alcoholics and drug dependents can and do stop using for periods of time; thus the ability to "quit" is not the measure of the overall prognosis. Rather, the ability to maintain abstinence is the best single predictor of prognosis.

Most well-designed studies in adults have demonstrated clearly that alcoholics cannot drink alcohol in a controlled fashion. To recommend moderation in alcohol or drug consumption in the elderly alcoholic is contraindicated. Moreover, after the detoxification period the use of benzodiazepines and other sedative-hypnotic drugs is also contraindicated because it frequently induces a relapse to alcohol as well as a dependence on the same drugs.

References

Adams RD, Victor M: The Principles of Neurology, 4th edition. New York, McGraw-Hill, 1986

American Psychiatric Association: Diagnostic and Statistical Manual of Mental Disorders, 3rd Edition, Revised. Washington, DC, American Psychiatric Association, 1987

Atkinson JH, Schuckit MA: Geriatric alcohol and drug misuse and abuse. Advances in Substance Abuse 3:195–237, 1983

Atkinson RM, Turner JA, Kofoed LL, et al: Early versus late onset alcoholism in older persons. Alcoholism: Clinical and Experimental Research 9:513–515, 1985

Baum C, Kennedy DL, Forbes MB: Drug utilization in the geriatric age group, in Geriatric Drug Use—Clinical and Social Perspectives. Edited by Teal TW, Moore SK. New York, Pergamon Press, 1985, pp 63–69

Beardsley RS, Gardocki GL, Larson DB, et al: Prescribing of psychotropic medication by primary care physicians and psychiatrists. Arch Gen Psychiatry 45:1117–1119, 1988

Beers M, Avorn JA, Sounerai SB, et al: Psychoactive medication use in intermediate care facility residents. JAMA 260:3016–3024, 1988

Bienenfeld D: Substance abuse in the elderly, in Verwoerdt's Clinical Geropsychiatry, 3rd Edition. Edited by Bienenfeld D. Baltimore, MD, Williams & Wilkins, 1990

Curtis JR, Geller G, Stokes EG, et al: Characteristics, diagnosis, and treatment of alcoholism in elderly patients. J Am Geriatr Soc 37:310–316, 1989

Gitlow SE, Peyser HS: Alcoholism: A Practical Treatment Guide, 2nd edition. New York, Grune & Stratton, 1988

Goodwin DW: Alcoholism and geriatrics: the sins of the father. Arch Gen Psychiatry 42:171–174, 1985

Hartford JT, Samorajski T: Alcoholism in the geriatric population. J Am Geriatr Soc 30:18–24, 1982

Koch H, Knapp DE: Highlights of drug utilization in office practice, National Ambulatory Medical Survey, 1985. Advance Data From Vital and Health Statistics, No. 134. (DHHS pub no. (PHS) 87-1250) Hyattsville, MD, National Center for Health Statistics, 1987

Kosen TR, Rounsaville BJ, Kleber HA: Parental alcoholism in opioid addicts. J Nerv Men Dis 173:461–468, 1987

Lieber CS: Medical Disorders of Alcoholism: Pathogenesis and Treatment. Philadelphia, PA, WB Saunders, 1982

Mellinger GD, Balter MB, Uhlenhuth EH: Prevalence and correlates of the long-term regular use of anxiolytics. JAMA 251:375–379, 1984

Miller NS, Gold MS: Suggestions for changes in DSM-III-R criteria for substance abuse disorders. Am J Drug and Alcohol Abuse 2:223–230, 1989a

Miller NS, Gold MS: Identification and treatment of benzodiazepine abuse. Am Fam Physician 40:175–183, 1989b

Miller NS, Gold MS, Cocores JA, et al: Alcohol dependence and its medical consequences. NY State J Med 88:476–481, 1988

Perry PJ, Alexander B: Sedative/hypnotic dependence: patient stabilization, tolerance, testing, and withdrawal. Drug Bulletin of Clinical Pharmacology 20:532–537, 1986

Robins LN, Helzer JE, Przybeck TR, et al: Alcohol disorders in the community: a report from the Epidemiologic Catchment Area, in Alcoholism: Origins and Outcome. Edited by Rose R, Barret J. New York, Raven, 1988, pp 15–29

Schuckit MA: A clinical review of alcohol, alcoholism, and the elderly patient. J Clin Psychiatry 43:396–399, 1983

Schuckit MA: Genetic and clinical implications of alcoholism and affective disorder. Am J Psychiatry 143:140–147, 1986

Schweizer E, Case WG, Rickles K: Benzodiazepine dependence and withdrawal in elderly patients. Am J Psychiatry 146:529–531, 1989

Small P, Stockwell T, Canter S, et al: Alcohol dependence and phobic anxiety states, I: a prevalence study. Br J Psychiatry 144:53–57, 1984

Stephens RC, Haney CA, Underwood S: Psychoactive drug use and potential misuse among persons aged 55 years and older. J Psychoactive Drugs 13:185–193, 1981

Vaillant GE: The Natural History of Alcoholism. Boston, MA, Harvard University Press, 1983

Whitcup SM, Miller F: Unrecognized drug dependence in psychiatrically hospitalized elderly patients. J Am Geriatr Soc 35:297–301, 1987

CHAPTER 20

Charles F. Reynolds III, M.D.

Sleep Disorders

Complaints of disturbed nocturnal sleep and daytime sleepiness are common among older Americans in general and are very important symptoms in late-life psychiatric disorders, particularly depression and dementia. Further, as I will review in this chapter, the prevalence of sleep medication use increases steadily with advancing age, as does the prevalence of many types of sleep-related behavioral disturbances. These disturbances, including nocturnal wandering, confusion, and agitated behavior, are not well tolerated by caregivers (Sanford 1975) and may thus trigger a family's decision to institutionalize an older, often demented relative (Pollak and Perlick 1987). It is not surprising that the prescription of sedating medication is highly prevalent among the institutionalized elderly (James 1985; U.S. Public Health Service 1976). Finally, as recent epidemiologic work has indicated, complaints of disturbed sleep are frequent among the community-residing elderly, particularly those who live alone, are unemployed, or are depressed or bereaved (Ford and Kamerow 1989; Rodin et al. 1988).

Clinical Epidemiology of Late-Life Sleep Disorders

Earlier epidemiologic surveys reported that as many as 30% of the older population (i.e., persons aged 60 and older) suffer from and complain of poor sleep quality on a chronic basis (e.g., see Miles

This work was supported in part by NIMH grants MH-00295, MH-37869, and AG-06836.

and Dement 1980). The National Institute of Mental Health (NIMH) and The National Institute on Aging Epidemiologic Catchment Area (ECA) study of 7,954 respondents (who were questioned between 1981 and 1985, at baseline and 1 year later) found that 10.2% reported persistent insomnia and 3.2% reported persistent hypersomnia at the first interview (Ford and Kamerow 1989). Rates of prevalent and incident insomnia complaints were highest among the 1,801 respondents aged 65 and older: 12.0% and 7.3%, respectively. By contrast, rates of prevalent and incident hypersomnia complaints in the elderly were lower than complaints of insomnia. Thus, 1.6% of those aged 65 and older had complaints of persistent hypersomnia at the initial interview ("prevalent" hypersomnia), and an additional 1.8% of elderly respondents complained of hypersomnia at the follow-up interview 1 year later ("incident" hypersomnia). It is important that the risk of developing new major depression was much higher in those respondents (of any age) who had insomnia at both interviews versus those without insomnia (odds ratio: 39.8) and those whose insomnia had resolved by the second visit (odds ratio: 1.6). This finding led Ford and Kamerow (1989, p. 1479) to raise the intriguing suggestion that early recognition and treatment of sleep disturbances may prevent future psychiatric disorders. In this context, the authors found that "those with sleep complaints were more likely to have received services from both the general medical and specialty mental health sectors." Other surveys of nighttime sedation in community-resident elderly have shown that 20% to 25% regularly use sleeping pills (Drugs and Insomnias 1984). Older patients frequently complain that their sleep is nonrestorative and that they have difficulty maintaining sleep, whereas younger subjects are more likely to complain of difficulty initiating sleep. Trouble maintaining alertness during the day is also a frequent complaint in the elderly, and, consistent with this complaint, sleep laboratory studies have demonstrated an increase in sleepiness during the day in late life. Most sleep researchers believe this increase reflects unmet sleep need, in turn a reflection of nocturnal sleep fragmentation (Carskadon et al. 1982).

Sleep-related behavioral disturbances (including nocturnal agitation, night wandering, shouting, and incontinence) are particularly important among the institutionalized elderly with dementing disorders. It is likely that the widespread use of tranquilizing medication in nursing home residents reflects in part the clinical importance of "sundowning" (agitated verbal or physical behavior at the time of sunset) and related nocturnal agitation, wandering, and screaming. An earlier survey of physicians' prescribing practices in nursing homes and other institutional settings suggested that as many as 90% of patients in nursing homes may receive medication for sleep on a regular basis (US PHS 1976). A more recent report by James (1985) estimated that 35% receive tranquilizing medication.

Finally, sleep disturbance is a major and debilitating symptom of bereavement, particularly following the death of a spouse. For example, Clayton and colleagues (1972) found that complaints of sleep disturbance were about as prevalent at 13 months (48%) as at 1 month following the loss of a spouse. The frequency of spousal death has been estimated at 1.6% and 3.0% yearly for older men and women, respectively (Murrell et al. 1984). Given the large number of spousally bereaved elderly, the strong likelihood of concurrent sleep disturbance, and the risk for developing major depression posed by persistent sleep disturbance (see Ford and Kamerow 1989), the public health import of sleep disturbance in late-life bereavement is clear. It also seems plausible to suggest that persistent sleep loss in bereavement may lead not only to bereavement-related depression, but also to self-medication with alcohol and sleeping medication.

Rodin and associates (1988) examined the relationship among aging, sleep, and depression by focusing on "how the frequency of depressed affect over time related to poor sleep" in the community-residing elderly ($n = 264$, aged 62 or older). The frequency of depressed affect over a 3-year period was "related positively to sleep disturbance, even when subjects' age, gender, and health status were considered simultaneously." Further, the authors noted that "early morning awakening was the sleep symptom most consistently related to depressed mood over the course of study. Poor health and female gender showed positive but less consistent relationships to the sleep complaints than depressed affect." Sleep laboratory studies of elderly depressed patients have confirmed the correlation between severity of depression and early morning awakening (Reynolds et al. 1985), as well as the predictive validity of early morning awakening in distinguishing depression from dementia (Reynolds et al. 1989).

Diagnosis

In this section the two major categories of dyssomnia (sleep disorder) will be reviewed: the insomnias (disorders of initiating and maintaining sleep) and the hypersomnias (disorders of excessive daytime sleepiness). The importance of these categories to psychiatry is underscored by the NIMH ECA data cited previously (Ford and Kamerow 1989). Specifically, 40% of respondents with persistent insomnia and 46.5% of those with hypersomnia had a psychiatric disorder, as determined by the Diagnostic Interview Schedule. Thus psychopathological disorders are of major importance in the differential diagnosis of the dyssomnias. However, they do not exhaust the differential diagnostic possibilities.

In the following discussion the terms "nonrapid eye movement" (NREM) and "rapid eye movement" (REM) sleep are used. These terms denote two very different operating states of the central nervous system during sleep: REM sleep represents an activated brain, and NREM sleep, a quiescent brain. Also, during REM sleep, heart rate, respiratory rate, and blood pressure tend to increase relative to NREM sleep, and ventilatory response to increased concentrations of inhaled carbon dioxide is decreased compared with NREM sleep. Further, the onset of REM sleep is mediated by the firing of cholinergic cells in the pontine tegmentum, whereas NREM sleep depends on the basal forebrain area and the midbrain raphe. Further, REM sleep represents the circadian component of sleep-wake regulation, occurring near the low point of the circadian temperature rhythm. NREM sleep (and particularly the slow-wave sleep component) represents the homeostatic component of sleep-wake regulation. It is particularly slow-wave sleep that diminishes with age. For further discussion of the physiological dimensions of sleep and sleep regulation, see Kryger et al. (1989).

The key symptoms in the diagnosis of late-life sleep disorders are complaints of insomnia; nonrestorative sleep; excessive daytime sleepiness; a shift in the timing of the major sleep period; frequent periods of sleep and wakefulness during the 24-hour day (rather than consolidation of major sleep and wake periods); and decrements in mood, performance, and alertness related to the foregoing symptoms.

The initial aim of clinical assessment is to determine the duration of the patient's complaint and likely contributing factors. Transient disturbances, lasting less than 2 to 3 weeks, are usually situationally determined; more persistent disturbances, lasting longer than a month, often indicate more serious underlying medical or psychiatric problems and thus may require more detailed medical, physiological, and psychiatric evaluation (1983 NIH Consensus Conference on Drugs and Insomnia). Sources of diagnostic information should include interviews with both the patient and a bed partner, as well as a sleep-wake log kept daily over a 2-week period to determine the distribution and quality of the patient's sleep during the 24-hour day. The usefulness of such a log is enhanced if daily data concerning scheduling of sleep and naps as well as social activities are obtained, together with information about the timing of meals, medications, exercise, and other indicators of social rhythms. Further assessment should attend to physician- and self-prescribed drug use.

Sleep disturbances in late life reflect the following factors:

- Age-dependent decreases in the ability to sleep ("sleep decay").
- An increased prevalence of sleep-disordered breathing (sleep apnea) and nocturnal myoclonic activity of lower extremities.
- Sleep-phase alterations, particularly advancement of the major sleep period to an earlier time of day.
- Psychiatric disorders, such as depression, dementia, anxiety, and paranoid disorders.
- Medical disorders, particularly those involving nocturia, pain, and limitation of mobility.
- Poor sleep habits, particularly the tendancy to spend excessive amounts of time in bed.
- Iatrogenic factors, particularly the use of sedating medications during the daytime.
- Adverse environmental factors, such as inadequate lighting that may encourage sleeping at the "wrong" time of the 24-hour day, or excessive heat or noise.
- Psychosocial factors, such as loneliness, inactivity, and boredom.

Bearing these factors in mind, the clinician should investigate the following differential diagnostic possibilities:

- Irregular sleep-wake scheduling, including spending excessive amounts of time in bed (more than 7 or 8 hours per 24 hours).
- Evening self-medication, especially with nicotine, alcohol, or caffeinated beverages.
- Obsessive worry about sleep and the use of the bed for the activities not conducive to sleep.
- Dependency on sleeping pills.
- Temporal redistribution of the major sleep period to an earlier time in the 24-hour day.
- Heavy snoring or obstructive breathing during sleep, which may indicate the presence of sleep apnea.
- Feelings of restlessness in the legs at sleep onset, which may indicate nocturnal myoclonus.
- The presence of an affective, psychotic, anxiety, or dementing disorder.
- Medical disorders known to be specifically exacerbated by sleep

(parasomnias), such as nocturnal angina, congestive heart failure, and esophageal reflux.
- The use, timing, and dosage of other medications known to have psychotropic effects, such as antihypertensives, antihistamines, and antiparkinsonian drugs. (For example, propranolol may lead to insomnia, alpha-methyldopa to daytime sedation, and L-dopa to insomnia or nightmares.)

Sleep laboratory evaluation (polysomnography) can be helpful to the elderly person with a sleep disorder and is indicated if the physician suspects sleep apnea (suggested particularly by the presence of heavy snoring and excessive daytime sleepiness) or nocturnal myoclonus (suggested by complaint of restless legs or akathisialike sensations in the legs interfering with sleep onset). Sleep laboratory evaluation should also be considered if routine treatment measures have not resolved the problem. In this context, routine treatment should include 1) consistent attention to the sleep-wake schedule and a comfortable sleep environment, with limiting time in bed to approximately 7 hours nightly (temporal control); 2) reduction or omission of self-medication with nicotine, alcohol, or excessive liquid ingestion; 3) use of the bedroom for sleep and intimacy only, with avoidance of activities not conducive to sleep (stimulus control); 4) careful attention to the timing of physical activity, meals, medication, and sleep periods (including naps); 5) detoxification from depressant or stimulant drugs; and 6) appropriate behavioral treatment for insomnia.

Etiology and Pathogenesis of Late-Life Sleep Disorders

There is an age-dependent decrease in the ability to sleep, which reflects both the aging process per se and the impact of concurrent physical and psychiatric disorders. The most important age-dependent decrements in the ability to sleep include 1) a decreased continuity of sleep, manifested particularly by an increase in the number of microarousals (3–15 seconds in duration); 2) decreased slow-wave sleep (the deepest level of NREM sleep and perhaps the most restorative sleep); 3) a tendency for the major sleep period to occur earlier in the night (phase advancement); 4) a tendency for REM sleep to occur earlier in the night; 5) increased napping during the day; and 6) a general tendency to spend more time in bed, which may be a response to poor sleep but only tends to perpetuate the problem and make sleep quality worse.

Other age-associated changes in sleep include a decrement in growth-hormone secretion (which typically is maximal during the first 2 hours of sleep, in association with NREM sleep stages 3 and 4), decreases in sleep-associated prolactin and testosterone, increases in plasma norepinephrine levels, and increases in cortisol secretion (particularly in depressed elderly). A general reference on age-dependent changes in sleep, biological rhythms, and sleep-related neuroendocrine activity is provided by Roth and Roehrs (1989).

Sleep researchers generally agree that it is the ability to sleep, rather than the need for sleep, that diminishes with age. The belief that many older people have unmet sleep need is substantiated by findings of increased daytime sleepiness among the elderly. This unmet sleep need of late life probably results from sleep fragmentation, loss of sleep depth, and redistribution of sleep in the 24-hour period. In essence, the nocturnal sleep of many older people is brittle and shallow, characterized by numerous transient arousals and by decrease or total loss of the deepest levels of NREM (slow-wave) sleep.

Previous reports of sleep in the healthy elderly have also noted gender-related differences in sleep continuity and slow-wave sleep, with elderly men having more impaired sleep maintenance and less slow-wave sleep than elderly women. Paradoxically, however, older women are more likely than men to complain of sleep disturbance and to receive sleeping pills. Possibly, older women may be more sensitive to sleep quality and sleep losses than older men, particularly to the mood-disrupting effects of sleep loss (Reynolds et al. 1986).

With respect to observable behaviors during sleep in late life, snoring has received considerable attention. Koskenvuo and colleagues (1985, 1987) found habitual, severe snoring in 9% of men ($n = 3,847$) and 3.6% of women ($n = 3,664$) aged 40 to 67. Snoring was more prevalent in men and women with hypertension (relative risks of 1.91 and 3.19, respectively) and in men ($n = 4,388$) with ischemic heart disease (relative risk, 1.91) or stroke (2.38). Clinically, it is believed that severe snoring is likely to reflect frank or complete occlusion of the airway during sleep, leading to sleep apnea.

Numerous studies have now shown that sleep-disordered breathing increases with advancing age, more so in men than in women. The best epidemiologic work in this area has been done by Ancoli-Israel and colleagues (1985, 1989), who have shown an overall prevalence for sleep disordered breathing of about 25% among a large sample of community-residing elderly in San Diego.

From a sleep physiological perspective, both major depression and dementia of the Alzheimer's type are associated with characteristic changes in the organization and intensity of sleep (Reynolds et al. 1988). The sleep physiological correlates of late-life depression include 1) short REM sleep latencies; that is, diminished time between sleep onset and REM sleep onset; 2) prolonged first REM sleep periods with enhanced density of rapid eye movements; 3) shifting of electroencephalogram slow-wave activity from the first to the second NREM sleep period; and 4) early morning awakening. By contrast, sleep in Alzheimer's dementia deteriorates as the dementia progresses, with the development of an arrhythmic, polyphasic sleep-wake pattern, gradual loss of all phasic activity (i.e., decreased spindles and K-complexes in stage 2, decreased rapid eye movements in stage REM), normal or prolonged REM sleep latency, and increased prevalence of sleep apnea (Prinz et al. 1982). Sleep physiological alterations in depressive pseudodementia are similar to those of endogenous depression, including transient antidepressant response to all-night sleep deprivation and a robust REM sleep rebound during recovery sleep after acute sleep deprivation (Buysse et al. 1988). Patients afflicted with primary degenerative dementia and secondary depression do not show an antidepressant response to acute total sleep deprivation or a REM sleep rebound during the recovery sleep that follows sleep deprivation. As recently reviewed by Wu and Bunney (1990), more than half of patients with depression experience transient improvement in symptoms of depression after a night of sleep deprivation. The authors also reported that more than 80% of these patients, if unmedicated with thymoleptics, would relapse after one night of sleep.

Generalized anxiety disorder and panic disorder are characterized by sleep continuity disturbances, such as sleep onset and sleep maintenance difficulties, but generally lack the REM sleep stigmata of major or endogenous depression. Sleep in mania and psychotic depression are characterized by extreme sleep fragmentation and early-onset REM sleep. (For further review see Vogel et al. 1989.)

The occurrence of "sundowning" has been empirically studied by Evans and associates (1987) and found to be associated with a diagnosis of dementia and/or fluid or electrolyte abnormalities; it occurred more frequently in patients recently admitted to a nursing facility, in patients whose rooms had been changed in the past month, and in patients who participated in fewer daytime activities. Sundowning has been linked to sensory deprivation, loneliness, diminished social and physical time cue (e.g., visits, lighting), partial arousal from REM sleep (Feinberg et al. 1967), and sleep apnea (Hoch et al. 1989). Thus, it appears that sundowning may be the final common expression of numerous different underlying mechanisms, some related to changes in sleep-wake rhythmicity and some to the physical and psychosocial time cues that impinge on "internal clocks."

In the context of internal clocks, the circadian temperature rhythm exerts powerful effects on the regulation of sleep. Conversely, sleep disturbances such as insomnia are associated with diminished amplitude in the body temperature rhythm. The body temperature cycle is the generally accepted "marker" or output of the circadian clock, which drives the daily cycle (Weitzman et al. 1982). REM sleep is most likely near the low point of the daily temperature rhythm. It is now generally accepted that human temperature rhythms tend to flatten and shorten with age. This reduction in amplitude appears to result from an increase in its daily low point. There may also be a change with age in circadian "type." Thus, older people tend to prefer earlier bedtimes and wake-up times than their younger counterparts and tend to be rated as "larks" (morning types) rather than as "owls" (evening types). This shift in circadian type from owl to lark may be related to an age-dependent shortening in the duration or period of the circadian temperature rhythm.

It is likely that lifestyle changes play an important contributory role in late-life sleep disorders. For example, the fact that many older people spend increased time in bed may reflect a feeling that they have little reason to get up, including few opportunities for social and physical activity as well as loss of important social time cues that may attend retirement. Among the institutionalized elderly, environmental factors such as temperature, noise, and lighting undoubtedly provide important and perhaps deleterious changes in time cues for the circadian regulation of sleep and wakefulness.

Treatment of Late-Life Sleep Disorders

Elderly persons and their families may need to be told that some sleep disturbance, particularly insomnia, may be an unavoidable consequence of aging—not that less sleep is needed, but rather that ability to sleep may diminish with age. Reinforcement of a regular sleep-wake schedule, together with limiting time in bed to no more than 7 or 8 hours nightly, may counteract the age-related tendency to lose the consolidation of sleep and to develop a poly-phasic sleep-wake cycle. In practical terms, the elderly person with a complaint of insomnia should be encouraged to go to bed only when sleepy, get up at the same time each morning, reduce naps to no more than 30 to 45 minutes daily, and limit nightly time in bed to 7 hours (all examples of temporal control). The older patient with the complaint of sleep disturbance, particularly insomnia, should also be instructed to maintain "stimulus control" by not using the bedroom for activities not conducive to sleep. Stimulus control serves to keep the bed as a powerful stimulus to sleep. In practice, strengthening temporal and stimulus control, together with education and reassurance, help the older person achieve a sense of increased control and diminished need for medication.

Although controlled data are lacking, there is reason to believe that regular exercise, particularly if it leads to improved aerobic fitness, may enhance the quality and depth of sleep in late life. There is also reason to believe that the use of a behavioral technique called sleep restriction therapy may be particularly useful among elderly insomniacs. As developed by Spielman and colleagues (1987), sleep restriction therapy teaches the patient to spend less time in bed at night in order to create a modest sleep debt, which then overrides sleep fragmentation.

With respect to the use of sleeping pills in late life, diagnosis is the most salient of all clinical considerations. Most sleep disorder experts agree that sedatives-hypnotics have a place in 1) the management of transient or situational insomnia; 2) persistent sleep loss that is associated with bad habits and does not respond to behavioral interventions; and 3) persistent insomnia associated with nonpsychotic psychiatric disorders. Additional clinical considerations include 1) a review of the relative indications and contraindications for using low-dose sedating antidepressants, benzodiazepines, or antipsychotic compounds; 2) age-dependent changes in the rate of metabolism; 3) effects on daytime alertness and performance; 4) concurrent medications that might potentiate the effects of sedative hypnotics; and 5) the potentially exacerbating effect on borderline and full-blown sleep apnea syndrome.

There are few controlled trials of sedative hypnotics in well-diagnosed samples of geriatric patients. In a recent review of this area, only six controlled studies of sedative use in elderly patients with dementia or organic brain syndromes had been published during the past 15 years (Reynolds et al. 1989). These studies involved a total of 134 inpatients, some with mild to moderate dementia and others diagnosed with "organic brain syndrome" with agitation. None of the studies employed sleep laboratory or objective methods to assess drug effects, but all did employ a placebo control and were double blind; nursing observations of sleep onset time, sleep duration, and duration of arousals were the main dependent measures. In general, the studies reported that compared with placebo, the use of active compounds was associated with nurses' observations of increased sleep time (less time to sleep onset and fewer intermittent wakenings). The drugs investigated included butabarbital, nitrazepam, flurazepam, chloral hydrate, lorazepam, temazepam, hydroxyzine, and thioridazine. With the exception of thioridazine, all compounds were associated with significant and negative side effects, such as increased daytime sleepiness, drug withdrawal insomnia, and diminished capability for performing activities of daily living (e.g., see Linnoila and Viukari 1976).

These findings strongly suggest that benzodiazepines do not offer a viable long-term strategy for successful management of sleep disturbance in dementia. Further, given the finding that sleep apnea appears to occur significantly more often in dementia than in the general elderly population (Hoch et al. 1989), the use of sleeping pills might exacerbate sleep apnea and thereby increase the burden of cognitive deterioration in dementia. Accordingly, it may be preferable to use an antipsychotic compound, such as perphenazine (4–8 mg), thioridazine (25–50 mg), or haloperidol (0.5–1 mg), for patients with marked behavioral disturbances at night who have dementia associated with psychosis and/or nocturnal wandering or agitated behavior. The use of such medications in the elderly necessitates monitoring for orthostatic blood pressure changes, extrapyramidal symptoms, and tardive dyskinesia.

In other older patients with chronic insomnia who cannot function without maintenance sleep-promoting medication, the use of a low dose of sedating antidepressant, such as 25 to 50 mg of trazodone or trimipramine, may be preferable to using a benzodiazepine on a long-term basis. Antidepressants may retain their sedating effects longer than benzodiazepines, without the development of tolerance, daytime sequelae, or withdrawal symptoms. However, orthostatic blood pressure changes during therapy must be monitored. Moreover, such patients often have diagnosable affective disorders, and they frequently have low-grade sleep apnea that might be diminished by a tricyclic antidepressant but exacerbated by a benzodiazepine. When prescribed to patients with major depression, tricyclic antidepressants usually prolong REM sleep latency and suppress REM sleep to between 8% and 10%. More sedating antidepressants such as amitriptyline also shorten sleep latency and decrease intermittent wakefulness and early morning awakening. (The atropinic side effects of amitriptyline may make it unsuitable for use in most geriatric patients.) Maintenance benzodiazepine therapy should be considered in chronic insomnia associated with a diagnosable anxiety disorder, if there is no sleep apnea.

When using benzodiazepines in the elderly, probably the key pharmacokinetic issue is the elimination half-life of the compound (Carskadon et al. 1983). Long-acting benzodiazepines (e.g., flurazepam) are likely to produce daytime sedation or "hangovers." Benzodiazepines with shorter elimination half-lives (e.g., temazepam 15 mg, lorazepam 0.5–2 mg, and triazolam 0.125 mg) tend to be better tolerated by the elderly. [Editor's note: Triazolam, however, has been associated with anterograde amnesia, which could lead to confusional syndromes in the elderly; compare Chapter 22.] (Table 20-1 shows the range of elimination half-lives for commonly prescribed benzodiazepines.) A physician who determines that a benzodiazepine is indicated for an elderly patient should establish the smallest effective dose, often one-third to one-half that prescribed for middle-aged patients. The patient should take the medication about 30 minutes before bedtime. Daytime consequences should be monitored, particularly daytime sleepiness and amnestic episodes. The patient should be followed regularly, with an effort to limit the use of the benzodiazepine to less than 20 doses per month over a period of not more than 3 months. At the same time, the clinician should teach the patient to use nonpharmacologic approaches to sleep disturbance, in order to avoid the long-term use of these compounds.

Table 20-1. Elimination half-lives of various benzodiazepines

Drug	Usual range of elimination half-life (hours)
Diazepam	20–70
Alprazolam	8–15
Lorazepam	10–20
Oxazepam	5–15
Flurazepam	36–120
Temazepam	8–20
Triazolam	1.5–5
Clonazepam	30–60

Source. Adapted from Greenblatt and Shader 1987.

Diphenhydramine (25–50 mg) has long been used to promote sleep in elderly people. Its effectiveness as a sedative hypnotic is not as great as benzodiazepines, and its usefulness in cholinergically brittle older patients may be limited. Similarly, although L-tryptophan (500–2,000 mg) may induce sleep, there is no evidence that it maintains sleep, the major problem for elderly insomniacs. In January 1990 the Food and Drug Administration recalled L-tryptophan for clarification of safety issues.

If it is determined that the period of leg jerks during sleep (nocturnal myoclonus) is a major factor in the patient's complaint of insomnia (a judgment that depends on the results of sleep laboratory evaluation), then the use of a benzodiazepine may be helpful. The cause of nocturnal myoclonus is unknown; although benzodiazepine therapy does not suppress myoclonus, it overrides the arousal effect of periodic leg jerks, allowing the maintenance of sleep continuity. In an elderly sleeper, the use of benzodiazepines with shorter elimination half-lives is generally preferable (see Table 20-1).

The judgment that sleep disturbance is related to sleep apnea also depends on the findings of sleep laboratory evaluation. The causes of sleep apnea are multiple, complex, and imperfectly understood; hypotonus of upper airway muscles leading to airway occlusion is probably an important element in the pathogenesis. The decision whether to treat and, if so, how to intervene is also complex and depends on the severity and type of apnea together with its physiological and behavioral sequelae. Interventions range from the behavioral (e.g., weight loss, training the patient to sleep on the side) and the prosthetic (e.g., continuous positive airway pressure) to the pharmacologic (e.g., acetazolamide) and surgical (e.g., uvulopalatopharyngoplasty or tracheotomy). For detailed reviews of therapy for nocturnal myoclonus and sleep apnea, the reader is referred to Kryger et al. (1989).

Prognosis and Outcome

Most clinicians believe that late-life sleep disturbance tends to be a chronic and intermittent problem. However, there are relatively few studies of the natural history of sleep disorders in late life. It is reasonable to assume that the prognosis of sleep disturbance is related to that of the associated medical and psychiatric conditions.

A major aspect of the clinical and epidemiologic importance of sleep duration in late life is its well-established relationship to mortality. In analyzing data on more than 1 million adults interviewed by the American Cancer Society in 1959–60, Kripke and colleagues (1979, p. 103) observed that "men who reported usually sleeping less than four hours were 2.80 times as likely to have died within six years as men who reported 7.0 to 7.9 hours of sleep." Ancoli-Israel's reexamination of the Kripke data indicated that 86% of the deaths associated with reported short (less than 7 hours) or long (more than 8 hours) sleep periods occurred among respondents over 60 years of age (Ancoli-Israel 1989).

In reviewing the data available from epidemiologic surveys of sleep complaints in later life, Webb (1989, p. 285) issued an important caveat:

> Sleep disorders, in the sense of pathologic conditions which interfere with vital and life style functioning in the aged will be present in the midst of "sleep difficulties" which are associated with aging. It is important that the latter not be elevated to the status of "disorders" or be permitted to distract from the detection and treatment of a more profound and threatening sleep problem.

References

Ancoli-Israel S: Epidemiology of sleep disorders. Clin Geriatr Med 5:347–362, 1989

Ancoli-Israel S, Kripke DF, Mason W, et al: Sleep apnea and periodic movements in an aging sample. J Gerontol 40:419–425, 1985

Buysse DJ, Reynolds CF, Kupfer DJ, et al: EEG sleep in depressive pseudodementia. Arch Gen Psychiatry 45:568–576, 1988

Carskadon MA, Brown ED, Dement WC: Sleep fragmentation in the elderly: relationship to daytime sleep tendency. Neurobiol Aging 3:321–327, 1982

Carskadon MA, Seidel WF, Greenblatt DJ, et al: Daytime carryover of triazolam and flurazepam in elderly insomniacs. Sleep 5:361–371, 1983

Clayton PJ, Halikas JA, Mauria WL: The depression of widowhood. Br J Psychiatry 120:71–78, 1972

Drugs and insomnias, the use of medications to promote sleep. JAMA 251:2410–2414, 1984

Evans LK: Sundown syndrome in institutionalized elderly. J Am Geriatr Soc 35:101–108, 1987

Feinberg I, Koresko RL, Heller N: EEG sleep patterns as a function of normal and pathological aging in men. J Psychiatr Res 5:107–144, 1967

Ford DE, Kamerow DB: Epidemiological studies of sleep disturbances and psychiatric disorders: an opportunity for prevention? JAMA 262:1479–1484, 1989

Hoch CC, Reynolds CF, Nebes RD, et al: Clinical significance of sleep-disordered breathing in Alzheimer's disease: preliminary data. J Am Geriatr Soc 37:138–144, 1989

James DS: Survey of hypnotic drug use in nursing homes. J Am Geriatr Soc 33:436–439, 1985

Koskenvuo M, Kaprio J, Partinen M, et al: Snoring as a risk factor for hypertension and angina pectoris. Lancet 1:893–896, 1985

Koskenvuo M, Kaprio J, Telaviki T, et al: Snoring as a risk factor for ischemic heart disease and stroke in men. Br Med J 294:16–19, 1987

Kripke DF, Simons RN, Garfinkel L, et al: Short and long sleep and sleeping pills: is increased mortality associated? Arch Gen Psychiatry 36:103–116, 1979

Kryger MH, Roth T, Dement WC (Eds): Principles and Practice of Sleep Medicine. Philadelphia, PA, WB Saunders, 1989, pp 413–430

Linnoila M, Viukari M: Efficacy and side effects of nitrazepam and thioridazine as sleeping aides in psychogeriatric inpatients. Br J Psychiatry 128:566–569, 1976

Miles LE, Dement WC: Sleep and aging. Sleep 3:119–220, 1980

Murrell SA, Norris, F, Hutchins G: Distribution and desirability of life events in older adults: population and policy implications. Journal of Community Psychology 12:301–311, 1984

1983 NIH Consensus Conference on Drugs and Insomnia. Drugs and insomnia: the use of medications to promote sleep. JAMA 251:2410–2414, 1984

Pollak CP, Perlick D: Sleep problems and institutionalization of the elderly. Sleep Research 16:407, 1987

Prinz P, Peskind ER, Vitaliano PP, et al: Changes in the sleep and waking EEGs of nondemented and demented elderly subjects. J Am Geriatr Soc 30:86–93, 1982

Reynolds CF, Kupfer DJ, Taska LS, et al: EEG sleep in healthy elderly depressed, and demented subjects. Biol Psychiatry 20:431–442, 1988

Reynolds CF, Kupfer DJ, Hoch CC, et al: Sleep deprivation in healthy elderly men and women: effects on mood and on sleep during recovery. Sleep 9:492–501, 1986

Reynolds CF, Hoch CC, Monk TH: Sleep and chronobiologic disturbances in late life, in Geriatric Psychiatry. Edited by Busse EW, Blazer DG. Washington, DC, American Psychiatric Press, 1989, 475–488.

Robins LN, Helzer JE, Croughan J, et al: National Institute of Mental Health Diagnostic Interview Schedule: its history, characteristics and validity. Arch Gen Psychiatry 38:381–389, 1981

Rodin J, McAvay G, Timko C: Depressed mood and sleep disturbances in the elderly: a longitudinal study. J Gerontol 43:45–52, 1988

Roth T, Roehrs TA (Eds): Clin Geriatr Med 5(2), 1989

Sanford JRA: Tolerance of debility in elderly dependents by supporters at home: its significance for hospital practice. Br Med J 3:471–473, 1975

Spielman A, Saskin P, Thorpy MJ: Treatment of chronic insomnia by restriction of time in bed. Sleep 10:45–56, 1987

U.S. Public Health Service: Physician's drug prescribing patterns in skilled nursing facilities (PHS Publ No 76-50050). Bethesda, MD, U.S. Department of Health, Education and Welfare, 1976

Vogel GW, Reynolds CF, Akiskal HS, et al: Psychiatric disorders, in Principles and Practice of Sleep Medicine. Edited by Kryger MH, Roth T, Dement WC. Philadelphia, PA, WB Saunders, 1989, pp 413–430

Webb WB: Age-related changes in sleep. Clin Geriatr Med 5:275–287, 1989

Weitzman ED, Moline ML, Czeisler CA, et al: Chronobiology of aging: temperature, sleep/wake rhythms, and entertainment. Neurobiol Aging 3:299–309, 1982

Wu JC, Bunney WE: The biological basis of an antidepressant response to sleep deprivation and relapse: review and hypothesis. Am J Psychiatry 147:14–21, 1990

CHAPTER 21

Domeena C. Renshaw, M.D.

Sexuality

Disbelief, condescending humor, silence, and benign neglect have pervaded the topic of geriatric sexual expression through the centuries. In ancient times, fertility and virility were so deeply linked that when King David (Book of Kings) was unable to provide an heir, Adonijah took the throne. Nothing is mentioned about the aging queen, perhaps because at the time childbearing and sexuality were considered synonymous. Since those bygone days sexual disenfranchisement of the aged has continued despite laboratory studies (Masters and Johnson 1966) and subjective reports (Brecher 1983; Butler and Lewis 1977; Kinsey et al. 1948) that sexual interest, activity, fantasy, and arousal may continue for both sexes, to at least age 96 (my oldest patient).

Technology can now document sexual responses and test for anatomical, vascular, hormonal, and tissue changes. By the mid-1950s, silicone penile implants were being used, and in the 1970s a new bionic era dawned with the dramatic development of the first inflatable penile prosthesis (Krauss et al. 1987). Since then, despite litigation risks, the United States has witnessed what is in fact a thriving penis industry that includes "chemical erections" by injections (Virag 1982). There are hundreds of impotence clinics in large and small hospitals across the country; "potency fairs" display treatment options; Impotence Anonymous and similar self-help groups advertise and attract elderly men and their partners, contrary to predictions that privacy concerns would deter this age group.

Sexual Dysfunctions After Age 50

Over a 10-year period, only 3% of the patients of the Johns Hopkins Sex Clinic were aged older than 60 years, and none was over 70 (Wise 1983). Erectile disorder was the predominant presenting complaint in 70% of patients. According to a 15-year study of 1,285 couples seen at Loyola Sex Therapy Clinic, about 20% were aged older than 50, with 240 over 65 years and several in their eighties (Renshaw 1988b). The final diagnoses are listed in Table 21-1. The duration of the symptom varied from 3 to 40 years. At times the partner was more upset about a sexual problem than the patient (Renshaw 1979).

Concurrent physical problems included hypertension, diabetes, poststroke, postprostatectomy, postmastectomy, and postcoronary bypass. Most patients were literate, middle-class white or black (6%), and Catholic (32%), Protestant (30%), or Jewish (25%).

In the Kinsey and associates (1948) interviews, 125 of 5,000 men were aged over 60. Subjective complaints of erection problems came from 2% of 40-year-olds, 7% of 50-year-olds, 18% of 70-year-olds, and 80% of 80-year-olds. In the mailed response to Consumer's Union (Brecher 1983), 44% of those over 50 reported less firm erections than in their younger days and 32% reported frequent lost erections during sexual activity. Neither study was clinical.

Table 21-1. Erectile disorders in aging patients (Loyola Sex Therapy Clinic study)

Males (n = 251)	
Erectile disorder	128
No sexual symptom	42
Hypoactive sexual desire	33
Erectile disorder + premature ejaculation + hypoactive sexual desire	22
Erectile disorder + premature ejaculation	16
Inhibited orgasm (delayed ejaculation)	10
Females (n = 251)	
Inhibited orgasm	108
No sexual symptom	71
Hypoactive sexual desire	46
Dyspareunia	13
Inhibited orgasm + dyspareunia	9
Hypoactive sexual desire + dyspareunia	4

Source. Renshaw 1988b.

A small group of cognitively impaired persons came to clinical attention in one study because of inappropriate sexual behaviors (Boller and Frank 1982). Although some of these were young (e.g., with developmental disabilities or head injury), there were some older men and women with chronic neurologic or psychiatric illness who required assistance at home, in day hospitals, or in long-term settings. Family, neighbors, and staff may become upset, rejecting, or severely punitive when sexual behavior occurs in public or intrudes on weaker, younger, or unwilling partners. However, clinical experience suggests that therapy is possible and effective through sex education and directive techniques that help implement external controls, allaying observer anxiety and improving the care of the afflicted men and women (Renshaw 1988a).

Brief Sex Therapy

Brief therapy for any sexual dysfunction is individualized, but there are several general steps that are usually taken. Table 21-2 lists the DSM-III-R diagnostic categories of sexual dysfunctions (American Psychiatric Association 1987).

Once an individual or a couple determines that there is a problem, the first step is to seek help from a physician who has had

Table 21-2. DSM-III-R diagnostic categories of sexual dysfunctions

Specify:	Psychogenic only, or psychogenic and biogenic (Note: If biogenic only, code on Axis III)
Specify:	Lifelong or acquired
Specify:	Generalized or situational
Sexual desire disorders	
302.71	Hypoactive sexual desire disorder
302.79	Sexual aversion disorder
Sexual arousal disorders	
302.72	Female sexual arousal disorder
302.72	Male erectile disorder
Orgasm disorders	
302.73	Inhibited female orgasm
302.74	Inhibited male orgasm
302.75	Premature ejaculation
Sexual pain disorders	
302.76	Dyspareunia
302.51	Vaginismus
302.70	Sexual dysfunctions not otherwise specified

Source. American Psychiatric Association 1987.

some training in sexual medicine. It is best for sexual partners to go for diagnosis together.

The doctor first takes an explicit history of the sexual complaint and both partners' reactions to it, followed by a routine medical, personal, family, and marital history. Some persons are more articulate on paper and can express their feelings to the partner that way with less embarrassment. Asking each partner to review accomplishments of past years in writing can be personally integrating and can enhance bonding. The therapist then selects, facilitates, interprets, and shares such a letter to enhance closeness and encourage honesty and so improve communication.

Psychological evaluation begins with an in-depth interview regarding the present problem, early and current family life, illness, and both partners' dating, love, and sexual relationships. The reasons for administering psychological tests as part of sex therapy are 1) for each partner to know himself or herself better, 2) for partners to know each other better, 3) to determine how each regards the relationship, and 4) to exclude organicity, particularly in situations of head injury or mental changes. There is no "standard test battery" as part of sex therapy.

Much sexual distress may relate to uncertainties and needless guilt, which breed anxiety. The way an explicit sexual history is taken, therefore, can be educative and therapeutic; for example, one may say, "Masturbation has been studied and found to be natural, not at all abnormal, and practiced privately by nearly everyone. However, people worry about it. How often per month do you masturbate? Do you have any questions about it?" With such basic sex education the relief to the patient may be profound, as illustrated in a letter 2 years after examination from a 62-year-old woman who said, "You will never know what it meant for me to hear that the clitoris was solely a pleasure organ. For over 50 years I secretly worried that I was weird." Sex education, of itself, provides powerful sex therapy by cognitive correction of restrictive misinformation. This process of sex education may be further reinforced by relevant readings (Brecher 1983; Butler and Lewis 1977; Masters et al. 1986).

A thorough physical and genital examination for both partners is needed to carefully exclude, or take into account, overt physical problems. Visible or palpable genital abnormalities, the strength of male peripheral pulses, and local causes for vaginal or pelvic pain (atrophic vaginitis) may be diagnosed during such an examination. If the problem is not found from such examination, further tests might be needed (Table 21-3 outlines common causes of impotence, 60% arise from organic causes). If there are no gross abnormalities, the next step may be a diagnostic trial of brief sex therapy, that is, sex education, relationship therapy, and direction for sexual activities at home. This therapy may occur while further investigation is progressing.

At home the couple is instructed in use of sensate focus technique (nongenital foreplay), which allows them to learn to relax, discover how highly erotic the skin is, and enjoy this loving foreplay while they delay intercourse (Masters et al. 1986). Both are encouraged to be open and honest and to use private sexual fantasy to stimulate erections and vaginal lubrication. The younger woman is often helped by such foreplay because her arousal response, on the average, takes four times longer than a man's, although after age 50, the male lasts longer and the time difference is shortened. This "foreplay only" approach may relieve some males of performance and penetration pressures.

Cooperative patients risk change and take the time at home for playful touching, kissing, sexual surprises, laughter, showering together, and enjoying their own and each other's total bodies rather than focusing only on genitals and genital arousal; for them, positive, even surprising sexual responses may occur, often recapitulating the affection that they shared in courtship. Such a bonding, therapeutic approach is a modified Masters-Johnson technique, and it may bring about a high rate of symptom reversal in rela-

Table 21-3. Common etiology of erectile disorders

Organic
  Vascular: arteriosclerosis, pelvic trauma/surgery
  Postsurgical: prostatectomy, cystectomy; abdominoperineal resection of rectum
  Neurological: diabetes mellitus; cord trauma; demyelinating lesions; pituitary adenoma
  Chemical: alcohol; tranquilizers; antihypertensives; diuretics; beta-blockers; antidepressants
  Hormonal: hyperprolactinemia; low testosterone; high estrogen
  Carcinoma: prostatic; radiotherapy, chemotherapy
Somatopsychic
  Some mild organic changes with heavy psychogenic overlay
Psychological
  Anxiety; anger; conflict; sexual trauma; depression; inhibitions; job/financial loss; deliberate control; situational potency

tively few visits (Masters et al. 1986). In the Loyola study, symptom reversal to coitus occurred in 72% of patients after 7 weeks of therapy (Renshaw 1988a).

In itself, sex therapy may be entirely effective, so that further expensive laboratory studies may be unnecessary. If sex therapy does not solve the problem, further workup may be indicated to discover relevant physical or psychological problems.

Impotence or Erectile Disorder

Impotence or erectile disorder is the persistent inability to obtain or maintain a penile erection suitable for sexual intercourse. In the United States, it is estimated that 10 million men are chronically impotent.

Every man aged over 50 years needs to know that, because of general and peripheral arteriosclerotic vascular changes and diminished connective tissue elasticity, partial erections are normal, natural, and predictable. With increasing age, there are decreases in the amount of semen and the intensity of orgasm, while the postejaculatory refractory phase increases (Masters and Johnson 1966). This is not impotence. With longer, stronger, direct-on-the-penis foreplay, the erection improves so that penetration and climax can follow.

Although more and more sophisticated diagnostic procedures for the evaluation of erectile disorders have evolved since 1980, they are still not entirely conclusive. To exclude endocrine causes of impotence, a medical workup includes fasting blood sugar and levels of testosterone, luteinizing hormone, prolactin, estradiol thyroid-stimulating hormone, and T_4. Diabetes, thyroid, and pituitary pathology must be excluded. Because reduced blood flow may be a factor, special, noninvasive tests of the penis are undertaken, which include measurement of nonerect penile blood pressure (normally 80% of brachial pressure). Penile pulse is measured by a Doppler amplification device. Penile width during sleep erections may be measured in a test called a nocturnal penile tumescence study, which must include an electroencephalogram to identify the sleep stages. Vascular problems may be sought with arteriography studies. Injection of dye into the vas deferens, followed by masturbation and X-rays of the penis, can exclude rare, but surgically correctable, congenital crural "leakage points" (Wagner and Green 1981). Evaluation of afferent and efferent innervation of the penis may be tested with sacral evoked potential studies. Many medications as well as alcohol have side effects that may lead to impotence (Buffum et al. 1981).

There are specific "high risk for impotence" situations, which may be superimposed on a very moderate organic change. For example, divorce or death of a spouse may lead to potency loss. Erections are commonly vulnerable to emotional pressure, pain, loss, and personal financial loss. Marital conflict, marriage breakdown, and bereavement may lead to secondary impotence, and resolution of the sexual disorder may be delayed because of unresolved emotional and interpersonal conflict. Even in the ugliest divorce or the profoundest grief, the possibility of a physical cause for impotence must not be ignored. It would be a great injustice to suggest a psychological etiology, when, for example, reduced penile blood flow is responsible for the impotence. Physical and psychological causes are not mutually exclusive.

The more extensive, time-consuming, and often quite costly tests for impotence may be appropriate in cases when the patient 1) reports he has never been functional in intercourse (male virgin), 2) was formerly functional but now reports recurrent or frequent erectile failure with intercourse, or 3) has "soft tip" erections (i.e., rigidity is insufficient for penetration of the vagina), or a course of brief sex therapy fails despite the cooperation of both partners.

Treatment

Chemical Treatment. From the days of alchemy, aphrodisiacs have been sought but none has scientifically materialized. The latest—papaverine injections into the penile corpora—became widely used in the United States by 1987 and went beyond diagnostic use (Virag 1982; Zorgniotti and Lafleur 1985). The injections were popularized for home use as giving an instant chemical erection. Abuse has resulted in "group papaverine parties." Complications so far have included one unexpected death, nonresponse, local infections, crural scarring, and priapism that may require emergency chemical or surgical reduction.

Surgical Treatment. Surgical treatment for impotence due to physical causes is very widely available and includes several types of inflatable or semirigid, surgically implanted penile prostheses (Krauss 1987). These devices have made headlines in the past decade, heralding an era of "bionic sex." Such an implant, nonetheless, may not ensure satisfactory intercourse for its owner if his relationship with his partner is conflictual or if the partner is not interested. Nor are penile devices free of complications such as mechanical failure, local infection, and tissue erosion of the device. For obvious reasons, both partners therefore must consider such surgery carefully. If a man's partner is receptive, the implant may afford great sexual pleasure and closeness. The implant does not, however, give the man a climax or an ejaculation. It provides an erectile splint plus assurance that penetration is possible.

Mechanical Devices. Vacuum erection devices are noninvasive and have been perfected to the point of being useful to some impotent men, including the elderly, who are not interested in surgery or injections (Nadig et al. 1986). A pump builds a vacuum in the long plastic cylinder covering the penis at the perineum. Blood is thus drawn into the penis, and then a wide rubber band is slipped onto the penile root (to be removed not more than 30 minutes later). The cost in 1990, with a safety valve for rapid deflation, was $295. A willing partner, a sense of humor, and patience improve its value.

Premature Ejaculation

Premature ejaculation (PE) as the sole symptom rarely presents in the older age group but, rather, along with or prior to secondary impotence in inhibited sexual desire. Very few cases of PE have biologic or chemical causes. A major medical workup is rarely indicated. PE self-corrects in some men when practice and confidence reduce sexual anxiety. Sexual self-esteem declines unless PE is corrected, and secondary impotence often follows because of the pervasive fear of recurrence of instant ejaculation. In a young man, a thorough, explicit sexual history may reveal that rapid (less than 1 minute) erection plus ejaculation is a new or transient symptom. If the physical-genital examination is normal, then the physician can inquire about possible recent causes of PE, such as high excitement; a new, awkward, or unfamiliar setting; fear of being seen; return to sex after a long abstinence; or infrequent coitus. Such psychosocial causes of occasional premature ejaculation respond well to reassurance and directives from the physician to make love in a relaxed atmosphere. For men aged older than 60, these same questions can establish whether, underneath the erectile disorder or hypoactive sexual desire, there was earlier PE. PE usually responds readily to sex education, reassurance, and sex therapy techniques practiced at home alone or with a cooperative partner.

Contrary to popular belief, masturbation does not cause premature ejaculation. In fact, masturbating to ejaculation before intercourse might assist in early correction of the problem, because the second erection lasts longer. It is worth telling this to a patient of any age. The squeeze technique is a frequently prescribed sex therapy exercise. During foreplay, the partner (when told ejaculatory inevitability has almost been reached) squeezes the penis at the coronal ridge for 15 seconds. The erection is then allowed to subside. They wait 50 seconds, play again, squeeze again, and repeat several times to gain confidence in controlling his orgasm before actual intercourse. This procedure usually occurs with the man supine and the woman on top (Masters et al. 1986). There are many variations.

Inhibited Male Orgasm (Delayed or Absent Ejaculation)

A medical workup for this problem begins with a careful history of alcohol use, needed medication, or other chemical intake. Physical and genital examinations are accompanied by explicit questions about whether the symptom is "selective" or situational (only with intercourse or after alcohol indulgence or the taking of medications) or generalized (with both intercourse and masturbation and apparently unrelated to chemical ingestion).

If the symptom is generalized, then mechanical factors that could obstruct the flow of semen must be sought, for example, congenital absence of seminal vesicles; an inflammation obstructing the urethra; problems in the neck of the bladder; or problems that arise after prostate surgery, leading to retrograde ejaculation into the bladder. The latter may be quite compatible with good erections, intercourse, and climax. If the patient becomes aware of and understands his internal ejaculation, he may be able to enjoy it differently. Because about 30% of men over 60 have a prostatectomy, this diagnostic question is an important one (Wennenberg et al. 1988). Neurological and some endocrine lesions may affect ejaculation; therefore a neurological exam and blood hormone tests (as for impotence) may be indicated, because early diabetic neuropathy, for example, may cause retrograde ejaculation. Vasectomy, which causes a barely noticeable reduction in volume of ejaculate, is not the cause of delayed or absent ejaculation.

Female Sexual Dysfunction

Inhibited orgasm may be primary (never attained a climax in any way—not by hand, mouth, vibrator, or coitus), secondary, or situational. Sexual pain disorders include dyspareunia and vaginismus. Dyspareunia is pain on intercourse. Vaginismus is spasm of the vaginal pubococcygeus muscles.

For any female sexual problem, a full physical and genital-pelvic examination should follow an explicit history. The examination should be educative, with instruction from the physician about the position of the clitoris and its attachments and the circular pubococcygeus muscle of the lower vagina, which a woman can voluntarily contract and relax. During the examination, she may be given a hand mirror for viewing her genitals and offered accurate education about her genital anatomy so that she can explore at home on her own or with her partner.

The sexological examination is standard practice in sex therapy. It may be done with the partner present, so he may learn from the sex education (Masters et al. 1986). If there is physician concern about litigation, a nurse chaperone should be present and her presence and name charted.

Standard sex therapy home exercises for anorgasmia include self-stimulation to orgasm. A woman thus finds where her pleasure areas are and can direct her partner (if she has one) or find release and normal relaxation on her own at any time. Brief sex therapy with home massage and foreplay is helpful regardless of age, and women in their fifties to late seventies have thus had the satisfaction of at last experiencing their very first orgasm.

At menopause or after an early, total hysterectomy, the vaginal wall may be thin or dry and less elastic because of reduced estrogen. Orgasm may be less intense (Masters and Johnson 1966). Hormonal replacement treatment (unless contraindicated because of risk of cancer) may be indicated, because many older women remain interested in sexual activity. The older women responds rapidly and well to estrogen alone or combined with progesterone but needs regular gynecology follow-up every 6 months. If there is a vaginal infection, a culture may be done and specific medications prescribed. When there is localized or focal vaginal pain, a minor vestibular area may be infected and require excision under local anesthetic if it has not responded to antibiotics.

Hypoactive Sexual Desire

Explicit sex history questions determine whether the hypoactive sexual desire (HSD) is situational (relating to sex with a specific partner or to sex under particular circumstances) or generalized (at all times). If it is generalized, then hormonal blood tests may be indicated, because (for example) underactive thyroid gland, pituitary problems, or secondary prolactinemia may be causative. In some uncommon cases neurological problems can be diagnosed with a computed tomography scan for intracranial pathology, underscoring the need for careful medical evaluation as an integral part of the overall treatment of a sexual problem at any age. Postbypass coital fears must be routinely addressed (Renshaw 1987).

The most common but not age-specific underlying causes of selective HSD have to do with fatigue, career, financial, or time pressures; major depression; medications; alcohol; and conflict between partners. If both partners are motivated to change, sex therapy can be effective, often combined with other approaches such as marital or individual psychotherapy or antidepressants. Relaxed, rested, early morning love play is often best for high-pressure-stressed, fatigued, or disabled persons. Pleasurable closeness can encourage open, honest communication, avoidance of blame, and respect for normal libido differences. Patients are advised to take turns giving and receiving affection with sustained touch, so that both may be emotionally nurtured and pleasurable sexual exchange restored. Outcome data of efficacy in those over 65 are not available.

Libido Differences

Libido differences are so common in marriages and in relationships that they are not considered to be a diagnostic category. They are individual differences—neither good nor bad, simply differences. When a couple is unable to negotiate a compromise between themselves in their frequency of sexual encounters, then the issue may become a crisis. Negotiation may be open or there may be veiled threats ("I'm going to look for it elsewhere") or taunts ("It's fine with me—go find someone else").

Distress about discrepant sexual desire is coded as an adjustment disorder when a couple seek help with libido differences as their presenting complaint. The wife may be upset enough to call, but in older couples it is more common for a husband to do so.

For example, a 64-year-old man on the verge of retirement said, "I want more than golf; it's time she stops being so frigid." The pejorative term was, of course, upsetting to his coitally compliant wife. Mary, 63, was a "good wife" who waited for his initiation, felt "good" about intercourse, could "take it or leave it, but I look forward to being held." She was nonorgasmic, yet she blossomed when sex therapy provided massage, cuddling, baths together, and permission to use sexual fantasy. She said, "The bedroom has gone from mechanical to marvelous." Despite her newfound pleasure, she still could not be a sexual initiator. "I still can't do that," she said. "What if he doesn't want to? It's a man's role. I'm 64 next month."

Special Circumstances

If a minor is molested by an older person, careful evaluation must include search for a previous history of such behavior, because young pedophiles, exhibitionists, and voyeurs become old ones (MacNamara and Sagarin 1977). However, organic mental disorders can also lead to sexually deviant behavior.

Even if cognitive impairment is documented by the physician, a report to child protective authorities may be mandatory by law. When organicity is present, usually the patient's family can be given custody by the court. Family, neighbors, and children must be educated about the sexual disinhibition sometimes associated with cognitive pathology.

When an institutionalized, cognitively impaired, elderly patient displays inappropriate or disinhibited public sexual behavior, caregivers may feel needless panic about being raped, although coercive sexual behavior is rare in cognitively impaired elders. They are usually too frail and uncoordinated to rape. Much more common are verbal obscenities or clumsy sexual overtures to staff or to other impaired patients. Although realistic danger is minimal, staff still may become fearful.

Management consists of evaluating mental status, noting the sexual behaviors, open staff discussion of these behaviors, and modification by behavioral techniques: extinction (nonattention if

possible), firm limit setting, privilege reduction, or positive reinforcement for appropriate behavior.

Caregivers are instructed in specific steps they may take to deal
with inappropriate sexual situations, including anticipating repetition of the behavior, defining staff members' roles, verbally defining the sexual problem to the patient while it is occurring, and
using outside controls if the initial steps prove ineffectual. Adjunctive use of small daily doses of liquid haloperidol may enhance
management of the difficult situation.

References

American Psychiatric Association: Diagnostic and Statistical Manual of
    Mental Disorders, 3rd Edition, Revised. Washington, DC, American
    Psychiatric Association, 1987

Boller F, Frank E: Sexual Dysfunction in Neurological Disorders: Diag-
    nosis, Management, and Rehabilitation. New York, Raven, 1982

Brecher EM, Editors of Consumer Reports Books: Love, Sex, and Aging.
    Boston, MA, Little, Brown, 1983

Buffum J, Smith DE, Moser C, et al: Drugs and sexual function, in Sexual
    Problems in Medical Practice. Edited by Lief H. Monroe, WI, American
    Medical Association, 1981, pp 211–242

Butler R, Lewis M: Sex After Sixty. New York, Harper & Row, 1977

Kinsey AC, Pomeroy WB, Martin CE: Sexual Behavior in the Human Male.
    Philadelphia, PA, WB Saunders, 1948

Krauss DJ: Management of impotence, II: selected surgical procedures:
    penile prostheses. Clin Ther 9:149–156, 1987

MacNamara, DE, Sagarin E: Sex, Crime and the Law. New York, Free
    Press, 1977

Masters WH, Johnson VE: Human Sexual Response. Boston, MA, Little,
    Brown, 1966

Masters WH, Johnson VE, Kolodny RC: Sex and Human Loving. Boston,
    MA, Little, Brown, 1986

Nadig PW, Ware JC, Blumoff R: Noninvasive device to produce and main-
    tain an erection-like state. Urology 2:126–131, 1986

Renshaw DC: Wives of impotent men. Consultant 19(8):41–48, 1979

Renshaw DC: Sex after coronary bypass surgery. Cardio 4(8):46–48, 1987

Renshaw DC: Sex and cognitively impaired patients. Consultant
    28(3):133–137, 1988a

Renshaw DC: Profile on 2,376 patients treated at Loyola sex clinic be-
    tween 1972 and 1987. Sexual and Marital Therapy 3:111–117, 1988b

Scott FB, Bradley WE, Timm GW: Management of erectile impotence: use
    of implantable inflatable prosthesis. Urology 2:80–82, 1973

Virag R: Intracavernous injection of papaverine for erectile failure. Lancet
    2:938, 1982

Wagner G, Green R: Differential Diagnosis of Erectile Failure. Impotence, Physiological, Psychological, Surgical Diagnosis and Treatment. New York, Plenum Press, 1981, pp 114–118, 123–127, 151

Wennenberg JE, Mulley AG, Hanley D, et al: An evaluation of prostatectomy for benign urinary tract obstruction: geographic variations and the assessment of medical care outcomes. JAMA 259:3027–3030, 1988

Wise TN: Sexual disorders in medical and surgical conditions, in Clinical Management of Sexual Disorders. Edited by Meyer JK, Schmidt CW, Wise TN. Baltimore, MD, Williams & Wilkins, 1983, pp 317–332

Zorgniotti AW, Lafleur RS: Auto-injection of the corpus cavernosum with a vasoactive drug combination for vasculogenic impotence. J Urol 133:39–41, 1985

SECTION 4

Treatment

CHAPTER 22

Robert C. Young, M.D.
Barnett S. Meyers, M.D.

Psychopharmacology

General Principles

Geriatric psychopharmacology is a broad and therefore potentially intimidating field. However, it is also a relatively new discipline, and the amount of clinically relevant empirical information
available is limited. Some texts (Jenike 1985; Salzman 1984) and
review articles (Meyers and Kalayam 1989; Rockwell et al. 1989;
Shamoian 1988; Wragg and Jeste 1988) are helpful, as are discussions focusing on psychopharmacologic issues from the perspectives of age and age-related disease effects on particular organ systems (Jarvik 1989; Jefferson and Greist 1979; Roose et al. 1987).
Finally, some discussions of general psychopharmacology include
mention of geriatric issues (Schatzberg and Cole 1986).

An initial, thorough medical and neurologic history and examination are essential to the management of elderly patients. Physical illnesses and the drugs used to manage them can produce psychiatric signs and symptoms. Psychopathology may be treated or
alleviated by treating previously undiagnosed physical illness or
eliminating (when possible) offending drugs; these steps should be
attempted, when appropriate, prior to pharmacotherapeutic intervention. Thorough evaluation is also necessary for identification of
disease and drug factors that may complicate drug treatment.

The approach to pharmacotherapy in the elderly has much in
common with that in younger patients. For example, all classes of
drugs useful in younger patients have been used effectively and
safely in elderly patients. Nevertheless, certain issues are highlighted by age-related factors. In the elderly, the selection of class

of drug and the selection of specific agents within classes require particularly careful risk-benefit analysis. Consideration of dosage and duration of treatment are also critical.

Drug selection needs to be informed by a thorough history of previous drug use including agents and doses used, efficacy and side effects, duration of unsuccessful or successful treatments, and serum-plasma concentrations. This inquiry should clarify whether trials of particular agents have been adequate or whether they have been compromised by intolerance of side effects or by noncompliance. A history of current use of prescribed and over-the-counter (OTC) medications must be obtained.

Treatment efforts are directed to acute symptom reduction, continuation of improvement, and prevention of relapse. The latter is particularly important in the elderly, because they are at high risk for further morbidity. Late-life paranoid disorders, for example, are chronic illnesses (Kay 1962; Post 1966), and chronicity and recurrence of affective disorders are commonly encountered in the elderly (Alexopoulos et al. 1989; Post 1972; Zis and Goodwin 1979); however, studies comparing illness course in elderly and young patients are needed, because other data are somewhat contradictory (cf. Chapter 16). The juxtaposition of indications for chronic use with increased sensitivity to adverse reactions complicates decisions about long-term use of neuroleptics and thymoleptics in elderly psychiatric patients.

Compliance of the elderly patient with drug regimens, particularly among ambulatory outpatients living independently, can be compromised by lack of information, cognitive dysfunction, physical disability, dissatisfaction with side effects, and complex drug regimens. When possible, once-daily or at most twice-daily doses, with the fewest possible number of drugs, should be prescribed. This approach is feasible because of the long half-lives of many psychopharmacologic agents, which may be prolonged with increasing age. Drugs with long half-lives, however, may be undesirable in view of prolonged side effects (e.g., long-acting benzodiazepines).

Finally, the psychiatrist must be cognizant of each medication's side effects and how they change as a function of age. Thus, older patients are less likely to develop acute dystonias from neuroleptics but are more vulnerable to bradykinesia and tremor (Salzman et al. 1970). Similarly, anticholinergic activity of low-potency neuroleptics and tricyclics can lead to severe constipation, fecal impaction, and (more rarely) paralytic ileus in older patients who have less physical activity and decreased bowel motility.

Pharmacology of Aging

Pharmacokinetics can be described as the effect of a patient on a drug. By contrast, pharmacodynamics is the effect of a drug on a patient (Meyers 1989).

Pharmacokinetics and Aging

Pharmacokinetic factors determine concentration of drug in body compartments over time. Consideration of pharmacokinetics precedes attributing differences in drug effects to pharmacodynamic differences, because much of the interindividual differences in response to drugs in mixed-age populations is accounted for by pharmacokinetic differences. In pharmacokinetics are included the component processes of absorption, metabolism, distribution, and excretion.

Absorption. Psychotropic drugs are well absorbed from the gastrointestinal tract. They are absorbed by diffusion. Although a number of physiologic changes that occur with aging would theoretically decrease drug absorption (see Table 22-1) and the rate of absorption of lipid soluble drugs may decrease with age, there is no evidence that, in the absence of gastrointestinal disease, a clinically significant decrease in total absorption of psychotropic drugs occurs with normal aging (Israili and Wenger 1981).

Metabolism. The liver is the principal site for metabolic transformation of lipid-soluble psychotropic drugs. Metabolites can be pharmacologically active or inactive. Metabolic pathways include demethylation, ring hydroxylation, and acetylation. (Glucuronidation of parent compound or metabolites generates inactive, water-soluble forms that are renally cleared). These processes are mediated by microsomal enzymes. The activity of these enzymes varies widely among individuals and is determined genetically. Some drugs are metabolized largely on the initial transit through the hepatic circulation—the "first pass effect."

Age-associated effects on hepatic metabolism, outlined in Table 22-1, can influence drug pharmacokinetics in the elderly. Some metabolic pathways (e.g., demethylation) may be slowed by age, and these effects may contribute to raising blood levels of specific psychopharmacologic agents, for example, tertiary amine tricyclics (Nies et al. 1977) and benzodiazepines with active metabolites (Greenblatt and Shader 1981). However, it is difficult to sepa-

Table 22-1. Effects of age on pharmacokinetics

Component	Effect	Consequence
Absorption	Decreased gastric pH, motility; decreased intestinal surface area and blood flow	None known
Metabolism	Decreased hepatic blood flow	Not known
	Decreased enzyme activity	May decrease demethylation of tertiary amine tricyclics and benzodiazepines with active desmethyl metabolites
Distribution	Increase in fat-lean body ratio	Increased concentration of plasma lithium and hydrophilic drug metabolites; decreased plasma concentration of lipid soluble drugs but increased total distribution and prolonged half-life
	Decrease in albumen	Increased free benzodiazepine
Excretion	Decrease in renal function	Decreased clearance of lithium; decreased clearance of polycyclic antidepressant metabolites

rate the effects of altered metabolism from effects of changes in distribution and excretion on drug plasma concentration and half-life.

Distribution. Drugs are distributed throughout the body in three compartments: fat tissue, body water, and plasma proteins. Volume of distribution indicates how widely a particular drug is distributed in the body.

The distribution of particular drugs is determined in part by their lipid solubility. Most psychotropic drugs are highly lipid soluble; the notable exception is lithium, which is a hydrophilic cation. The increase in proportion of body fat to water with increasing age (Hollister 1981) increases the volume of distribution of nearly all psychotropic agents in elderly patients.

Psychotropic drugs, with the exception of lithium salts, are extensively bound to plasma proteins. Polycyclic antidepressants are extensively bound to alpha acid glycoprotein, whereas benzodiazepines are bound predominantly to albumen. Aging is associated with changes in body composition and plasma proteins that can alter drug distribution (see Table 22-1).

Excretion. Psychotropic drugs are mainly eliminated by the kidneys. Renal excretion of lipid-soluble drugs occurs mainly as hydrophilic metabolized forms that are glucoronide conjugated or unconjugated. For tricyclic antidepressants, hepatic hydroxylation followed by renal excretion is the major pathway of elimination. The decrease in glomerular filtration that is associated with aging (Rowe 1980) accounts for part of the increased accumulation of hydrophilic metabolites in some elderly patients (Young et al. 1984). This age-related decrease also leads to a slower clearance of lithium in elderly patients (Chapron et al. 1982; Hardy et al. 1987).

Related terms. *Clearance* refers to the volume of blood from which all drug is removed per unit of time. The *half-life* of a drug is the time required for half of an amount of drug to be eliminated. This time is directly proportional to the volume of distribution and inversely proportional to clearance. *Steady-state* concentrations are obtained when the amount of a drug entering plasma on repeat administration balances its clearance. Such concentrations are directly proportional to dose, at a given dosing interval, and inversely proportional to clearance. Steady-state concentrations are achieved after five or six half-lives of repeated administration. Age-related prolongation of the half-life of certain drugs increases the time to steady state. For most psychotropic drugs, steady-state concentrations have a linear relationship to dose in a particular individual.

Physical Illness Effects on Pharmacokinetics. Elderly patients frequently have one or more physical illnesses, which can modify pharmacokinetics by decreasing absorption, altering the concentration of plasma proteins that bind drugs, and diminishing renal clearance (see Table 22-2). Drugs and restricted diets used for management of physical disorders can interact with psychotropic medications. Such interactions can occur at a pharmacokinetic level; the concentration of either the psychotropic or the nonpsychotropic, or of both drugs, can be affected. The influences on psychotropics may or may not be clinically significant; they can include

Table 22-2. Effects of illness on pharmacokinetics

Component	Type of illness or surgery	Consequence
Absorption	Gastric or small bowel resection; heart failure	Possibly decreased absorption
Metabolism	Liver disease; heart failure	Decreased metabolism of antidepressants
Distribution	Inflammatory states	Increased alpha acid glycoprotein causing increased plasma "total" antidepressant levels
	Malnutrition	Decreased albumen and alpha acid glycoprotein
Excretion	Renal failure; heart failure	Decreased clearance of lithium and drug metabolites

decreases or delays in absorption, increases or decreases in hepatic metabolism, displacement from binding proteins, and decreases in renal excretion. Salzman's text (1984) provides a listing of interactions. Important examples are given in Table 22-3 and described in sections discussing specific medications.

Pharmacodynamics and Aging

In addition to individual differences in pharmacokinetics, individuals may differ in tissue response to a given concentration of drug; this phenomenon is called *pharmacodynamics*. Age-associated changes occur in both peripheral and central neurotransmitter systems, and these changes may alter the therapeutic and toxic effects of the agents. Table 22-4 lists morphologic, biochemical, and physiologic changes at the synaptic level. The significance of such changes for neuroendocrine function and behavior remains to be elucidated, however.

Age effects on neuroendocrine and other responses to acute administration of pharmacologic agonists and some psychotropic agents have been reported. These effects include a blunted prolactin response to neuroleptics, presumably related to dopaminergic neurotransmission (Rolandi et al. 1982); decreased response of peripheral beta-adrenergic receptors to agonist drugs (Vestal et al. 1979); and decreased noradrenergic response to desipramine administration (Bickford-Wimer et al. 1987).

Table 22-3. Examples of pharmacokinetic drug interactions

Interactions	Consequence
Phenothiazines, tricyclics, or benzodiazepines with antacids	Decreased absorption
Anticholinergic tricyclics with methylphenidate	Decreased tricyclic metabolism
Tricyclics or benzodiazepines with cimetidine	Decreased metabolism
Tricyclics with barbiturates	Enhanced metabolism of tricyclics
Lithium carbonate with proximal loop diuretics	Decreased lithium excretion
Lithium carbonate with nonsteroidal anti-inflammatory agents	Decreased lithium excretion
Monoamine oxidase inhibitors with meperidine	Release of serotonin and inhibition of metabolism causes serotongergic crisis

There is very limited empirically derived information concerning possible differences among age groups in behavioral response to pharmacologic challenge. Increased sensitivity of elderly patients to cognitive dysfunction after receiving diazepam has been reported (Pomara et al. 1985; Reidenberg et al. 1978).

Most psychotropic drugs interact with many neurotransmitter systems. Considerations of pharmacodynamics are also complex because these neurotransmitter systems themselves interact. Furthermore, biologic consequences of drug action change as a function of time during chronic administration.

The concept of increased "sensitivity" of older persons to toxic effects of psychotropic drugs administered at conventional doses and present in usual concentrations has evolved out of case reports of adverse reactions; systematic studies of this question are lacking. It is possible, but also remains to be demonstrated, that elderly patients have a narrower margin between therapeutic and toxic doses and concentrations. Similarly, the clinical lore that therapeutic effects of psychotropic drugs occur at lower doses and concentrations in the elderly have not been documented by empirical studies. We do not know that elderly patients treated with a broad range of plasma concentrations of tricyclic antidepressants or lithium have the same concentration-response relationship as

Table 22-4. Effects of age on psychotropic substrates at synaptic level

Substrate	Age effect	Example
Neurotransmitter synthesis		
Neuron number	Decrease	Nigrostriatal pathway; cholinergic pathways
Precursor availability	Unknown	
Synthetic enzymes	Decreased activity	Tyrosine hydroxylase; dopa decarboyxlase; dopamine-B-hydroxylase; choline acetyltransferase
Neurotransmitter concentration	Decreased	Dopamine; norepinephrine
Synaptic release		
Presynaptic neurotransmitter receptors	Possible decreased binding	Alpha$_2$-adrenergic
Presynpatic drug receptors	Unknown	—
Neurotransmitter inactivation		
Reuptake (presynaptic)	Unknown	—
Degradative enzymes	Increased or decreased	Monoamine oxidase B increased; catechol-o-methyl transferase increased or decreased
Metabolite	Increased	Homovanillic acid; 5-hydroxyindoleacetic acid
Postsynaptic receptors		
Neurotransmitters	Decreased density	Muscarinic; GABA; dopamine D$_2$; β-adrenergic
	Decreased sensitivity	
Drug receptors	Increased density	Benzodiazepine
Intraneuronal messengers		
Phosphodiesterase	Unknown	—
Protein kinase	Unknown	—

younger adults. Studies showing that elderly patients do respond to concentrations comparable to those effective in young adults will be discussed in sections related to the specific agents.

Physical-Neurologic Illness Effects on Pharmacodynamics. Certain brain disorders in the elderly can further alter age-related neuronal changes and thereby influence drug effects. Such illnesses include Parkinson's disease, cerebrovascular disease, and primary degenerative dementia. Evidence for central disruption of biogenic amine and acetylcholine neurotransmitter systems by these disorders has been summarized by Addonizio (1989), Young (1989), and Meyers and Young (1989). (This information is outlined in Table 22-5.) Clinically relevant manifestations include increased sensitivity of patients with Parkinson's disease to neuroleptic-induced exacerbation of motor dysfunction and to anticholinergic delirium (Figiel et al. 1989), and the sensitivity of patients with cerebrovascular disease and degenerative dementia to central anticholinergic drug effects (Sunderland and Silver 1988). The psychiatrist who prescribes a neuroleptic to treat the agitation or psychosis of a patient with Parkinson's disease must recognize that this treatment will worsen the functional dopamine deficiency and increase neuromuscular symptoms; the alternative approach of lowering dosage of an antiparkinsonian medication that could be causing the psychiatric disorder should be considered.

Drug-Drug Interaction at the Pharmacodynamic Level. Drugs for medical or neurologic disorders can interact with psychotropics at the pharmacodynamic level. (Examples of such interactions are provided in Table 22-6.) They include instances in which drug interactions are additive (e.g., increased anticholinergic effects from low-potency neuroleptics add to those of antiparkinsonian drugs), and those in which there is inhibition of the effect of one class of agents by those of another (e.g., guanethidine and phenothiazines or tricyclics).

Overview of Drug Classes

Thymoleptic Agents

Among antidepressant agents, the tricyclic antidepressants (TCAs) have been first-line agents for pharmacotherapy of depressive syndromes in older as well as younger patients. In recent years other polycyclic antidepressants have been introduced in the U.S. mar-

Table 22-5. Alterations of central neurotransmitter-related measures in brain disorders compared to same-age controls

System	Parkinsonism	Cerebrovascular disease (stroke, multi-infarct dementia)	Degenerative dementia
Acetylcholine	Decreased cortical enzyme; decreased cortical synthetic enzyme	—	Decreased cell number
Dopamine	Decreased nigrostriatal mesocortical and mesolimbic neurons	Decreased cerebrospinal fluid metabolite concentrations in dementia	Decreased neurotransmitter and metabolite concentrations
Norepinephrine	Decreased cell loss	—	Decreased cell number and increased metabolite concentrations
Serotonin	Decreased cell loss	Decreased cerebrospinal fluid metabolite concentrations in dementia	Decreased cell numbers and decreased metabolite concentrations
GABA	—	—	Decreased synthetic enzyme and decreased **GABA**

ket. Monoamine oxidase inhibitors (MAOIs) have received renewed attention as clinically useful alternatives. Stimulant drugs are occasionally used in depressed patients, but systematic studies of efficacy are unavailable.

Lithium salts are first-line antimanic agents in patients of all ages; they also have other indications in the elderly. Other antimanic and mood stabilizing compounds, such as antiepileptics, also have been used in the elderly.

Neuroleptics

These compounds are first-line agents in the elderly for the management of psychotic symptoms. They also have a role in the man-

Table 22-6. Examples of pharmacodynamic drug interactions

Drug interaction	Consequence
Tricyclics, neuroleptics, or benzodiazepines with other sedative drugs	Additive sedative effect
Tricyclics or low-potency neuroleptics with antihypertensives	Increased vulnerability to orthostatic hypotension
Tricyclics and phenothiazine with guanethidine	Blockade of neuronal uptake prevents activity of either agent
Tricyclics with clonidine	Competition at alpha-2 receptor interferes with activity of either agent
Lithium with neuroleptics	Increase in parkinsonian side effects
Tricyclics with quinidine	Additive Type I antiarrhythmic effects decreasing cardiac conduction

agement of behavioral disturbances accompanying organic mental syndromes (Sunderland and Silver 1988). For current purposes they can be viewed as a single group of drugs that differ primarily in their side-effect profiles. Even less information on dose-response relationships is available for neuroleptics than for thymoleptic agents; these medications should be prescribed empirically, in the lowest effective dose. The absence of systematic data on dosage, the heterogeneity of indicators for neuroleptic use in elderly patients, and the increased sensitivity of this population to specific adverse reactions suggest a conservative approach.

Antianxiety Agents and Sedatives-Hypnotics

The primary antianxiety agents are the benzodiazepines. This class also includes glycol derivatives (meprobamate), antihistamines, and buspirone.

The sedatives-hypnotics include benzodiazepines, barbiturates, and other agents such as halogenated hydrocarbons (chloral hydrate). Barbiturates are not recommended because of their potential risk of respiratory suppression in overdose and their high potential for dependence and for drug-drug interactions. Others such as glutethamide, methaqualone, and ethylchlorvynol should also be avoided. Meprobamate can be problematic because it induces the metabolism of other medications, has a narrow margin between toxic and therapeutic doses, and is associated with dependence and life-threatening withdrawal reactions. Unfortunately, the recent requirement by some states of special prescriptions for benzodiazepines may lead to an increased use of agents that carry greater risk but are less restricted.

Clinical studies reported for patients aged older than 65 generally are based on small samples; consequently the clinician needs to maintain an attitude of healthy skepticism with regard to the literature on treatment outcome (efficacy, side effects, and toxicity) for any specific drug.

General Baseline Assessment

Treatment History

A history of previous successful or unsuccessful drug treatment provides guidelines for selection of drug class and of particular agents within classes. Adequacy of prior treatment efforts needs to be assessed by noting drug dose, duration of administration, and (in the case of thymoleptics) drug plasma levels if available. Therapeutic response needs to be judged, and any treatment-limiting side effects need to be noted.

Clinical Assessment

Clinicians can make use of psychopathology rating scales as an adjunct in monitoring change during treatment. However, some of these "observer-rated" scales require specific training in their use; for example, the Hamilton Rating Scale for Depression (Hamilton 1960) is applicable for rating depressive signs and symptoms in cognitively intact patients, whereas the Cornell Scale (Alexopoulos et al. 1988) is useful for elderly patients with cognitive impairment. The 30-item Geriatric Depression Rating Scale is a self-report instrument with established reliability and validity for identifying geriatric depression (Yesavage et al. 1983).

Cognitive function should be evaluated before and during treatment. Although it has limited sensitivity, the Mini-Mental State Exam (Folstein et al. 1975) is a convenient and widely used instrument for screening. If indicated, more sensitive and detailed instruments can be used, for example, the Dementia Rating Scale (Mattis 1988). (See also Chapter 8.)

Further, the importance of an initial complete "review of systems" drives from the fact that many "side effects" are related to psychopathologic state. In evaluating physical complaints during drug treatment it is critical to be able to compare these to complaints before treatment in order to judge whether they represent drug toxicity.

Blood pressure assessment should include determination of orthostatic change, especially if antidepressants and/or low-potency neuroleptics are to be used. This side effect can be particularly risky in elderly patients with osteoporosis and coronary artery disease. Orthostatic hypotension is not correlated with age per se (Glassman et al. 1979); however, orthostatic hypotension can be more severe and have serious consequences in patients with decreased cardiac output and/or those treated with diuretics or beta-blockers (Glassman et al. 1979). Baseline measurement of orthostatic blood pressure change is especially important because pretreatment orthostatic changes are correlated with changes that occur during TCA treatment (Glassman et al. 1979). Administration of neuroleptics should be preceded by assessment of neuromuscular function; this approach enables the clinician to identify neuroleptic-induced side effects of parkinsonism and tardive dyskinesia. Elderly patients have an increased vulnerability to both forms of adverse reactions (Ayd 1976; Jeste et al. 1987). A simple screening instrument such as the Abnormal Involuntary Movement Scale (Whittier 1969) can characterize and quantify baseline functioning.

Laboratory Assessment

This generally includes an electrocardiogram (ECG). Ischemia, dysrhythmia, rate disturbance, and conduction abnormalities need to be assessed in planning antidepressant pharmacotherapy. TCAs may increase rate and thereby can increase ischemia. Their quinidinelike Type I antiarrhythmic effects delay conduction through the His-Purkinje system and can produce heart block in patients with underlying conduction abnormalities (Roose et al. 1987). Less is known about the newer heterocyclics, but the lower anticholinergic and alpha-1 adrenergic antagonist potencies of these agents may make them safer in patients with cardiac disease. The limited data available for TCAs indicate prolongation of conduction peaks after 3 or 4 weeks of treatment (Glassman and Bigger 1981); this suggests that patients with borderline conduction defects before treatment should have weekly ECGs for the first 4

weeks on TCAs, after which time routine monitoring can be re-
sumed.

A baseline ECG to assess for sinus functioning is also indicated
prior to use of lithium, because of the reported development of sick
sinus syndrome (Roose et al. 1979a). This complication might be
encountered particularly in older patients with coronary artery
disease that has compromised the sinus node.

In patients to be treated with lithium salts, baseline evaluation
should also include thyroid and renal function tests. Serum creatinine is not a sensitive index of renal function; patients with renal
insufficiency who require careful monitoring and for whom collection of 24-hour urine is not feasible can have creatinine clearance
approximated from age, body weight, and serum creatinine (Friedman et al. 1979). Assessment of thyroid status, including thyroid-
stimulating hormone (TSH), is especially important in the elderly.
Lithium's antagonizing effect on thyroid gland function, in combination with the diminished thyroid reserve that accompanies aging (Sawin et al. 1985), makes this population vulnerable to developing hypothyroidism during lithium treatment.

Patients treated with carbamazepine should have baseline and
followup hematologic assessment.

Use of Thymoleptics

These drugs are of central importance in primary mood disorders,
both unipolar (major depression) and bipolar. Although switching
between agents with different types of neurotransmitter activity
(e.g., from desipramine, which is nonadrenergic, to fluoxetine,
which is serotonergic) has theoretical appeal, it is not supported
by clinical trials. Switching to another class of agents (e.g., from a
TCA to an MAOI) can be effective, but the conservative approach of
waiting 2 weeks between discontinuation of the TCA and starting
the MAOI is recommended. The use of lithium augmentation prior
to making this change assures that there is an active mood stabilizer "on board" during the pharmacologic waiting period.

Thymoleptics have a role in the treatment of mood disorders
secondary to medical or neurological disorders, especially if the
physical condition has been treated specifically (e.g., stroke, hypothyroidism) but the mood disorder persists. The risk of orthostatic
hypotension complicates treatment of poststroke depression; however, according to one study, most patients with this syndrome tolerate and respond to doses of nortriptyline that are comparable to

those used to treat young adult depressives (Lipsey et al. 1984). Methylphenidate was found in a retrospection study by Lingam et al. 1988 to be effective for elderly patients with poststroke depression.

The frequency of recurrence and chronicity in elderly depressives (Alexopoulos et al. 1989) and the increased risk of suicide (Blazer et al. 1986), occurring in conjunction with vulnerability to adverse reactions, complicate decisions concerning duration of medication treatment after recovery from a depressive episode. The concurrence of depression and dementia (Reifler et al. 1982) and poststroke depression (Robinson and Price 1982) are clinical problems with special relevance to geriatric psychiatry.

A recent study showing that Alzheimer's patients can tolerate and benefit from vigorous treatment with a tertiary amine TCA (Reifler et al. 1989) disputes the clinical lore that the use of these agents is contraindicated in patients who have central cholinergic lesions. Case reports previously indicated that MAOIs can be used safely and effectively in Alzheimer's patients (Jenike 1986).

Delusional symptoms are relatively common among elderly with major depression. The pharmacologic treatment approach to the delusionally depressed elderly patient is not well studied. Mixed-age, delusionally depressed adults treated with TCAs alone respond less well than do nondelusional patients. Combination of neuroleptic and antidepressant drugs is necessary for optimal response in many of these patients, and response rates to combined treatment can approach those in patients treated with electroconvulsive therapy (ECT) (Nelson and Bowers 1978; Perry et al. 1982; Spiker et al. 1985). However, elderly patients may not tolerate the toxicity associated with two drugs, and therefore clinicians may initially try neuroleptic or antidepressant alone and proceed promptly to ECT (cf. Chapter 23).

Tricyclic Antidepressants and Monoamine Oxidase Inhibitors

Secondary amine TCAs, specifically nortriptyline and desipramine, have advantages over tertiary amine TCAs for use in the elderly. They have less anticholinergic and sedative potency, which may be related to diminished affinities for muscarinic, histaminic, and adrenergic receptors (Richelson 1982). Notriptyline has a relatively low potential for inducing orthostatic hypotension (Roose et al. 1981). The use of protriptyline is complicated by its long half-life.

The patient is started at a low dose, which is increased gradually. In most cases the target dose can be achieved within 2 weeks, but each patient's tolerance of side effects must be considered. Gradual increments allow patients to become accustomed to side effects and may increase compliance. There is no systematic evidence that divided dose administration is more effective than single dose; however, it may reduce side effects. A single nighttime dose is usually well tolerated and improves sleep, except that orthostatic hypotension presents a major risk in patients who get up during the night.

Duration of treatment required for adequate response in elderly patients with depressive syndromes may be somewhat longer than in younger adults (Georgotas et al. 1986), although early reduction in symptoms may predict good outcome (Jarvik and Mintz 1987). Some patients may require at least 6 weeks for symptoms to resolve. Duration of treatment for optimal response and prophylaxis in the elderly has not been sufficiently studied.

The acute efficacy of phenelzine in ambulatory elderly with major depression having an "endogenous" symptom profile is superior to placebo and comparable to nortriptyline (Georgotas et al. 1986). Although the fact that platelet and brain MAO activity can increase with increasing age (Robinson 1981) is consistent with the use of MAOIs in geriatric patients, the clinical significance of such changes is unknown.

Therapeutic response to phenelzine in elderly depressives can occur at dosages comparable to those employed with younger depressed patients (Georgotas et al. 1986). Systematic data on dose-response relationships in the elderly are unavailable. Plasma levels of phenelzine may be higher in elderly patients versus younger patients receiving equivalent doses (Robinson 1981); whether this possibility has clinical significance is not known.

Tranylcypromine is also effective for elderly patients, but systematic studies assessing its use in this population are not yet available.

The optimal target dose for elderly patients is not well delineated for any agent. Clinical studies show that older patients respond to doses and steady-state plasma levels of nortriptyline and desipramine that are comparable to those effective in younger adults (i.e., 50–150 ng/ml of nortriptyline and more than 125 ng/ml of desipramine [Georgotas et al. 1986; Nelson et al. 1985]). In patients showing a good response, low steady-state plasma levels should not be "treated," however. Hydroxylated metabolites of secondary amine TCAs, which are cleared by the kidneys, may reach increased levels in elderly depressed patients; these compounds have pharmacodynamic activity that can increase toxicity and may influence efficacy (Young et al. 1984).

An early study using imipramine in outpatient major depressives suggested response at low dosage (Gerner et al. 1980), but this investigation was hampered by high dropout rate, low response rate, and lack of plasma levels. In contrast to secondary amine TCAs, for which plasma concentrations of the parent compound per milligram dose are equivalent to those in younger patients, tertiary amine TCA concentrations may be increased per milligram dose in elderly patients. Relationships to clinical response are not delineated.

Potentiation of a TCA with thyroid hormone can be considered after determining that subclinical hypothyroidism (elevated TSH with normal T_3 and T_4 values) is present. This state can present as depression and be resistant to TCAs. The elderly patient's cardiac status is of special concern before the use of thyroid potentiation, for it can worsen preexisting coronary insufficiency by increasing the heart rate. Consultation with the patient's cardiologist prior to instituting treatment is indicated.

Special concerns with MAOIs include the need for dietary restriction of tyramine-rich foods and avoidance of drug-drug interactions, particularly with sympathomimetic agents and meperidine. In the elderly, compliance may be reduced by cognitive and physical deficits. Analysis of the tyramine content of commonly prohibited foods suggests the lists usually given to patients are overrestrictive (McCabe and Tsuang 1982; Shulman et al. 1989; Sullivan and Shulman 1984). The availability of clear, easy-to-follow guidelines is especially relevant to treatment of elderly depressives, who must frequently depend on others for shopping or food preparation. The rare spontaneous hypertensive crises that have been reported may have greater potential morbidity in elderly patients, but whether advanced age increases vulnerability to such reactions is uncertain.

MAOIs have weak anticholinergic activity and do not have quinidinelike effects. Their principal side effect, orthostatic hypotension, emerges more slowly than with TCAs but is more profound (Kronig et al. 1983). Pedal edema, presumably due to the vasodilating property of these agents, can complicate treatment; whether this adverse reaction is more common in elderly patients than young adults is not clear.

Other Antidepressants

Some more recently available polycyclic antidepressants are potentially useful alternatives to TCAs or MAOIs in the elderly. All have the limitation of less clinical experience. They may also be effective in fewer patients than are TCAs and MAOIs, because of a narrower spectrum of pharmacologic actions. They include trazodone, fluoxetine, and buproprion. Specific data about the use of these agents in the elderly are still sparse because of limited clinical experience. Some studies of efficacy and toxicity of the newer antidepressants in the elderly have involved comparisons with tertiary amine TCAs. In an early outpatient study involving trazodone (Gerner et al. 1980), the response rates for both trazodone and imipramine versus placebo were low, presumably because of the high dropout rate at the doses used. Comparisons of new compounds with placebo and with secondary amine TCAs in the elderly are awaited.

The sedating property of trazodone can be useful if it is prescribed at bedtime and the dosage is gradually increased to prevent oversedation. Although trazodone lacks anticholinergic toxicity and quinidinelike effects, it does have alpha-adrenergic blocking effects. Orthostatic hypotension, premature ventricular contractions, and priapism have been associated with use of trazodone.

Fluoxetine is a relatively selective serotonin reuptake inhibitor. Its main active metabolite, norfluoxitine, has a long half-life (1–2 weeks). Metabolism of fluoxetine or norfluoxitine appears to be unaffected by aging (Lemberger et al. 1985). The drug has low propensity for cardiovascular and anticholinergic side effects, but fluoxetine can increase anxiety, motor restlessness, and insomnia. There is a potentionally lethal interaction between fluoxetine and MAOIs. Administration of fluoxetine to potentiate the antidepressant effects of TCAs has been reported (Weilburg et al. 1989). The clinician using this approach must be aware that fluoxetine can markedly increase TCA levels (Aranow et al. 1989).

Bupropion has an unusual pharmacologic profile. As with fluoxetine, h.s. dosing should be avoided to minimize disruption of sleep. The spectrum of side effects is narrower than for TCAs. The association of seizures with bupropion should be considered. Although age does not appear to increase the occurrence of seizures in patients treated with bupropion, a history of prior seizure does (Davidson 1989). Both fluoxetine and bupropion offer the advantages of diminished anticholinergic and cardiovascular side effects; their disadvantage is that they have been only recently marketed and less is known about their efficacy and their drug-disease and dose-response relationships in elderly depressive patients.

Stimulants

Stimulants (dextroamphetamine, methylphenidate, pemoline) have reportedly been helpful in some elderly patients with "apathy" or depressive syndromes (Chiarello and Cole 1987). Systematic literature on efficacy is extremely limited. A recent review of controlled studies using stimulants (Satel and Nelson 1989) concluded that most studies in patients with primary depression do not demonstrate greater efficacy with stimulant treatment than with placebo. The use of stimulants in patients with organic brain disease or physical illness has special relevance to geriatric psychiatry. Although increased energy and improved mood have been noted in both populations, emergent agitation and cognitive deterioration may limit treatment in patients with organic brain disease. Activation can lead to prompt behavioral improvement in physically ill patients, but this improvement is not equivalent to the reversal of depression (Satel and Nelson 1989). Controlled studies in the cognitively and medically impaired are required to clarify the appropriate indications for stimulant treatment in older patients.

Lithium Salts

Despite clinical lore that the therapeutic effects of lithium occur in geriatric patients at plasma lithium levels below those needed for younger patients, lower need has not been empirically demonstrated. However, elderly patients are more likely to develop a fine tremor (Murray et al. 1983) or even myoclonus at "therapeutic" levels; the altered pharmacodynamic sensitivity to neurologic side effects, combined with the decreased renal clearance of lithium that is associated with aging, is consistent with beginning at low doses in the range of 150 mg to 600 mg per day and making increments slowly while monitoring plasma levels. Anecdotally, levels of 0.3 to 0.6 meq. have been clinically effective. The dose necessary to achieve a targeted blood level is usually one-half to two-thirds of that required in younger adults (Hardy et al. 1987).

The half-life for lithium approximates 24 hours in patients aged older than 70 without renal disease (Chapron et al. 1982; Hardy et al. 1987). The plasma level obtained 5 days after a patient has started a specific dose of lithium does not change significantly unless medical illness or use of medications that influence lithium excretion supervene (see Tables 22-2 and 22-3).

Salt depletion, caused by vomiting and diarrhea or a low-sodium diet, increases renal reabsorption of lithium and can raise plasma levels (Jefferson and Griest 1979). The presence of renal disease does not preclude use of lithium; despite persistent controversy, there is no clear evidence that lithium causes or accelerates the course of renal failure (Meyers 1989).

The potential for concurrent use of agents that diminish lithium clearance is of special concern. Thiazide diuretics block reabsorption of sodium in the proximal loop, leading to increased distal reabsorption of both sodium and lithium and an increase in lithium plasma levels by 33% or more. Potassium-sparing diuretics may have a similar, although less profound, effect. Furosemide, which acts distally, is not associated with significant accumulation of lithium (see review by Jefferson and Griest 1979).

Nonsteroidal anti-inflammatory medications are used commonly by the elderly. Some of these agents diminish renal clearance of lithium by nearly 50% (Jefferson et al. 1981). Availability of OTC forms of these agents (e.g., ibuprofen) makes it incumbent on the psychiatrist to instruct elderly patients not to begin a new medication without prior discussion.

In young adult manic patients treated with lithium, features such as masked severity, dysphoric mood, negative family history, and high frequency of episodes have been associated with diminished lithium responsiveness; comparable studies have not been completed with geriatric patients. Although preliminary findings in predominantly young patients suggest that increased age may be associated with some attenuation of treatment response (Young et al. 1989), lithium continues to be the first-line treatment of mania in the elderly.

Shulman and Post's study (1980) of elderly patients with mania showed more than 40% had late-onset bipolar illness, and many of these cases had coarse brain pathology. Of the late-onset cases, 24% had overt brain disease. Lithium was well tolerated and effective, but doses and levels were not reported. Himmelhoch and associates (1980) found that neurologic status (including extrapyramidal syndromes and dementia, but not age) was associated with delayed and/or poor treatment response, including lithium-induced neurotoxicity; lithium levels were not specified. Black et al. (1988) reported that "complicated" manias (i.e., those with coexisting nonaffective psychiatric illness or with serious medical illness) had poorer immediate response to lithium treatment. Shukla and colleagues (1987) also reported that in nongeriatric patients, "secondary manias" had a relatively poor acute response.

In summary, lithium is an effective treatment for episodes of primary mania in elderly patients. Lithium may be less effective in patients with mania occurring in the context of neurologic, medical, or other psychiatric disorder, perhaps partly because these patients have an increased sensitivity to neurotoxic reactions.

Patients with bipolar disorder who have a depressive syndrome respond to antidepressant treatment. If patients are taking lithium carbonate or other mood stabilizer, the adequacy of this treatment needs to be documented with plasma levels, and dose adjusted if necessary. If symptoms persist, the usual clinical approach is continuation of the mood-stabilizing drug and addition of an antidepressant.

Acute lithium toxicity includes tremor, ataxia, gastrointestinal distress, cognitive impairment, and severe polyuria. Roose and associates (1979) reported more instances of toxicity in elderly bipolar outpatients compared with younger patients in a maintenance treatment program, including development of the specific adverse reaction of a sick sinus syndrome—presumably through the interaction of lithium and a sinus node previously damaged by coronary artery disease; two of the reported cases had lithium levels within the therapeutic range. The identification of sinus node dysfunction on a baseline EKG can be considered a relative contraindication to the use of lithium. Although elderly patients are more likely to develop fine tremor at "therapeutic" levels of lithium, the occurrence of polyuria and polydipsia apparently does not increase with age (Murray et al. 1983).

Concern over long-term adverse reactions to lithium involves impact on renal and thyroid function. Despite some persistence of controversy, damage to glomerular function from prolonged lithium use has not been established after more than 40 years of use, including more than 18 years in the United States (Meyers 1989). Conservative management, however, indicates twice-yearly monitoring of renal function. Diminished renal function does not preclude the use of lithium, but careful consideration must be given to the benefit of continued use versus the possibility that lithium has contributed to the renal pathology in these patients. Similarly, thyroid function should be assessed twice yearly, particularly if there is a change in the course of affective illness or physical health. If TSH increases, the increase can be managed with thyroid hormone. Although potentiation of TCAs or MAOIs with lithium has not been specifically studied in elderly depressives, lithium augmentation should be considered in poor responders.

Carbamazepine, clonezapam,or valproic acid can be used as alternatives to lithium in elderly patients who do not tolerate or respond to lithium salts. There is, however, no systematic information available concerning their use in the elderly. Effective lithium augmentation of fluoxetine has been reported (Pope et al. 1988).

Continuation and Maintenance Treatment

Although patients do occasionally fail to respond to an antidepressant that was effective previously, there is no body of evidence that "tolerance" to therapeutic effects develops after prolonged use. Most patients fail to respond because they have not been treated adequately (Lydiard 1985). The possibility that an undiagnosed medical condition is presenting as a clinical depression must be reconsidered. Lack of response to adequate blood levels for 4 to 6 weeks can be classified as treatment resistance. Reviews of approaches used to overcome this clinical impasse in young adult (Extein 1989) and elderly depressives (Goff and Jenike 1986) are available.

Continuation treatment is designed to prevent relapse of the index episode during the first 6 months of therapy; maintenance treatment is use of medication longer than 6 months to prevent the occurrence of new episodes. Georgotas and colleagues (1988) prospectively treated recovered elderly major depressives for 4 to 8 months with nortriptyline at an average dose of 80 mg per day or phenelzine at 54 mg per day. Only 17% of the patients completing nortriptyline continuation and 24% of those completing phenelzine suffered relapses. Patients in a subgroup were randomly assigned to nortriptyline, phenelzine, or placebo as maintenance treatment for another year. During the second year, phenelzine continued to demonstrate a strong prophylactic effect, but this time compared with both nortriptyline and placebo; more than half the patients who received the latter treatments relapsed.

The efficacy of lithium for prophylaxis has received little study in elderly bipolar patients. Abou-Saleh and Coppen (1983) noted no difference in affective morbidity over an average of 5 years in elderly versus younger patients maintained on comparable lithium levels. In a prospective study, Murray and associates (1983) reported greater manic psychopathology, although no more frequent hospitalizations, among the older patients from a mixed-age sample. Both studies used maintenance levels between 0.6 and 1.0

meq/L. These results are consistent with the conclusions that bipolar illness does not "burn out" and that lithium prophylaxis continues to play a crucial role as these patients age.

Although lithium carbonate has demonstrated efficacy in preventing recurrence of unipolar illness in young adults, the use of lithium to prevent recurrence in elderly unipolar depressives has not been studied specifically.

Neuroleptics

The occurrence of behavioral disturbance and psychotic symptoms in patients suffering from dementia is receiving increasing attention. Caregivers seeking professional assistance to cope with dementia patients residing in the community report that approximately 70% of these patients demonstrate disturbed behavior and nearly 50% have psychotic symptoms (Rabins et al. 1982). Furthermore, the number and type of behavior problems have been correlated with the severity of the dementia (Teri et al. 1988); 18% of mildly impaired Alzheimer's patients reported no behavior problems compared with only 4% of patients with severe cognitive dysfunction (Mini-Mental State Exam score of less than 10); 38% of patients with severe dementia had agitation, compared with 10% with mild impairment; the corresponding rates for the presence of hallucinations were 30% and 10%, respectively. This issue has special public health relevance because persistently unmanageable and disruptive behavior is the principal reason reported by caregivers for seeking institutionalization (Ferris et al. 1985). Cohen-Mansfield (1986) applied a 13-item agitated-behavior scale to nursing home residents and found that 73% of individuals assessed demonstrated a minimum of one agitated behavior at a frequency of several times a day; 56% of these individuals were receiving neuroleptics.

Three reviews have addressed the efficacy of neuroleptic treatment for behavior disturbances (e.g., agitation, assaultiveness, and wandering) and for psychotic symptoms in patients with dementia (Raskind et al. 1987; Sunderland and Silver 1988; Wragg and Jeste 1988). They pointed to the dearth of controlled studies and suggested the following conclusions: 1) neuroleptics are superior to placebo in controlling agitation and psychosis in patients with dementia; 2) the efficacy of neuroleptics appear to be proportional to the degree of disturbance; 3) there is no evidence for the superiority of one neuroleptic or class of agents over another; 4) neuroleptics improve behavioral symptoms but do not abolish them; and 5) amelioration of behavioral and psychotic symptoms has an uncertain relationship to improvement in cognitive functioning.

The latter issue is especially important because on theoretical grounds patients with Alzheimer's disease should be highly sensitive to the anticholinergic properties of low-potency neuroleptics (Raskind et al. 1987; Sunderland and Silver 1988). Two studies reported contradictory findings regarding the impact of neuroleptics on cognitive functioning. One noted improved cognitive functioning in a mixed sample with Alzheimer's and multi-infarct dementia receiving loxapine or thioridazine versus placebo (Barnes et al. 1982). The other (Devenand et al. 1989) found that higher doses of haloperidol (nearly 5 mg versus about 1 mg) increased improvement in behavior but worsened cognitive performance. Thus, unanswered questions remain.

In late-life paranoid disorders, neuroleptic treatment has proven more effective than placebo or no treatment (Post 1966) in open trials. Raskind and colleagues (1979) noted that depot fluphenazine was more effective than oral haloperidol in the ongoing outpatient management of elderly patients with schizophrenia; however, blood levels were not determined and noncompliance could have contributed to these results.

Studies of dose-response relationships using neuroleptics to treat behavioral dyscontrol due to dementia or chronic paranoid states are lacking. There are also no studies of the relationships among efficacy, toxicity, and plasma concentrations of neuroleptics in the elderly.

Neuroleptics can be placed on a continuum with low-potency drugs (e.g., thioridazine and chlorpromazine) on one end and high-potency agents (e.g., fluphenazine and haloperidol) on the other. Low-potency agents possess greater anticholinergic, alpha-1-adrenergic antagonism, and antihistaminic activities (Richelson 1982): these agents have a greater potential for causing sedation, confusion, and orthostatic hypotension. The high-potency agents have greater dopamine 2 receptor blocking action and produce more extrapyramidal side effects; whether these drugs increase the risk of tardive dyskinesia or neuroleptic malignant syndrome remains to be studied. Elderly patients receiving neuroleptics are at increased risk for falls and related morbidity (Ray et al. 1987); low-potency agents may contribute to falls by increasing confusion and cardiovascular instability, whereas high-potency agents may cause falls through drug-induced parkinsonism. Selecting a particular neuroleptic must be recognized as choosing a particular set of side effects.

The neuroleptic malignant syndrome (involving extrapyramidal symptoms, delirium, hyperpyrexia, and autonomic dysfunction) can also occur in the elderly. A literature search completed in 1987 identified 18 reported patients aged over 65 (Addonizio 1987). Although the relative vulnerability of elderly patients to this life-threatening reaction to neuroleptics is not known, the possibilities that age masks the phenomenology of the syndrome and that dementia confounds diagnosis (Wragg and Jeste 1988) must be recognized.

Although controversy persists (Moleman et al. 1986), the predominance of evidence indicates that elderly patients, particularly those with dementia (Peabody et al. 1987), have an increased vulnerability to developing extrapyramidal reactions to neuroleptic treatment; more than 50% of geriatric patients who receive these agents have parkinsonian side effects (Ayd 1976; Salzman 1984). These side effects could result from degeneration of nigrostriatal pathways associated with aging (Meyers and Kalayam 1989), higher plasma levels per dose of neuroleptics, or a longer duration of drug exposure (Wragg and Jeste 1988).

The pattern of extrapyramidal side effects of neuroleptics appears to change as a function of increased age. Acute dystonic reactions, commonly seen in young men, are very rare; conversely, resting tremor, cogwheeling rigidity, and bradykinesia are more common than in young patients (Salzman et al. 1970).

Akathisia occurs across a broad range of ages. The behavioral manifestations of this adverse reaction are thought to result from an internal sense of restlessness (Crane and Naranjo 1971). The diminished ability of demented patients to vocalize their sensations could lead to underdiagnosis in this population (Wragg and Jeste 1988). An unfortunate cycle in which motor restlessness leads to increasing doses of neuroleptic, which cause worsening of akathisia, can ensue. Alternatively, considering "agitated behavior" as a possible expression of akathisia and attempting to decrease the dose of neuroleptic reverses this form of iatrogenic suffering in some patients.

Jeste and Wyatt's (1987) summary on tardive dyskinesia and aging concluded that 40% of elderly inpatients with histories of prolonged treatment with neuroleptics suffer from this syndrome. They summarized the literature as indicating that the elderly have a stronger predominance of orofacial over limb dyskinesia than younger patients, that tardive dyskinesia tends to be more severe with increasing age, and that increased intensity and/or duration of neuroleptic exposure, including altered pharmacokinetics, does not explain the greater vulnerability of elderly patients to this syndrome. Elderly patients with dementia may be at even greater risk (Wragg and Jeste 1988). Finally, fewer than 50% of elderly patients with tardive dyskinesia recover after discontinuation of neuroleptics versus 80% of young adults (Smith and Baldessarini 1980). The differential diagnosis of tardive dyskinesia must include the rare and mild spontaneous dyskinesia that can accompany aging and the oral dyskinesic movements caused simply by loose-fitting dentures (Jeste and Wyatt 1987).

Antianxiety Agents and Sedative-Hypnotics

The acute efficacy of antianxiety agents has received limited investigation in the elderly. Greater efficacy compared to placebo in reducing anxiety and insomnia has been reported for oxazepam (Koepke et al. 1982) and alprazolam (Cohn 1984).

Benzodiazepines have a limited place in the management of demented patients. In such patients, diazepam has been found more calming than thioridazine, but thioridazine was associated with greater improvement of behavioral disturbance (Kirven and Montero 1973). Lorazepam has also been found effective in reducing agitation, wandering, and restlessness in demented patients (Sizaret et al. 1974). These studies do not distinguish sedation from an anxiolytic action of benzodiazepines. Although anxiety can be a concomitant of dementia, demented patients may be agitated but not appear anxious. Benzodiazepines may increase the cognitive impairment of demented patients and precipitate falls.

The indications for benzodiazepine use in elderly patients without dementia are analogous to those in younger adults. They include generalized anxiety, panic disorder, and short-term use in the treatment of disturbed sleep. The association of anxiety with depression after middle age deserves special attention. Nearly one-third of older depressed patients continue to have morning anxiety more than a year after discharge from hospital treatment; two-thirds of these have symptoms of anxiety at other times (Blazer et al. 1989). Many of these patients may use anxiolytic agents despite uncertain benefits and potential risks of long-term use.

Toxic doses of anxiolytics can produce sedation, ataxia, and impaired cognitive performance. Even "therapeutic" doses of benzodiazepines can decrease memory consolidation in this population (Jenike 1985a; Pomara et al. 1984; Rickels et al. 1987). "Paradoxical" reactions to benzodiazepines can also occur (Pomara et al. 1984); these involve increased irritability, agitation, and loss of behavioral control. The triazolobenzodiazepines may have greater potential for producing this disinhibition, which if present generally occurs during the first week of treatment. Whether age influences the vulnerability to such reactions is not known.

Tolerance to the effects of benzodiazepines can occur. Furthermore, dependence can become a problem with long-term use.

As described previously, pharmacokinetic and pharmacodynamic concomitants of aging make older patients especially vulnerable to adverse reactions. The twofold to threefold increase in half-life of long-acting agents with active metabolites (diazepam, chlordiazepoxide, flurazepam) over short-acting compounds (lorazepam, oxazepam, temazepam, triazolam) in elderly patients versus young adults (Greenblatt et al. 1982; Salzman et al. 1983) argues for the use of the latter group of medications in the elderly.

Also there are apparent pharmacodynamic differences among benzodiazepines. For example, the very short half-life of triazolam must be weighed against the drug's propensity for causing anterograde amnesia (Scharf et al. 1988). This effect could lead to confusional syndromes in elderly patients. Also, very short half-life is associated with high peak levels.

In summary, benzodiazepines have a legitimate role in the therapeutic arsenal of geriatric psychiatrists. The indications appear to be narrow, and the dangers of dependence and toxicity are of sufficient concern that therapeutic trials should be undertaken with careful monitoring on a time-limited basis.

References

Abou-Saleh MT, Coppen A: The prognosis of depression in old age: the case for lithium therapy. Br J Psychiatry 143:527–528, 1983

Addonizio G: Neuroleptic malignant syndrome in elderly patients. Journal American Geriatrics Society 35:1011–1012, 1987

Addonizio G: The patient with Parkinson's disease, in Treatments of Psychiatric Disorders: A Task Force Report of the American Psychiatric Association, Vol 2. Edited by Karasu TB. Washington, DC, American Psychiatric Association, 1989, pp 860–867

Alexopoulos GS, Abrams RC, Young RC, et al: Cornell scale for depression in dementia. Biol Psychiatry 23:271–284, 1988

Alexopoulos GS, Young RC, Abrams RC, et al: Chronicity and relapse in geriatric depression. Biol Psychiatry 26:551–564, 1989

Aranow RB, Hudson JI, Pope HG, et al: Elevated antidepressant plasma levels after addition of fluoxetine. Am J Psychiatry 146:911–913, 1989

Ayd FJ: A survey of drug-induced extrapyramidal reactions. JAMA 175:1045–1060, 1976

Barnes R, Veith R, Okimoto J, et al: Efficacy of antipsychotic medications in behaviorally disturbed dementia patients. Am J Psychiatry 139:1170–1174, 1982

Bickford-Wimer PC, Parfitt K, Hoffer BJ, et al: Desipramine and noradrenergic neurotransmission in aging: Failure to respond in aged laboratory animals Neuropsychopharmacology 26:597–605, 1987

Black SW, Winokur D, Nasrallah A, et al: Complicated mania: comorbidity and immediate outcome in the treatment of mania. Arch Gen Psychiatry 45:232–236, 1988

Blazer DG, Bachar JR, Manton KG: Suicide in late life. J Am Geriatr Soc 34:519–525, 1986

Blazer DG, Hughes DC, Fowler N: Anxiety as an outcome symptom of depression in elderly and middle-aged adults. International Journal of Geriatric Psychiatry 4:273–278, 1989

Chapron DJ, Cameron IR, White LB, et al: Observations on lithium disposition in the elderly. J Am Geriatr Soc 30:651–655, 1982

Chiarello RJ, Cole JO: The use of psychostimulants in general psychiatry. Arch Gen Psychiatry 44:296–295, 1987

Cohen-Mansfield J: Agitated behaviors in the elderly, II: preliminary results in the cognitively deteriorated. J Am Geriatr Soc 34:722–727, 1986

Cohn JB: Double-blind safety and efficacy comparison of alprazolam and placebo in the treatment of anxiety in geriatric patients. Curr Ther Res 35:100–112, 1984

Crane GE, Naranjo ER: Motor disturbances induced by neuroleptics. Arch Gen Psychiatry 24:179–184, 1971

Davidson J: Seizures and bupropion: a review. J Clin Psychiatry 50:256–261, 1989

Devanand D, Sakheim HA, Brown RP, Mayeuy R, et al: A pilot study of haloperidol treatment of psychosis and behavioral disturbance in Alzheimer's disease. Arch Neurol 46:854–857, 1989

Ferris SH, Steinberg G, Shulman E, et al: Institutionalization of Alzheimer's patients: reducing precipitating factors through family counseling. Arch Found Thanatol 12:7, 1985

Figiel GS, Krishnan KRR, Breitner JC, et al: Radiologic correlates of antidepressant-induced delirium: the possible significance of basal-ganglia lesions. Journal of Neuropsychiatry and Clinical Neurosciences 1:188–190, 1989

Folstein MF, Folstein SE, McHugh PR: Mini-Mental State: a practical method for grading the cognitive state of patients for the clinician. J Psychiatr Res 12:189–198, 1975

Friedman JR, Norman DC, Yoshikawa TT: Correlation of estimated renal function parameters versus 24-hour creatinine clearance in ambulatory elderly. J Am Geriatr Soc 37:145–149, 1989

Georgotas A, McCue RE, Hapworth W, et al: Comparative efficacy and safety of MAOIs versus TCAs in treating depression in the elderly. Biol Psychiatry 21:1155–1166, 1986

Georgotas A, McCue RE, Cooper TB, et al: How effective and safe is continuation therapy in elderly depressed patients? Arch Gen Psychiatry 45:929–932, 1988

Gerner R, Estabrook W, Steuer J, et al: Treatment of geriatric depression with trazodone, imipramine, and placebo: a double-blind study. J Clin Psychiatry 41:216–220, 1980

Glassman AH, Bigger JT Jr: Cardiovascular effects of therapeutic doses of the tricyclic antidepressants: a review. Arch Gen Psychiatry 38:815–820, 1981

Glassman AH, Bigger JT Jr, Giardina EV, et al: Clinical characteristics of imipramine-induced orthostatic hypotension. Lancet 1:468–472, 1979

Goff DC, Jenike MA: Treatment-resistant depression in the elderly. Journal American Geriatrics Society 34:63–70, 1986

Greenblatt DJ, Shader RJ: Benzodiazepine kinetics in the elderly, in Clinical Pharmacology in Psychiatry. Edited by Usdin E. New York, Elsevier, 1981, pp 174–181

Greenblatt DJ, Sellers EM, Shader RI: Drug disposition in old age. N Engl J Med 306:1081–1088, 1982

Hamilton M: A rating scale for depression. J Neurol Neurosurg Psychiatry 23:56–62, 1960

Hardy BG, Shulman KI, Mackenzie SE, et al: Pharmacokinetics of lithium in the elderly. J Clin Psychopharmacol 7:153–158, 1987

Himmelhoch JM, Neil JF, May SJ, et al: Age, dementia, dyskinesias and lithium response. Am J Psychiatry 137:941–944, 1980

Hollister LE: General principles of treating the elderly with drugs, in Clinical Pharmacology and the Aged Patient. Edited by Jarvik L, Greenblatt DJ, and Harman D. New York, Raven, 1981, pp 1–9

Israili ZH, Wenger J: Aging, gastrointestinal disease, and response to drugs, in Clinical Pharmacology and the Aged Patient. Edited by Jarvik L, Greenblatt DJ, and Harman D. New York, Raven, 1981, pp 131–155

Jarvik LF, Mintz J: Treatment of Depression in Old Age: What Works? in Disturbed Behavior in the Elderly. Edited by Awad AG, Durost H, Mayer HMR, and McCormick WO. New York, Pergamon Press, 1987, pp 51–57

Jefferson JW, Griest JH: Lithium and the kidney, in Psychopharmacology Update. Edited by David JM, Greenblatt D. New York, Grune & Stratton, 1979, pp 81–104

Jefferson JW, Greist JH, Baudhuin M: Lithium: interactions with other drugs. J Clin Psychopharmacol 1:124–131, 1981

Jenike MA: Handbook of Geriatric Psychopharmacology. Littleton, MA, PSG Publishing, 1985a

Jenike MA: Monoamine oxidase inhibitors as treatment for depressed patients with primary degenerative dementia (Alzheimer's disease). Am J Psychiatry 142:763–764, 1985b

Jeste DV, Wyatt RJ: Aging and tardive dyskinesia, in Schizophrenia and Aging. Edited by Miller NE, Cohen GD. New York, Guilford, 1987

Kay DWK: Outcome and cause of death in mental disorders of old age: a long-term follow-up of functional and organic psychoses. Acta Psychiatr Scand 38:149–276, 1962

Kirven LE, Montero EF: Comparison of thioridazine and diazepam in the control of nonpsychotic symptoms associated with senility: double-blind control study. J Am Geriatr Soc 21:545–551, 1973

Koepke HH, Gold RL, Linden ME, et al: Multicenter controlled study of oxazepam in anxious elderly patients. Psychosomatics 23:641–645, 1982

Kronig MH, Roose SP, Walsh BP, et al: Blood pressure effects of phenelzine. J Clin Psychopharmacol 3:307–310, 1983

Lemberger L, Bergstron RF, Wolen RL, et al: Fluoxetine: clinical pharmacology and psychologic disposition. J Clin Psychiatry 46(3, sec 2):14–19, 1985

Lingam VR, Lazarus LW, Groves L, et al: Methylphenidate in treating poststroke depression. J Clin Psychiatry 49:4,151–153, 1988

Lipsey JR, Robinson RG, Pearlson GD: Nortriptyline treatment of poststroke depression: a double-blind study. Lancet 1:297–300, 1984

Lydiard BR: Tricyclic-resistant depression: treatment resistance or inadequate treatment? J Clin Psychiatry 46:412–417, 1985

Mattis S: Dementia Rating Scale. Odessa, FL, Psychological Assessment Resource, 1988

McCabe B, Tsuang MT: Dietary consideration in MAO inhibitor regimens. J Clin Psychiatry 43:178–181, 1982

Meyers B: The patient with renal disease, in Treatments of Psychiatric Disorders: A Task Force Report of the American Psychiatric Association, Vol 2. Edited by Karasu TB. Washington, DC, American Psychiatric Association, 1989, pp 915–930

Meyers B, Kalayam B: Update in geriatric psychopharmacology, in Advances in Psychosomatic Medicine, Vol 19. Basel, Karger, 1989, pp 114–137

Meyers B, Young RC: Dementia of the Alzheimer type, in Treatments of Psychiatric Disorders: A Task Force Report of the American Psychiatric Association, Vol 2. Edited by Karasu TB. Washington, DC, American Psychiatric Association, 1989, pp 965–979

Moleman P, Janzen G, von Bargen BA, et al: Relationship between age and incidence of parkinsonism in psychiatric patients treated with haloperidol. Am J Psychiatry 143:232–234, 1986

Murray N, Hopwood S, Balfour JK, et al: The influence of age on lithium efficacy and side-effects in out-patients. Psychol Med 13:53–60, 1983

Nelson JC, Bowers MB: Delusional unipolar depression. Arch Gen Psychiatry 35:1321–1328, 1978

Nelson JC, Jatlow P, Mazure C: Desipramine plasma levels and response in elderly melancholic patients. J Clin Psychopharmacol 5:217–220, 1985

Nies A, Robinson DS, Friedman MJ, et al: Relationship between age and tricyclic antidepressant levels. Am J Psychiatry 134:790–793, 1977

Peabody CA, Warner D, Whiteford HA, et al: Neuroleptics and the elderly. J Am Geriatr Soc 35:233–238, 1987

Perry PJ, Morgan DE, Smith RE, et al: Treatment of unipolar depression accompanied by delusions. J Affective Disord 4:195–200, 1982

Pomara N, Stanley B, Block R, et al: Adverse effects of single therapeutic doses of diazepam on performance in normal geriatric subjects: relationship to plasma concentrations. Psychopharmacology 84:342–346, 1984

Pope HG, McElroy SL, Nixon RA: Possible synergism between fluoxetine and lithium in refractory depression. Am J Psychiatry 145:1292–1294, 1988

Post F: Persistent Persecutory States of the Elderly. Oxford, Pergamon Press, 1966

Post F. The management and nature of depressive illnesses in late life. Br J Psychiatry 121:393–404, 1972

Price LH: Lithium augmentation in tricyclic-resistant depression, in Treatment of Tricyclic-Resistant Depression. Edited by Extein I. Washington, DC, American Psychiatric Press, 1989, pp 51–79

Rabins PV, Mace NL, Lucas MJ: The impact of dementia on the family. JAMA 248:333–335, 1982

Raskind MA, Risse SC, Lampe TH: Dementia and antipsychotic drugs. J Clin Psychiatry 485, suppl:16–18, 1987

Raskind MN, Alvarez C, Herlin S: Fluphenazine enanthate in the outpatient treatment of late paraphrenia. J Am Geriatr Soc 27:459–469, 1979

Ray WA, Griffin MR, Schaffner W, et al: Psychotropic drug use and the risk of hip fracture. N Engl J Med 316:363–369, 1987

Reidenberg MM, Levy M, Warner H, et al: Relationship between diazepam dose, plasma level, age, and central nervous system depression. Clin Pharmacol Ther 23:371–374, 1978

Reifler BV, Larson E, Hanley R: Coexistence of cognitive impairment and depression in geriatric outpatients. Am J Psychiatry 139:623–626, 1982

Reifler BV, Teri L, Raskind M, et al: Double-blind trial of imipramine in Alzheimer's disease in patients with and without depression. Am J Psychiatry 146:45–49, 1989

Richelson E: Pharmacology of antidepressants in use in the United States. J Clin Psychiatry 43:4–13, 1982

Rickels K, Schweizer E, Lucki I: Benzodiazepine side effects, in Psychiatry Update: American Psychiatric Association Annual Review, Vol 6. Washington, DC, American Psychiatric Press, 1987, pp 781–801

Robinson DS: Monoamine oxidase inhibitors and the elderly, in Age and the Pharmacology of Psychoactive Drugs. Edited by Raskin A, Robinson DS, Levine J. New York, Elsevier, 1981, pp 149–161

Robinson RG, Price TR: Post-stroke depressive disorders: a follow up study of 103 patients. Stroke 13:635–641, 1982

Rockwell E, Lam RW, Zisook S: Antidepressant drug studies in the elderly. Psychiatr Clin North Am 11:215–233, 1988

Rolandi E, Magnani G, Sannia A, et al: Evaluation of Prl secretion in elderly subjects. Acta Endocrinol 42:148–151, 1982

Roose SP, Nurnberger J, Dunner D, et al: Cardiac sinus node dysfunction during lithium treatment. Am J Psychiatry 136:804–806, 1979a

Roose SP, Bone S, Haidorfer C, et al: Lithium treatment in older patients. Am J Psychiatry 136:843–844, 1979b

Roose SP, Glassman AH, Siris SG, et al: Comparison of imipramine and nortriptyline-induced orthostatic hypotension: a meaningful difference. J Clin Psychopharmacol 1:316–319, 1981

Roose SP, Glassman AH, Giardina EGV, et al: Tricyclic antidepressants in patients with cardiac conduction disease. Arch Gen Psychiatry 44:273–275, 1987

Rowe JW: Aging and renal function. Ann Rev Gerontol Geriatr 1:161–179, 1980

Salzman C: Clinical Geriatric Psychopharmacology. New York, McGraw-Hill, 1984

Salzman C, Shader RI, Pearlman M: Psychopharmacology and the elderly, in Psychotropic Drug Side Effects. Edited by Shader RI, DiMascio A. Baltimore, MD, Williams & Wilkins, 1970

Salzman C, Shader RI, Greenblatt DJ, et al: Long versus half-life benzodiazepines in the elderly: kinetics and clinical effects of diazepam and oxazepam. Arch Gen Psychiatry 40:293–297, 1983

Satel SL, Nelson JC: Stimulants in the treatment of depression: a critical overview. J Clin Psychiatry 50:241–249, 1989

Sawin CT, Castelli WP, Hershman JM, et al: The thyroid: thyroid deficiency in the Framingham study. Arch Intern Med 145:1386–1388, 1985

Scharf MB, Fletcher K, Graham JP: Comparative amnestic effects of benzodiazepine hypnotic agents. J Clin Psychiatry 49:4, 1988

Schatzberg AF, Cole JO: Manual of Clinical Psychopharmacology. Washington, DC, American Psychiatric Press, 1986, pp 249–251

Shamoian CA: Somatic therapies in geriatric psychiatry, in Essentials of Geriatric Psychiatry. Edited by Lazarus LW. New York, Springer, 1988, pp 173–188

Shukla S, Hoff A, Aronson T, et al: Treatment outcome in organic mania. Paper presented at New Research Program, Annual Meeting, American Psychiatric Association, 1987

Shulman K, Post F: Bipolar affective disorders in old age. Br J Psychiatry 136:26–32, 1980

Shulman KI, Walker SE, MacKenzie S, et al: Dietary restrictions, tyramine, and the use of monoamine oxidase inhibitors. J Clin Psychopharmacol 9:397–402, 1989

Sizaret P, Versavel MC, Engel G, et al: Clinical investigation of lorazepam. Psychol Med 6:591–598, 1974

Spiker DG, Weiss JC, Dealy RS, et al: The pharmacological treatment of delusional depression. Am J Psychiatry 141:430–436, 1985

Sullivan EA, Shulman KI: Diet and monoamine oxidase inhibitors: a reexamination. Can J Psychiatry 29:707–711, 1984

Sunderland T, Silver MA: Neuroleptics in the treatment of dementia. International Journal Geriatric Psychiatry 3:79–88, 1988

Teri L, Larson EB, Reifler BV: Behavioral disturbances in dementia of the Alzheimer's type. JAGS 36:1–6, 1988

Vestal RE, Wood AJ, Shand DG: Reduced beta adrenergic receptor sensitivity in the elderly. Clin Pharmacol Ther 26:181–186, 1979

Weilburg JB, Rosembaum JF, Biederman J, et al: Fluoxetine added to non-MAOI antidepressants converts nonresponders to responders: a preliminary report. J Clin Psychiatry 50:447–449, 1989

Whittier JR: Psychotropic Drugs and Dysfunctions of the Basal Ganglia. Edited by Crane GE, Nardner RJ Jr. Washington, DC, United States Public Health, 1969, 26

Wragg RE, Jeste DV: Neuroleptics and alternative treatments: management of behavioral symptoms and psychosis in Alzheimer's disease and related conditions. Psychiatr Clin North Am 11:195–213, 1988

Yesavage JA, Brink TL, Rose TL, et al: The geriatric depression rating scale: comparison with other self-report and psychiatric rating scales, in Assessment in Geriatric Psychopharmacology. Edited by Crook T, Ferris S, Bartus R. New Canaan, CT, Mark Powley Associates, 1983, pp 153–165

Young RC: Multi-infarct dementia, in Treatments of Psychiatric Disorders: A Task Force Report of the American Psychiatric Association, Vol 2. Edited by Karasu TB. Washington, DC, American Psychiatric Association, 1989, pp 961–964

Young RC, Falk JR: Age, manic psychopathology and treatment response. International Journal Geriatric Psychiatry 4:73–78, 1989

Young RC, Alexopoulos GS, Shamoian CA, et al: Plasma 10-hydroxy-nortriptyline in elderly depressed patients. Clin Pharmacol Ther 35:540–544, 1984

Young RC, Alexopoulos GS, Shamoian CA, et al: Plasma 10-hydroxy-nortriptyline and ECG changes in elderly depressives. Am J Psychiatry 142:866–868, 1985

Zis AP, Goodwin FK: Major affective disorder as a recurrent illness: a critical review. Arch Gen Psychiatry 36:835–839, 1979

CHAPTER 23

Donald P. Hay, M.D.

Electroconvulsive Therapy

Overview

With more than half a century of use of electroconvulsive therapy (ECT) worldwide, and with many clinical and research studies completed, it is evident that ECT is a remarkably safe and effective treatment for several psychiatric illnesses, especially for depressive disorders (American Psychiatric Association 1978; Fink 1979; Palmer 1981; Abrams and Essman 1982; NIMH Consensus Conference 1985; Abrams 1988; American Psychiatric Association 1990). Lack of familiarity with information regarding ECT has allowed fear and apprehension to continue among many people regarding the treatment. However, inroads are being made in educating both the public and professionals regarding this often poorly understood procedure (Endler and Persad 1988; Hay and Hay 1989).

The frequency with which depression is encountered by psychiatrists, the increased vulnerability of older patients to side effects from pharmacotherapeutic agents, and the demonstrated safety and efficacy of ECT make this treatment especially suitable for use in the elderly (Avery and Winokur 1976; Fraser and Glass 1980; Yesavage 1980; Fraser 1981; Bidder 1981; Gaspar and Samarasinghe 1982; Salzman 1982; Weiner 1982; Karlinsky and Shulman 1983; Weiner 1983; Raskind 1983; Alexopoulos et al. 1984; Mielke et al. 1984; Burke et al. 1985; Meyers and Mei-tal 1985; Regestein and

The author expresses sincere appreciation to Barry Blackwell, M.D.; Barnett Meyers, M.D.; Richard Weiner, M.D., Ph.D.; Larry Lazarus, M.D.; and Joel Sadavoy, M.D., for helpful comments on the manuscript.

469

Reich 1985; Godber et al. 1987; Benbow 1987; Burke et al. 1987; Fogel 1988; Hay 1989; Alexopoulos et al. 1989).

The low risk of complications from ECT must be considered along with findings suggesting that depression itself can increase the mortality rate in elderly medical inpatients with severe physical illness (Koenig et al. 1989). Finally, it has been reported by some that elderly patients with major depressive illness respond to ECT as well as, or better than, younger individuals (Stromgren 1973; Hesche et al. 1978; Benbow 1987).

With the efficacy of ECT in the elderly having been well established, the primary concern becomes that of evaluating the relative safety of the procedure for older individuals. The increased number of medical problems as well as the pharmacotherapy for these coexistent illnesses does, in theory, place these older individuals at higher risk for side effects or complications from ECT. Nonetheless, ECT is frequently considered the safest procedure for this population, especially when careful attention is given to the patient's medical state (Bidder 1981; Alexopoulos et al. 1984, 1989; Regestein 1985; Weiner and Coffey 1988; Hay 1989; Huang et al. 1989).

Indications

The indications for ECT in the elderly are essentially the same as those for younger patients. The APA Task Force on ECT, in 1978, listed affective disorders and certain forms of schizophrenia (e.g., schizoaffective and catatonic schizophrenia) as two of the primary indications for ECT (APA 1978). Indications for use of ECT, which are currently being defined by the latest APA Task Force, include severe organic affective psychoses in addition to major depression and mania. This task force reports that the efficacy of ECT does not diminish with advancing age, and that ECT may be generally less risky than pharmacotherapy in this group. Major depressive disorder is by far the illness most frequently treated with ECT in the elderly population.

The efficacy of ECT in the treatment of major depressive disorder has been studied extensively, with comparison trials of ECT versus tricyclics, versus monoamine oxidase inhibitors (MAOIs), versus sham ECT, and in patients in whom antidepressant medications were ineffective. The APA Task Force on Treatments in Psychiatry summarized the literature and found that ECT is as effective for depression as, if not more effective than, all other treatment modalities (Welch 1989).

The syndrome of "depressive pseudodementia" with symptoms of disorientation and impaired cognition is often misdiagnosed as senile dementia. Such individuals may respond well to a course of ECT and frequently tolerate this treatment better than antidepressant medications (Abrams 1988).

The clinical features predicting good outcome for ECT in the depressed elderly include mood disorder, guilt, psychomotor retardation, and coexistent symptoms of agitation and anxiety (Fraser and Glass 1980; Fraser 1981). Other indications for ECT in the depressed elderly include nonresponsiveness to psychotropic medication, serious suicidal risk, refusal to eat or drink resulting in malnutrition, dehydration, insomnia, history of better response to ECT than to other treatment, and the presence of delusions. A long duration of depressive illness correlates with a poorer outcome of both ECT and pharmacotherapy (Gaspar and Samarasinghe 1982; Salzman 1982; Karlinsky and Shulman 1983; Zorumski et al. 1988). A less favorable response has also been noted in depressed individuals with other preexisting psychiatric syndromes, especially if the preexisting condition is dementia or somatization disorder (Zorumski et al. 1988).

The issue of whether ECT would be safer or more effective as the first choice of treatment for depression has been reviewed, but not answered. For patients with delusional depressions, tricyclics alone have been found to be effective less than half the time, and although tricyclic-neuroleptic combinations can approach the efficacy of ECT in young adults (Spiker et al. 1986), these combinations are riskier and less well tolerated by the elderly because of their greater vulnerability to orthostatic hypotension, tardive dyskinesia, drug-induced parkinsonism, and other side effects. Therefore, ECT can be considered a first choice for the delusionally depressed older patient (Fogel 1988; Welch 1989).

Similarly, nondelusional depression with somatic preoccupation and profound agitation may respond better and more rapidly to ECT than to antidepressants. Other psychiatric disorders in the elderly that may benefit from ECT include depression with vegetative signs but without the cognitive verbal expression of dysphoria, such as may occur in Alzheimer's disease or poststroke disorders (Fogel 1988). Agitated depressed patients with moderate to severe dementia and patients with parkinsonism accompanied by psychosis and paraphrenia represent other clusters of symptoms for which ECT may be effective (Fogel 1988). However, these indications remain controversial, and systematic studies are needed to establish the efficacy and safety of ECT for such patients.

Risks

As with younger adult populations, there are few absolute contraindications to ECT, and the decision whether to proceed with
this treatment balances the risks of ECT with the dangers of the
continuing depression and of the alternate treatments. Specific
conditions that have traditionally been of concern for the psychiatrist considering ECT include depression with coexisting cardiac
illness, especially recent myocardial infarction, congestive heart
failure, conduction abnormalities, hypertension, and impaired
pulmonary function; these illnesses may require specific medical
measures prior to ECT in order to lessen the risk of complications.
One study in the elderly identified major risk factors to be cardiac
failure, myocardial infarction in the previous year, angina, stroke
in the preceding 2 years, chronic renal failure, and significant arrhythmias or conduction disturbances (Gaspar and Samarasinghe
1982). Subsequent studies, however, have shown that most contraindications to ECT are relative rather than absolute; ECT has
been given successfully to elderly poststroke patients within 1
month of the stroke (Murray et al. 1986). Although older age per se
does not predispose to increased complications from ECT, the
above-mentioned comorbid conditions occur with much greater
frequency in the elderly.

Increased intracranial pressure, such as that caused by a brain
tumor, is considered an absolute contraindication to ECT (Chen et
al. 1989; Welch 1989).

Adverse Effects

The mortality due to ECT has been estimated at approximately
three or four deaths per 100,000 treatments or per 10,000 patients
treated (Fink 1979; Abrams 1988), and it may be even lower (Kramer 1985). The death rate from ECT is not too dissimilar from that
of anesthetic induction alone (Fink 1979; Abrams 1988). The leading cause of death associated with ECT was cardiovascular complication.

Rarely, ECT treatments lead to prolonged seizure activity, status epilepticus, or other unusual behavioral manifestations. Although such consequences are unusual, a pretreatment electroencephalogram (EEG) is useful for comparison in patients with
histories of seizures or unusual neurologic responses to ECT.

Confusion after treatments differs from patient to patient, and the extent of any confusion depends on the variables of electrode placement, type of stimulus, length of seizure activity, number of previous treatments, and spacing between treatments. Most reports have described less postictal confusion after unilateral than bilateral electrode placement, and it has also been reported that reorientation always occurred earlier after brief-pulse stimulation than after sine-wave stimulation (Abrams 1988).

Memory problems have been difficult to assess in depressed patients receiving ECT because of the effect of the depression itself on memory. This area is a sensitive one in the elderly, who are vulnerable to memory deficits due to multiple systems problems. It is important to be aware of the fact that treatment of depression often results in improved memory; therefore preexisting memory impairment need not be considered a contraindication to ECT in the elderly (Salzman 1982). Numerous reports have revealed that bilateral ECT results in a greater degree of memory loss than unilateral ECT, and brief-pulse right unilateral ECT appears to produce the least impairment (Abrams 1988).

Procedures

Consent

Obtaining informed consent from the elderly patient may be complicated, especially if the patient is exhibiting symptoms of psychotic major depressive illness. If the patient expresses reluctance to consent to ECT, treatment cannot begin. Legal assistance is required when patients are considered incompetent to give informed consent and refuse to do so, especially if delaying much-needed treatment is life threatening. A court order, as a lifesaving intervention, may be required. More frequently, however the patient does not refuse ECT but is perceived as possibly not having full cognition and appreciation of the procedure. In situations such as these, further in-depth discussions with the patient and his or her family may become essential to ensure adequate understanding by all. Guardianship or durable power of attorney may need to be obtained. Risks, benefits, and treatment alternatives are explained, and the discussions are recorded in the patient's chart. The use of written descriptive information regarding ECT as well as of informed consent videotapes may be helpful. A second or third opin-

ion from a psychiatrist who is not involved in the patient's care
may also be helpful.

Assessment

Pretreatment assessment should include all of the laboratory evaluations routinely done for younger adults including (when indicated) chemistry screening panel, thyroid function tests, urinalysis, electrocardiogram, chest X ray, and physical and neurological
(optional) examination; the primary care physician's opinion regarding medical stability for ECT should be recorded in the patient's chart. Specific evaluations can include complete spinal X
rays to apprise the psychiatrist of fractures, osteoporosis, or significant spinal degeneration in the elderly patient requiring closer attention or precautionary measures (e.g., increased amounts of succinylcholine or increased support of the head and neck). Such X
rays also serve to document preexisting lesions. Occasionally cal-
cified abdominal aortic aneurysms have been noted on spinal X
rays, allowing the clinician to determine whether further evaluation or intervention is required, although several published reports
have noted no untoward effects in patients receiving ECT with
either treated or untreated aneurisms (Abrams 1988).

In the presence of neurologic findings, a computed tomography
brain scan or magnetic resonance imaging scan alerts the practitioner to recent or old infarctions or other central nervous system
lesions that may be contributing to the depression or post-ECT
cognitive dysfunction.

Obtaining an EEG prior to ECT is occasionally useful, although
the yield from this procedure is limited. Once the ECT series is initiated, the changes brought about by treatment (generalized slowing with increased amplitude) do not allow a reference baseline
EEG until at least 30 days after the series ends (Abrams 1988).

Careful evaluation of the dentition of the elderly patient prior
to ECT is essential, because many patients have several loose or
missing teeth as well as partial or full dentures. If there are no
loose teeth and only a few teeth missing, then one can proceed
safely with the use of a rubber semicircular bite block, which helps
to distribute the pressure of contraction of the masseter (the
strongest muscle in the body). A semicircular bite block should be
used rather than a padded or rubberized tongue blade because direct stimulation of the temporalis muscles may not be blocked by
succinylcholine, and in the elderly patient there is a greater risk of

further loosening teeth if jaw pressure is focused at only one point (Abrams 1988).

Full or partial denture plates should be removed prior to ECT to prevent damage. However, there can be instances in which a partial plate surrounds and supports only a few or even just one tooth and its removal might result in damage to the unsupported teeth during the ECT. In situations such as these, a consultation with a dental specialist can help determine the best way to proceed. It is usually preferable to keep a strong and intact partial dental plate in place during the procedure to support the existing permanent teeth. Also, the assistance of the anesthesiologist to hold the jaw up against the bite block at the time of administering the stimulus is helpful; this measure prevents sudden slapping of the jaw against the maxilla and the potential for dental damage and biting of the lip.

If there is any question of the patient's physical status prior to ECT, a consultation should be obtained from the appropriate specialist. Depending on the patient's physical state, consultation with a cardiologist, neurologist, anesthesiologist, orthopedist, rheumatologist, or other specialist may be indicated. If there is any question regarding appropriateness for ECT, another psychiatrist skilled in the use of ECT can be consulted.

Electrical Stimulus

Efficacy of ECT is predicated on the assumption that the electrical stimulus delivered to the brain functions only to produce a seizure; there is no indication that the electrical stimulus itself contributes to improvement. In fact, an electrical stimulus significantly beyond that which is necessary to initiate the seizure may contribute to side effects of confusion and memory loss (Abrams 1988). Recent reports, however, indicate that for most patients, especially the elderly, higher energy levels than seizure threshold are now preferred (Fink 1989).

Regarding the waveform of electrical stimulation, most studies to date indicate that the brief-pulse, square-wave stimulus is preferable to the sine-wave stimulus, because the latter is thought to contribute to confusion and memory loss but not to the therapeutic effect (Abrams 1988). Research on waveform and stimulus intensity in ECT for the elderly has been recommended, especially because older patients have a higher seizure threshold and may have different patterns of physiological response to particular stimulus parameters (Fogel 1988).

Laterality of Stimulation

A controversy has continued for years regarding unilateral versus bilateral ECT with respect to efficacy and side effects. Although bilateral ECT is viewed by many to be the most effective form of treatment (Abrams et al. 1983), unilateral treatments are said by some to be just as effective but without the side effects of memory loss and confusion (Fraser and Glass 1980; Salzman 1982; Welch 1982; Kroessler 1985). Many, but not all, studies have reported equal efficacy of unilateral and bilateral ECT (Fogel 1988). In 29 depressed elderly patients receiving randomly assigned unilateral or bilateral ECT, no significant differences were noted (Fraser and Glass 1980). Another study in the elderly showed equal improvement but found the rate of recovery of respiration, consciousness, and orientation to be prolonged with bilateral treatments (Fraser 1981). One study of 122 elderly patients who received bilateral ECT with few problems argued that those who do not respond to unilateral treatment should be given bilateral ECT (Benbow 1987). Other studies indicate a greater number of missed seizures or a higher relapse rate associated with unilateral ECT; and some experts have recommended bilateral ECT as the treatment of choice for severely agitated, psychotic, and suicidal patients (Fogel 1988). The issue remains unresolved. Unilateral ECT can be initiated in nonemergency cases with a change to bilateral treatment if improvement does not begin rapidly, although more recent reports indicate that bilateral electrode placement is preferred, especially in the elderly; unilateral placement is reserved for those patients who exhibit cognitive worsening during the course of treatment (Fink 1989).

Dosage

Seizure threshold increases with age; conversely, seizure duration decreases with age and with number of treatments in the series, and therefore, stimulus needs to be increased accordingly (Abrams 1988).

The frequency of treatments varies; most practitioners in the United States and Canada provide three treatments per week on alternate days, whereas in Great Britain treatments have traditionally been given twice a week (Fogel 1988). A double-blind study comparing the two methods reported the actual number of treatments required to reach improvement to be the same, with improvement occurring more rapidly in the three-times-per-week group (Shapira et al. 1989). Some studies have reported that multiple treatments of ECT during one treatment session—"multiple-monitored ECT" (MMECT)—may achieve the same degree of clinical improvement with the advantages of shorter treatment duration, fewer sessions of general anesthesia, and lower dosages of anesthetic agents, as well as a reduction in the time the patient is at risk for suicide (Yesavage and Berens 1980). Others have reported that it is no better than singly monitored ECT (Salzman 1982). However, a study of 44 elderly patients with severe depression found MMECT to be as safe and efficacious for elderly as for younger patients and that the elderly tolerate many seizures as well as the nonelderly; this finding suggests that MMECT could be used safely with the elderly (Mielke et al. 1984). The question of whether this approach is more effective or, conversely, might be more toxic on a cardiovascular or neurologic basis requires further study.

The total number of ECT treatments required in a series is usually 6 to 9 for the elderly, although they often need 12 or more treatments for complete remission (Fogel 1988). In deciding to continue any ECT series, the potential for greater improvement must be weighed against the risk of anesthetic complications (Fogel 1988). Typically, treatment continues until the patient is symptom free unless side effects of confusion or significant memory loss supervene.

Medications and Anesthesia

Premedication with an anticholinergic agent, atropine, or glycopyrrolate is generally recommended to diminish or block the direct vagal effects on the heart during and immediately after the electrical stimulus (Abrams 1988). The advantages of lycopyrrolate (a synthetic agent that does not enter the central nervous system) are low likelihood of inducing postictal confusion (Kramer et al. 1986; Abrams 1988) and reduced frequency of cardiac arrhythmias (Swartz and Saheba 1989). Regarding the necessity of atropinic premedication (Wyant and MacDonald 1980), a case report of cardiac arrest in an elderly patient who received a beta-blocker unopposed by pretreatment with an atropinic agent (Decina et al. 1984) suggests an atropinic drug should be used if a beta-blocker may be administered during ECT.

The anesthetic agent most commonly used is methohexital. It reportedly induces fewer cardiac arrhythmias than thiopental (Pitts et al. 1965; Abrams 1988). Methohexital also induces a shorter sleep time and less postanesthetic confusion (Egbert and Wolfe 1960; Osborne et al. 1963; Woodruff et al. 1968).

Adequate muscle relaxation during ECT is necessary to prevent strain on the cardiovascular system, prevent fractures in osteoporotic patients, and limit increases in blood pressure and heart rate (Salzman 1982). The muscle relaxant of choice is succinylcholine. It is given intravenously by rapid bolus push after the anesthetic at a dosage of 0.5 to 1.0 mg per kilogram of body weight (Abrams 1988). For the elderly patient with a greater potential for fractures, higher doses of succinylcholine may be required, but the benefit needs to be weighed against potential complications from prolonged respiratory paralysis.

After administration of the succinylcholine, the treatment team observes for muscle fasciculations, which begin in the neck region and travel to the legs and feet. One must be careful to observe the fasciculations in the gastrocnemius and in the toes; otherwise, those unaware of the fact that in the elderly the circulation is often slow may proceed to give ECT to patients who are not sufficiently paralyzed, placing them at greater risk for fracture. It is therefore important, in addition to observing the course and cessation of fasciculations, to establish the absence of the patellar deep tendon reflex and facial or radial nerve reflex (by means of a hand-held nerve stimulator) as well as to watch for abdominal relaxation (Baker 1986; Hay 1989).

Because the elderly are more likely to exhibit an elevated seizure threshold, which often increases as the treatment series continues, it is critical to determine that a seizure has been induced, and if not, to re-treat with different settings or electrode placement while the anesthetic and muscle relaxant are still exerting their full effect. Failure to check for this may result in missed seizures, which may lead to the erroneous conclusion that the ECT series was ineffective.

The cuffing-off of an extremity prior to administration of succinylcholine to observe the presence of the seizure in the cuffed-off limb is, therefore, extremely important, even if the ECT apparatus has a built-in EEG recording device. At times it is difficult to tell by way of EEG alone if a seizure has occurred, and the peripheral seizure has a different duration (usually shorter) than the centrally recorded one.

Oxygenation with 100% oxygen is essential, because cerebral oxygen requirements are increased during a seizure (Abrams and Essman 1982; Abrams 1988). Pretreatment oxygenation also tends to minimize side effects of memory loss and cardiac arrhythmias

(Salzman 1982). It is not uncommon for elderly patients requiring ECT to have chronic obstructive pulmonary disease, emphysema, or asthma (Fawver and Milstein 1985). It is important, therefore, to carefully evaluate respiratory function before proceeding with ECT. Consultation with an internist—and, if necessary, with a pulmonologist—and the anesthesiologist may be helpful. The use of a pulse oximeter during ECT is becoming increasingly frequent. A case of status epilepticus as a complication of concurrent ECT and theophylline therapy has been reported (Peters et al. 1984).

The most significant physiological stress of ECT is to the cardiovascular system; tachycardia and hypertension develop in most patients, and cardiac work increases severalfold during the seizure. At the end of the seizure there can be an abrupt shift to bradycardia and occasional potentially dangerous bradyarrhythmias can develop (Welch 1989). Various strategies of premedication have been proposed to prevent the development of hypertension, tachycardia and the rebound hypotension, bradycardia, and bradyarrhythmias. These premedications include nitroprusside, propranolol, and diazoxide (Weiner 1983; Regestein and Reich 1985; Fogel 1988). Other recommended pre-ECT antihypertensives found to be advantageous because of their relatively short duration of action include labetalol and esmolol (Hay 1989).

Some elderly patients referred for ECT exhibit cardiac arrhythmias. Pretreating the patient with lidocaine may cause an elevation of the seizure threshold and prevent the induction or shorten the duration of a seizure (Abrams 1988). Most arrhythmias are relatively benign premature ventricular contradictions (PVCs) and need not be treated. PVCs are sometimes anxiety induced and tend to disappear after ECT. If they persist or worsen after the treatment, lidocaine or another antiarrhythmic such as verapamil can be administered. If the arrhythmia is of concern and treatment of the arrhythmia appears to be indicated before ECT is initiated, cardiac consultation may be requested (Hay 1989).

It is the responsibility of the psychiatrist who administers the ECT to alert the anesthesiologist and the rest of the treatment team (recovery room nurses, psychiatric nurses from the patient's unit, nurse anesthetists) to the special needs of the elderly patient and to encourage the use of the techniques conducive to a good and safe outcome: adequate preoxygenation, rubber bite block as opposed to padded tongue blade, adequate amounts of succinylcholine, observation for fasciculations and absence of patellar and other reflexes, and cuffing-off of the distal portion of an extremity before administration of succinglcholine (Hay 1989).

Management of Concurrent Medication

Elderly patients referred for ECT are sometimes receiving anticoagulation therapy. The question arises whether to continue warfarin during the ECT treatment or to switch to intermittent bolus heparin before and after, but not during, ECT. Recent studies suggest that it is preferable to continue warfarin anticoagulation throughout the ECT series; there is no evidence that it increases the risk for cardiovascular problems (Tancer and Evans 1989; Hay 1987, 1989).

Concurrent administration of ECT and various medications may pose problems. Lithium coincident with ECT may prolong the muscular blockade of succinylcholine, and it has been implicated in the causation of acute confusional states (Abrams 1988).

Although some reports indicate that the use of antidepressants during the ECT treatments does not increase the antidepressant effect and may even reduce affective improvement (Abrams 1975; Price et al. 1978; Siris et al. 1982), one report suggests that outcome may be improved for those patients who receive tricyclic antidepressant drugs concurrent with ECT (Nelson and Benjamin 1989).

Benzodiazepines increase the seizure threshold (Abrams 1988) and therefore should be tapered and discontinued, if possible, prior to ECT.

The use of MAOIs during ECT has been avoided in the past, given concern for interaction of the MAOI with anesthesia. Some authors suggest this precaution may be unnecessary (Abrams 1988), but they add that no therapeutic advantage has been noted from combining ECT and MAOIs.

Many older patients referred for ECT exhibit coexistent movement disorders of idiopathic Parkinson's disease, neuroleptic-induced parkinsonism, dystonias, akathisia, and tardive dyskinesia. Various studies have reported improvement not only in the affective illness being treated by ECT, but also of the movement disorder as well (Fink 1988).

Maintenance ECT

Because it is well substantiated that ECT is an effective and safe treatment for elderly patients with psychiatric illnesses, how to avoid relapse following completion of a series of ECT treatments is an important clinical issue. A customary approach is to place patients on an antidepressant drug or lithium. At the conclusion of the ECT series, maintenance ECT provided as an outpatient procedure is recommended for patients who have shown adequate improvement with a prior course of ECT and relapsed within 6 months despite adequate maintenance antidepressant therapy (Abrams 1988). Maintenance ECT is begun approximately 1 week after the initial series is completed, and thereafter the interval is increased and the frequency of treatment decreased. The first maintenance ECT treatment is given approximately 1 week after the last of the series, the second treatment is given 2 weeks later, the third 3 or 4 weeks later, and so on; the interval is steadily increased so that the patient usually receives approximately four to six treatments over the 6-month period after the series.

Summary

After 50 years of experience with ECT, it has been found to be effective, safe, and at times a lifesaving procedure. The treating psychiatrist must identify those individuals whose symptoms are valid indicators for ECT and administer ECT in such a manner as to keep side effects at a minimum. One needs to continue to be familiar with modern techniques of administering ECT, including delivery of the stimulus, anesthesia, and muscular relaxation, as well as ways of minimizing stress to the cardiovascular system.

ECT can be especially valuable for geriatric patients who have failed to respond to pharmacotherapy, those intolerant to the side effects of antidepressant drugs, the delusionally depressed, and patients (such as the suicidal and malnourished) who need immediate relief from a life-threatening psychiatric illness.

References

Abrams R: Drugs in combination with ECT, in Drugs in Combination With Other Therapies. Edited by Greenblatt M. New York, Grune & Stratton, 1975, pp 157–164

Abrams R: Electroconvulsive Therapy. New York, Oxford University Press, 1988

Abrams R, Essman W: Electroconvulsive Therapy: Biological Foundations and Clinical Applications. New York, Spectrum Publications, 1982

Abrams R, Taylor MA, Faber R, et al: Bilateral versus unilateral electroconvulsive therapy: efficacy in melancholia. Am J Psychiatry 140:463–465, 1983

Alexopoulos G, Shamoian C, Lucas J, et al: Medical problems of geriatric psychiatric patients and younger controls during electroconvulsive therapy. J Am Geriatr Soc 32:651–654, 1984

Alexopoulos G, Young R, Abrams RC: ECT in the high-risk geriatric patient. Convulsive Therapy 5:75–87, 1989

APA Task Force Report on Electroconvulsive Therapy. Task Force No. 14. Washington, DC, American Psychiatric Association, 1978

APA Task Force Report on Electroconvulsive Therapy: The Practice of ECT: Recommendations for Treatment, Training and Priviledging. Washington, DC, American Psychiatric Association, 1990

Avery D, Winokur G: Mortality in depressed patients treated with electroconvulsive therapy and antidepressants. Arch Gen Psychiatry 33:1029–1037, 1976

Baker NJ: Electroconvulsive therapy and severe osteoporosis: use of a nerve stimulator to assess paralysis. Convulsive Therapy 2:285–288, 1986

Benbow S: The use of electroconvulsive therapy in old age psychiatry. International Journal of Geriatric Psychiatry 2:25–30, 1987

Bidder T: Electroconvulsive therapy in the medically ill patient. Psychiatr Clin North Am 4:391–405, 1981

Burke W, Rutherford J, Zorumski C, et al: Electroconvulsive therapy and the elderly. Compr Psychiatry 26:480–486, 1985

Burke W, Rubin E, Zorumski C, et al: The safety of ECT in geriatric psychiatry. J Am Geriatr Soc 35:516–521, 1987

Chen LS, McNamara JO, Maltby DA, et al: Affect of intranigral application of clinically affective anti-convulsants on electroshock induced seizure. Neuropharmacology 28:781–786, 1989

Decina P, Malitz S, Sackeim HA, et al: Cardiac arrest during ECT modified by beta-adrenergic blockade. Am J Psychiatry 141:298–300, 1984

Egbert LD, Wolfe S: Evaluation of methohexital for premedication in electroshock therapy. Anesth Analg 39:416–419, 1960

Endler NS, Persad E: Electroconvulsive Therapy: The Myths and the Realities. Toronto, Hans Huber Publishers, 1988

Fawver J, Milstein V: Asthma/emphysema complication of electroconvulsive therapy: a case report. Convulsive Therapy 1:61–64, 1985

Fink M: Convulsive Therapy: Theory and Practice. New York, Raven, 1979

Fink M: ECT for Parkinson's disease? Convulsive Therapy 4:189–191, 1988

Fink M: Editorial—an adequate treatment? Convulsive Therapy 5:311–313, 1989

Fogel B: Electroconvulsive therapy in the elderly: a clinical research agenda. International Journal of Geriatric Psychiatry 3:181–190, 1988

Fraser R: ECT and the elderly, in Electroconvulsive Therapy: An Appraisal. Edited by Palmer R. New York, Oxford University Press, 1981

Fraser RM, Glass IB: Unilateral and bilateral ECT in elderly patients. Acta Psychiatr Scand 62:13–31, 1980

Gaspar D, Samarasinghe A: ECT in psychogeriatric practice—a study of risk factors, indications, and outcome. Compr Psychiatry 23:170–175, 1982

Godber C, Rosenvinge H, Wilkinson D, et al: Depression in old age: prognosis after ECT. International Journal of Geriatric Psychiatry 2:19–24, 1987

Hay DP: Anticoagulants and ECT. Convulsive Therapy 3:236–237, 1987

Hay DP: Electroconvulsive therapy in the medically ill elderly. Convulsive Therapy 5:8–16, 1989

Hay DP, Hay LK: The role of ECT in the treatment of depression, in Depression: New Directions in Research, Theory, and Practice. Edited by McCann CD, Endler NS. Toronto, Wall and Emerson, Inc, 1990, pp 255–272

Heshe J, Roeder E, Theilgaard A: Unilateral and bilateral ECT: a psychiatric and psychological study of therapeutic effect and side effects. Acta Psychiatr Scand 275:1–180, 1978

Huang KC, Lucas LF, Tsueda K, et al: Age-related changes in cardiovascular function associated with electroconvulsive therapy. Convulsive Therapy 5:17–25, 1989

Karlinsky H, Shulman K: The clinical use of electroconvulsive therapy in old age. J Am Geriatr Soc 32:183–186, 1983

Koenig H, Shelp F, Goli V, et al: Survival and health care utilization in elderly medical inpatients with major depression. J Am Geriatr Soc 37:599–606, 1989

Kramer BA: Use of ECT in California. Am J Psychiatry 142:1190–1192, 1985

Kramer BA, Allen RE, Friedman B: Atropine and glycopyrrolate as ECT preanesthesia. J Clin Psychiatry 47:199–200, 1986

Kroessler D: Relative efficacy rates for therapies of delusional depression. Convulsive Therapy 1:173–182, 1985

Meyers B, Mei-tal V: Empirical study on an inpatient psychogeriatric unit: biological treatment in patients with depressive illness. Int J Psychiatry Med 15:111–124, 1985–1986

Mielke D, Winstead D, Goethe J, et al: Multiple-monitored electroconvulsive therapy: safety and efficacy in elderly depressed patients. J Am Geriatr Soc 32:180–182, 1984

Murray GB, Shea V, Conn DK: Electroconvulsive therapy for post-stroke depression. J Clin Psychiatry 47:258–260, 1986

Nelson JP, Benjamin L: Efficacy and safety of combined ECT and tricyclic antidepressant drugs in the treatment of depressed geriatric patients. Convulsive Therapy 5(4)321–329, 1989

NIMH Consensus Conference: Electroconvulsive therapy. JAMA 254:2103–2108, 1985

Osborne RG, Tunakan B, Barmore J: Anaesthetic agent in electroconvulsive therapy: a controlled comparison. J Nerv Ment Dis 137:297–300, 1963

Palmer R: Electroconvulsive Therapy: An Appraisal. New York, Oxford University Press, 1981

Peters SG, Wochos DN, Patterson GC: Status epilepticus as a complication of concurrent electroconvulsive and theophylline therapy. Mayo Clin Proc 59:568–570, 1984

Pitts FN, Desmaris GM, Stewart W, et al: Induction of anesthesia with methohexital and thiopental in electroconvulsive therapy. N Engl J Med 273:353–360, 1965

Price TR, Mackenzie TB, Tucker GJ, et al: The dose response ratio in electroconvulsive therapy: a preliminary study. Arch Gen Psychiatry 35:1131–1136, 1978

Raskind M: Electroconvulsive therapy in the elderly. J Am Geriatr Soc 32:177–178, 1983

Regestein QR, Reich P: Electroconvulsive therapy in patients at high risk for physical complications. Convulsive Therapy 1:101–114, 1985

Salzman C: Electroconvulsive therapy in the elderly patient. Psychiatr Clin North Am 5:191–197, 1982

Shapira B, Kindler S, Lerer B: Treatment schedule and rate of response to ECT. Biol Psychiatry 25:106A-107A, 1989

Siris SG, Glassman AH, Stetner F: ECT and psychotropic medication in the treatment of depression and schizophrenia, in Electroconvulsive Therapy: Biological Foundations and Clinical Applications. Edited by Abrams R, Essman WB. New York, Spectrum, 1982, pp 91–112

Spiker DG, Dealy RS, Hanin I, et al: Treating delusional depression with amitriptyline. J Clin Psychiatry 47:243–245, 1986

Stromgren LS: Unilateral versus bilateral electroconvulsive therapy: investigations into the therapeutic effect in endogenous depression. Acta Psychiatr Scand 240:8–65, 1973

Swartz CM, Saheba NC: Comparison of atropine with glycopyrrolate for use in ECT. Convulsive Therapy 5:56–60, 1989

Tancer M, Evans D: Electroconvulsive therapy in geriatric patients undergoing anticoagulation therapy. Convulsive Therapy 5:102–109, 1989

Weiner R: The role of electroconvulsive therapy in the treatment of depression in the elderly. J Am Geriatr Soc 30:710–712, 1982

Weiner R: ECT in the physically ill. Journal of Psychiatric Treatment and Evaluation 5:457–462, 1983

Weiner R, Coffey CE: Indications for use of electroconvulsive therapy, in American Psychiatric Press Review of Psychiatry, Vol 7. Edited by Frances AJ, Hales RE. Washington, DC, American Psychiatric Press, 1988, pp 458–481

Welch CA: The relative efficacy of unilateral nondominant and bilateral stimulation. Psychopharmacol Bull 18:68–70, 1982

Welch CA: Electroconvulsive therapy, in Treatments of Psychiatric Disorders: A Task Force Report of the American Psychiatric Association. Edited by Karasu TB. Washington, DC, American Psychiatric Association, 1989, 3:1803–1813

Woodruff RA, Pitts FN, Jr., McClure JN: The drug modification of ECT. Arch Gen Psychiatry 18:605–611, 1968

Wyant GM, MacDonald WB: The role of atropine in electroconvulsive therapy. Anaesth Intensive Care 8:445–450, 1980

Yesavage J, Berens ES: Multiple monitored electroconvulsive therapy in the elderly. J Am Geriatr Soc 28:206–209, 1980

Zorumski C, Rubin E, Burke W: Electroconvulsive therapy for the elderly: a review. Hosp Community Psychiatry 39:643–647, 1988

CHAPTER 24

Lawrence W. Lazarus, M.D.
Joel Sadavoy, M.D.
Pauline R. Langsley, M.D.

Individual Psychotherapy

The data on geriatric psychotherapy are based largely on clinical consensus and single-case studies, with some empirical data available in specific areas: cognitive (Gallagher and Thompson 1982); behavioral, group, and milieu (Sadavoy and Robinson 1989); institutional treatment (Goldfarb and Turner 1953); and brief psychotherapy (Lazarus et al. 1987). Gallagher and Thompson (1983) compared cognitive-behavioral, and brief relational and insight therapies in 30 depressed patients (15 endogenous and 15 nonendogenous). All three modalities produced positive results, comparable to studies of tricyclic antidepressants in similar populations.

Apparently contradictory opinions that arise in the literature about geriatric psychotherapy are generally the result of observations made in different age cohorts. The contradictions frequently can be resolved if the therapist applies appropriate principles of psychotherapy to appropriate subgroups of the elderly, avoiding erroneous attempts to homogenize the aged population. Age per se defines neither indications nor contraindications for specific therapies. (Nemiroff and Colarusso 1985a; Myers 1984; and Leszcz 1987; Rechtschaffen 1959; Steuer 1982; Yesavage and Karasu 1982).

Innovative psychiatric outpatient programs were developed in the late 1960s to encourage older patients in the community to avail themselves of treatment. The Langley Porter Neuropsychiatric Institute (Feigenbaum 1973) publicized its special outpatient program, and within 3 years the proportion of elderly patients doubled. Furthermore, it was the clinical impression of the therapists that the improvement of elderly patients was similar to that of younger patients. The San Francisco Geriatric Screening Project (Simon and Lowenthal 1970) demonstrated in an uncontrolled study that early detection, evaluation, and treatment of psychiatrically impaired elderly persons in the community reduced the admission rate of elderly patients to state mental hospitals.

Psychotherapeutic goals, indications, techniques, and process are best defined based on a functional, rather than chronological, perspective. Function in old age may be conceptualized as a continuum between two poles: normative aging at one extreme and physical and mental frailty at the other (Kahana 1979). Within these two extreme poles, or boundaries, is a transitional period of development characterized by a variety of life stressors, some presenting as crises, others as chronic strain (Figure 24-1).

Barriers to Psychotherapy

The elderly, according to a study by Eisdorfer and Stotsky, comprise only about 2% to 4% of patients seen in psychiatric outpatient clinics and even a smaller percentage of most private psychiatric practices. Reasons for this low use of outpatient services can be understood from the perspective of the patient, the family, the physician, and the health care system (Gaitz 1974).

Raised in an era when shame and embarrassment were associated with seeing a psychiatrist, older people may shun such intervention and become indignant when family or physician suggests it. Negative beliefs about psychiatry, common to their sociocultural milieu and geographical locale, reinforce this hesitation. Some aging individuals believe that depression and anxiety are to be expected with aging or attribute the symptoms to medical rather than psychiatric causes. Moreover, the psychiatric prob-

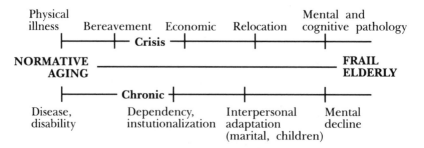

Figure 24-1. The continuum of functioning in old age.

lems themselves, such as depression with its associated helplessness and apathy, are often deterrents to treatment.

Additional barriers include such practical problems as arranging transportation, and interruptions of therapy because of medical illnesses. Adult children of aging parents may harbor the same negative, stereotypic attitudes about psychiatry as their parents, and they may minimize or deny their parent's psychiatric symptoms. The family may fear that disapproval and anger would result if treatment were suggested. Conscious and unconscious resentment or ambivalence toward an aging parent or concerns about assuming financial responsibility may act as deterrents to advocating adequate psychiatric care.

Primary care physicians may question the value of psychiatric intervention for frail, debilitated, elderly patients and may believe that their shortened lifespan renders them unsuitable for psychotherapy. Difficulty convincing elderly patients and their families of the usefulness of psychiatric treatment may be an additional deterrent.

General Principles of Individual Psychotherapy

The therapist of the elderly patient individualizes interventions in a flexible manner (Blau and Berezin 1975; Yesavage and Karasu 1982) and takes into account the need to change to another therapeutic approach because of crises, health changes, and so on.

The therapist often uses psychotherapy when appropriate, either as a primary or as an adjunctive treatment, in combination with medications, social and environmental manipulation, and patient advocacy. No single technique, principle, or rule of psychotherapy adequately addresses the heterogeneous geriatric population.

The complex interplay of medical, psychological, and sociocultural problems confronting the frail elderly requires flexibility and ingenuity on the part of the therapist. The therapist may be called on to function in different roles with the same patient, such as family therapist, psychopharmacotherapist, primary care physician, and, at times, coordinator of the patient's treatment team. The psychiatrist is also concerned about previously undiagnosed medical problems and medication side effects that may be masquerading as, or aggravating, a psychiatric disorder. The initial office visit usually requires more than an hour to complete a comprehensive assessment of biopsychosocial factors and, when indicated, to spend some time with the patient's family. For a somatically oriented patient, beginning an initial interview in a medically oriented manner may have the advantage of familiarity and place the patient at ease.

Therapists need to be aware of concurrent physical problems that may be a cause of psychiatric referral, and ensure that psychotherapy or any other treatment has been preceded by a thorough medical workup. Family often may have to be involved to obtain important collateral information not attainable from the patient and to gain their support and cooperation with the treatment plan, particularly when dealing with the frail elderly. However, the therapist should take care to respect the competent patient's wishes in this regard, as in others. Setting realistic psychotherapeutic goals helps patient and therapist to avoid mutual frustration and a sense of failure.

The identified elderly patient is usually interviewed first alone, to convey respect for the patient's individuality and to elicit information that may not be obtainable in the family's presence. Some elderly patients are apprehensive about seeing a psychiatrist, and so careful exploration of reactions and resistances to therapy often is best followed by empathic explanations and realistic reassurances. When the patient and/or family is highly anxious or hopeless, the therapist adopts an active stance in working through patient and family resistances to therapy, demonstrating a willingness to help, and aiding patient and family to experience benefits from the very first interview; for example, explaining a treatment plan or offering an expression of valid hope is conducive to further therapy.

Goals of Psychotherapy

Normative Elderly

At the normative end of the continuum, structural change in psychoanalysis or psychoanalytic psychotherapy may be a realistic goal for some patients (Grotjahn 1955; Grunes 1987; Kahana 1987b; Myers 1984; Sadavoy and Leszcz 1987; Sandler 1982; Wheelright 1959; Zinberg 1963); as frailty increases, the goals of intensive psychotherapy become less achievable. These goals include psychological mastery over the past, leading to enhancement of current adaptation; formation and working through of conflicts in the therapeutic transference; resolution of childhood and adult sources of unconscious conflicts associated with shame, guilt, and humiliation; working through of unresolved grief reactions that were inhibited by earlier conflicts, thereby releasing restricted creativity and capacities for intimacy—in Pollock's (1987) terminology, mourning-liberation; resolution of current interpersonal conflict stemming from earlier, often unconscious, conflicts; working through loss, and finding substitute sources of self-esteem; and coming to terms with failure to achieve ideal aspirations, as retirement and other forms of disengagement are imposed by life circumstance (Pollock 1987).

Crisis

When psychological defenses are overwhelmed by crisis, the first goal of therapy is aiding the patient to return to his or her current best level of function, rather than attempting structural or intrapsychic change. During and after the crisis, patients often require help to identify new, more realistic levels of function and to work toward them. Specific goals of psychotherapy during the crisis phases of old age, whether at the normative or frail end of the continuum, include mourning for lost capacities (if a patient retains enough ego strength to work through his or her losses); redirection of energy and creativity to realistic levels of functioning; redefinition of interpersonal relationships and acceptance of an appropriate level of dependency; acceptance and/or working through of separation and disengagement conflicts and fears; reengagement with new sources of gratification, for example, new relationships with other patients and caregivers; control of regression and lessened need for using such defenses as splitting, projection, primitive denial, and magical thinking (Sadavoy 1987); and reestablishment of adaptive defenses to promote feelings of control and mastery (Goldfarb and Sheps 1954). Practical consequences of crisis therapy are improved adaptation to stress, including more appropriate use of the health care and social support systems.

Frail Elderly

The closer the patient's function to the more impaired end of the aging continuum, the more explicit, restricted, and focused become the goals of psychotherapy.

At the more debilitated, frail end of the developmental continuum, therapeutic goals are often focused on narrowly defined behavioral change. Psychodynamic formulations, however, remain useful and serve to humanize the patient and enhance the staff's comprehension of him or her. The goal of therapy is to strengthen the roles of necessary caregivers and family and alter the environmental response, so that it is in keeping with the patient's psychological and other needs (Cohen 1989).

The goals of therapy with the frail elderly deal with problem-oriented resolution of specific issues, such as the role status imposed by sudden bereavement, physical illness or relocation, acute psychosis, danger of suicide, psychiatric complications of dementia and confusional states, and terminal illness. The anxiety of family members over the deterioration of an elderly family member may focus therapy on the caregivers as well as, or instead of, the identified patient.

The goal of helping the aged work through anxieties and fears associated with death, although sometimes important (Segal 1958), is less clinically relevant than one might think. The elderly, especially the very old, do not seem to express much death anxiety (Berezin 1972, 1987; Pollock 1987; Weisman and Hackett 1967). Indeed, death-related anxiety and conflict may be much more a phenomenon of earlier adult life (Jacques 1965; Yalom 1980). The elderly who are confronting illness or decline often tend to be preoccupied with fears of pain, disability, abandonment, and dependency.

Indications for Individual Psychotherapy

Insight-oriented, intensive psychotherapy is indicated most frequently for the normative-aging cohort and is most productive if the patient is motivated; has a capacity for self-observation, insight, and mourning; is able to tolerate painful affects without excessive regression; and has demonstrated a capacity for productive work, intimacy, and pleasure (Pollock 1987).

Adaptation to the stresses and losses associated with aging can be accompanied by a variety of conflicts that may be indications for individual psychotherapy directed toward structural change. These issues include adaptation to loss; conflicts over feared or actual sexual decline; loss of identity and the accompanying narcissistic gratification as a productive worker; marital conflict; fears of dependency; failure to achieve goals that often arose from an idealized self-perception (classically termed "ego ideal" or, more recently, the self psychology term "grandiose self"); and coming to grips with mortality and the imminence of death (King 1980).

As aging progresses, crises often become the entrée to therapy and crisis intervention techniques may be helpful. Supportive therapy is generally indicated until the patient's defenses and adaptive capacities can reconstitute. Psychotherapy in these circumstances is often an adjunct to medical, pharmacological, and environmental support (Kahana 1987b). Although brief psychotherapy and cognitive therapy are particularly useful, long-term therapy may follow in selected cases. However, caution is necessary, because defenses should not be challenged by interpretative therapy unless the patient retains a capacity to replace the lost defenses with new, adaptive, and fulfilling mechanisms for bolstering narcissistic supplies, protecting against damaged self-esteem, and replacing selfobject relationships (Yesavage and Karasu 1982).

Neugarten (1979) suggested that expectable and age-appropriate crises are handled more easily than crises that are temporally out of phase with an individual's life; for example, coming to terms with the death of a middle-aged child may be exceedingly difficult because it is out of phase with the normal chronology of expectable life events. Psychotherapy is indicated when the individual is unable to master and adapt to the psychological impact of the crisis. Vulnerability is enhanced if there is a history of serious, early-life deprivation; long-standing reliance on rigid and/or primitive defenses; overreliance on the selfobject component of intimate relationships; previous unmourned losses; multiple or unbearably intense assaults on the individual's life circumstance—as may occur, for example, during war or severe deprivation; breakdown of ego capacities because of physical and/or emotional pathology; and inability of caregivers, especially family, to tolerate the individual's pain.

Frailty usually interferes with the capacity to tolerate intensive psychotherapy and in general severely restricts or contraindicates its use. However, even in the frail elderly group, focal therapy focused on specific, here-and-now issues can use techniques of insight and interpretation (Rosenthal 1985)—termed "adaptive intervention" by Kahana (1987b)—in conjunction with cognitive, supportive, and educational techniques. Psychotherapy specifically adapted to the frail and institutionalized elderly (Aronson 1958; Goldfarb 1956; Sadavoy and Dorian 1983; Sadavoy and Robinson 1989) has been used successfully. The more limited and frail the patient, the greater the indication for problem-oriented interventions, such as behavioral therapies and environmental manipulation.

Often, the frail patient welcomes a more familiar relationship with the therapist: sitting closer, physical contact, first names. However, this wish is not universal among geriatric patients and can be experienced as unprofessional or disturbing, especially by those in the normative-aging phases. The therapist must take pains to individualize his or her approach.

Themes and Issues Discussed in Psychotherapy

One of the most common issues discussed by elderly patients is that of loss. Many psychotherapists believe that a major developmental task for the aging individual is to find restitution for the myriad biopsychosocial losses associated with this stage of the life cycle (Cath 1976; Meissner 1975). What appears to be so devastating for some elderly persons is the rapidity and cumulative effect of repeated losses before sufficient time has passed to allow for mourning and resolution.

Erikson (1968) conceptualized the last phase of life as the struggle to attain and maintain ego integrity, with failure to do so leading to a state of despair and disgust. Cath (1976) characterized the middle and later years as a balance between factors that support a person's self-esteem, such as wisdom derived from life experience, and attainment of a satisfying philosophical and religious world view and past accomplishments, versus factors leading to emotional depletion, such as failing health and cognitive impairment. Cath asserts that, given adequate ego resources and a sustaining environment, most elderly people master the challenges of later life. Atchley (1982), a sociologist, stated that persons who lose self-esteem in late life do so because they have lost a feeling of control over their environment to such a degree that they feel defenseless, because self-esteem had previously been too dependent on work or social roles and/or because physical deterioration had become so extensive that the person must accept a less desirable self-image. The elderly, according to Atchley, defend themselves against a negative self-image by choosing to interact with people who provide an egosyntonic experience, refusing to apply negative societal myths about aging to themselves, discounting messages that do not fit with their existing self-image, and focusing on past successes.

Transference

The literature on geriatric psychotherapy generally endorses the premise of the timelessness of the unconscious leading to the persistence of unconscious attitudes and fantasies from early life (Berezin 1972). These factors determine much of the content of the transference. There is little clinical evidence to support strongly the concept of a highly age-specific transference, although the stressors inherent in old age tend to mobilize certain reactions more often than others. Further, developmental theory suggests that the transference derives not only from unconscious ties to significant childhood figures, but also contains elements of significant object relationships acquired (internalized) during adult life, for example, spousal, child, (or filial) and peer transferences (Nemiroff and Colarusso 1985a). Table 24-1 summarizes some of the age-related conflicts that tend to be associated with certain transferences that arise in therapy.

Frail elderly, struggling with various fears and conflicts (including abandonment to institutions by their adult children and helpless reliance on caregivers) easily develop parental transferences with hopes for an idealized, magical protector and savior. The self in the transference constellation is experienced as weak and helpless, while the other (e.g., physician or nurse) is powerful and protective. At times the patient, especially when disappointed, may angrily reject the therapist and relate to the therapist as an abandoning parent, child, or spouse.

Narcissistic assaults inherent in lost beauty, power, and physical prowess often promote an idealizing and/or mirror transference to the therapist. The patient experiences himself or herself as a powerful, admired person just as the patient perceives the therapist as powerful and admired. The patient unconsciously believes that the therapist is admiring and beneficent to him or her and basks in the fantasized approval attributed to the therapist. Frail patients, often institutionalized and having to cope with pain, illness, and lost capacity, are prone to these transference constellations.

Bereavement and grief, especially for a lost spouse, may lead the patient to unconsciously turn to the therapist as a wished-for replacement leading to spousal or "lover" transference that may be eroticized. The patient identifies with a much more youthful self-image and sees himself or herself as sexually appropriate for the therapist (Crusey 1985). Similar eroticized transference may be mobilized as the patient becomes aware of his or her sexual decline

Table 24-1. Age-related conflicts associated with transference

Age-related conflict	Developmental stage	Transference
Giving up of ideal goals (Kahana 1987a)	Normative	Sibling rivalry; envy; jealousy; peer; mirror
Sexual decline/ unavailability	Normative	Erotic
Loss of roles	Normative	Sibling rivalry; idealized filial or peer
Conflict over death and mortality (Segal 1958)	Whole spectrum	Idealized protector, negative filial, or parental
Conflicts with adult children (Meerloo 1955; Myers 1984)	Whole spectrum	Filial
Bereavement (Levin 1965b)	Normative/crisis	Spousal, erotic, or peer
Narcissistic assaults (Grunes 1987; Lazarus 1980, 1988)	Normative/frail	Mirror, idealized, or peer; rivalry; envy
Dependency/abandonment (Levin 1965a)	Frail/crisis	Parental
Vulnerability/helplessness (Goldfarb 1956)	Frail/crisis	Idealized; magical savior
Pain, illness, lost capacity to adapt (Gitelson 1981)	Frail/crisis	Parental, idealized, or filial

and the unavailability of sexual objects. This normative stage of self-awareness may also lead to intense negative feelings toward the therapist, who may be perceived as unable or unwilling to restore to the patient his or her lost youth and sexuality. Beneath the anger lies depressive loss of self-esteem.

Classical oedipal conflicts also arise in the transference, leading the patient to experience libidinal or aggressive feelings toward the therapist associated with anxiety and neurotic behavior generated by the unconscious neurotic conflict.

The normative giving up of occupation through retirement can lead to loss of self-esteem and an angry or depressive sibling rivalry transference. The patient may begin to feel like the devalued, unloved child, while perceiving the therapist as the successful, valued child. Conscious or unconscious conflicts over death and mortality may cause the patient to view the therapist as an idealized, magical protector with parental, filial, or spousal qualities, who will ward off the inevitability of death. The realistic inability of the therapist to provide the needed comfort and protection may then induce negative, angry feelings toward the perceived, disappointing parental, spousal, or filial transference figure.

Geriatric patients may develop "apparent" transference resistances to therapy in which they challenge the therapist, for example, as being too young and inexperienced and therefore incapable of understanding the old. This defensive stance, however, often is the patient's initial defense against deeper fears of lost self-esteem. In this version of the so-called reverse transference (Grotjahn 1955; Levin 1965; Myers 1984), the patient adopts the "old-experienced" self-perception, whereas the therapist is seen as young and therefore in need of help and education. Another version of the reverse transference may be evident when the patient adopts a kindly parental stance. However, beneath the surface interaction, whether positive or negative, often lurk feelings of helplessness and inferiority and fears of decline.

Countertransference

Therapists often do not advise or think of psychotherapy for the elderly (Ford and Sbordone 1980). Countertransference (unconscious reactions to the patient) and counterreactions (conscious reactions) may account for much of this apparent avoidance (Butler and Lewis 1977). Counterreactions include feeling that the elderly are unattractive, unproductive, close to death, chronic, unchangeable, and unrewarding. These ideas about therapy of the elderly are not supported by clinical experience.

The frail elderly, especially those who are institutionalized, are more likely to mobilize the therapist's own unresolved conflicts about aging, including unconscious fears of illness, decline, and death (Nemiroff and Colarusso 1985a; Yesavage and Karasu 1982). Therapists may become anxious about their patient's apparent helplessness and dependency, which promote fears of engulfment and can lead to withdrawal from, or rejection of, the patient. Conversely, in the face of the patient's decline, therapists may act on a grandiose need to conquer the forces of aging (Myers 1984). The therapist's narcissism is easily at risk in these circumstances, and he or she may experience depression or unreasonable anger (Nemiroff and Colarusso 1985a). When the therapist overidentifies with the patient's problems, feelings of pity and sadness may arise (Hiatt 1971) that block accurate empathy and realistic exploration of the possibilities for change. Conversely, the therapist may unconsciously avoid the pain of accurately empathizing with the patient's loneliness and loss. If overwhelmed by the patient's problems, the therapist may avoid termination, because of the conviction that he or she is keeping the patient alive, so that continuing therapy becomes a defense to ward off the patient's death (King 1980).

With geriatric patients, especially in the normative-aging group, therapists (particularly those who are younger and inexperienced) may be shocked and/or repelled when they encounter erotic countertransference feelings in themselves. Belief in the asexuality of the aged (Meerloo 1953) can act as a defense against unresolved conflicts over parental sexuality or oedipal conflicts (Myers 1984; Nemiroff and Colarusso 1985a; Zinberg and Kaufman 1963).

Therapy with older patients may mobilize countertransference feelings associated with unresolved conflicts with parents more readily than with younger patients (King 1980; Myers 1986). For example, unresolved hostility to his or her parent may lead the therapist to a defensive idealization of the patient or inappropriate reliance on superficial, supportive modes of intervention—either way, avoidance of deeper areas of psychological conflict is permitted (Grotjahn 1955; Lazarus and Weinberg 1980). Similar feelings may lead to an unconscious wish to dominate the patient (parent) and promote an overmedicalized or controlling stance.

Use of Defenses

In general, the dramatic defensive maneuvers of youth—such as promiscuity, self-destructive actions like self-mutilation, and antisocial behaviors—seem to abate in old age (Sadavoy 1987), although long-term follow-up and study of the elderly with regard to these behaviors has not yet been done. The frail elderly are more likely to use defenses of withdrawal, infirmity, and physical preoccupation to deal with intrapsychic conflict and anxieties. Therapeutic involvement may be avoided, with claims of illness or immobility, or patients may take refuge in past accomplishments, overusing reminiscence and avoiding the present, including the transference. The normative group demonstrates a fuller range of defenses, which, however, take on an age-related coloration, for example, denial of aging by attempts at youthful dress, seductiveness, or physical activity. In crises or periods of decline, regression may be intense.

Defenses and other unconscious material are expressed in a variety of forms, including dreams (Myers 1984) and acting out (Kahana 1987a, 1987b; Miller 1987; Nemiroff and Colarusso 1985a; Sadavoy and Leszcz 1987).

Termination

In general, clinical evidence suggests that open-ended therapeutic relationships are often necessary in psychotherapy of the elderly because of the frequency of recurrent crises in the life of the aging patient. Conflicts associated with issues of remaining life span and mortality, loneliness, abandonment, and dependency are mobilized by termination. However, the older patient with good interpersonal supports and ego strengths often will be able to work through disengagement conflicts (Cath 1975).

Specialized Approaches to Psychotherapy of the Elderly

Psychotherapy With the Cognitively Impaired

Psychodynamic issues remain important in the cognitively impaired and influence interpersonal relationships, behavior expression, and response to treatment (Cohen 1989). Psychotherapeutic interventions with this group address the remaining reflective capacity of the individual patient while at the same time using psychodynamic understanding to intervene at the level of environmental manipulation and family and caregiver education and support. Often therapy is directed at minimizing "excess disability" (Brody et al. 1971; Kahn 1965).

A wide variety of psychotherapy techniques has been employed with these patients, most often in institutions. Cognitive-behavioral techniques often focus on changing specific target behaviors. Goals of therapy include increasing the patient's level of participation in activities of daily living; enhancing social interest and interaction; and improving skills in communication and such concrete tasks as toileting, bathing, ambulation, and feeding (Hussian 1984). Studies suggest that behavior therapies are most effective when integrated with milieu and other individual techniques (Sadavoy and Robinson 1989; Tobin 1989). Similar results have been shown for reality orientation techniques, that is, the more interactive and "person centered" the interventions, the greater the improvement (Hanley et al. 1981).

Individual psychotherapy may be useful for the cognitively impaired if employed judiciously and with well-defined goals (Cohen 1989; Sadavoy and Robinson 1989), although no controlled studies are yet available. Occasional references to intensive psychotherapy are made in the literature (Grotjahn 1940; Hollos and Ferenczi 1925; Sadavoy and Robinson 1989), but these efforts are best viewed as investigative rather than of practical value.

Goldfarb and Turner (1953) pioneered a useful and practical psychotherapeutic intervention to bolster self-worth and a sense of mastery in the institutionalized elderly. This method is based on the patient's need for sustaining selfobject relations and self-esteem enhancement (Lazarus 1980, 1988). During once-weekly, 15-minute sessions, the therapist encourages an idealizing transference, enhancing the patient's sense of control and self-esteem by encouraging him or her to identify with and "borrow" the therapist's apparent power and prestige. The therapist tries to carry out a patient's request, thus fostering the patient's sense of mastery, control, and power over the therapist. Goldfarb's open, uncontrolled study showed this method to be effective if patients had neither psychosis nor major depression. Of 59 patients divided into three groups—psychosis without brain damage ($n = 5$), neurosis and personality disorder ($n = 13$), and chronic brain syndrome ($n = 41$)—28 improved and 18 stabilized using this method; only 15 of these cases were seen for more than 10 sessions.

Communication with the cognitively impaired patient begins with a basic understanding and knowledge of both his or her behavior as well as its psychodynamic underpinnings. Behavior and verbal expression may be otherwise unintelligible to the uninformed caregiver (Cohen 1989; Sadavoy and Robinson 1989).

The more advanced the cognitive decline, the greater the patient's need to interact on a nonverbal level, for example, through activity, movement, or music. Frequently, cognitive impairment is accompanied by delusions. Gentle redirection of the patient's attention to another focus, or simple distraction of the patient's attention may be helpful (Cohen 1989), as is empathic reintroduction of reality and "jogging" the patient's memory, especially with use of memory aids such as pictures and memorabilia (Sadavoy and Robinson 1989). However, aggressive reality orientation can exacerbate psychosis or increase the patient's agitation. For the most frail, individual therapy often is most effective and efficient when brief, frequent contact is used 5 to 10 minutes several times a week, focused on day-to-day issues. Questions are brief, focused, and concrete rather than abstract. The flow of communication commonly is slow, and therapists give the patient ample time to respond, while avoiding being too reflective or unstructured.

The therapist is most helpful if able to tolerate the often ambiguous, impoverished, repetitive, and sometimes bizarre verbal interactions with these patients. Such patients often have a need to idealize the therapist, who must be able to tolerate the idealization despite his or her knowledge of therapeutic limitations.

Reminiscence or Life Review Therapy

Some authors have suggested that the realization of one's mortality leads the aging person to reflect on and reminisce about the past—a process that helps the person to conceptualize his or her life over time and to give it significance and meaning (Butler 1963). Reminiscence is characterized by the expression of memories of past experiences, especially those that were meaningful or conflictual.

To varying degrees, most patients in therapy, including the elderly, reminisce about the past, seek meaning for their life, and strive for some resolution of interpersonal and intrapsychic conflicts. The purpose of life review therapy is to enhance this process and make it more conscious and deliberate. Lewis and Butler (1974) reported that this technique helps to resolve old problems; increases tolerance of conflict; relieves guilt and fears; and enhances creativity, generosity, and acceptance of the present. Normative aspects of reminiscence and life review are more fully discussed in Chapter 5.

Life review therapy includes encouraging the patient to return to places of earlier experiences, write or tape his or her autobiography, reunite with family and old friends, review memorabilia, and attempt verbal or written summations of his or her life. However, despite its usefulness, this therapy may be contraindicated for patients who have realistic or overwhelming guilt about the past or who otherwise cannot cope with unmourned or unresolvable past disappointments and losses.

Brief Psychodynamic Psychotherapy

A brief psychodynamic therapy approach can be considered for elderly patients with clearly defined, circumscribed problems that can be expected to resolve within a limited amount of time. Examples of problems amenable to brief psychotherapy include adjustment disorder, grief reaction, and traumatic stress disorder that has not become chronic and entrenched. Setting a time limit on therapy reinforces the patient's confidence in his or her ability to resolve the problem, focuses and accelerates the therapeutic process, diminishes the patient's fear of protracted dependency on the therapist, and considers the patient's limited finances.

A recent, preliminary, uncontrolled study of the process and outcome of brief, psychodynamic psychotherapy with eight elderly outpatients used individually constructed outcome scales for each patient (Lazarus et al. 1987). Seven of the eight outpatients (ranging in age from 63 to 77) met the DSM-III (American Psychiatric Association 1980) criteria for either an adjustment disorder with depressed mood or dysthymic disorder, and one patient had a panic disorder. Patients received 15 therapy sessions, and each was videotaped for subsequent outcome ratings by researchers. Analysis of variance for measuring outcome on seven scales for each patient at the end of treatment and at 6-month follow-up demonstrated that seven of the eight subjects showed significant lessening of their presenting symptoms ($p < .01$) and some resolution of their focal conflict. The four women showed greater improvement earlier, and maintained the improvement longer than the men did.

Study of the process of therapy with these elderly outpatients revealed that patients often used the therapeutic relationship to reestablish a sense of self over time and/or to consolidate diverse and disparate aspects of the self into a more positive sense of self. The therapist was used by the patient for validation of competency and normalcy and for restoration of feelings of mastery and self-esteem.

The generalizability of the results of this preliminary study to other elderly outpatients is limited by the small sample size and reliance on unvalidated, individualized scales.

Cognitive Psychotherapy

Cognitive psychotherapy (Beck et al. 1979) is a brief therapy approach that uses interpretations, explanations, and practical information to correct the depressed patient's stereotypic, self-defeating thoughts and dysfunctional attitudes. The goal is to promote integration of positive perceptions and thinking patterns and thereby diminish depression. Patients learn to reverse their negative cognitive sets by the following five processes: 1) learning to monitor negative thoughts, 2) recognizing connections between negative thoughts and feelings of depression, 3) examining the evidence for and against specific automatic thoughts, 4) learning to identify and alter dysfunctional beliefs that sustain these negative cognitions, and 5) developing more reality-oriented and adaptive strategies for coping with depression.

Modifications of cognitive therapy have been suggested to address the special problems of elderly depressed patients (Gallagher and Thompson 1982). These modifications include 1) acclimatizing patients for therapy (e.g., presenting therapy as a way to learn to adjust to the stress of life, and encouraging active participation in the therapeutic process); 2) enhancing learning capabilities (e.g., by empathically understanding the patient's hesitation to try therapeutic suggestions); and 3) terminating therapy gradually (e.g., anticipating future problems and leaving the door open for the patient to return). If patients complain they are "too old to change," the therapist may respond, "Perhaps it is true that you cannot learn new ways of thinking about your problems, but how will you know this for certain unless you try?" If the patient complains that the therapist is "too young to help," the therapist can encourage temporary suspension of this belief so that a trial of therapy can proceed.

Clinical studies and experience to date indicate that cognitive therapy is especially efficacious for cognitively intact, motivated elderly patients with minor and major depressions. A comparison of three brief therapy approaches—cognitive, behavioral, and psychodynamic—for elderly outpatients with major depression found that all three were equally efficacious at the completion of therapy (the overall positive response rate for the three therapies was 70%; 52% had complete remission and 18% showed significant symptomatic improvement). There was a trend at follow-up for those treated with either cognitive or behavioral therapy to maintain their improvement more than those treated psychodynamically (Thompson et al. 1987). Age was not a predictor of outcome: very elderly patients responded as well as younger elderly patients to all three treatment modalities. Patients with major depression who tended to be unresponsive to all three treatment modalities had many endogenous signs, a concomitant personality disorder, and low expectations of improvement (Thompson et al. 1988).

Karasu (1986) reviewed therapeutic factors accounting for change in various psychotherapies. He believed that the positive aspects of cognitive therapy in adult patients (which may have application to the elderly) include its structured procedures and time-limited nature, expectation of positive change, consideration of limited financial resources, support of higher-level defense mechanisms, encouragement of the patient's active participation, and potential for integration with other treatment modalities (e.g., behavioral or psychodynamic). Shortcomings include its restricted application to depression and less severely impaired patients and the potential (when used as the sole treatment modality) to produce overintellectualization and (if applied mechanically) to foster isolation of the patient's feelings. As noted by Thompson and colleagues (1988), patients with many endogenous signs were less responsive to cognitive therapy.

Personality Disorders

Elderly patients with a Cluster B (DSM-III-R) personality disorder (American Psychiatric Association 1987) tend to be excessively demanding, extremely sensitive, emotionally labile, and impulsive, and they may engage in destructive, acting-out behavior. They often have few or inadequate support systems because of their propensity for unstable relationships. Therapists may become frustrated because of the preponderance of demands and expectations.

Similar signs and symptoms are present in the personality-disordered elderly patient that are present in the younger adult but with modifications brought on by age-relevant factors, such as confinement to a nursing home and physical infirmities. These elderly patients, because of impaired motoric behavior and generalized "slowing down," are less likely than their younger counterparts to flagrantly act out with criminality or promiscuity. Passive-dependent behavior, social withdrawal, apathy, and vulnerability to depression may be prominent. Whereas the elderly patient without significant character pathology shows some resiliency and flexibility in dealing with change and traumata associated with aging, the personality-disordered patient remains rigid, overwhelmed, and unable to adapt to age-related stresses.

Presentation

The elderly patient with a personality disorder in the dramatic, Cluster B spectrum carries with him or her psychopathology established in early stages of intrapsychic development. Sadavoy (1987) pointed to five unresolved intrapsychic maldevelopments that affect the elderly patient with a personality disorder: 1) fear of abandonment or loneliness; 2) real or fantasied narcissistic injury to self-esteem and failure of self and selfobject relationships; 3) impaired affect tolerance; 4) failure in the development of modulators of rage, which in turn leads to increased use of splitting; and 5) loss of self-cohesion induced by age-associated stressors, which may be so extreme as to cause brief psychotic episodes.

Dysfunction of intrapsychic structure can impair mourning and ability to cope with grief. This issue is a particularly familiar and difficult one to address in geriatric treatment because elderly patients are routinely faced with the task of dealing with losses.

As at other ages, these patients express their personality disorders in many ways. Most frequent is their pathological way of relating to family and other caregivers. The patient may become increasingly helpless (Breslau 1987) and exhibit panicky behavior, for example, calling family members for unreasonable reassurances. Patients may make incessant demands that interfere with family obligations, expecting that others will change plans and cancel activities in order to respond to their requests. Such behavior eventually angers and frustrates family, caregivers, and/or staff. Treatment of concomitant anxiety can often lessen the patient's demands and acting out. A second presentation consists of exaggerated somatic complaints that cannot be alleviated by reassurance.

A third presentation is depressive withdrawal. Some of these patients exhibit anhedonia, apathy, anorexia, and loss of the will to live. In these cases, life-threatening depressions may be superimposed on the personality disorder, and they require vigorous treatment.

Treatment

In developing a treatment plan, consideration is given to the patient's pathological behavior, to the stresses on the family and health care team, and to the patient's ability to engage in individual psychotherapy. Various treatment strategies have been suggested, although no formal studies of effectiveness have been undertaken to date. Sadavoy and Dorian (1983) described a psychodynamic approach that incorporates behavioral techniques for use in a long-term care setting. He enlists the help of the family and/or other caregivers in preparing a written statement of expected behavior from the patient. This approach takes into account the patient's underlying psychodynamics as evident, for example, in his or her need for a sense of control, as well as recognizing the limitations of the staff's tolerance of the patient's unreasonable demands, acting out, and other disturbing behavior. The staff sets nonpunitive limits on verbal and physical acting out, specific requirements for participation in prescribed activities, adherence to medication schedules, and conditions for privileges. With a clearly spelled-out contract, a working alliance may be established that includes family and caregivers who work together to strive for mutually established goals.

In individual therapy with these patients, the therapist adjusts the frequency of sessions, titrating the intensity of therapy against the patient's sensitivity to rejection and forestalling the patient's feeling overwhelmed with rage and anxiety. Therapy focuses on helping the patient to connect feelings to causal events, thus promoting maintenance of self-esteem and self-cohesion. Developmental history is largely used for understanding the patient's needs and actions; Sadavoy limits the emphasis on past unresolvable losses and mourning during the earlier phases of treatment, focusing instead on current issues. This technique employs clarification and confrontation instead of deeper interpretations. In some cases, as a working alliance develops, a measure of working through of unresolved mourning may be attempted.

Gabbard (1989) addressed the issue of "splitting," a common defense of the adult patient with a personality disorder, which is also found in elderly patients. The reality of the caregiver's efforts is distorted by the disordered intrapsychic self of the patient. The caregiver is perceived as either good or bad, as defined by split-off, internal representations from the patient's past. For example, the patient may willingly accept medication from one caregiver but not from another. Thus, the same situation provokes either compliant or negativistic reaction, depending on the patient's intrapsychic assessment of a particular caregiver, despite the fact that each caregiver may behave in a similar fashion toward the patient. The psychotherapist deals with the internal world of the patient by using explanations, clarifications, and sometimes interpretations, with the goal of minimizing splitting of internal self and object representations. Staff intervention addresses the integration and moderation of the external world of the patient.

Use of Medication

Medication is often an important component of the comprehensive treatment plan. Patients' compliance with medication may be compromised because of distrust of the physician and staff, susceptibility to side effects, and negative beliefs and attitudes about these medications on the part of the patient, family, and other care-givers (Lazarus and Mershon 1987).

Summary

Many clinical reports and a limited number of outcome studies support the contention that elderly patients are very responsive to various modalities of psychotherapy. Individual psychotherapy with the elderly is distinguished from that with younger adults by 1) attention to specific developmental tasks and challenges associated with aging; 2) the need for especially active therapeutic intervention to overcome patient, family, and health care system barriers to treatment; 3) the nature of the transference and counter-transference reactions and resistances; and 4) the need to employ specialized psychotherapeutic approaches for the frail, demented, and personality-disordered patient. The therapist of the elderly maintains a flexible approach because the patient's changing clinical status may require a shift from one treatment approach to another. For many elderly patients, insight-oriented psychotherapy provides an opportunity to resolve new and old conflicts while helping to give meaning to a lifetime of experience. For the frail elderly, supportive psychotherapy and environmental manipulation can shore up healthy defenses; provide for a caring, protective environment; help preserve self-respect and self-esteem; and provide understanding and guidance to an often bewildered family.

References

American Psychiatric Association: Diagnostic and Statistical Manual of Mental Disorders, 3rd Edition. Washington, DC, American Psychiatric Association, 1980

American Psychiatric Association: Diagnostic and Statistical Manual of Mental Disorders, 3rd Edition, Revised. Washington, DC, American Psychiatric Association, 1987

Aronson MJ: Psychotherapy in a home for the aged. Arch Neurol Psychiatry 79:671–674, 1958

Atchley RC: The aging self. Psychotherapy: Theory, Research, and Practice 9:338–396, 1982

Beck A, Rush J, Shaw BF, et al: Cognitive Therapy of Depression. New York, Guilford, 1979

Berezin M: Psychodynamic considerations of aging and the aged: an overview. Am J Psychiatry 128:12, 33–41, 1972

Berezin M: Reflections on psychotherapy with the elderly, in Treating the Elderly With Psychotherapy: The Scope for Change in Later Life. Edited by Sadavoy J, Leszcz M. Madison, CT, International Universities Press, 1987, pp 45–63

Blau D, Berezin MA: Neurosis and character disorders, in Modern Perspectives in the Psychiatry of Old Age. Edited by Howells JG. New York, Brunner/Mazel, 1975, pp 201–233

Breslau L: Exaggerated helplessness syndrome, in Treating the Elderly With Psychotherapy: The Scope for Change in Later Life. Edited by Sadavoy J, Leszcz M. Madison, CT, International Universities Press, 1987

Brody E, Kleban MH, Lawton MP, et al: Excess disabilities of mentally impaired aged: impact of individualized treatment. Gerontologist Summer, Part I: 124–134, 1971

Butler RN: The life review: an interpretation of reminiscence in the aged. Psychiatry 26:65–70, 1963

Butler RN, Lewis MI: Aging and Mental Health: Positive Psychosocial Approaches. St. Louis, MO, Mosby, 1977

Cath SH: Some dynamics of middle and later years: a study in depletion and restitution, in Geriatric Psychiatry: Grief, Loss, and Emotional Disorders in the Aging Process. Edited by Berezin MA, Cath SH. New York, International Universities Press, 1975, pp 21–72

Cath SH: Functional disorders: an organismic view and attempt at reclassification, in Geriatric Psychiatry. Edited by Bellak L, Karasu TB. New York, Grune & Stratton, 1976

Cohen GD: Psychodynamic perspectives in the clinical approach to brain disease in the elderly, in Psychiatric Consequences of Brain Disease in the Elderly. Edited by Conn D, Grek A, Sadavoy J. New York, Plenum Press, 1989, pp 85–99

Crusey J: Short-term psychodynamic psychotherapy with a sixty-two-year-old man, in The Race Against Time. Edited by Nemiroff RA, Colarusso CA. New York, Plenum Press, 1985

Eisdorfer C, Stotsky BA: Intervention, treatment and rehabilitation of psychiatric disorders, in The Handbook of the Psychology of Aging. Edited by Birren JE, Schaie KW. New York, Van Nostrand Reinhold, 1977

Erikson EH: The human life cycle, in International Encyclopedia of the Social Sciences. Edited by Sills DL. New York, Macmillan, 1968, pp 286–292

Feigenbaum E: Ambulatory treatment of the elderly, in Mental Illness in Later Life. Edited by Busse EW, Pfeiffer E. Washington, DC, American Psychiatric Association, 1973

Ford CV, Sbordone RT: Attitudes of psychiatrists toward elderly patients. Am J Psychiatry 137:571–575, 1980

Gabbard GO: Splitting in hospital treatment. Am J Psychiatry 146:444–451, 1989

Gaitz GM: Barriers to the delivery of psychiatric services to the elderly. Gerontologist 14:210–214, 1974

Gallagher DE, Thompson LW: Differential effectiveness of psychotherapies for the treatment of major depressive disorders in older adult patients. Psychotherapy: Theory, Research and Practice 19:482–490, 1982

Gallagher DE, Thompson LW: Effectiveness of psychotherapy for both endogenous and non-endogenous depression in older adult outpatients. J Gerontol 38:707–712, 1983

Gitelson MA: The emotional problems of elderly persons, in Readings in Psychotherapy with Older People. Edited by Steury S, Blank ML. Washington, DC, National Institute of Mental Health, 1981, pp 8–17

Goldfarb AI: Psychotherapy of the aged: The use and value of an adaptational frame of reference. Psychoanalytic Review 43:168–181, 1956

Goldfarb AI, Sheps J: Psychotherapy of the aged. Psychosom Med 16:209–219, 1954

Goldfarb AI, Turner H: Psychotherapy of aged persons, II: utilization and effectiveness of "brief" therapy. Am J Psychiatry 109:916–921, 1953

Grotjahn JM: Psychoanalytic investigation of a 71-year-old man with senile dementia. Psychoanal Q 9:80–97, 1940

Grotjahn M: Analytic psychotherapy with the elderly. Psychoanal Rev 42:419–427, 1955

Grunes JM: The aged in psychotherapy: psychodynamic contributions to the treatment process, in Treating the Elderly With Psychotherapy: The Scope for Change in Later Life. Edited by Sadavoy J, Leszcz M. Madison, CT, International Universities Press, 1987, pp 31–44

Hanley IG, McGuire RJ, Boyd WD: Reality orientation and dementia: a controlled trial of two approaches. Br J Psychiatry 138:10–14, 1981

Hiatt H: Dynamic psychotherapy with the aging patient. Am J Psychother 25:591–600, 1971

Hollos S, Ferenczi S: Psychoanalysis and the Psychic Disorder of General Paresis. New York, Nervous and Mental Disease, 1925

Hussian RA: Behavioral Geriatrics. Progress in Behaviour Modification, Vol 16. New York, Academic Press, 1984, pp 159–183

Jacques E: Death and the mid-life crisis. Int J Psychoanal 46:502–514, 1965

Kahana R: Strategies of dynamic psychotherapy with the wide range of older individuals. J Geriatr Psychiatry 12:71–100, 1979

Kahana R: Discussion: The Oedipus complex and rejuvenation fantasies in the analysis of a seventy-year-old woman. J Geriatr Psychiatry 20:53–60, 1987a

Kahana R: Geriatric psychotherapy: beyond crisis management, in Treating the Elderly With Psychotherapy: The Scope for Change in Later Life. Edited by Sadavoy J, Leszcz M. Madison, CT, International Universities Press, 1987b, pp 233–263

Kahn RS: Comments, in Proceedings of the York House Institute on the Mentally Impaired Aged. Philadelphia, PA, Philadelphia Geriatric Center, 1965

Karasu TB: The specificity versus nonspecificity dilemma: toward identifying therapeutic change agents. Am J Psychiatry 143:687–695, 1986

King PMH: The life cycle as indicated by the nature of the transference in the psychoanalysis of the middle-aged and elderly. Int J Psychoanal 61:153–159, 1980

Lazarus LW: Self psychology and psychotherapy with the elderly: theory and practice. J Geriatr Psychiatry 13:69–88, 1980

Lazarus L: Self-psychology—its application to brief psychotherapy with the elderly. J Geriatr Psychiatry 21:109–125, 1988

Lazarus LW, Mershon S: Psychiatric drugs and the elderly, in Handbook of Applied Gerontology. Edited by Lesnoff-Caravaglia G. New York, Human Sciences Press, 1987, pp 119–126

Lazarus LW, Weinberg J: Treatment in the ambulatory-care setting, in Handbook of Geriatric Psychiatry. Edited by Busse EW, Blazer DG. New York, Van Nostrand Reinhold, 1980, pp 427–452

Lazarus LW, Groves L, Guttman D, et al: Brief psychotherapy with the elderly: a study of process and outcome, in Treating the Elderly With Psychotherapy: The Scope for Change in Later Life. Edited by Sadavoy J, Leszcz M. Madison, CT, International Universities Press, 1987, pp 265–293

Levin S: Some comments on the distribution of narcissistic and object libido in the aged. Int J Psychoanal 46:200–208, 1965a

Levin S: Depression in the aged, in Geriatric Psychiatry: Grief, Loss, and Emotional Disorders in the Aging Process. Edited by Berezin MA, Cath S. New York, International Universities Press, 1965b, pp 203–225

Lewis MI, Butler RN: Life-review therapy: putting memories to work in individual and group psychotherapy. Geriatrics 29:11, 165–169, 172–173, 1974

Meerloo JAM: Contribution of psychoanalysis to the problem of the aged, in Psychoanalysis and Social Work. Edited by Hermann M. New York, International Universities Press, 1953, pp 321–337

Meerloo JAM: Transference and resistance in geriatric psychotherapy. Psychoanal Rev 42:72–82, 1955

Meissner WW: Normal psychology of the aging process revisited, I: discussion. Paper presented at the Annual Scientific Meeting of the Boston Society of Gerontologic Psychiatry, 1975

Miller E: The Oedipus complex and rejuvenation fantasies in the analysis of a seventy-year-old woman. J Geriatr Psychiatry 20:29–51, 1987

Myers WA: Dynamic Therapy of the Older Patient. New York, Jason Aronson, 1984, p 6

Myers WA: Transference and countertransference issues in treatments involving older patients and younger therapists. J Geriatr Psychiatry 19:221–239, 1986

Nemiroff RA, Colarusso CA: The literature on psychotherapy and psychoanalysis in the second half of life, in The Race Against Time. Edited by Nemiroff RA, Colarusso CA. New York, Plenum, 1985a, pp 25–43

Nemiroff RA, Colarusso CA: Discussion, in The Race Against Time. Edited by Nemiroff RA, Colarusso CA. New York, Plenum, 1985b, pp 117–120

Neugarten B: Time, age and the life-cycle. Am J Psychiatry 136:887–894, 1979

Pollock GH: The mourning-liberation process: ideas on the inner life of the older adult, in Treating the Elderly With Psychotherapy: The Scope for Change in Later Life. Edited by Sadavoy J, Leszcz M. Madison, CT, International Universities Press, 1987, pp 3–29

Rechtschaffen A: Psychotherapy with geriatric patients: a review of the literature. J Gerontol 14:73–84, 1959

Rosenthal HM: The use of psychoanalytic principles in the treatment of older people. Am J Psychoanal 45:119–134, 1985

Sadavoy J: Character disorders in the elderly: an overview, in Treating the Elderly With Psychotherapy: The Scope for Change in Later Life. Edited by Sadavoy J, Leszcz M. Madison, CT, International Universities Press, 1987, pp 175–229

Sadavoy J, Dorian B: Treatment of the elderly characterologically disturbed patient in the chronic care institution. J Geriatr Psychiatry 16:223–240, 1983

Sadavoy J, Leszcz M (eds): Treating the Elderly With Psychotherapy: The Scope for Change in Later Life. Madison, CT, International Universities Press, 1987

Sadavoy J, Reiman-Sheldon E: General hospital geriatric psychiatric treatment: a follow-up study. J Am Geriatr Soc 31:200–205, 1983

Sadavoy J, Robinson A: Psychotherapy and the cognitively impaired elderly, in Psychiatric Consequences of Brain Disease in the Elderly. Edited by Conn D, Grek A, Sadavoy J. New York, Plenum, 1989, pp 101–135

Sandler AM: A developmental crisis in an aging patient: comments on development and adaptation. J Geriatr Psychiatry 15:11–32, 1982

Segal H: Fear of death (notes on the analysis of an old man). Int J Psychoanal 39:178–181, 1958

Simon A, Lowenthal MF: Crisis and Intervention: The Fate of the Elderly Mental Patient. San Francisco, CA, Jossey-Bass, 1970

Steuer J: Psychotherapy with the elderly. Psychiatr Clin North Am 5:199–213, 1982

Thompson LW, Gallagher D, Breckenridge JS: Comparative effectiveness of psychotherapies for depressed elders. J Consult Clin Psychol 55:385–390, 1987

Thompson LW, Gallagher D, Czirr R: Personality disorder and outcome in the treatment of late-life depression. J Geriatr Psychiatry 21:133–153, 1988

Tobin SS: Issues of care in long-term settings, in Psychiatric Consequences of Brain Disease in the Elderly. Edited by Conn D, Grek A, Sadavoy J. New York, Plenum, 1989, pp 163–187

Weisman AD, Hackett TP: Denial as a social act, in Psychodynamic Studies on Aging, Creativity, Reminiscing, and Dying. Edited by Levin S, Kahana RJ. New York, International Universities Press, 1967, pp 79–110

Wheelright JB: Some comments on the aging process. Psychiatry 22:407–411, 1959

Yalom I: Existential Psychotherapy. New York, Basic Books, 1980

Yesavage JA, Karasu TB: Psychotherapy with elderly patients. Am J Psychother 36:41–55, 1982

Zinberg NE: The relation of regressive phenomena to the aging process, in Normal Psychology of the Aging Process. Edited by Zinberg NE, Kaufman I. New York, International Universities Press, 1963, pp 123–137

Zinberg ME, Kaufman I: Cultural and personality factors associated with aging: an introduction, in Norman Psychology of the Aging Process. Edited by Zinberg NE, Kaufman I. New York, International Universities Press, 1963, pp 17–71

CHAPTER 25

Marion Goldstein, M.D.

Family Therapy

Overview

The practice of family therapy with elderly individuals—whether based on family systems theory, family developmental theories, or intergenerational approaches—will continue to take on considerably more prominence regardless of whether resources increase for the elderly and their providers of care. If resources increase, more elderly couples and families will be able to avail themselves of such therapy. If resources do not increase, the acute, intermittent and chronic problems and disabilities that occur during the aging process will require even more creative coping strategies on the part of families. Help with coping strategies becomes a necessity in an era of federal, state, and local budget deficits, whereas formal resources such as access to psychiatric hospitalization, clinics, respite care, home health care, long-term care, and flexibility in the workplace become entitlements in an era of affluence.

As early as 1966, Brody suggested that the total family, rather than the aged individual alone, should be considered the patient-client when an elderly person is brought for professional help (Brody 1966).

There is usually an interval of many years before theory and research findings are translated into clinical practice. For example, despite the importance and efficacy of family therapy, there is yet no Medicare procedure code for family therapy. Family members of the elderly who are insured by health maintenance organizations may require referral by primary care physicians who have not been trained in assessing the need for such a psychiatric refer-

513

ral. In such a situation, a self-referral for psychiatric care leads to lack of insurance coverage. Many family members themselves require education in order to become aware of the potential effectiveness of family therapy and require time to overcome resistance to participation.

Family therapy can facilitate arrival at a level of filial maturity that will enhance appropriate role definition and more comfortable adaptation to midlife and late-life developmental stages (Goldstein 1989c). The family therapist can contribute substantially to increased motivation among family members and to personal well-being, while attending to conflicts between connectedness versus separateness and autonomy versus dependence. Attention to these issues can lead to emotional growth of each participating family member. Acceptance of the process of redefinition of roles as conditions and circumstances require can contribute to survival of the family unit regardless of geographic proximity or distance.

Researchers have found that the family is the most important social group for older people and that families in general do not abandon their elder members (Comptroller General of the United States 1977; Shanas 1979a, 1979b; Horowitz 1985; Doty 1986; Stone et al. 1987). Family contacts remain especially frequent in the early and later parts of the life cycle. Powerful feelings and attitudes prevail, especially in times of crisis, and resurgence of past unresolved conflicts can occur. Unfinished developmental tasks from early life affect behaviors and family interactions in later life.

Demographic changes, especially increasing longevity and the greater frequency of divorces, have an impact on family relationships (Cicirelli 1983a). It is important to note that 73% to 93% of persons 65 years of age or older have at least one living brother or sister (Brubaker 1983). Vaillant and Vaillant (1990) have shown the increasing importance of sibling ties with advancing age. For the 4% to 6% of elderly who never married, it is often a niece or nephew who assists in dealing with the bureaucracy of support systems on behalf of the elderly relative (Brubaker 1983).

Marital status—besides physical and mental health, age, and gender—has considerable bearing on the role of the elderly person in the family setting. In the 1970s, one in five first marriages reached their 50th anniversary, with couples staying together regardless of the positive or negative nature of the relationship (Ade-Ridder 1983). Divorce and remarriage among the elderly is rising (Uhlenberg and Myers 1981). Retirement has the potential of affecting the quality of marital relationships either positively or negatively. Divorce, remarriage, and the reconstituted family in one or more generations contribute to the complexities of the modern family. Table 25-1 highlights the increasing percentage of widowed women with increasing longevity. Widowed women are the group of elderly who require the most care, and this is most often provided by daughters or daughters-in-law (Troll 1986).

Eighty percent of persons aged 65 and older have surviving children (Cicirelli 1983b). The number of children in a family is declining, and this trend is expected to continue. Fifty years ago, 50% of women had four or more children; now, however, only 25% of women have four or more children (Brubaker 1983). Elderly men are more likely to live with their children than elderly women (40% vs. 13.4%) (Brubaker 1983). Five percent of elderly aged 65 and older live in institutional settings, as do 20% of those over 80 years of age. Ten percent of persons over 65 have living parents (a situation of the old helping the very old or at times vice versa). With the high risk of disabilities and acute and chronic illness in this age group, the need for extrafamilial supports is escalated.

Table 25-1. Distribution of men and women aged 55 years and older by age group and marital status (March 1981)

	Male		Female	
Age and marital status	Number (thousands)	%	Number (thousands)	%
55–64				
Married, spouse present	8,275	81.7	7,762	67.1
Married, spouse absent	310	3.1	371	3.2
Widowed	410	4.0	2,128	18.4
Divorced	615	6.1	827	7.1
Never married	520	5.1	486	4.2
65–74				
Married, spouse present	5,429	80.6	4,247	48.3
Married, spouse absent	159	2.4	154	1.7
Widowed	551	8.2	3,524	40.1
Divorced	261	3.9	389	4.4
Never married	333	4.9	475	5.4
75 and older				
Married, spouse present	2,354	69.7	1,263	21.8
Married, spouse absent	75	2.2	84	1.4
Widowed	745	22.1	3,949	68.2
Divorced	83	2.4	133	2.3
Never married	119	3.5	359	6.2

Source. U.S. Bureau of the Census 1981.

The elderly are generally members of multigenerational families. Seventy percent of people over 65 have grandchildren, and 40% have great-grandchildren (Hagsted 1985). We do not know how family solidarity, intimacy, and conflicts prevail in and among sets of related generations.

Assessment of Family and Indications for Family Therapy

Indications for family therapy occur often during life transitions or at times of mental and physical illness of one or more family members. One of four of Medicare's 30 million beneficiaries enters the hospital annually. Early and immediate family assessment for need of further interventions or periodic follow-up should be available for each family member of a geriatric admission. In situations where staffing patterns do not allow such a service routinely, assessment is required at least for family members of geriatric patients who are unable to articulate their own needs. It is important that the assessment address the need and nature of care for the patient as well as for involved family members. Goals of assessment are many, but they include preventing the medical and mental health care of the elderly and their family members from being fragmented, and determining the nature and severity of the stress, and burden on and satisfaction of the caregivers.

Although the impact of family dynamics among family members on symptom formation and outcome of illness is not usually the presenting complaint, family assessment should be integrated into an optimal treatment plan for the elderly patients and their families.

Events of midlife and other life transitions that may precipitate need for family therapy are children leaving, retirement, widowhood, relocations, grandparenthood, losses of relationships through relocations, illness and death, and illness and disabilities. More than 80% of people older than 65 have at least one chronic medical problem, and multiple conditions are common (Taeuber 1983). The presence of disability complicates adaptation to normal aging processes on the part of the elderly individual and his or her family. On-time, normative incidents (Neugarten 1977) do not usually result in emotional crisis. However, incidents perceived as normative by individuals, family units, or society may vary with family value systems, generational differences, and contemporary social and ethnic trends.

Mental health concerns that require urgent assessment for family therapy are elder neglect, abuse or exploitation, late-life paranoia, depression, suicide, acute behavioral disturbance associated with dementia, alcohol and medication abuse, and psychosis. Elder abuse is perpetrated most frequently by stressed family members for whom insufficient supports and resources are available (Goldstein 1989a).

Different perceptions and misperceptions among family members about the condition of the elderly and the possible etiologies of the condition can contribute to conflict, lead to nonparticipation in care, and result in criticism of one another and the professionals involved. When these issues are not addressed they can fester and become chronic, hindering adequacy of care (Goldstein, unpublished observations).

Research has shown that changes in the mental health status of an elderly family member tend to be more bewildering and anxiety provoking to others in the family than physical impairments that cause loss of independence and autonomy (Grad and Sainsbury 1966; Deimling and Bass 1986). The effects of mental and/or physical disabilities of the elderly on the mental health of family members must be addressed. Decline of physical activities of daily living (bathing, feeding, dressing, toileting) or instrumental activities of daily living (doing laundry and household chores, managing money, traveling, shopping) requires not only modification of the lifestyle of other family members but also access to community resources. Any change in the condition of an elderly family member that provokes symptomatic resentment or anger, apprehension or fear, distrust, depression, worry or anxiety, guilt, ambivalence, or martyrdom in other family members is an indication for assessment for family therapy. Both the nature of the disability of the elderly and the reaction or lack thereof by one or more family members are indications for family therapy and follow-up. The acquisition by family members of a common knowledge base about the elderly person's condition is a first step in the family therapy process.

Sibling rivalry (Ross and Milgram 1982) and unresolved resentments about the past can increase when a parent can no longer live independently and the family has to decide about a new living arrangement. Clinging behavior of a disabled—and at times not-so-disabled—elderly family member can be a source of irritation to the rest of the family. The clinician should be aware that one out of four elderly, before reaching age 15, has experienced the death of a parent. Parent loss at a young age may contribute to current fears of abandonment, severe separation anxiety, and recurrences of depression, although some data do not support this assertion. In Vaillant and Vaillant's study of normative aging (1990), parental death per se did not predict later-life depression. These experiences in the family of origin can adversely affect the relationships with the family of procreation when resultant behaviors are misperceived and taken personally and out of context.

Another commonly recurring theme in the course of assessing the indications for family therapy is the issue of appropriate money management by the elderly. The effects of having lived through the Great Depression and two world wars and now living on a fixed income must be taken into consideration. Here also, family therapy is indicated early in the course of a disability of the elderly patient. Mere education of patient and family members is usually not enough. For example, education about eligibility criteria for Medicaid can lead to premature acceptance of welfare and subsequent surrender of the choices only financial independence assures. Among these are choice of physician, choice of home health care, choice of long-term care facility if needed, and choice of length of time of maintaining the long-term-care bed during visits or hospitalizations. Limitations on these potential choices vary from state to state. The burdens of unresolved, intrapsychic conflicts from previous stages of development must be faced in conjunction with current reality. Well-meaning progeny's unwitting perpetuation of an elderly parent's maladaptive attitudes about spending money for personal care should be brought to consciousness at the time of consultation, and motivation for alternative approaches should be assessed.

In the course of assessment for family therapy, the following issues also need to be addressed: the incongruence between mental and physical capacity and social demands made of the elderly person; conflict between his or her own expectations and the expectations of significant others; discrepancies in family ideologies and historical sociocultural changes that may be affecting the family (e.g., adherence to ethnic, religious, linguistic, or other traditions may vary from generation to generation as well as within one generation); varying levels of adaptation to contemporary society within a family, which can create conflicts to be assessed during the initial family evaluation; and overall medical and mental health status of the elderly person as well as the primary caregiver and other significant others. Caregiving strain is manifested by symptoms of depression, anxiety, somatization, social isolation, and impaired personal growth and development. "Informal caregivers" were found to visit physicians more often on their own behalf and take more medications than matched controls who did not have caregiving responsibilities (Brody 1989). Hence, the assessment process is not complete without taking into account the condition of the caregivers.

In the course of assessment for family therapy with the elderly, evaluation of the individual patient precedes assessment of the family members' perceptions of the elderly relative's condition. Psychiatric evaluation of the spouse, adult children, grandchildren, and other kin who contribute to or detract from the elderly patient's quality of life needs to focus on conflicts that jeopardize the mental and physical health of each person involved. In the course of this initial assessment, family members who have not yet assumed an active positive role can be invited to participate.

Family members of the elderly frequently are seen only to obtain "collateral information." However, failure to assess family members for family therapy on their own behalf may lead them to enter mutual support groups rather than a therapeutic experience. Family therapy can explore and attempt to resolve such conflict-ridden topics as sexuality, money management, caregiver depletion, the right to die, and adapting to life after an impaired elderly relative dies—topics rarely raised or thoroughly discussed in mutual support groups (Hepburn and Wasow 1986). Although mutual support groups generally do not contribute to the resolution of family and marital conflict, they do diminish isolation of the caregivers. Mutual support groups can be a valuable adjunct to family and marital therapy (Goldstein, in press). Referral may be made, when indicated, during the initial family assessment.

Theoretical Models of Family Structure and Development

Several theoretical models of family structure and development that are based on models used for families with emotionally disturbed children, adolescents, or young adults have been adapted for the elderly. For example, the family research project in Palo Alto, which began in the 1950s with participants such as Bates, Haley, Weakland, and Jackson, focused initially on problems of children and young adults but has subsequently expanded its studies to families of the elderly (Herr and Weakland 1979). Borszor-menyi-Nagy and Spark (1973) analyzed the underlying sources of intergenerational conflict in terms of loyalty, entitlement, ledger balance, justice, and legacy for posterity. For further elaboration of these concepts and a longitudinal, intergenerational case description, the reader is referred to Ginsberg-McEwan (1987). Another theoretical model is Bowen's theory of re-relating with family members and redefining intergenerational roles, applied to families with an aging family member (Quinn and Keller 1981). Solomon (1973) suggested five stages of family development and postulated that unless each stage is worked through in due time, the remaining stages are burdened by unresolved conflicts from the previous stage. The first stage is marriage followed by the birth of the first child. A basic task of the second stage is the maintenance of the roles of husband and wife, which must be protected from being overshadowed by parenting commitments. In stage three the child becomes independent, and the fourth stage begins when the child departs from the family. The tasks of the fifth stage are resolution of losses (economic, social, and physical) and dealing with possible dependence on children.

A "resource theory" emphasizes the evolution of power in families over the course of the life cycle (Hesse-Bibers and Williamson 1984). This theory may be useful in family therapy, because shifts of resources among spouses and between generations require considerable adaptation and coping skills.

Jarvik and Small (1988) suggested a six-step, self-observation, common-sense guide to improving relationships with elderly parents. These six steps are 1) monitoring mood, 2) reflecting on the intensity of reactions, 3) planning constructive strategies, 4) reassessing the situation, 5) listening and negotiating, and 6) planning compromise. The family therapist can be a facilitator of this process. Setting appropriate limits on a parent in the negotiating process requires a role reversal and level of filial maturity that is difficult for many adult children to attain.

Unfortunately, at present there is a lack of research-validated outcome studies in marital and intergenerational family therapy with the elderly.

Practical Aspects

Family therapy is facilitated if the psychiatrist engages the family from the outset. The following sample telephone dialogue is a practical, capsule demonstration of one method to begin this process.

The adult child of the prospective patient begins: "My mother has stopped going out with her friends. She is getting more forgetful and has lost some weight. I think her medication has to be changed. Her family doctor says it's just old age."

The psychiatrist could reply: "Who is your mother's physician? Please have all records sent to me. Who does your mother live with? Does she know you want her to see a psychiatrist? Is she willing to come? Who else is in the family? Who will bring her?" The caller's replies are usually quite lengthy; probably at least 15 minutes will be required to deal with the entire call. The psychiatrist continues: "Of course I will see your mother. However, since *you* are calling, you may have some concerns of your own that need attention. Please set up an appointment for your mother and one for yourself. Other family members may also wish to participate. If so, they should set up appointments as well. However, we'll discuss that further when I see you."

The frequency and regularity of visits recommended for the family who brings a child for therapy are modified when a family requests help for an impaired elderly relative. Unlike the family of procreation, the family of origin rarely lives together. The elderly individual may not necessarily be included in the family therapy session each time. Whether the elderly patient should be present depends on the goals of therapy, the wishes of the elderly patient and family members, the elderly's cognitive and functional capacity and frequency and length of contacts with family members, and the availability of formal community resources and informal support networks for the elderly. When the elderly patient participates in family therapy, reminiscing about past experiences can enhance the patient's self-esteem and contribute to redefining the roles in the family into a perspective that is compatible with current reality. If increased dependence occurs in later life, efforts to maintain optimal autonomy without jeopardizing safety need to be encouraged.

An individual assessment of each family member contributes to understanding the developmental level attained by that individual and his or her defense mechanisms—information that is useful in conducting family therapy. Each family member needs reassurance that there will be nonjudgmental recognition of his or her feelings and views of the situation. Once individual family members have identified specific problems as each perceives them, they may then be brought together. Those who come the first time are not necessarily the same ones who come other times. The goals of family therapy should be clarified early in the process and the need established for a common basis of information about the physical and mental condition of the elderly patient, family conflicts, finances, accessibility of community resources, and family value systems. The therapist clarifies the problems in words the family can understand and explains clinical issues, the rationale for psychiatric medications, and the prognosis.

Ground rules for family therapy are set early in the process regarding location and length of sessions and participating members. Meeting times may be changed to accommodate various family members' schedules. Identification of whose time schedule the family revolves around is important. Those family members who are most accommodating may also be those most resentful because others in the family are perceived as having a limited commitment. The family therapist may be the first one to question this status quo and assist family members to consider alternative attitudes toward their time commitments.

Grouping together of families who come to visit elderly relatives in a hospital or other institutional setting such as a nursing home and engaging them in family therapy can be an efficient way to address common themes. Optimally, skilled family therapists should be available in hospitals and nursing homes.

Much conflict resolution and problem solving is done by family members themselves. Identification of problems and facilitation of the family's coping strategies can take place during the most intense periods of family crises. After the family crisis resolves, follow-up appointments to monitor family functioning can be scheduled several months later. Lengthening the intervals between subsequent appointments is often more appropriate than termination, especially in very impaired families. The family therapist assists in consolidating gains, summarizes work done and to be done, and expresses confidence in the ability of the family to do the work while giving credit for what has been done. Out-of-town relatives can be included in the process and encouraged to come for visits at the time of family therapy. This approach has the potential of identifying and reducing critical attitudes and unsupportive behaviors on the part of less involved family members. Disappointments and impatience with an idealized parent's frailties or a spouse's diminished capacity to nurture and provide, as well as the therapist's limitations, are repetitive themes that require ongoing attention. In the absence of adequate resources for the family and their elderly relative, the family and therapist can assume some aspects of the role of patient advocate and case manager.

Marital Therapy

A marital focus is often important in therapy of the elderly. Often when one spouse is seen by a psychiatrist, the other is expected to wait dutifully in the waiting room. However, separating the couple in this way deprives them of the opportunity for individual and marital growth. The unique problems of marriage in late life are explored, taking into account the relationship between past and present conflicts as they relate to sexual, financial, recreational, and social roles; retirement; and disabilities. Problems in sharing may have their etiology in each partner's past and may have been dormant earlier in the life cycle or taken a different expression while there was different interaction with family members and friends. Now that the couple spends many more hours of the day together, resentments of the past have the potential for creating intolerable situations, alienation, and isolation. Frustration, impatience, and intolerance of one's own and the spouse's frailties can be addressed in the course of marital therapy. Optimally, the couple comes to know each other better than before and each learns to appreciate, or at least tolerate, the other's differences as these emerge in late life. The family-oriented therapist can facilitate a redefinition of roles and focus on discrepancies between expectations and actual behaviors.

The presence of hearing deficits must be identified, discussed, and addressed to improve communication between the couple. For example, resistance to getting or using a hearing aid may be part of a power struggle between the two; professional intervention has the potential to eliminate this pathological focus of the conflict over control.

Summary

Just as the role of family members requires redefinition in later life, the role of the psychiatrist in the treatment of the elderly and their families needs ongoing definition and redefinition. The modern family is complex and the role of the elderly in the family is still poorly defined. The modern psychiatrist needs to be versed in clinical assessment and treatment of the elderly from a biopsychosocial perspective, which includes assessment and treatment of family members. Theoretical models of individual, marital, and family psychodynamics and therapy, as well as research findings by epidemiologists and gerontologists in psychology and sociology, need to be integrated into a common-sense approach for the relatives of our elderly patients.

References

Ade-Ridder L: Family relationships in later life, Part I in Quality of Long-Term Marriages. Edited by Brubaker TA. Beverly Hills, CA, Sage, 1983, pp 21–30

Borszormenyi-Nagy IA, Spark GM: Invisible Loyalties: Reciprocity in Intergenerational Family Therapy. Hagerstown, MD, Harper & Row, 1973

Brody EM: The aging family. Gerontologist 6:201–206, 1966

Brody EM: Family at risk, in Alzheimer's Disease; Treatment and Family Stress. Edited by Light E, Lebowitz B. (DHHS Publication No. (ADM) 89–1569) Rockville, MD, National Institute of Mental Health, 1989, pp 2–49

Brubaker TH: Family Relationships in Later Life. Beverly Hills, CA, Sage, 1983

Cicirelli VG: A comparison of helping behavior to elderly parents of adult children with intact and disrupted marriages. Gerontologist 23:619–625, 1983a

Cicirelli VG: Adult children and their elderly parents, in Family Relationships in Later Life. Edited by Brubaker T. Beverly Hills, CA, Sage, 1983b, pp 31–46

Comptroller General of the United States: Report to Congress on Home Health: The Need for a National Policy to Better Provide for the Elderly (GAO publ HRD 78–19). Washington, DC, December 30, 1977

Deimling GT, Bass DM: Symptoms of mental impairment among elderly adults and their effects on family caregivers. J. Gerontol 41:778–784, 1986

Doty P: Family care of the elderly: the role of public policy. Milbank Quarterly 64(1), pp 34–75, 1986

Ginsberg-McEwan E: The whole grandfather: an intergenerational approach to family therapy, in Treating the Elderly With Psychotherapy. Edited by Sadavoy J, Leszcz M. Madison, CT, International Universities Press, 1987, pp 295–324

Goldstein MZ: Elder neglect, abuse, and exploitation, in Family Violence: Emerging Issues of a National Crisis. Edited by Dickstein LJ, Nadelson CC. Washington, DC, American Psychiatric Press, 1989a, pp 101–124

Goldstein MZ: Parent care, in Family Involvement in the Treatment of the Frail Elderly. Edited by Goldstein MZ. Washington, DC, American Psychiatric Press, 1989c, pp 1–22

Goldstein MZ: The role of mutual support groups and family therapy for caregivers of demented elderly. J Geriatr Psychiatry (in press)

Grad J, Sainsbury P: Problems of caring for the mentally ill at home. Proceedings of the Royal Society of Medicine Section on Psychiatry 59:20–23, 1966

Hagsted GO: Continuity and connectedness, in Grandparenthood. Edited by Bengston VL, Robertson J. Beverly Hills, CA, Sage, 1985

Hepburn K, Wasow M: Support groups for family caregivers of dementia victims: questions, directions, and future research, in The Elderly and Chronic Mental Illness, New Directions for Mental Health Services No. 29, San Francisco, CA, Jossey Bass, 1986, pp 83–92

Herr JJ, Weakland JH: Counseling elders and their families, Practical Techniques for Applied Gerontology. New York, Springer, 1979

Hesse-Bibers S, Williamson J: Resource theory and power in families: life cycle considerations. Fam Process 23:261–278, 1984

Horowitz A: Family caregiving to the frail elderly, in Annual Review of Gerontology and Geriatrics, Vol 5. Edited by Eisdorfer MP, Lawton MP, Maddox GL. New York, Springer, 1985, pp 194–246

Jarvik L, Small G: Parent Care. New York, Crown Publishers, 1988

Neugarten BL: Adaptation and the life cycle, in Counseling Adults. Edited by Schlossberg NK, Entine AD. Monterey, CA, Brooks/Cole, 1977

Quinn WH, Keller JF: A family therapy model for preserving independence. American Journal of Family Therapy 9:79–84, 1981

Ross HG, Milgram JJ: Important variables in adult sibling relationships, in Sibling Relationships: Their Nature and Significance. Edited by Lamb ME, Sutton ME. Hillsdale, NJ, Erlbaum, 1982

Shanas E: Social myth as hypothesis: the case of the family relations of old people. Gerontologist 19:3–9, 1979a

Shanas E: The family as a social system in old age. Gerontologist 19:169–174, 1979b

Solomon MA: A developmental conceptual premise for family therapy. Family Process 12:179–188, 1973

Stone R, Cafferata GL, Sangi J: Caregivers of the frail elderly: a national profile. Gerontologist 27:616–626, 1987

Taeuber CM: America in transition: an aging society. Current Population Reports, Series P-23, No 128, U.S. Bureau of the Census. Washington, DC, U.S. Government Printing Office, 1983

Troll LE: Family Issues in Current Gerontology. New York, Springer, 1986

Uhlenberg P, Myers MAP: Divorce and the elderly. Gerontologist 21:276–282, 1981

U.S. Bureau of the Census: Marital status and living arrangements. Current Population Reports, Series P-20, No 372. Washington, DC, U.S. Government Printing Office, 1981

Vaillant GE, Vaillant CO: Natural history of male psychosocial health, XII: a 45-year study of predictors of successful aging at age 65. Am J Psychiatry 147:31–37, 1990

CHAPTER 26

Molyn Leszcz, M.D.

Group Therapy

Overview

The appropriate application of group treatments to the elderly requires knowledge of the range of patients, settings, and techniques
associated with this age group (Burnside 1978; MacLennan et al.
1988). Homogenization may result in misapplication of techniques
and models appropriate for one patient population to another. The
designation "geriatric" fails to denote differences in age, ego function, education, sociocultural background, ethnic variables, and
the degree of psychological-mindedness.

A key concept in this chapter is the requirement that the therapist be flexible in conducting the group. Differences between supportive and insight-oriented groups, and between depth and nondepth groups, are frequently blurred. Many geriatric patients in
fact are treated in some modified group that contains both insight-
oriented and supportive approaches commingled. In almost every
instance, the therapist's awareness of both psychodynamic and
process considerations—as well as specific, structured techniques
and content considerations—enhances therapeutic efficacy. Similarly, a realistic therapeutic perspective that recognizes the scope
for growth or restoration of lost interpersonal, emotional, and cognitive capacities is essential. Maintaining this perspective in the
face of patient demoralization, societal myths about aging, and the
elderly individual's real impairment and loss is an ever-present
challenge to the group leader.

Examination of the themes that emerge in group therapy (see
Table 26-1) illustrates that many of the psychological concerns of

Table 26-1. Themes in group therapy

Loss of significant relationships
Loss of physical and cognitive capacities
Loss of functions and tasks
Loss of self-worth and self-esteem
Loneliness and isolation
Depression and demoralization
Dependency-autonomy conflicts
Interpersonal conflict with spouse and family
Hopelessness, helplessness, and purposelessness
Wish for restoration of a sense of competence and mastery

Table 26-2. Objectives of treatment

Restoration of a sense of self-esteem and self-worth
Reduction of isolation and promotion of interpersonal engagement
Symptom reduction and mastery
Acquisition of coping skills and interpersonal skills
Grieving and adaptation to loss
Appropriate acceptance of dependency and rational use of available re-
    sources

the elderly are generated by age-induced losses and changes, and by the patient's difficulty in negotiating the late-life developmental challenge of maintaining a sense of self that is continuous in the present with the past (Leszcz 1987). These themes shape the overall objectives of the group therapies with the elderly, as noted in Table 26-2.

Group Therapy Approaches

Table 26-3 summarizes the types of group therapy currently employed with geriatric patients.

Verbal-Centered Groups for the Cognitively Intact Elderly

Psychodynamic Psychotherapy. Kohut's (1984) conceptualization of narcissism and self psychology has greatly influenced the conduct of individual and group psychotherapy with the elderly because of the understanding it provides of the internal and subjective experience of the elderly individual (Lazarus 1980). This conceptualization is particularly relevant to the individual faced

Table 26-3. Group therapy approaches for the elderly

Verbal-centered groups for the cognitively intact
    Psychodynamic psychotherapy groups
    Life review groups
    Cognitive-behavioral groups
    Homogeneous groups (e.g., widows, postretirement and relocation
        groups)
    Burdened caregivers groups

Verbal-centered groups for the cognitively impaired
    Resocialization and remotivation groups
    Reality orientation groups

Activity- and creativity-centered groups
    Dance movement therapy groups
    Project groups
    Nutrition groups
    Drama, art, or poetry groups

Settings
    Outpatient groups
    Acute hospital groups
    Institutional settings (i.e., chronic hospital groups, nursing home
        groups)

with the challenge of maintaining the sense of self in the face of the narcissistic injuries of aging and the loss of central functions, capacities, and selfobject relationships. This conceptualization also augments and facilitates the use of the standard psychodynamic group therapeutic mechanisms described by Yalom (1985).

Group therapy provides a self-esteem, self-sustaining treatment matrix in which the narcissistic injuries to the self may be addressed through the feeling of group cohesion, and the providing of relationships that serve necessary selfobject functions, in addition to providing real objects for relatedness and support (Schwartzman 1984). The selfobject transference may be to the other individuals, the group as a whole, or the therapist, and it serves to restore a sense of self-stability and vitality by providing one or more of the three central elements of self (Kohut 1984): 1) mirroring selfobjects that value, praise, and admire the individual; 2) idealized selfobjects in whose presence the individual feels safe, protected, and worthwhile; and 3) alter ego or twinning selfobjects with whom the individual can feel an essential alikeness and resonance through the process of pairing with another person (Lothstein and Zimet 1988). The emphasis on empathic recognition of the subjective experience of the elderly in the group deepens the therapist's understanding of the processes of relationships, interactions, and resistances in the group. With a self psychology perspective it becomes more possible to understand the interpersonal phenomena of defensive withdrawal, haughty devaluation, grandiose exhibitionism, monopolization, idealization, and the pursuit of special relatedness as attempts to protect or stabilize the vulnerable sense of self (Stone and Whitman 1977). Opportunities for interpersonal learning are thereby enhanced.

Life Review Group Therapy. The process of reminiscing, or life review (Butler 1974; Poulton and Strassberg 1986), has been employed in a variety of ways in psychotherapy groups. Conceptualized as a developmentally appropriate and natural process of review through which elderly persons organize and evaluate their lives, it has been used to promote reintegration of individuals' sense of who they are, by having them reconnect to what they were. The life review has been used as a technique to enhance the development of cohesion in beginning groups and groups experiencing demoralization in the face of group developmental difficulties (Leszcz et al. 1985). In addition, it has been used effectively as an organizing principle in group psychotherapy for more impaired patients (Lesser et al. 1981).

In practice, the process of reminiscing may be used adaptively or maladaptively, correlated with the way it is experienced by the group members and managed by the group therapist. At its best, the reminiscing process fleshes out individuals in the group and makes them three-dimensional people rather than one-dimensional objects of projection for one another. It restores feelings of worth, stature, and competence through the articulation of past successes and the recollection of prior credentials. What has been of greatest importance to any individual often cannot be assumed without confirmation, and subjective valuation may be very different from objective valuation. The reminiscing about previous challenges that have been mastered helps soothe the apprehension about facing the unknown future. Further, appropriate grieving and conflict resolution may be facilitated, promoting better engagement in the current environment.

However, with profoundly depressed or withdrawn patients, reminiscing may result in a further preoccupation with the past; guilt over irreparable errors; and a heightened, morbid self-absorption that results in social alienation. In such instances, group cohesion can be seriously undermined and the therapist needs to determine if the reminiscing is serving the intended purpose of deepening the group members' understanding of one another, strengthening feelings of group cohesion and universality, and promoting both a sense of mastery and willingness to engage. Benefits can be maximized and risks reduced if the therapist establishes a group norm that all reminiscing, and the experience of talking about, listening to, and sharing the life review, be brought back into the here and now of the group and examined at the interpersonal level (Poulton and Strassberg 1986).

Cognitive-Behavioral Group Therapy. Cognitive-behavioral group therapy emphasizes conscious cognition and learning, adapting behavioral strategies and the cognitive therapy model to the group setting. Central elements include the identification of dysfunctional attitudes and cognitive distortions that engender depression. This process includes 1) helping patients identify their reactions in particular situations; 2) confronting and correcting distortions by realigning the attributions of meaning made by the individual; 3) determining the basic assumptions and themes that shape these reactions; 4) practicing alternative cognitive and behavioral responses to anticipated stresses, by encouraging patients to tackle ever-increasing challenges; and (5) achieving mastery and maintenance of positive affects that breed alternative and more correct and objective assumptions (Rush 1983). Reframing and focusing attention on partial positive outcomes as a way to counteract cognitive distortions of global negative outcome is an example of this process. Patients are taught to reevaluate their situation by looking at pros and cons in a conscious, behavioristic fashion. They are taught to monitor negative thoughts and solve problems with group support.

In this model, the repetitive, maladaptive, depressogenic behaviors and cognitions are viewed as automatic. They reflect a form of learned behavior that is blind to other options. Psychodynamic considerations and questions of motivation are viewed as irrelevant.

Social isolation and the lack of alternative input exacerbate negative, self-devaluing, and self-blaming assumptions and make some elderly individuals particularly prone to distortions in attributing meaning (Parham et al. 1982). The exchange and feedback that occur in a group are particularly well suited to confronting such assumptions and distortions. Treatment promotes the realignment and objectification of cognitive assumptions and the attribution of meaning to events and experiences.

More focused behavioral approaches (Gallagher 1981) employ

modeling, role playing, didactic discussions, and feedback about
each group member's efforts in using skills required to reengage
with pleasurable experiences. The focus is on external and observable behavior only. The aim of treatment is to break the vicious
cycle of depressed mood resulting in reduced interaction and reduced stimulation of positive interpersonal reinforcement, further
social withdrawal, and the consequent erosion of social skills. The
group serves as a supportive laboratory for prescribed behavioral
practice. Patients identify pleasurable and unpleasurable activities and learn how to engage in pleasurable ones. Relaxation techniques and problem-solving skills as well as time management,
self-assertion, and self-expression are taught. Depression is demys-
tified and there is a strong emphasis on the acquisition of behavioral skills.

Integrated Verbal-Centered Group Therapy.   In clinical practice,
the three models (psychodynamic, life review, and cognitive-
behavioral) may be effectively integrated into an approach that
capitalizes on the strengths of each. Focusing on the elaboration of
affect and self-disclosure is useful in gaining an understanding of
the individual, and the life review further fleshes out this understanding. However, patients highly value skill acquisition (Gallagher and Thompson 1982). It aids in mastery, restoration of competence, and generalization of gains, and it amplifies the very
important therapeutic factor of group cohesion by virtue of the
feeling of shared achievement in the group. On the other hand, disregard for the group process or the subjective experience of the individual can result in the group's assuming an unempathetic,
alienating, superficial, "pick yourself up by the bootstraps" orientation. In place of role playing and modeling, maladaptive interpersonal skills and interpersonal distortions can be addressed directly, in vivo, in a more interactive group that focuses on the
interpersonal relationships created in the here and now of the
group.
     In an integrated model, individuals have the opportunity of ex-
amining their experience of isolation and loneliness in the group,
exploring what they do that minimizes and maximizes their isolation and loneliness, and practicing new skills and risk taking. A
productive and logically consistent synthesis is formed of the patients' subjective experience and the specific importance of their
interpersonal relatedness, the historical context of the individuals
and their relationships, and the interpersonal contributions to
their own success and failure, coupled with the challenging of cog-

nitive and interpersonal distortions and the direct behavioral practices of successful relating.

Homogeneous Groups. There is a broad range of such groups, which generally meet for a short-term contract of 8 to 20 sessions; their composition is generally determined by a particular common problem, characteristic, or developmental issue. A relevant model is that of postretirement groups (Salvendy 1989). Such groups emphasize mutual support, countering the isolation and the loss of self-esteem induced by loss of the status of employment.

Groups for Burdened Caregivers. Caregiver groups have developed in response to the increasing number of cognitively impaired and dementing individuals cared for at home by their families (Kahan et al. 1985; Lazarus et al. 1981; Saul 1988). The rationale for these groups stems from the recognition that caregivers often are highly burdened, isolated, and frequently depressed. The absence of social supports exacerbates the caregivers' strain (Zarit et al. 1980). Homogeneity of situation promotes rapidly cohesive groups with much self-disclosure and mutual support. Extragroup contact is endorsed, and the self-help nature of the group is supported as well. A central psychological issue is the working through of the pain of providing care for a loved one who may have lost the capacity not only to express gratitude, but even to recognize the caregiver, or whose intermittent periods of recognition and lucidity may confuse the caregiver.

Objectives of these groups include 1) education about the dementing process and learning ways of interacting with the patient and providing care; 2) working through grief, promoting appropriate disengagement, and allowing institutional placement if necessary; 3) legitimizing the needs of the caregiver, thereby promoting self-care and regard to counter isolation and self-neglect; 4) working through relationships with health care professionals; and 5) working through the anger and guilt that often stem from the wish to believe that something could have been done to avoid the dementing process.

Verbal-Centered Groups for the Cognitively Impaired

Resocialization and Remotivation Groups. The objectives of verbal groups with the cognitively impaired stem from Linden's (1953) concept of "psychological senility." This term refers to the reversible picture of regressed dependency, morbid self-absorption, and disengagement arising from repeated losses and devaluation by society. Group therapy aims at stimulation, and reengagement through leader- or patient-originated discussion and interaction, melded with the providing of as much sensory stimulation as possible. These groups focus on members' strengths and fundamental humanness and, although highly structured, do have a group process that needs to be attended to and understood by the therapist. These groups achieve interpersonal engagement more through the structure and content than through the process. As is the case in group therapy with the cognitively intact, engagement is prompted and reinforced.

The broader the array of content offered, the greater the likelihood of effective activation and engagement. The leader may increase or decrease the amount of attention placed on process or activity according to patient needs. Cognitive exercises; activity and word games; life review; discussions; and participation in music, art, baking, and physical exercise are all components of these groups. The range is virtually limitless, but in each instance the emphasis should be on sensory stimulation, improved ego function, reality orientation, memory, judgment, problem solving, and interaction (Burnside 1978; Saul 1988).

Reality Orientation Groups. Objectives of treatment (Drummond et al. 1975) are the reversal of disengagement and of the decreased use of cognitive functions by continual stimulation and reorientation in an interactive environment. There is substantial overlap between reality orientation groups and remotivation and resocialization groups. Reality orientation thereby occurs in two modes. The chief mode is a 24-hour milieu approach to provide consistent and persistent orientation of the individual, making the milieu as rational and knowable as possible. The second mode is classroom or group reality orientation. The reality orientation group room contains a full array of multisensory stimuli. Every opportunity is capitalized on to elucidate and remind individual patients of the who, where, what, and why of what is going on in a firm, friendly, nondemanding fashion, repeatedly bringing the patient back to the here and now. Reinforcement for successful reorientation can be interpersonal or behavioral (Miller 1977) and can be linked to all activities of daily living. Small group reality orientation enhances the 24-hour program but appears to be of minimal use in the absence of the more comprehensive milieu approach. Without active therapeutic input and reinforcement, no generalization occurs and learning is readily extinguished.

Activity- and Creativity-Centered Groups

There is a broad range of activity- and creativity-centered groups, and there is substantial interplay among them (MacLennan et al. 1988). They provide opportunities for patients, whose verbal skills may be diminished, to express and rekindle a sense of self through the artistic or creative process, enhanced by working together and creating. Both pleasure and mastery may be stimulated, and in some instances the nonverbal expression may be deeper than the verbal. The objective is not only to experience art, but to create it. These modalities are additionally important vehicles to retain a sense of self in the midst of institutional life with its tendency toward homogenization and the blurring of individual differences. Creative expression is used as a form of engagement with the world as well as an expression of self.

Dance movement therapy focuses on the integration of the self through reconnection of the individual with his or her own body (Samberg 1988). It is not task oriented like physical exercise, but rather is process oriented, promoting the opportunity to study the relationship between mood and movement and physical sensations. In the same way that cognitive therapy challenges cognitive distortions and improves depression by altering the way in which one thinks, dance movement therapy aims at ameliorating depression and demoralization by evoking positive and pleasurable bodily expressions. The therapy involves challenging assumptions of the self, its restrictions, and its limitations, and increasing one's sense of physical mastery.

Indications for Group Therapy

As with every treatment modality, no particular therapy for the elderly is equally effective with all individuals. In every instance, however, effective psychotherapy can proceed only with a clear anti-ageism bias—that the psychological difficulties of the elderly person are treatable and reversible until proven otherwise.

Social isolation, interpersonal alienation, maladaptive interpersonal skills, diminished self-worth, depressive disengagement, and withdrawal are common presenting features. Group therapy is an effective treatment in addressing this clinical constellation, either as the sole treatment or adjunctive to pharmacotherapy or individual therapy. When treatments are provided conjointly, they must be offered in an integrated and coherent fashion; the therapeutic right hand must know what the therapeutic left hand is doing. Because depression in the elderly is often a chronic, relapsing disorder, even with initially effective pharmacological treatment (Murphy 1983), the importance of the psychosocial therapies is underscored. Although it remains unclear whether social isolation and lack of social supports cause depression, or whether depression-induced loss of social skills results in isolation, it is clear that the depressed elderly are indeed more likely to have both diminished social supports and diminished social skills (Gallagher 1981; Grant et al. 1988). What is cause and what is effect is often unclear, but this reverberation can be interrupted at either point. The group therapies are indicated for both these deficits. Regressive feelings related to dependency can also be diminished, and group therapy may be more acceptable and less anxiety provoking than individual therapy. In addition, the concrete opportunity for behavioral change and practice that occurs in all groups may hold special appeal for these older persons who are less able to deal with abstract psychological issues.

In some instances, these objectives can be met entirely by the manifest content of the interaction around group activities. In other instances, these benefits can be accessed only by addressing the process of the group and effectively working through the patients' resistance to engagement. The ideal treatment setting offers the broadest range of group modalities—a form of therapeutic "buffet." Resistance to engagement and severity of presenting symptoms often determine the relative indications for verbal- or activity-centered groups. Depression is unlikely to be treated effectively by an activity- or creativity-centered group alone, and the resistive, devaluing patient is unlikely to connect effectively in such a setting. Activity-centered groups serve useful maintenance and prophylactic functions, and for the highly motivated individual, participation in such groups may be all that is required to maintain psychological integration. The more depressed or functionally impaired patient may use activity-centered groups to good effect following a period of more intensive treatment. Referral to these groups should be linked to the special interests and talents of the patients. These observations derive from clinical experience, but empirical outcome data are sparse.

Group composition should be homogeneous for level of ego function, intellect, and degree of cognitive functioning. Age generally is not a determining factor. In fact, the active elderly may be treated effectively in psychotherapy groups with younger patients. Such groups provide a rich opportunity to work through issues of feeling old and inadequate in a youthful society. On the other hand, even in homogeneous geriatric settings, mixing cognitively intact and impaired patients together can result in the former feeling an unwillingness to engage and the latter being unable to engage. Even in groups that are designed for the cognitively impaired, similarity in level of function is optimal. The cognitively inaccessible patient does not benefit from the group and is likely to discourage participation by other members who may see in the grossly impaired patient their worst fear of personal decline.

Homogeneous groups are more likely to become cohesive quickly and generally are more supportive. Feelings of universality are enhanced, but there is a risk that excessive homogeneity may result in a lack of contrasting perspective that may diminish the possible range of problem solving. In general, the importance to group members of being able to identify positively with one another should be recognized in the selection and composition of groups. Individuals who are significantly deviant from the group norm are likely to be early dropouts.

Group therapy is contraindicated for patients who are in acute crisis or who are suicidal; patients with drug or alcohol abuse; paranoid or violently aggressive patients; patients with persistent inability to attend to the process of the group because of severe cognitive impairment, sedation, irremediable hearing loss, or differences in language; and difficult, characterologically disturbed patients who persistently attack and devalue others in maladaptive efforts to bolster their own self-esteem. These contraindications are relative and are intended to serve as guidelines to maintain the viability and effectiveness of the group, as well as to avoid negative outcomes to any individual patient, such as group rejection or extrusion. A strong, well-established, and mature group is better able to contain a difficult patient than a beginning, developmentally immature group. The group therapist needs to evaluate whether a particular group and a particular patient can benefit from one another at a particular point in time. Unlike the individual setting, in the group setting the therapist's selection of patients not only commits him or her to the patient, but also commits each of the other group members to a relationship with that patient.

Preparation and pretraining of patients prior to entry into group therapy has not been specifically researched with the elderly, but the evidence for its utility in other patient populations is overwhelming (Yalom 1985). Explaining the rationale of psychotherapy demystifies an otherwise anxiety-provoking situation, helps establish a therapeutic alliance, and sets group norms re-

garding regular attendance, confidentiality, and extragroup socialization. Effective pretraining results in enhanced group tenure,
task adherence, increased hopefulness, reduced anxiety, and increased interaction and self-disclosure, thereby increasing the
chances for successful treatment. Dropout rates for group therapy
with young patients range between 10% and 50%, and with the elderly the frequency rate is at least the same (Steuer et al. 1984).
The likelihood of a premature dropout is increased with the severity of depression, presence of a severe physical illness, and a char-
acterological style that devalues, externalizes, and blames.

In institutional settings, group therapy is indicated, further, to
provide a forum to deal with the imposed accommodations to
changes in life situation and the reduced feelings of autonomy. The
opportunity to work through and reconcile interpersonal difficulties may enhance the quality of life available to residents in institutions. In addition, some settings have a heavy preponderance of
female residents and staff, and group therapy may provide an opportunity for the relatively few men in the institution to meet together, stimulating models of identification with male figures in
the matriarchal environment typical of many nursing homes
(Leszcz et al. 1985).

Technical Applications of Group Therapy

General Considerations

The objectives and indications of the various geriatric group therapies necessitate certain adaptations in therapeutic technique.
The elderly are often resistant to group psychotherapy and behave
in ways that interfere with the development of group cohesion, especially when depressed. Withdrawal, devaluing self and others,
hopelessness, and blaming generally are not conducive to group
cohesion. It is striking that, regardless of the model of group therapy used (ranging from psychodynamic to behavioral) the recommended therapist posture and attitude is the same (Gallagher
1981). The therapist's posture of respect, hopefulness, genuine
warmth, and empathy appears to be as important as his or her
theoretical rationale (Tross and Blum 1988).

In general, the group leader carries a greater burden of responsibility to initiate and activate a geriatric group than is the case
with groups of younger patients. The group leader anchors the
group, ensuring the psychological integrity of each individual and
the logistical and functional integrity of the group as a whole. De-

termining a set and inviolate time for the group in an inviolate and comfortable location, free from time conflicts with other appointments, is essential. Active outreach by the group leaders to reduce fluctuations in composition of the group is a prerequisite for effective treatment. A cohesive group may not form spontaneously, and waiting for the group to activate itself is likely to result in a contagion of demoralization and group dropouts.

In view of the difficulty which some elderly persons have in getting started in the morning and the requirements of arranging transportation, it may be preferable to select a late morning or mid-afternoon time for the group. Normally, such a time would foredoom a younger person's group, but with the elderly it may be ideal, for it also promotes the opportunity for extragroup contact around lunch and coffee. In younger persons' groups, extragroup contact is generally prohibited because it often leads to subgrouping and, ultimately, to fragmentation in the group. In the geriatric population, however, extragroup contact may be fostered, with the goal of providing opportunities for real relatedness, because the elderly do experience a realistic reduction in opportunities for such engagement. Furthermore, in institutional settings, extragroup contacts are a fact of life. The key to successful management of this extragroup contact or subgrouping is to diminish the boundary of secrecy around the relationships and bring these interactions into the purview of the group, even if it is only to endorse and not to interpret them (Lothstein and Zimet 1988). Extragroup contact can be a rich source of feedback about the individuals in the group, reducing treatment blind spots while providing an opportunity to practice interpersonal skills learned in the group proper.

Verbal-Centered Groups

Verbal-centered groups function best with 6 to 10 patients and generally meet weekly in ambulatory settings or as frequently as daily in institutional settings. Activity- and creativity-centered groups may function quite well with much larger numbers and may benefit from multiple leaders. The cognitively intact patients may use the group meeting for one to one-and-a-half hours, whereas cognitively impaired patients generally make better use of briefer time frames (45 minutes) in light of their reduced attention and concentration.

The group therapist should ensure that the therapy is a nonfailure experience for each member. A related task is that of protecting

the group from fragmentation and rupture—a function more easily achieved when the therapist empathically recognizes the subjective experience of each group member. Awareness of what is
subjectively important to each individual provides the therapist
with a direction for the treatment and safeguards against the individual's loss of identity through group homogenization. Supporting even small gains and steps toward self-assertion and self-expression is essential.

Face-to-face interaction, direct contact, mutual support, and
interaction in the here and now of the group need to be reinforced
repeatedly by the therapist, as does any progroup cohesive interaction or feedback. Yalom and Terrazas (1967) advocated a model
of "ego enhancement." They recommended that therapists always
search for the central vulnerability, interpersonal core, or adaptive
focus in every interchange. Externalization of blame for failures in
the self, and projections of devaluation and denigration pose particular therapeutic challenges, for they are often quite ego syntonic
and valued by the patient (Lazarus and Groves 1987). The therapist who focuses on inviting desired behavior rather than rebuffing
what is undesirable enhances group cohesion and the opportunities for the group to feel effective, without damaging its members
through hostile confrontation. For example, trying to access the
loneliness that may reside beneath overt hostility makes each
member of the group more accessible and comprehensible to his or
her peers.

The relevance of each patient's comments and communications
should be noted. The group language and metaphors should be familiar and resonant to the group members and voiced in a cultur-
ally acceptable form. At times the therapist has to reframe, integrate, translate, summarize, and underscore, ideally in a fashion
that is not excessively gratifying of dependency needs but continues to respectfully insist on patients being accountable for themselves. In those instances when sensory impairment is prominent,
the use of audio aids such as FM amplifying systems is an additional consideration, but it will be of little use if the hearing impairment is being used defensively to achieve isolation and disengagement.

Activity-Centered Groups

Activity-centered groups and verbal groups for the cognitively impaired also require substantial therapist activity. Structured exercises and activities cannot be prescribed without the therapist's

own active and genuine participation, to safeguard against the group's feeling patronized. In resocialization and remotivation groups, patient initiative and responsibility enhance the group functions, and such groups are experienced as more cohesive than leader-dependent groups in which there is little patient initiation.

Special Problems

A broad range of countertransferential reactions may emerge in the treatment of the elderly, as noted elsewhere in this volume. Along with the countertransferential issues faced by the individual therapist, the group leader is personally more exposed. Because of group pressures, the group leader is more vulnerable to a complementary response to the group's depressive demoralization. "What can a bunch of old, useless people do for one another?" is a common statement of patients in geriatric groups. If the therapist begins to identify with a position of hopelessness, therapeutic perspective is lost. Warning signs include the therapist's own boredom, lateness, or cancellation of meetings with the rationalization that the group members will not miss the meeting. In fact, the opposite is true. Geriatric groups are exquisitely sensitive to feeling devalued and diminished, although their reaction and protest may be more silent than angry.

Conversely, the therapist may be an idealized object, the recipient of patients' projections of lost successes, health, and competence. The idealization is contained by the therapist more readily if he or she can recognize its transferential, selfobject roots and not feel personally overstimulated (Leszcz et al. 1985). Alternatively, if the idealization fails to strengthen and comfort group members but leaves them feeling bereft of any of their own power or efficacy, it needs to be actively confronted.

Resistances to intimacy and, frequently, inexperience in verbalization may slow the group work and make it more arduous than group work with younger patients. The therapist may feel devalued in identification with patients who devalue themselves. Consultation, supervision, and cotherapy serve to diminish these potential countertransferential difficulties. The burden of activating the group and engaging resistant patients is decreased by sharing the responsibility between coleaders. Mixed-sex cotherapy teams may also evoke greater wishes for engagement among the group members (Linden 1953). In addition, cotherapy ensures that the group meets regularly, despite therapists' vacations or illness, and reduces threats to the group's cohesiveness.

In institutional settings it is useful if at least one of the coleaders is a regular team member of the ward or floor staff, to facilitate exchange of information and treatment planning. The group program should be experienced as an integrated and integral part of the overall treatment. Without administrative and institutional support, logistical obstacles to attendance emerge. Both depth and nondepth approaches need to be valued; otherwise, interdisciplinary rivalries produce subtle devaluation of various parts of the group treatment, which is detected by the patients and leads to reluctance on their part to participate.

Group therapy both influences and is influenced by its setting, and generally staff morale is enhanced on wards where there is an opportunity for active psychological treatment (Reichenfeld et al. 1973). The group may function as a psychological biopsy of the larger milieu, allowing exploration of the status of the larger milieu by exploring the smaller group process (Levine 1980).

An additional challenge in group therapy with the elderly is the presence of physical illness. Physical illness is negatively correlated with successful outcome in treatment of depression (Parham et al. 1982), despite the fact that real deficits may become the focus of specific skill acquisition. Secondly, physical impairment requires some adaptations of techniques in recognition of limitations placed on certain behavioral interventions by an individual's physical impairment (Gallagher 1981). Physical impairment interferes logistically with attendance and participation in the group and may result in group attrition. Steuer and Hammen (1983) similarly commented on the slower pace of cognitive approaches with elderly patients, and their tendency to be more concrete and less abstract than younger patients.

The interplay among real and excess disability, true restriction, and treatment resistance is complex and requires diligence and patience in sorting out. The group is vulnerable to demoralization because of physical illness and impairment, but if contained effectively, the presence of real illness and real physical threats provides an opportunity for group members to address issues of quality of life, death, and dying.

Outcome of Group Therapy

Small sample size, brief time frames, study of nonpatient populations, lack of consensus on outcome measures, patients receiving more than one form of treatment at a time, and ethical difficulties in maintaining a nontreatment control group hamper evaluation of the outcome of group treatments (Parham et al. 1982; Steuer et al. 1984). Many reports are anecdotal and clinical. Nonetheless, there is sufficient outcome research to point with optimism to a number of conclusions about the usefulness and efficacy of group therapies with the elderly.

Cognitively Intact Patients

Although group psychotherapy is significantly superior to no treatment (Tross and Blum 1988), group therapy alone is less effective than psychopharmacotherapy in relief of depression (Steuer and Hammen 1983). However, it can play a strong adjunctive role, and in some instances psychotherapy may be the only treatment patients can tolerate medically. All models of group therapy—be they structured and cognitive-behavioral, or interactional and psychodynamic—are equally and significantly effective in reducing symptoms of depression, improving interpersonal and social functioning, and bolstering self-esteem (Gallagher 1981; Steuer et al. 1984; Sweet et al. 1989). Group therapy decreases anxiety and enhances group members' ability to deal with emotions verbally and to use the present more than the past to sustain self-esteem (Lieberman and Gaurash 1979). There is some evidence to suggest that specific skill acquisition is directly linked to significantly improved outcome at follow-up 1 year after treatment cessation (Gallagher and Thompson 1982).

Tentative outcome research on groups for burdened caregivers indicates that participants in these groups show improved feelings of self-control and self-direction; an increased ability to consider separation from the ill members of their family with increased capacity to grieve; and (quite important) an increased capacity to care for themselves (Kahan et al. 1985; Lazarus et al. 1981).

In their extensive review in the American Group Psychotherapy monograph on geriatric group psychotherapies, Tross and Blum (1988) concluded that all consistent and rational group psychotherapies for the elderly are equally efficacious as long as patients stay engaged in treatment for the prescribed time. Successful outcome is linked to tenure; therefore, ensuring treatment maintenance, as described earlier, is essential. Severe physical illness and chronicity of depression are negatively correlated with successful outcome (Gallagher 1981; Steuer et al. 1984).

Cognitively Impaired Patients

Early outcome studies (Linden 1953) based on populations of institutionalized, chronic, psychogeriatric patients treated in remotivation and resocialization groups documented improved discharge rates, hygiene and grooming, socialization, and participation in hospital activities. Reichenfeld and associates (1973) also documented statistically significant increases in discharge rates and reductions in behavioral deterioration. Those who were physically more ill or more cognitively impaired at the outset improved less. Behavioral improvement is linked not only to the specifics of reality orientation techniques but also to the behavioral engagement and reinforcement of more adaptive functions. Exposure to reality orientation techniques is insufficient without actual interaction, encouragement, and reinforcement by the staff. Staff's enthusiasm, realistic hopefulness, and behaviorally consistent response are also essential (Katz 1976). These therapies have been shown to produce statistically significant improvement in patients in group behavior and in socially adaptive behaviors inside and outside the group (Bower 1967).

References

Bower HM: Sensory stimulation and the treatment of senile dementia. Med J Aust 22:1113–1119, 1967

Burnside IM: Working With the Elderly: Group Process and Techniques. North Scituate, MA, Duxbury Press, 1978

Butler R: Successful aging and the role of the life review. J Am Geriatr Soc 22:529–535, 1974

Drummond L, Kirchhoff L, Scarbrough DR: A practical guide to reality orientation: a treatment approach for confusion and disorientation. Gerontologist 18:568–573, 1975

Gallagher D: Behavioral group therapy with elderly depressives: an experimental study, in Behavioral Group Therapy. Edited by Upper D, Ross SM. Champaign, IL, Research Press, 1981

Gallagher DE, Thompson LW: Treatment of major depressive disorder in older adult outpatients with brief psychotherapies. Psychotherapy: Theory, Research, and Practice 19:482–490, 1982

Grant I, Patterson TL, Yager JC: Social supports in relation to physical health and symptoms of depression in the elderly. Am J Psychiatry 145:1254–1258, 1988

Kahan J, Kemp B, Staples FR, et al: Decreasing the burden in families caring for a relative with a dementing illness: a controlled study. J Am Geriatr Soc 33:664–670, 1985

Katz MM: Behavioral change in the chronicity pattern of dementia in the institutional geriatric resident. J Am Geriatr Soc 11:522–528, 1976

Kohut H: How Does Analysis Cure? Chicago, IL, University of Chicago Press, 1984

Lazarus LW: Self psychology and psychotherapy with the elderly: theory and practice. J Geriatr Psychiatry 13:69–88, 1980

Lazarus LW, Groves L: Brief psychotherapy with the elderly: a study of process and outcome, in Treating the Elderly With Psychotherapy: The Scope for Change in Later Life. Edited by Sadavoy J, Leszcz M. Madison, CT, International Universities Press, 1987, pp 265–293

Lazarus LW, Stafford B, Cooper K, et al: A pilot study of an Alzheimer patients' relatives discussion group. Gerontologist 21:353–358, 1981

Lesser J, Frankel R, Havasy S: Reminiscence group therapy with psychotic geriatric inpatients. Gerontologist 21:291–296, 1981

Leszcz M: Group psychotherapy with the elderly, in Treating the Elderly With Psychotherapy: The Scope for Change in Later Life. Edited by Sadavoy J, Leszcz M. Madison, CT, International Universities Press, 1987, pp 325–349

Leszcz M, Feigenbaum E, Sadavoy J, et al: A men's group: psychotherapy of elderly men. Int J Group Psychother 35:177–196, 1985

Levine HB: Milieu biopsy: the place of the therapy group on the inpatient ward. Int J Group Psychother 30:77–93, 1980

Lieberman MA, Gaurash N: Evaluating the effects of group changes on the elderly. Int J Group Psychother 29:283–304, 1979

Linden M: Group psychotherapy with institutionalized senile women: study in gerontologic human relations. Int J Group Psychother 3:150–170, 1953

Lothstein LM, Zimet G: Twinship and alter ego selfobject transferences in group therapy with the elderly: a reanalysis of the pairing phenomenon. Int J Group Psychother 38:303–317, 1988

MacLennan BW, Saul S, Weiner MB: Group Psychotherapies for the Elderly. American Group Psychotherapy Association Monograph no 5. Madison, CT, International Universities Press, 1988

Miller E: The management of dementia: a review of some possibilities. British Journal of Social and Clinical Psychology 16:77–83, 1977

Murphy E: The prognosis of depression in old age. Br J Psychiatry 142:111–117, 1983

Parham JA, Priddy MJ, McGovern TU, et al: Group psychotherapy with the elderly: problems and prospects. Psychotherapy: Theory, Research, and Practice 19:437–447, 1982

Poulton JL, Strassberg DS: The therapeutic use of reminiscence. Int J Group Psychother 36:381–398, 1986

Reichenfeld HF, Csapo KG, Carriere L, et al: Evaluating the effect of activity programs on a geriatric ward. Gerontologist 13:305–310, 1973

Rush AJ: Cognitive therapy of depression. Psychiatr Clin North Am 6:105–127, 1983

Salvendy JT: Brief group psychotherapy at retirement. Group 13:43–52, 1989

Samberg S: Dance therapy groups for the elderly, in Group Psychotherapies for the Elderly. American Group Psychotherapy Association Monograph no 5. Edited by MacLennan BW, Saul S, Bakur Weiner M. Madison, CT, International Universities Press, 1988

Saul SR: Group therapy with confused and disoriented people, in Group Psychotherapies for the Elderly. American Group Psychotherapy Association Monograph no 5. Edited by MacLennan BW, Saul S, Bakur Weiner M. Madison, CT, International Universities Press, 1988, pp 199–208

Schwartzman G: The use of the group as selfobject. Int J Group Psychother 34:229–242, 1984

Steuer JL, Hammen CL: Cognitive-behavioral group therapy for the depressed elderly: issues and adaptations. Cognitive Therapy Research 7:285–296, 1983

Steuer JL, Mintz J, Hammen CL, et al: Cognitive-behavioral and psychodynamic group psychotherapy in treatment of geriatric depression. J Consult Clin Psychol 52(4):80–89, 1984

Stone WN, Whitman RM: Contributions of the psychology of self to group process and group therapy. Int J Group Psychother 27:343–359, 1977

Sweet M, Stoler N, Kelter R, et al: A community of builders: support groups for veterans forced into early retirement. Hosp Community Psychiatry 40:172–176, 1989

Tross S, Blum JE: A review of group therapy with the older adult: practice and research, in Group Psychotherapies for the Elderly. American Group Psychotherapy Association Monograph no 5. Edited by MacLennan BW, Saul S, Bakur Weiner M. Madison, CT, International Universities Press, 1988

Yalom ID: The Theory and Practice of Group Psychotherapy. New York, Basic Books, 1985

Yalom ID, Terrazas F: Group therapy for psychotic elderly patients. Am J Nurs 1690–1694, 1967

Zarit SH, Reever KE, Bach-Peterson J: Relatives of the impaired elderly: correlates of feelings of burden. Gerontology 6:649–655, 1980

CHAPTER 27

Sharon M. Curlik, D.O.
Deborah Frazier, PH.D.
Ira R. Katz, M.D., PH.D.

Psychiatric Aspects of Long-Term Care

Nursing homes provide care to injured, disabled, or sick patients who require medical, nursing, or rehabilitation services. Depending on the level of care provided, they may be skilled nursing facilities (SNFs) or intermediate care facilities (ICFs); a given institution may include either or both types of facilities. Nursing homes may provide convalescent care during a period of recovery from acute illness or injury, or long-term care for chronic illness and disability. Knowledge of the psychiatric disorders of nursing home residents is expanding rapidly as the result of intensive research in a number of centers. At the same time, the delivery of services is being shaped by federal legislation and evolving regulations. These developments emphasize both the importance of, and the problems in, this area. In this chapter we first discuss the evolving federal regulations and then the relevant clinical issues.

Federal Regulations

The Nursing Home Reform Act of the Omnibus Budget Reconciliation Act of 1987 deals specifically with the psychiatric aspects of long-term care. One section of the Act mandates preadmission screening of potential nursing home residents and screening of current residents, to ensure that patients with mental illness are not admitted solely as a result of their psychiatric disorder to long-

This work was supported in part by Clinical Research Center grant MH-40380 from the National Institute of Mental Health.

term care facilities that receive federal financing. Patients cannot be admitted unless they require the level of services provided by a nursing facility and do not require "active treatment" for their mental illness that would not be available in the nursing home. For this purpose the Act states that an individual is considered to be "mentally ill" if the individual has a primary or secondary psychiatric diagnosis of mental illness (as defined in DSM-III-R [American Psychiatric Association 1987]) and does not have a primary diagnosis of dementia (including Alzheimer's disease or a related disorder [Nursing Home Reform Act 1987]). In its discussion of the Act, the House Committee on the Budget stated, "Substantial numbers of mentally retarded and mentally ill residents are inappropriately placed at Medicaid expense in SNFs or ICFs. These residents often do not receive the active treatment or services that they need." The committee cited a General Accounting Office report that noted that the states have a strong financial incentive for placing the mentally ill and the mentally retarded in Medicaid-certified SNFs or ICFs, where the federal government participates in the cost of their treatment (Committee on the Budget 1987) (see also Chapter 34).

This section of the Act thus appears related to ongoing controversies about the process of deinstitutionalization and the question of who should bear the costs of treatment for the patient with severe, chronic psychiatric illness. Although these issues are relevant primarily for chronic schizophrenic patients, the Act applies to all patients with a primary or secondary psychiatric diagnosis. The impact of the requirement for preadmission screening will depend on the regulations to be issued by the Health Care Financing Administration (HCFA) and the individual states. At best, preadmission screening may help to ensure that patients with disability due in large part to treatable psychiatric disorders (such as depression) are not placed in long-term care facilities before receiving the benefits of adequate psychiatric treatment. At worst, it could prevent admission for patients with severe medical illness when they have psychiatric symptoms resulting from difficulties in adjusting to disease and disability. However, it is important to emphasize that nursing home residents' need for psychiatric services will remain in spite of any efforts to exclude patients with mental illness.

The value of psychiatric evaluation and treatment for patients with Alzheimer's disease and related disorders is well established. For other patients, who require admission as a result of medical or neurological illness, the same factors that necessitate nursing home admission (e.g., chronic disease, self-care deficits, sensory impairments) are also risk factors for psychiatric disorders such as depression. The risk of psychiatric disorders is further augmented by the consequences of admission, including changes in social status; disruption of the social network; and loss of privacy, independence, and autonomy. The patients with the greatest need for nursing home admission are those who also have the greatest need for psychiatric services.

Other sections of the Nursing Home Reform Act provide federal standards for the quality of care in nursing homes. Sections specifically relevant for psychiatry include those concerned with the use of restraints, psychopharmacological treatment, and the quality of life. Proposed HCFA regulations state, "The resident has the right to be free of and the facility must ensure freedom from physical restraints imposed or drugs administered for the purpose of discipline and convenience and not required to treat the resident's medical symptoms" (Health Care Financing Administration 1989). With respect to psychopharmacological treatment, the Nursing Home Reform Act states, "Psychopharmacological drugs may be administered only on the orders of a physician and only as a part of a plan detailed to eliminate or modify the symptoms for which the drugs are prescribed and only if, at least annually, an independent, external consultant reviews the appropriateness of the drug plan of each resident receiving such drugs." Although HCFA regulations are not yet available, the House Budget Committee's discussion provides insight into the rationale and the intent of this provision: "The Committee is concerned that psychotropic drugs are being used to manage residents for the convenience of nursing facility staffs in a manner that is wholly inconsistent with high quality care or an adequate quality of life. . . . The Committee amendment would require an annual review of the appropriateness of the drug plan . . . by an independent consultant in psychopharmacology" (Committee on the Budget 1987).

With respect to the quality of life, proposed HCFA regulations state that facilities must provide for each resident the necessary care and services to "attain or maintain the highest possible mental and physical functional status" and the "highest practicable physical, mental, and psychosocial well-being." They also state that the facilities must ensure that "a resident who displays psychosocial adjustment difficulty receives appropriate treatment and services to achieve as much remotivation and reorientation as possible" (Health Care Financing Administration 1989). The Act thus requires the screening of residents to identify those in need of mental health services and the providing of such services. Appropriate psychiatric diagnosis and psychosocial assessment are central to all of the concerns raised by the Act. Minimizing the use of restraints requires that psychotherapeutic and behavioral strategies be used whenever possible to manage disruptive or dangerous behavior. Obtaining expert psychopharmacological consultation in the nursing home requires the services of trained geriatric psychiatrists. Finally, optimizing the quality of life in the nursing home and providing treatment to improve psychosocial adjustment requires the services of experienced geriatric mental health professionals.

Nursing Home Demographics

The 1985 National Nursing Home Survey found that 5% of Americans aged 65 or older (1.5 million people) resided in more than 20,000 long-term care facilities and that 88% of all residents in nursing homes were 65 or older. One percent of the population aged 65 to 74, 3% of those 75 to 84, and 22% of those 85 or older lived in these settings. These institutions cared for a population that was both very old and functionally impaired: 91% of residents required assistance in bathing; 78% in dressing; 63% in both toileting and transferring; 40% in eating; and 55% were incontinent. Only 8% were independent in all activities of daily living. The average resident took 3.2 medications daily. Eighty-four percent of residents were without spouses and 57% had been transferred to the setting from another health care facility, most commonly a hospital. The mean length of stay in a nursing home was 2.5 years; 67% of current residents had lived in a home for at least 1 year. One-half of elderly residents used their own or family finances to fund their first month in the nursing home. Most residents had exhausted their savings after only a few months (Benson and Gambert 1984; Campion et al. 1983; Hing 1987).

There are projections that 25% of Americans can now expect to spend part of their lives in nursing homes (Campion et al. 1983) and that the number of nursing home residents will more than triple by the year 2020 (McCarthy 1989). These figures, as well as the high prevalence of psychiatric illnesses and behavioral disturbances in this population, emphasize the need for the development of specifically trained personnel in geriatric mental health and for research on the psychiatric aspects of long-term care.

Epidemiology of Psychiatric Illness in
Nursing Home Residents

The literature uniformly reports a high prevalence of psychiatric illness in nursing home residents. One study that surveyed the vast majority of the residents of a large urban nursing home and confirmed diagnoses by clinical evaluation found DSM-III-R psychiatric disorders in 91% (Parmelee et al. 1989). Other investigations, based on psychiatric interviews of randomly selected samples, found prevalence rates of DSM-III (American Psychiatric Association 1980) or DSM-III-R disorders as high as 94% (Chandler and Chandler 1988; Rovner et al. 1986). Other studies have reported lower rates but appear to have used less rigorous methods or to have assessed only selected subpopulations of residents (Burns et al. 1988; Custer et al. 1984; German et al. 1986; Teeter et al. 1976).

In all studies, the most common psychiatric disorder is dementia, with prevalence rates from one-half to three-fourths of residents (Chandler and Chandler 1988; Katz et al. 1989; Parmelee et al. 1989; Rovner et al. 1986; Teeter et al. 1976). An Epidemiologic Catchment Area study reported a lower prevalence of cognitive impairment, but the more severely impaired patients who could not complete the testing were excluded (German et al. 1986). Alzheimer's disease (primary degenerative dementia) accounts for approximately one-half of cases; multi-infarct dementia, for approximately one-fourth (Barnes and Raskind 1980; Rovner et al. 1986). Other causes of dementia are reported with lower prevalence and greater variability between sites.

Patients with dementing illnesses are at high risk for secondary complications, including delirium, psychosis, and depression. Although delirium and other toxic or metabolic encephalopathies have not been systematically investigated in the long-term care setting, the available studies reported that approximately 6% to 7% of residents had been delirious at the time of evaluation (Barnes and Raskind 1980; Rovner et al. 1986). However, the number of patients with reversible components to their cognitive impairment was probably underestimated; one study found that nearly 25% of impaired residents had potentially reversible conditions (Sabin et al. 1982). Psychotic symptoms have been reported in approximately 25% to 50% of residents with a primary dementing illness (Berrios and Brook 1985; Chandler and Chandler 1988; Rovner et al. 1986; Teeter et al. 1976). Clinically significant depression has been seen in approximately 25% of demented patients;

one-third of these exhibited symptoms of a secondary major depression (Parmelee et al. 1989; Rovner et al. 1986).

Depressive disorders are the most common of the "functional" diagnoses and the second most common of all psychiatric diagnoses among nursing home residents. Most studies evaluating depression in long-term care settings report a prevalence range of 15% to 50%, which varies with the population studied and the instruments used, whether major depression or depressive symptoms are being reported, and whether primary depression and depression occurring secondary to dementia are considered together or separately (Chandler and Chandler 1988; Hyer and Blazer 1982; Katz et al. 1989; Lesher 1986; Parmelee et al. 1989; Rovner et al. 1986; Teeter et al. 1976). Studies from other countries have reported similar percentages (Mann et al. 1984; Snowdon 1986; Snowdon and Donnelly 1986). The risk of depressive illnesses is significantly higher than in the community elderly (Blazer and Williams 1980; Kramer et al. 1985). Approximately 6% to 10% of nursing home residents (or 20% to 25% of those residents who are cognitively intact) meet DSM-III or DSM-III-R criteria for major depression; the prevalence of other forms of depression is somewhat higher (Parmelee et al. 1989). Although the somatic and vegetative components of major depression are difficult to evaluate in the frail elderly, the symptoms of this disorder do characterize a group of patients with increased disability, medical morbidity, and mortality. Nursing home residents with symptoms of major depression commonly have medical illnesses and/or medications that can either cause depressive symptoms or complicate pharmacological treatment. In the evaluation and treatment of these patients, it is important to balance the need to seek out vigorously the treatable sources of distress and disability versus the need for caution in treating a highly vulnerable group of patients.

In contrast to prevalence data, little information is available on the incidence of depression in long-term care. One study has reported that 14% of patients not suffering from major depression at the time of an initial evaluation met diagnostic criteria after 6 months, with most of the new cases coming from those with depression of lesser degree at baseline. Ongoing assessment is indicated in this high-risk group (Katz et al. 1989).

As many as two-thirds of nursing home residents with psychiatric disorders may be improperly diagnosed (German et al. 1986; Sabin et al. 1982). Lack of diagnosis and misdiagnosis are of grave concern when one considers the prevalence rates, the numbers of patients involved, the risks of excess disability, and the impact on quality of life. Standardized screening instruments administered on a regular basis by nursing home staff may be of use in identifying patients in need of psychiatric consultation. Both the Mini-Mental State Exam (Folstein et al. 1975) and the Blessed Dementia Index (Blessed et al. 1968) have been used in screening for cognitive impairment. The Geriatric Depression Scale shows promise for use in identifying nursing home residents who need further evaluation for depression (Brink et al. 1982). When administered verbally, it remains reliable in screening for depression among those with a mild or moderate degree of dementia (Parmelee et al. 1989).

However, structured instruments cannot replace evaluation by experienced clinicians. Psychiatrists and other mental health professionals with expertise in geriatrics must become increasingly involved both in providing services in these settings and in educational outreach to physicians and nursing home staff. They can assist administrators and caregivers in implementing screening procedures to detect psychiatric disorders and in establishing services for treatment.

Behavioral Symptoms

The majority of psychiatric consultations in long-term care settings are for the evaluation and treatment of behavioral disturbances, primarily in patients with dementia. These symptoms cause distress for patients, families, and caregivers and often create therapeutic dilemmas for the clinician. The most common behavioral difficulties include pacing and wandering, verbal abusiveness, disruptive shouting, physical aggression, and resistance to necessary care. At least one such symptom may be present in as many as two-thirds of residents, and more than one such behavior occurred in nearly half (Chandler and Chandler 1988; Cohen-Mansfield 1986; National Center for Health Statistics 1979; Rovner et al. 1986; Zimmer et al. 1984). Risk factors for behavioral disturbances include both dementia and psychotic symptoms. Patients with psychotic symptoms are more demented and more behaviorally disturbed than the remainder of the population; the association between psychosis and behavioral disturbance remains, even after controlling for cognitive impairment (Rovner et al. 1986). Other causes of agitation and hyperactivity may include agitated depression, delirium, occult physical illness, pain, urinary retention, and adverse drug effects including akathisia due to neuroleptics. The presence of behavioral disturbances calls for a careful evaluation of causative factors with interventions directed, where possible, to the basic etiology of the disturbance. When patients require symptomatic treatment, it is important to consider all available options including environmental manipulations, psychosocial and activity modifications, and behavioral strategies, as well as psychopharmacologic agents (Cohen-Mansfield and Billig 1986).

Use of Psychotropic Medication

There is widespread concern regarding the overuse of psychotropic drugs in nursing home residents. In general, studies report that approximately 50% of residents have orders for these agents, with 20% to 40% taking neuroleptics, 10% to 40% taking anxiolytics or hypnotics, and 5% to 10% taking antidepressants (Avorn et al. 1989; Beers et al. 1988; Buck 1988; Burns et al. 1988; Cohen-Mansfield 1986; Custer et al. 1984; DeLeo et al. 1989; Ray et al. 1980; Teeter et al. 1976; Zimmer et al. 1984). This high prevalence means that a substantial proportion of nursing home residents are at risk for adverse drug effects.

Psychotropic drugs are, in general, prescribed without adequate input from psychiatry. One study reported that only 15% of residents receiving psychotropic drugs had received a psychiatric consultation (Zimmer et al. 1984). Others have reported that mental health services were available to fewer than 5% of those with a known psychiatric illness and that 21% of patients with no psychiatric diagnosis received psychotropic medication (Burns et al. 1988), that physicians' caseloads (rather than patient characteristics) predicted drug dosage (Ray et al. 1980), and that psychotropic drugs were often prescribed in the absence of any charted reference to patients' mental status (Avorn et al. 1989). The concerns expressed about psychotropic drugs in the Nursing Home Reform Act are well founded. Given the high prevalence of psychiatric disorders among nursing home residents, it is difficult, a priori, to estimate what constitutes overuse of psychotropic medication. The goal of nursing home reform should be the creation of services designed to ensure that each patient receives appropriate treatment, not just an across-the-board decrease in the use of medication.

The use of neuroleptic drugs for the control of behavioral symptoms may present the greatest potential for abuse. There is a pressing need for research on alternative treatments. Although there is evidence of the efficacy of neuroleptics in managing agitation and related symptoms in nursing home residents with dementia, the effects are often undramatic and placebo responses may be common (Barnes et al. 1982). Other medications (as well as behavioral or environmental treatments) may be equally effective. Nevertheless, prescription of neuroleptics is frequently necessary both to manage dangerous or disruptive symptoms and to facilitate diagnostic evaluations. Evaluating the response of the patient to such treatment in the long-term care setting requires an active collaboration between the psychiatrist and other caregivers including, as a rule, nursing staff and the patients' families.

It is important to note that all of the evidence for the efficacy of antipsychotic medications comes from short-term studies, but the medications are frequently prescribed for long-term treatment. One classic, double-blind, neuroleptic-withdrawal study showed that only 16% of patients who had been receiving medications on a chronic basis exhibited significant deterioration when they were withdrawn (Barton and Hurst 1966). A more recent withdrawal study in patients who had been receiving neuroleptics for several months ($n = 9$) found that 22% experienced increased agitation upon withdrawal, 22% were unchanged, and 55% actually showed improvement (Risse et al. 1987). Thus, it is important to reevaluate the need for neuroleptic treatment with trials of drug withdrawal on a regular basis.

Data from a recent unpublished survey conducted by Katz and associates at a large urban nursing home, demonstrated that the psychotropic drugs most commonly prescribed in this facility were the benzodiazepines. Twenty percent of a sample of 284 residents were receiving them on a regular basis and another 20%, p.r.n. Most of these prescriptions were given to assist sleep, most were for chronic use, and most were initially prescribed before the patients were admitted to the facility. In addition, many of the residents were taking other medications that could cause cognitive, affective, or behavioral symptoms: 14% of the residents were taking digoxin, 14% were taking H2-blockers, 9% were taking dopamine agonists for treatment of Parkinson's disease, 8% were taking a beta-blocker (alpha methyldopa or clonidine), and 20% were taking an anticholinergic drug on a regular or p.r.n. basis.

In light of these statistics, one important component of psychopharmacological treatment in the nursing home should be careful reevaluation of the risks versus the benefits of chronic treatment with hypnotic medication, with trials of drug withdrawal whenever possible. Another component should be monitoring for psychiatric symptoms occurring as adverse effects of drugs used for the treatment of medical disorders. All patients receiving centrally acting drugs, whether prescribed for the treatment of psychiatric disorders or medical illness, should be evaluated on a regular basis to determine whether the medications are causing cognitive, affective, or behavioral symptoms.

The problems related to the misuse of psychotropic drugs in the nursing home are not confined to overtreatment and the lack of recognition of adverse effects (Murphy 1989). Underdiagnosis and undertreatment of depression is another significant problem. The high prevalence of depression demonstrates the need for programs for both psychopharmacological and psychosocial treatment.

Mechanical Restraints

Discussion of the use of mechanical restraints for the control of behavior makes the most dramatic case for increased mental health services in the nursing home. The 1977 survey of American nursing home residents found that 25% of 1.3 million people were restrained by geriatric chairs, cuffs, belts, or similar devices (Department of Health, Education, and Welfare 1979). Other surveys have reported prevalence rates up to 85%. Patient factors predicting the use of restraints in nursing homes and other settings include age, cognitive impairment, risk of injuries to self or others (e.g., from falls or combative behavior), physical frailty, presence of monitoring or treatment devices, and the need to promote body alignment. Institutional and system factors include pressure to avoid litigation, staff attitudes, insufficient staffing, and the availability of restraint devices. Mechanical restraints are frequently used to control disruptive behavior. However, there has been little research devoted to evaluating the benefits versus the risks of the use of restraints or systematic investigations of alternatives. Potential adverse effects include an increased risk of falls and other injuries, functional decline, skin breakdown, physiological effects of immobilization stress, disorganized behavior, and emotional desolation. Cross-national studies suggest that it is possible to manage nursing home residents without them (Cape 1983; Innes and Turman 1983). Because mechanical restraints are used to control behavior, mental health professionals should be involved in decisions about their use, both in evaluating individual patients and in formulating institutional policy. To be able to do so, they must be knowledgeable both about the behavioral disorders of the elderly and about the nature of the physical and social environments in the long-term care facility (Evans and Strumpf 1989).

Psychosocial Aspects of Long-Term Care

If the major problem with psychopharmacology in the nursing home is misuse, the problem with respect to psychosocial treatment is neglect. There is a need for increased availability of both psychosocial treatment for specific psychiatric disorders and programs designed to improve the quality of life for all long-term care residents.

Lawton and Nahemow (1973) provided a theoretical framework for considering psychosocial treatment in the long-term care setting. The "ecological theory of aging and adaptation" postulated that the behavior and affect of any given resident are a function of the interaction between that person's competence and the environmental "press" or demands. When capability and demands are well matched there are positive affective and adaptive behavioral outcomes. Conversely, when personal capability and environmental demands are widely discrepant, the individual is likely to manifest negative affect and/or maladaptive behaviors. Immediately surrounding the ideal matching of the individual and the environment are zones in which there are mild discrepancies. When demands somewhat exceed competence, the individual can achieve maximum performance. When competence somewhat exceeds demands, the individual experiences maximum comfort and security. The less competent one is, the greater is the sensitivity to changes in environmental demands.

This model has clear and useful implications for interventions in the residential care facility. First, interventions can be targeted either to an individual or to the environment; interventions may range from purely intrapersonal (e.g., individual psychodynamic psychotherapy) to purely environmental (e.g., recommending a floor change), with many approaches integrating the two aspects. Second, the mental health effects of any large-scale environmental intervention (e.g., policy or structural changes) must be considered in terms of the impact on each individual and the interaction with his or her level of competence. Third, given that long-term care settings are homes as well as treatment settings, it is important to place a high value on comfort as well as on maximizing performance.

Psychotherapy

Individual Interventions

Individual psychotherapy is the most widely recognized and practiced form of mental health intervention. In terms of the Lawton-Nahemow model, it is designed to raise the individual's "competence" (i.e., psychological adjustment or cognitive capacity). In general, there has been little research conducted, either to refine the procedures for the individual therapies, or to establish their efficacy, specifically in the long-term care setting. Historically, psychodynamic or insight-oriented therapy was considered inappropriate for the elderly. More recently this assumption has been challenged as revealing age bias rather than empirically based findings (Levy et al. 1980), and numerous authors have recommended dynamic and supportive therapies with the elderly, although the evidence for efficacy is usually anecdotal (Butler and Lewis 1982; Goodstein 1982; Sadavoy and Leszcz 1987; Verwoerdt 1976). Modifications of psychotherapy that have been suggested for the elderly, especially those in long-term care, include a shorter duration, a more problem-oriented approach, a more active and directive therapist, and a behavioral as well as an intrapsychic focus of change (Sadavoy and Robinson 1989; Spayd and Smyer 1988).

Among the psychotherapies, cognitive and behavioral therapies have been the most thoroughly investigated in the elderly. The efficacy of these approaches, as well as of brief dynamic therapy, has been demonstrated (Gallagher and Thompson 1982; Thompson et al. 1987). Numerous other forms of individual therapy have been used with the depressed and/or disoriented elderly, including life review or reminiscence therapy, pet-assisted therapy, sensory stimulation, reality orientation, validation therapy, and cognitive rehabilitation. Although the efficacy of these forms in general has not been established in controlled studies in the nursing home setting, there is a large anecdotal literature describing their use.

Behavior therapy is a promising intervention for the treatment of agitated or socially inappropriate behavior. It looks at the individual in his or her environment and identifies the exact problem behaviors and their time of occurrence, frequency, and duration, as well as the components of the human and structural environment that may be inciting, exacerbating, or reinforcing the inappropriate behaviors. Strategies for interventions have been described for both behavioral excesses (shouting, cursing, aggression, stripping, wandering, and chronic complaints or excessive demands) and for behavioral deficits (ambulation, self-care, attendance at activities, and social interactions). While traditional techniques of behavior therapy (chaining, shaping, prompting, reinforcing, and time out) are used, the importance of stimulus control is elevated in the treatment of long-term care residents. Many behaviors such as wandering, stereotypies, self-stimulation, and disorientation do not fit neatly into a traditional behavior therapy analysis and may be viewed as "stimulus-free responding." Strategies for stimulus enhancement and stimulus control may be useful in the cognitively impaired elderly (Hussian and Davis 1985). Individual psychotherapy is discussed in detail in Chapter 24.

Group Therapy

Many authors have found significant therapeutic benefits from group therapy, but the differential efficacy of specific techniques or theoretical approaches remains controversial (Gatz et al. 1985). Groups carry the same benefits as with younger patients: cost-effectiveness, socialization, provision of positive role models for coping strategies, and lessening of the sense that problems are unique. (See Chapter 25).

Milieu Therapy

Milieu therapy or the establishment of a "therapeutic community" originated in work during the 1950s to create a more "normalized" setting in mental hospitals. The central focus is on preservation of maximum dignity and self-care through maintenance of work and social roles. An approach to characterizing the nursing home milieu has been described (Moos and Lemke 1985). Milieu interventions in nursing homes have included sheltered workshops (MacDonald and Settin 1978), day treatment programs, and increased opportunities to exercise control and responsibility (Langer and Rodin 1976; Rodin and Langer 1977). Examples of interventions designed to increase control include choosing a plant to care for, choosing when visits will occur, and being able to predict visiting schedules. Even such apparently minor areas of perceived control can produce significant improvements in resident well-being, at least during the time period of the investigation. Integration of such milieu programs into the ongoing design of the facility may be necessary for sustained benefits.

A somewhat different approach to the long-term care milieu takes the view that the nursing home is a community consisting of residents, families, and staff members (Smyer 1988). Based on this sort of model, interventions can be targeted to other members of the community, for example, job enrichment techniques to redesign the nursing home aides' role to include aspects of a mental health paraprofessional (Borchandt and Brannon 1988).

Conclusion

In a very real sense, nursing homes are psychiatric institutions, not because they house deinstitutionalized, chronic psychiatric patients, but because the frail, elderly patients who require nursing home care have profound needs for psychiatric services. Although all nursing homes should have the availability of psychiatric consultation, consultative services alone are not sufficient. There is a need to develop and evaluate 1) a liaison approach to the delivery of services in the nursing home and 2) models that integrate the services of psychiatry and other mental health professionals. Optimally, mental health services should include direct treatment (both psychopharmacological and psychosocial), development of screening programs for case identification, staff education, input into the design of activities and the therapeutic milieu, and administrative consultation. The state of the art with respect to research in the nursing home has been reviewed (Beardsley et al. 1988; Larsen et al. 1989; Rabins et al. 1987). Although there have been major recent advances, further research is essential. Finally, given the magnitude of the need for psychiatric services in long-term care, there is a necessity for the development of trained personnel, both in psychiatry and in the other mental health professions.

References

American Psychiatric Association: Diagnostic and Statistical Manual of Mental Disorders, 3rd Edition. Washington, DC, American Psychiatric Association, 1980

American Psychiatric Association: Diagnostic and Statistical Manual of Mental Disorders, 3rd Edition, Revised. Washington, DC, American Psychiatric Association, 1987

Avorn J, Dreyer P, Connelly K, et al: Use of psychoactive medication and the quality of care in rest homes. N Engl J Med 320:227–232, 1989

Barnes RD, Raskind MA: DSM-III criteria and the clinical diagnosis of dementia: a nursing home study. J Gerontol 36:20–27, 1980

Barnes R, Veith R, Okimoto J, et al: Efficacy of antipsychotic medications

in behaviorally disturbed dementia patients. Am J Psychiatry 139:
1170–1174, 1982

Barton R, Hurst L: Unnecessary use of tranquilizers in elderly patients.
Br J Psychiatry 112:989–990, 1966

Beardsley RS, Larsen DB, Lyons JS, et al: Health services research in
nursing homes: a systematic review of three clinical geriatric journals.
J Gerontology 41:30–35, 1988

Beers M, Avorn J, Soumerai SB, et al: Psychoactive medication use in in-
termediate-care facility residents. JAMA 260:3016–3020, 1988

Benson, D, Gambert SR: The impact of misdiagnosis on nursing home
placement. Psychiatr Med 1:309–316, 1984

Berrios GE, Brook P: Delusions and psychopathology of the elderly with
dementia. Acta Psychiatr Scand 75:296–301, 1985

Blazer D, Williams CD: Epidemiology of dysphoria and depression in an
elderly population. Am J Psychiatry 137:439–444, 1980

Blessed G, Tomlinson BE, Roth M: The association between quantitative
measures of dementia and of senile change in the cerebral grey matter
of elderly subjects. Br J Psychiatry 144:797–811, 1968

Borchandt L, Brannon D: Job design interventions for improving caregiving, in Mental Health Consultation in Nursing Homes. Edited by Smyer
MA, Cohn MD, Brannon D. New York, New York University Press, 1988

Brink TL, Yesavage JA, Lum O, et al: Screening tests for geriatric depression. Clinical Gerontologist 1:37–43, 1982

Buck JA: Psychotropic drug practice in nursing homes. J Am Geriatr Soc
36:409–418, 1988

Burns BJ, Larson DB, Goldstrom ID, et al: Mental Disorder Among Nursing Home Patients: Preliminary Findings from the National Nursing
Home Survey Pretest. International J Geriatric Psych 3:27–35, 1988

Butler RN, Lewis MI: Aging and Mental Health: Positive Psychosocial Approaches. St. Louis, MO, CV Mosby, 1982

Campion EW, Ban A, May M: Why acute-care hospitals must undertake
long-term care. N Engl J Med 308:71–75, 1983

Cape RD: Freedom from restraint. Gerontologist (special issue) 23:217,
1983

Chandler JD, Chandler JE: The prevalence of neuro-psychiatric disorders
in a nursing home population. J Geriatric Psychiatry and Neurology
1:71–76, 1988

Cohen-Mansfield J: Agitated behaviors in the elderly: preliminary results
in the cognitively deteriorated. J Am Geriatr Soc 34:722–727, 1986

Cohen-Mansfield J, Billig N: Agitated behaviors in the elderly: a conceptual review. J Am Geriatr Soc 34:711–721, 1986

Committee on the Budget, U.S. House of Representatives: Omnibus Budget Reconciliation Act of 1987. Report to Accompany H.R. 3545, Report
100-391, Part 1 of 2, 1987

Custer RL, Davis JE, Gee SC: Psychiatric drug usage in VA nursing home
care units. Psychiatric Annals 14:285–292, 1984

DeLeo D, Stella AG, Spagnoli A: Prescription of psychotropic drugs in geriatric institutions. International J Ger Psych 4:11–16, 1989

Department of Health, Education and Welfare: National Nursing Home Survey, 1977 (DHEW publ no (PHS)79-1794). Hyattsville, MD, National Center for Health Statistics, 1979

Evans LK, Strumpf NE: Tying down the elderly: a review of the literature on physical restraint. J Am Geriatr Soc 37:65–74, 1989

Folstein MF, Folstein SE, McHugh PR: Mini-Mental State: a practical method for grading the cognitive state of patients for the clinician. J Psychiatr Res 12:189–198, 1975

Gallagher D, Thompson LW: Treatment of major depressive disorders in older adult outpatients with brief psychotherapies. Psychotherapy: Theory, Research, and Practice 19:482–490, 1982

Gatz M, Popkin SJ, Pino CD, et al: Psychological interventions with older adults, in Handbook of the Psychology of Aging. Edited by Birren JE, Warner-Schaie K. New York, Van Nostrand Reinhold, 1985

German PS, Shapiro S, Kramer M: Mental Illness in Nursing Homes: Agenda for Research. Edited by Harper MS, Lebowitz BD. Rockville, National Institute of Mental Health, 1986, pp 27–40

Goodstein RK: Individual psychotherapy and the elderly. Psychotherapy: Theory, Research, and Practice 19:412–418, 1982

Health Care Financing Administration: Medicare and Medicaid; Requirements for Long Term Care Facilities: Final Rule With Request for Comments, Federal Register 54:5316–5373, 1989

Hing E: Use of Nursing Homes by the Elderly: Preliminary Data from the 1985 National Nursing Home Survey. Advance Data from Vital and Health Stat, no 135 (DHHS Pub. No. (PHS) 87-1250). Hyattsville, MD, National Center for Health Statistics, 1987

Hussian RA, Davis RL: Responsive Care: Behavioral Intervention With Elderly Persons. Champaign, IL, Research Press, 1985

Hyer L, Blazer D: Depressive Symptoms: Impact and Problems in Long Term Care Facilities. International J Behavioral Geriatrics 1:33–44, 1982

Innes EM, Turman WG: Evolution of patient falls. QRB 9:30–35, 1983

Katz IR, Lesher E, Kleban M, et al: Clinical features of depression in the nursing home. International Psychogeriatrics 1:5–15, 1989

Kramer M, German PS, Anthony JC, et al: Patterns of mental disorders among the elderly residents of Eastern Baltimore. J Am Geriatr Soc 33:236–245, 1985

Langer EJ, Rodin J: The effects of choice and enhanced personal responsibility for the aged: a field experiment in an institutional setting. J Per Soc Psychol 34:191–198, 1976

Larsen DB, Lyons JS, Hohmann AA, et al: A systematic review of nursing home research in three psychiatric journals, 1966–1985. International J Geriatric Psychiatry 4:129–134, 1989

Lawton MP, Nahemow L: Ecology and the aging process, in The Psychology of Adult Development and Aging. Edited by Eisdorfer C, Lawton MP. Washington, DC, American Psychological Association, 1973

Lesher E: Validation of the geriatric depression scale among nursing home residents. Clin Gerontol 4:21–28, 1986

Levy SM, Derogatis LR, Gallagher D, et al: Intervention with older adults and the evaluation of outcome, in Aging in the 1980s. Edited by Poon LW. Washington, DC, American Psychological Association, 1980

MacDonald ML, Settin JM: Reality orientation versus sheltered workshops as treatment for the institutionalized aging. J Gerontol 33:416–421, 1978

Mann AH, Graham N, Ashby D: Psychiatric illness in residential homes for the elderly: a survey in one London borough. Age and Ageing 13:257–265, 1984

McCarthy P: Why one nursing home and not another? Senior Patient May/June:97–102, 1989

Moos RH, Lemke S: Specialized living environments for older people, in Handbook of the Psychology of Aging. Edited by Birren JE, Warner Schaie K. New York, Van Nostrand Reinhold, 1985

Murphy E: Editorial: the use of psychotropic drugs in long term care. International J Geriatric Psychiatry 4:1–2, 1989

National Center for Health Statistics: The National Nursing Home Survey (DHEW Pub. (PHS) 79-1794). Washington, U.S. Government Printing Office, 1979

Nursing Home Reform Act. Omnibus Budget Reconciliation Act of 1987. Public Law 100-203, 1987

Parmelee PA, Katz IR, Lawton MP: Depression among institutionalized aged: assessment and prevalence estimation. J Gerontol 44:M22–M29, 1989

Rabins PV, Rovner BW, Larsen DB, et al: The use of mental health measures in nursing home research. J Am Geriatr Soc 35:431–434, 1987

Ray WA, Federspiel CF, Schaffner W: A study of antipsychotic drug use in nursing homes: epidemiologic evidence suggesting misuse. Am J Public Health 70:485–491, 1980

Risse SC, Cubberley L, Lampe TH, et al: Acute effects of neuroleptic withdrawal in elderly dementia patients. J Geriatric Drug Therapy 2:65–77, 1987

Rodin J, Langer EJ: Long-term effects of a control-relevant intervention with institutionalized aged. J Pers Soc Psychol 35:897–902, 1977

Rovner BW, Kafonek S, Filipp L, et al: Prevalence of mental illness in a community nursing home. Am J Psychiatry 143:1446–1449, 1986

Sabin TD, Vitug AJ, Mark VH: Are nursing home diagnosis and treatment inadequate? JAMA 248:321–322, 1982

Sadavoy J, Leszcz M: Treating the Elderly With Psychotherapy: Scope for Change in Later Life. Madison, CT, International Universities Press, 1987

Sadavoy J, Robinson A: Psychotherapy and the cognitively impaired elderly, in Conn D, Grek A, Sadavoy J. Psychiatric Consequences of Brain Disease in the Elderly. New York, Plenum, 1989, pp 101–135

Smyer MA: The nursing home community, in Mental Health Consultation in Nursing Homes. Edited by Smyer MA, Cohn MD, Brannon D. New York, New York University Press, 1988

Snowdon J: Dementia, depression, and life satisfaction in nursing homes. International J Geriatric Psychiatry 1986; 1:85–91

Snowdon J, Donnelly N: A study of depression in nursing homes. J Psychiatr Res 20:327–333, 1986

Spayd CS, Smyer MA: Individual interventions for nursing home residents, in Mental Health Consultation in Nursing Homes. Edited by Smyer MA, Cohn MD, Brannon D. New York, New York University Press, 1988

Teeter RB, Garetz FK, Miller WR, et al: Psychiatric disturbances of aged patients in skilled nursing homes. Am J Psychiatry 133:1430–1434, 1976

Thompson LW, Gallagher D, Breckenridge JS: Comparative Effectiveness of Psychotherapies for Depressed Elders. J Consult Clin Psychol 55:385–390, 1987

Verwoerdt A: Clinical Geropsychiatry. Baltimore, MD, Williams & Wilkins, 1976

Zimmer JG, Watson N, Treat A: Behavioral problems among patients in skilled nursing facilities. Am J Public Health 74:1118–1121, 1984

CHAPTER 28

David G. Folks, M.D.
F. Cleveland Kinney, M.D., PH.D.

Consultation-Liaison in the General Hospital

Overview

The geriatric population uses the largest proportion of health care resources in this country. Although patients over the age of 65 constitute approximately 12% of the U.S. population, this segment occupies one-third of all beds used in acute care hospitals and accounts for 30% of all expenditures for personal health care (Allen et al. 1986). Obviously, because the number of those persons over the age of 65 is expected to nearly double within the next 30 years, the health care needs of this hospital population will continue to grow. Undoubtedly psychiatric consultation requests will rise, and the organization and delivery of consultation services will need to be more efficient. Such care has been shown to have a significant impact on therapeutic outcome and helps to diminish morbidity (Ford and Folks 1985; Levitan and Kornfeld 1981).

Consultation psychiatry in the general hospital already involves a significant number of geriatric cases. Several studies report that 20% or more of referrals in teaching hospitals include patients aged 65 or older (Folks and Ford 1985; Popkin et al. 1984; Rabins et al. 1983). Most if not all of these patients exhibit medical, neurologic, or surgical illnesses with associated social, behavioral, physiological, and psychological components. These cases are initially encountered on the medical–surgical wards or in an ambulatory clinic, emergency department, or critical care setting.

General hospitals, complemented by ambulatory facilities, are preferred treatment settings for the elderly, especially because of their comprehensive services and easy access. Arie and Jolley (1982) described several factors pertinent to the value of a geriatric psychiatry service in the general hospital: 1) defining demographic and epidemiologic characteristics of the population to be served, 2) working with multiple professional disciplines, 3) making home visits available, and 4) providing comprehensive treatment, especially in those cases with overlap between "functional" and "organic" illnesses. The establishment of consultation-liaison services for the elderly is likely to be effective in producing coordinated networks among related services and health care providers.

Clinical Approach to the Elderly Medical-Surgical Patient

A comprehensive psychiatric consultation includes a number of elements that are placed in the patient's permanent record and represent the final product of a concerted effort. The consult note includes a title, date, time, and source of referral with an identifying statement as to the nature of the consult request, as well as the history, mental status examination, and pertinent physical and neurological findings. Personal and past history, laboratory and radiographic data, and other elements, including the current therapeutic regimen, serve to support the consultant's written diagnostic impression and formulation. The use of DSM-III-R (American Psychiatric Association 1987) and its multiaxial schemata provides diagnostic clarity. The diagnostic impression and the consultant's recommendations are the first and sometimes only comments read by the consultee. Thus, the written consultation concludes with a concise and clear statement of the question posed, a comprehensive approach to the clinical problem, and carefully delineated immediate and long-term management recommendations.

The consultation effort may include any or all of the following: 1) clarification of diagnosis; 2) recommendations for management, whether they be pharmacologic, psychosocial, psychotherapeutic, or crisis intervention; 3) need for social work intervention or ancillary treatment, such as occupational or physical therapy; 4) need for environmental manipulation or interventions that affect situational or psychological functioning; and 5) other recommendations for psychiatric management on the medical-surgical ward or for transfer for inpatient psychiatric care. A number of obstacles may be encountered in the consultation setting with respect to appreciation of the family and biopsychosocial systems. Conferences with family members or caregivers may be necessary, especially to obtain historical data from a reliable source. Issues must be addressed relevant to any possible therapeutic nihilism or ageism on the part of all concerned, including the patient.

These considerations together with direct communication with the primary or treating physician are of major importance. Such efforts often lay the groundwork for therapeutic endeavors with the patient's family. The consultant must appreciate those family members or caregivers who experience conflict with respect to their aging relative's deteriorating or debilitating health or who must address issues of role reversal, loss of autonomy, or nursing home placement. Comprehensive care is often required for older patients referred for psychiatric consultation; the consultant may need to indicate whether he or she should be considered for assuming primary responsibility for the case.

The "full" consultation effort is contrasted with a number of requests that may require only a limited response to a very focused question, or may simply represent a request for transfer for inpatient psychiatric care. Three final areas of general importance regarding psychiatric consultation include the clinical impact of a consultation, the concordance with recommendations (made by the consultant), and the relative effect of psychiatric disturbance on the patient's hospital course and/or therapeutic outcome.

Consultation-Liaison Psychiatry and Age-Related Considerations

The elderly suffer a disproportionate amount of disease and, as outlined in the previous section, now constitute a significant proportion of patients present in general hospitals. A high prevalence of psychiatric illness has been found in the medically hospitalized elderly; the more frequent, primary, psychiatric diagnoses include organic mental syndrome, anxiety, and depression (Folks and Ford 1985). Lipowski (1983) reported that as many as 50% of elderly patients on medical or surgical units have some significant psychiatric disturbances.

Arie and Jolley (1982) showed that the consulting geriatric psychiatrist needs to be familiar with the ambulatory medical facilities, local pattern of ancillary services, and community agencies that are involved with the hospitalized elderly, as well as the phenomenology and demographics of the population being served.

The geriatric psychiatrist practicing consultation-liaison psychiatry is knowledgeable about age-related medical, social, and psychological problems and is prepared to coordinate his or her efforts with the health care team. Furthermore, a geriatric psychiatrist who acts as a medical management coordinator is more than likely to appreciate both the medical and psychological needs of the elderly patient, as well as the impact of psychosocial factors and how these factors interact and influence diagnosis and management. A consulting geriatric psychiatrist is in an ideal position to continuously educate his or her medical-surgical colleagues about organic brain syndromes, mood disorders, and other psychiatric disturbances prevalent among the aged.

The Relationship Between Consultation-Liaison and Inpatient Psychiatry

The development of geriatric psychiatry as a specialized field in psychiatry has been facilitated by active consultation-liaison efforts in the general hospital setting and by subsequent development of specialized hospital units for medically and psychiatrically ill elderly patients (Arie and Jolley 1982). Reisberg and Ferris (1982) suggested that the consultation-liaison psychiatrist can effectively identify those elderly patients with a psychiatric disorder and determine whether an inpatient referral is indicated. In support, Lipowski (1983) suggested that consultation-liaison and geriatric psychiatry training programs are ideally suited for integration.

Starkman and Hall (1979) were the first to demonstrate that the consultation psychiatrist could offer easy movement from one mode of service delivery to another, i.e., inpatient, outpatient, partial hospitalization, as well as consultation. Thus, psychiatric consultation in the general hospital often results in an effective beginning for using a multidisciplinary approach, that is, teaching the biologic, psychologic, and experiential aspects of aging, and demonstrating the interaction of these biopsychosocial influences on medical or neurologic illnesses. This consultation approach facilitates the identification of those cases that require inpatient referral for intensive psychiatric treatment or evaluation. A close working relationship between the consultation-liaison and inpatient psychiatrists can lead to a more comprehensive approach to the geriatric medical-surgical patient.

Indications for Psychiatric Consultation and Use of Consultation Services

Despite the notable prevalence of psychiatric disorders in elderly hospitalized patients, several studies have shown that these patients are referred far less frequently for psychiatric consultation than are their nonelderly counterparts (Rabins et al. 1983). Several reports (Folks and Ford 1985; Koenig et al. 1988; Popkin et al. 1984; Rabins et al. 1983) have observed that the referral rate of hospitalized inpatients aged 65 and older was conspicuously less than the estimated prevalence of psychiatric morbidity in similar populations. In part, the negative attitudes and therapeutic nihilism displayed toward the aged (by both psychiatric and nonpsychiatric physicians) explain this phenomenon. In addition, a number of the psychiatric disturbances are simply unrecognized by the primary physician. For example, Folks and Ford (1985) reported a study of psychogeriatric consultations in which two-thirds of those referred for consultation had a previously unrecognized organic mental syndrome. Poynton (1988) studied psychiatric liaison referrals of elderly inpatients in a teaching hospital. Thirty-seven percent of referrals were diagnosed with an organic mental syndrome and 23% with depression. More than half of the above-mentioned patients were suffering from chronic medical illness, and a third or more—four of whom had primary alcohol abuse—gave a definitive past history of psychiatric disturbance. The overwhelming majority of cases were referred for symptoms of depression or acute confusion.

Despite disproportionately low referral rates for geriatric patients, the literature suggests that physicians are beginning to request consultations earlier in the course of hospitalization for older patients. Christie and Wood (1987) found that the increasing numbers of hospitalized elderly patients and demand for psychiatric follow-up were the two factors explaining greater physician awareness of psychiatric disturbances among the elderly. Greater use of consultation-liaison psychiatry in geriatric populations has strengthened the roles of both consultation and general psychiatrists in the general hospital (Allen et al. 1986; Thienhaus et al. 1988). A model of collaborative care in which the geriatric case is coordinated by a single identified team leader was proposed by Small and Fawzy (1988). This concept is quite practical and employs a method of improving consultation services in most general hospitals by instituting a central focus of four existing services: general medicine, consultation-liaison psychiatry, geriatric medicine, and geriatric psychiatry. The collaborative approach of these four groups presumably could result in significant clinical overlap between disciplines, thus resulting in meaningful collaboration and improved care and therapeutic outcome. Small and Fawzy's format affords the older patient an opportunity to receive specialized care from a geriatric psychiatrist or internist–family physician. Contact with a primary care physician is maintained, and existing general consultation-liaison hospital services may also be used. Because most hospitals do not have sufficient numbers of geriatric psychiatrists who regularly provide consultation to medical-surgical units, this collaborative model provides a format for efficient delivery of care to the psychiatrically disturbed, geriatric medical-surgical patient.

Emergency psychiatric consultations in the general hospital setting were examined by Perez and Blouin (1986), who compared the demographic and clinical characteristics and treatment recommendations for individuals aged older than 60 with those of younger patients. Eleven characteristics differentiated urgent consults for geriatric patients from those involving younger patients. The most notable was that the elderly experienced their chief complaint longer than the younger patients before an emergency referral was instituted by their primary care physician.

Older patients use traditional psychiatric emergency room services much less frequently than younger patients (Perez and Blouin 1986; Thienhaus et al. 1988). Geriatric cases seen in a traditional emergency setting have a higher prevalence of DSM-III (American Psychiatric Association 1980) affective disorders and psychological factors affecting their physical condition. Factors predictive of subsequent admission to a psychiatric unit include dementia and advanced age. Dementia (the single most frequent diagnosis seen in emergency room consultation) increases the likelihood of hospitalization only if the dementia exists in combination with another psychiatric diagnosis or behavioral disturbance. It is interesting that medical comorbidity appears to have no effect on whether an elderly patient is subsequently hospitalized in an emergency room consultation (Thienhaus et al. 1988).

Diagnostic Issues in Psychiatric Consultation

The differential diagnosis of psychiatric symptoms is a major consideration in hospitalized elderly patients. Dementia, a diffuse impairment that interferes with memory and interpersonal and higher intellectual functioning, must be distinguished from the fluctuating level of consciousness and confusional state that occurs with delirium. Rabins and Folstein (1982) documented that delirious patients had higher fatality rates at 1-year follow-up than did depressed, cognitively intact, or demented patients. Mood and anxiety disorders represent the highest percentage of "functional" psychiatric disturbances in patients referred for psychiatric consultation (Folks and Ford 1985; Koenig et al. 1988; Popkin et al. 1984; Rabins et al. 1983). Mood disturbances have been strongly associated with a number of medical illnesses and medical regimens (Folks and Ford 1985); they often lead to diagnostic problems and, if untreated, to therapeutic failure or prolonged hospitalization.

Depressive Syndromes

Depression, dysphoria, and other depressive spectrum disorders of late life are found in as many as 25% of hospitalized medical-surgical geriatric patients (Koenig et al. 1988). Numerous medical illnesses and medications are known to produce secondary depression or an organic mood disorder. Koenig and associates (1988) evaluated the ability of health professionals to detect and treat major depression in older, medically ill, hospitalized patients. These investigators observed that depression continues to be underdiagnosed and undertreated. One hundred and seventy-one patients admitted to the medical and neurology wards of a Veterans Administration medical center were evaluated for major depression. Twenty percent had depressive symptoms documented in their charts prior to the request for psychiatric consultation. Sadavoy and Reiman-Sheldon (1983) followed, for an average of 30.5 months, 52 geriatric patients who had been treated for major depression in a general hospital psychiatric unit. They concluded that many of these patients do poorly over long periods of time and that follow-up must be carefully arranged.

Accurately diagnosing a depressive disorder, correctly identifying a subtype, and initiating effective treatment (which does not complicate the patient's physical condition) are all difficult tasks for the consulting psychiatrist. Depression, irrespective of the patient's medical or surgical status, necessitates rigorous treatment, especially because both mortality and morbidity are increased by a clinical depression. A number of depressed patients relapse after an initial positive response to treatment, and follow-up by the consulting psychiatrist is needed (Sadavoy and Reiman-Sheldon 1983).

Grief, secondary either to significant losses or to a decline in health status, may significantly complicate the hospital course of a patient. Grief symptoms may be intense and often include gastrointestinal complaints, weight loss, difficulty sleeping, and/or a variety of somatic disturbances, including lethargy, fatigue, and emotional paralysis. Zisook, in a presentation at the 1990 annual meeting of the American Association for Geriatric Psychiatry in San Diego, CA, reported that grief symptoms and DSM-III-R criteria for major depression were indistinguishable. Although grief may represent a normal human response, persistence of severe symptoms beyond several months suggests a condition more serious than the normal grief process, such as a major depression (Brown and Stoudemire 1983). In essence, the consultation and clinical approach to these pathologic or prolonged episodes of grief are similar to the clinical approach to depression. Patients with prolonged grief are often responsive to psychotherapeutic intervention that includes mobilizing the psychosocial support system (Horowitz et al. 1984). In fact, the limited number of recent studies suggests that virtually all of those with pathologic or prolonged grief require attention to the psychological and psychosocial aspects of their illness. This need is in contrast to depressed, nongrieving individuals who may respond to somatic therapy alone. Antidepressant medication may also be indicated for patients with pathologic grief and coexistent core symptoms of major depression, for example, guilt, suicidal preoccupation, anhedonia, and/or vegetative disturbances (Brown and Stoudemire 1983; Cavanaugh 1984a; Folks and Ford 1985).

Major depression is notably characterized by persistently depressed mood or loss of interest with accompanying vegetative symptoms. However, in the consultation setting, patients may be especially prone to deny or minimize their depressed mood and present with preoccupation with somatic complaints and coexistent sleep disturbance, appetite disturbance, decreased libido, anhedonia, and/or inability to concentrate; these symptoms may suggest major depression. Patients whose mood disturbance is masked, that is, expressed in somatic complaints (somatizers) or symptoms of apparent dementia (depressive pseudodementia), are well described in the literature. Medically ill, depressed patients are notoriously poor historians, and it is often necessary, despite the inconvenience, to interview an ancillary source who has known the patient well and is familiar with his or her current mood and pertinent history. Moreover, it is sometimes difficult to distinguish the aforementioned vegetative symptoms of depression from the vegetative disturbances caused by a medical illness or its treatment (Cavanaugh 1984a). Particular emphasis may be placed on such psychological symptoms as hopelessness, helplessness, worthlessness, suicidal ideation, and anhedonia in order to distinguish the depressed medically ill from the medically ill who are suffering but not clinically depressed (Cavanaugh et al. 1983; Rodin and Voshart 1986). In addition, affectively disordered medical-surgical patients must be assiduously reassessed and evaluated periodically with specific questioning in order to determine whether the presence of depression is possible (Rodin and Voshart 1986).

In addition to grief and depressive disorders, many elderly patients are increasingly faced with life's vicissitudes and may present with chronic dysphoria. Long-standing and often pervasive unhappiness may be associated with character traits such as passive aggressiveness or frank personality disorders (Fogel and Martin 1987). Treatment is often difficult with some of these patients, and although these cases are sometimes partially responsive to antidepressant medication, most require social work referral or treatment with psychotherapy, psychosocial programs, or behavioral approaches (Cavanaugh 1984b; Sadavoy and Dorian 1983).

Other Psychiatric Conditions

Somatopsychic syndromes and hypochondriacal behavior manifested in late life frequently mask depression, anxiety, and other potentially treatable psychiatric syndromes. The frequency of hypochondriasis and other types of somatoform disorders in a geriatric consultation population is estimated at between 6% and 11% (Folks and Ford 1985; Folks et al. 1990)—a relatively low prevalence of the "pure form" of these disorders in hospitalized elderly patients. However, major and primary forms of somatization and corresponding disorders do extend to late life and can be most troublesome to diagnose and manage in older hospitalized patients. As somatizing patients grow older their behavior and manifest symptoms may or may not change significantly (a subject deserving further study). Behavioral manifestations of somatoform disorders are limited only by the patient's physiological status or psychosocial situation. Concurrent physical disease, perhaps iatrogenic, or the psychobiologic consequences of illness behavior may also be difficult to distinguish from functional complaints. Recommendations for diagnostic procedures in these somatizing patients is based on objective clinical data in order to avoid iatrogenic consequences (Folks et al. 1990).

Psychiatric consultation to hospitalized geriatric patients must often address problems, such as disturbances on the ward, refusal to cooperate with treatment, unresolved issues or conflicts in the family constellation, problems presented by community or governmental agencies, and questions of patient competency. A request for assessment of an elderly patient's competency is a particularly important task for the psychiatric consultant. Consultations involving competency in general must identify the specific area of competency in question (e.g., the capacity to consent to a treatment) and not seek to make a global assessment. Questions of competency can have an immediate impact on the treatment of the patient's medical condition (competency to give informed consent). Additional competency questions affect the patient's future in terms of capacity to manage financial or legal affairs; these questions also may ultimately change the patient's lifestyle and living situation. The patient's autonomy and control of his or her lifestyle and body are respected and preserved to the fullest extent possible. A comprehensive discussion of competency is provided in Chapter 32.

Application of Consultation Principles to the Geriatric Patient

Small and Fawzy (1988) examined psychiatric consultation for the medically ill, elderly, hospitalized patient and developed the previously mentioned model of collaborative care. This work confirmed the important differences between psychiatric consultations for younger and older patients and the findings of differences in types and frequencies of psychopathology. They showed that older patients have much higher rates of chronic medical illnesses, which impact on therapeutic planning and outcome; not unexpectedly they also found that the elderly have high rates of organic mental syndromes (46.6%), consistent with prior studies. This relative shift in the distribution of diagnostic problems found in psychiatric consultation among geriatric cases, together with the degree of intellectual and functional impairments suffered by the hospitalized elderly, may contribute to the lower rates of consultation referral for other mental disorders, for example, personality and adjustment disorders. Conversely, primary care providers may simply give less attention to milder psychiatric problems when they occur in geriatric cases.

The severity of problems encountered in the majority of geriatric cases referred for psychiatric consultation requires that a very thorough comprehensive assessment be performed. Transfer to a psychiatric or psychogeriatric unit may be an optimal choice for some patients, because these facilities are equipped to assist with clarifying multiple diagnoses, initiating psychiatric treatment, and coordinating further medical management, including plans for appropriate follow-up. The utility and appropriateness of transfer is an important consideration, especially because highly effective treatments for psychiatric disorders of the elderly are now available. Psychiatric and behavioral complications of dementia, other organic syndromes, and severe mood disturbances can be assiduously evaluated and treatment can be effectively applied. Adjunctive therapies (i.e., occupational, physical, or recreational therapy) can also be initiated in an attempt to restore or maintain the patient's functional capacity. The development of the medical-psychiatry unit has provided an ideal setting for addressing complicated psychiatric disorders, enabling relatively longer stays (as well as acute admissions) and leading to productive treatment while minimizing tension between psychiatry and medical-surgical disciplines. These settings may also provide an opportunity for the consultation psychiatrist to provide inpatient psychiatric care.

Outcome of Consultation to Geriatric Medical-Surgical Patients

Allen and associates (1986) examined house staff's compliance with recommendations made by a geriatric psychiatry consultation team. Recommendations formulated for 185 patients were randomized into intervention (performed by the geriatric consult team) and control (performed by the general consult team) groups; only 27.1% of the actions recommended by the control team versus 77% recommended by the intervention team were implemented independently by the house staff. Problems commonly neglected in association with control cases included polypharmacy, sensory impairment, confusion, and depression. These differences suggest that geriatric psychiatric expertise, or focus, resulted in an observed attitudinal shift regarding concordance between recommendations and implementation of treatment. The intervention group's highest compliance rates occurred 1) with cases where recommendations addressed functional impairment or falls and 2) with respect to discharge planning. This study revealed that consultation teams with emphasis on geriatrics contribute substantially to the care of older medical-surgical patients. Relatively high compliance can be achieved when recommendations are made by a team that emphasizes its expertise in geriatrics and its ability to provide needed follow-up, thus overcoming an important barrier to the establishment of comprehensive psychogeriatric care.

Koenig and colleagues (1988) reported that after referring physicians (house staff) were informed of the possibility of major depression in a referred case, only 27% of patients were subsequently referred for psychiatric consultation and only 13% had antidepressant medication treatment initiated. A relevant factor was that 87% of depressed patients under study were thought to have relative or absolute contraindications to antidepressant medication, including urinary obstruction, severe congestive heart failure, recent myocardial infarction, unstable angina, narrow-angle glaucoma, and/or current use of anticholinergic or other psychotropic drugs. Undoubtedly, the presence of chronic illness and functional disability among the hospitalized elderly represent important factors that impact significantly on a patient's adjustment to hospitalization and on prognostic outlook (Warshaw et al. 1982).

Liaison Functions of the Consulting Geriatric Psychiatrist

General psychiatrists practicing in an inpatient setting are sometimes isolated from medical-surgical services and as a result may be inadequately aware of the psychosocial and economic factors that can negatively impact on treatment outcome and undermine the patient's treatment plan. Thus, an integrated working relationship that is best coordinated by a consultation-liaison psychiatrist is conducive to therapeutic success; the consultant may also serve to minimize the effects of ageism and professional territory. Sadavoy and Reiman-Sheldon (1983) noted that the high relapse rates of depressed elderly after hospitalization were in part secondary to ineffective follow-up. Although there are few confirming data, most geriatric psychiatry consultants contend that home visits or follow-up visits soon after discharge are one means of preventing the "high level of rejection of the hospital treatment" that has been observed in elderly patients once contact is lost with the psychiatrist responsible for inpatient care (Sadavoy and Reiman-Sheldon 1983).

Several factors suggest that the consultation-liaison psychiatrist's relationship to inpatient psychiatry, and his or her ability to coordinate or provide direct inpatient psychiatric care, are exceedingly relevant to the outcome of cases referred for consultation. First, as many as 50% of elderly patients who exhibit prominent psychiatric symptoms have been shown to demonstrate a high prevalence of underlying physical illness (Folks et al. 1986). Ford (1984) also commented on the impact of overlapping symptoms that arise from physical illness and psychiatric disorders. Comorbidity contributes to the complexity of diagnosis and treatment of geriatric patients who are seen in psychiatric consultation or who are referred for inpatient psychiatric treatment. Thus, the hospital psychiatrist must remain cognizant of these complex, age-related factors and appreciative of the continuing potential for morbidity or poorer prognosis.

Second, the consultation psychiatrist has established a working relationship with his or her medical-surgical colleagues. Thus, in addition to the advantages of employing a biopsychosocial model adhered to by most consultation-liaison psychiatrists, interdisciplinary referral networks necessary for the practice of geriatric medicine remain open (Arie and Jolley 1982; Folks et al. 1986). The consultation psychiatrist who has a working knowledge of inpatient services can achieve the following aims: 1) prompt attention to requests for medical-surgical assessment, 2) close collaboration with other medical and ancillary disciplines, and 3) reliable availability of hospitalization or rehospitalization on the medical, neurological, or surgical services. The implications for outcome with an integrated psychogeriatric team, service, or program as previously outlined enable elderly patients with coexisting medical-surgical illness and psychiatric disorder to be optimally managed. Such liaisons can lead to direct referral for comprehensive psychiatric evaluation and treatment, ultimately providing or enabling easier access and more meaningful involvement with other medical disciplines.

Finally, family conferences, detailed observations of ward behavior, attention to psychotherapeutic issues, and an optimal disposition are difficult goals to achieve in hospitalized geriatric patients who have psychiatric disorders. Because psychiatric morbidity often goes unrecognized by a primary care or attending physician, the consulting psychiatrist must be actively involved in identifying those individuals who could benefit from psychotropic medication, psychotherapy, or other psychiatric interventions. Regarding the need for specialized services, "networking" efforts with community agencies are a focus in an integrated, consultative psychogeriatric approach. Also, the treatment milieu afforded by an integrated psychogeriatric approach is a more effective background for positive change in attitudes displayed toward the elderly medically ill. Functional disability has been found to impede recovery from physical illness, and the consulting psychiatrist should play an active role in identifying reversible physical limitations.

Efficacy of Psychiatric Consultation to Elderly Medical-Surgical Patients

Levitan and Kornfeld (1981) participated in the postoperative care of elderly patients who underwent surgery for fractured femurs. This classic study demonstrated that clinical outcomes for the consultation group (when compared to a control group who were not treated by a consultation-liaison psychiatrist) resulted in shorter length of stays (12 days). Furthermore, twice as many patients in the treatment group returned home as transferred to a nursing home or long-term care facility. This study provided substantial support for the role of consultation-liaison psychiatry in reducing the cost of medical care and in managing many of the methodological problems involved in psychiatric research in general hospital settings.

Major depression has significant impact on the course of medical illness and increases mortality rates through both "natural" and "self-induced" processes (Koenig et al. 1988). Mood disorders have adverse effects on compliance with medical therapy, and rehabilitative therapy and undoubtedly are associated with occult suicide (Allen et al. 1986). This association is perhaps best illustrated by those depressed patients who refuse life-sustaining therapy. The therapeutic nihilism often applied to the depressed hospitalized elderly patient not only is a result of ageism, but also is reflected when treatment is withheld because of concern about the severity of medical conditions and their potential interaction with antidepressants and other psychiatric medications. As previously cited in the study by Koenig and associates (1988), the question remains open whether the 87% of those elderly patients who had antidepressant treatment withheld would have actually benefited from treatment.

Summary

In this chapter I have outlined some of the current data and clinical aspects of geriatric consultation-liaison psychiatry in the general hospital. Unfortunately, there is a paucity of data concerning 1) the use of consultation and its efficacy or impact on prognosis and 2) the effect of coexisting psychiatric disturbance on medical-surgical patients. Studies of psychiatric intervention in other clinical settings may generalize to the hospital setting, and they certainly account for many of the diagnostic and therapeutic principles outlined in this chapter. As hospitalized elderly patients increase in numbers, greater overlap between consultation-liaison and geriatric psychiatry can be anticipated. The overlap between these areas will have important implications for educational programs and the future organization of clinical services. Thus, research of greater depth and validity may well be possible in the future.

References

Allen CM, Becker PM, McVey LJ, et al: A randomized, controlled clinical trial of a geriatric consultation team: compliance with recommendations. JAMA 255:2617–2621, 1986

American Psychiatric Association: Diagnostic and Statistical Manual of Mental Disorders, 3rd Edition. Washington, DC, American Psychiatric Association, 1980

American Psychiatric Association: Diagnostic and Statistical Manual of Mental Disorders, 3rd Edition, Revised. Washington, DC, American Psychiatric Association, 1987

Arie T, Jolley D: Making services work: organization and style of psychogeriatric services, in The Psychiatry of Late Life. Edited by Levy R, Post F. London, Blackwell Scientific Publications, 1982, pp 222–251

Brown JT, Stoudemire A: Normal and pathologic grief. JAMA 250:378–381, 1983

Cavanaugh SVA: Diagnosing depression in the hospitalized patient with chronic medical illness. Clin Psychiatry 45:13–16, 1984a

Cavanaugh SVA: Use of desipramine in the medically ill. J Clin Psychiatry 45:23–27, 1984b

Christie AB, Wood ER: Psychogeriatrics 1974 to 1984: expanding problems and fixed resources. Br J Psychiatry 151:813–817, 1987

Fogel BS, Martin C: Personality disorders in the medical setting, in Principles of Medical Psychiatry. Orlando, FL, Grune & Stratton, 1987, pp 253–270

Folks DG, Ford CV: Psychiatric disorders in geriatric medical/surgical patients, Part I: report of 195 consecutive consultations. South Med J 78:239–241, 1985

Folks DG, Franceschini JA, Freeman AM: Psychogeriatrics: the relationship between consultation-liaison and inpatient psychiatry, in Psychiatric Medicine. Edited by Hall RCW, Alarcon RD. Longwood, FL, Ryandic Publishing, 1986

Folks DG, Ford CV, Houck CA: Somatoform disorders, factitious disorders, and malingering, in Clinical Psychiatry for Medical Students. Philadelphia, JB Lippincott (in press)

Ford CV: Psychiatry and geriatric medicine, in Psychiatry Update: The American Psychiatric Association Annual Review, Vol 3. Edited by Grinspoon L. Washington, DC, American Psychiatric Press, 1984, pp 231–238

Ford CV, Folks DG: Psychiatric disorders in geriatric medical/surgical patients, II: review of clinical experience in consultation. South Med J 78:397–402, 1985

Horowitz MJ, Marmar C, Weiss DS, et al: Brief psychotherapy of bereavement reactions. Arch Gen Psychiatry 41:438–448, 1984

Koenig HG, Meador KG, Cohen HJ, et al: Detection and treatment of major depression in older medically ill hospitalized patients. Int J Psychiatry Med 18:17–31, 1988

Levitan SJ, Kornfeld DS: Clinical and cost benefits of liaison psychiatry. Am J Psychiatry 138:790–793, 1981

Lipowski ZJ: The need to integrate liaison psychiatry and geropsychiatry. Am J Psychiatry 140:1003–1005, 1983

Perez EL, Blouin J: Psychiatric emergency consultations to elderly patients in a Canadian general hospital. J Am Geriatr Soc 34:91–94, 1986

Popkin MK, Mackenzie TB, Callies AL: Psychiatric consultation to geriatric medically ill inpatients in a university hospital. Arch Gen Psychiatry 41:703–707 1984

Poynton AM: Psychiatric liaison referrals of elderly inpatients in a teaching hospital. Br J Psychiatry 152:45–47, 1988

Rabins P, Lucas MJ, Teitelbaum M, et al: Utilization of psychiatric consultation for elderly patients. J Am Geriatr Soc 31:581–585, 1983

Reisberg B, Ferris SH: Diagnosis and assessment of the older patient. Hosp Community Psychiatry 33:104–110, 1982

Rodin G, Voshart K: Depression in the medically ill: an overview. Am J Psychiatry 143:696–705, 1986

Sadavoy J, Dorian B: Treatment of the elderly characterologically disturbed patient in the chronic care institution. J Geriatr Psychiatry 16:223–240, 1983

Sadavoy J, Reiman-Sheldon E: General hospital geriatric psychiatric treatment: a follow-up study. J Am Geriatr Soc 31:200–205, 1983

Small GW, Fawzy FI: Psychiatric consultation for the medically ill elderly in the general hospital: need for a collaborative model of care. Psychosomatics 29:94–103, 1988

Starkman MN, Hall GG: Teaching medical gerontology: utilization of a psychiatry consultation program. J Med Educ 54:643–648, 1979

Thienhaus OJ, Rowe C, Woellert P, et al: Geropsychiatric emergency services: utilization and outcome predictors. Hosp Community Psychiatry 39:1301–1305, 1988

Warshaw GA, Moore JT, Friedman SW, et al: Functional disability in the hospitalized elderly. JAMA 248:847–850, 1982

CHAPTER 29

Marie-France Tourigny-Rivard, M.D.

Acute Care Inpatient Treatment

Overview

In the principles for good psychogeriatric care outlined by the World Health Organization (Skeet 1983), acute care inpatient treatment is seen as an important component of the comprehensive services that should be available to elderly psychiatric patients.

Some of the principles that allow for efficient running of such units include multidisciplinary staffing prepared to address the physical, psychological, and social needs of the patient; prehospitalization screening; a focus on returning the patient home as soon as possible; collaboration with community agencies; and efficient coordination of aftercare (Skeet 1983).

Multidisciplinary Staffing

The efficient running of a psychogeriatric service starts with a psychogeriatric team that has a special interest in the psychiatry of old age, is able to provide a full range of psychiatric skills, and has good knowledge of general medicine and social interventions (Pitt 1982). Multidisciplinary staffing is required to address concurrently the physical, psychological, and social problems that can contribute to the psychiatric illnesses of elderly patients. It is well recognized that there is a high prevalence of medical illnesses in the elderly: Williamson and associates (1964) found that 82% of a random sample of people aged older than 65 suffered from moderate or severe physical disabilities. Psychogeriatric patients admitted to hospital are reported to have similar high rates of physical illness: 78.4% had at least one of the common medical illnesses seen in old age in Conwell and colleagues' sample (1989), 75% in Harrison and associates' sample (1988), and 94% in a recently analyzed sample of 97 patients admitted to the author's acute care geriatric psychiatry unit in 1985. Weingarten and colleagues (1982) also emphasized the role of physical illness in precipitating psychiatric admissions and complicating treatment. Furthermore, many of the patients admitted to inpatient units have acquired multiple age- and disease-related deficits.

The inpatient treatment team needs to detect functional impairments through multidimensional assessments and orchestrate compensatory responses in an effort to restore, maximize, and maintain functional status and independence for as long as possible (Becker and Cohen 1984). The multidisciplinary team therefore includes members of the core mental health disciplines and other health professionals, including nonpsychiatric physicians, to assure that patients receive comprehensive needs assessment and care.

Prehospitalization Screening

"Screening evaluations" take place prior to hospitalization and are often most informative if done at the patient's residence to give a better idea of the physical and social assets or liabilities of the individual and to see how the person relates to his family and caregivers in the natural setting (Pitt 1982; Whanger and Busse 1975). This screening helps to establish proper prioritization, prevent unnecessary or inappropriate admissions, and prepare realistic plans for discharge.

Prompt Return Home

Another principle of acute inpatient treatment that is widely applied is that of returning patients home as quickly as possible. This principle is dictated not only by the economic pressures associated with this expensive form of treatment but also by the fear that the longer the hospital admission, the less likely that the patient will successfully return home, because of loss of supports and friends and the stigma attached to long psychiatric hospitalizations. Discharge from hospital care can occur sooner if 1) the unit is staffed in such a way as to allow intensive treatment by a team that is committed to getting the patient well enough to return home after as brief a hospitalization as possible; 2) relatives and friends are encouraged to visit and participate, as appropriate, in the care of the patient and are provided with useful information about psychiatric disorders and their treatment; 3) a well-organized network of integrated services operating in the community is prepared to receive the patient back into it and to give support to his or her family and caregivers; and 4) coordination and cooperation exist between the inpatient unit and community support services that will be required to help the patient after discharge (Skeet 1983).

Discharge Planning

Discharge planning starts at admission, with a good understanding of the patient's living situation prior to admission, maintaining the patient's community resources (living accommodation, support of family and friends), and dealing with potential obstacles to returning home as soon as possible. Advice to patients and families on the need for placement in supervised facilities or on the need for a change in residence is given only after an adequate inpatient evaluation is done and a clear prognosis established. This caution is particularly important for depressed patients who may feel hopeless and unable to care for themselves at the time of admission but have a good prognosis and should be able to return home after treatment. In fact, with good inpatient care, most patients improve enough to return to their preadmission residence, at least temporarily: Conwell and associates (1989) reported that 82% of their patients (n = 168) were discharged home alone or with relatives, 3.9% were transferred to other hospitals, and 14.4% were discharged to structured settings such as group homes and nursing homes. Harrison and colleagues (1988) reported that 54 of their 100 inpatients were discharged to the same level of accommodation or a more independent level. Spar and associates (1980) reported that 62% of their 122 inpatients were discharged home, 2.5% with relatives, and 35.5% to institutional care (7.5% were in institutions prior to admission); therefore approximately 70% of their patients were discharged to the same level of accommodation as on admission. Weingarten and associates (1982) reported that 71% of their 49 patients were discharged home, albeit with some additional support (day care or caretaker) in 18% of these cases.

Collaboration and Cooperation With Community Agencies

Collaboration with community agencies and coordination of aftercare are two important principles that help reduce hospital length of stay and readmission rates and make reinsertion into the community successful (Pitt 1982; Skeet 1983). Although collaboration and coordination are very difficult to measure and comparative studies of services with and without such support do not seem to exist, most papers related to psychogeriatric acute care units mention these two issues (Harrison et al. 1988; Spar et al. 1980) as important factors influencing length of stay and outcome of treatment. In summary, these principles emphasize the need to consider acute care inpatient treatment as part of a continuum of care that should be available to elderly patients with psychiatric problems.

Population Served

Diagnostic Categories

Redick and Taube (1980) reported on the diagnosis of all patients admitted to psychiatric facilities in the United States who were over the age of 65. Statistics related to private psychiatric hospitals and psychiatric inpatient units located in general hospitals likely describe the population that will require admission on acute geriatric psychiatry inpatient units. They found that 51.1% of patients admitted to private psychiatric hospitals and 46.1% of those admitted to general hospital psychiatric units had a diagnosis of depression, indicating that depression accounts for the majority of admissions to acute care inpatient units. Organic brain syndromes, excluding those related to alcohol and substance abuse, were the next most common diagnosis (25% and 28%), alcohol-related disorders came next with 7.5% and 6%, then schizophrenia (4.6% and 3.3%), psychoneuroses (2.7% and 5.1%), and other disorders (9%). Spar and colleagues (1980) and Weingarten and colleagues (1982) found that the most frequent diagnoses responsible for admission of elderly patients to acute care wards were depression (51.6% and 57%) and dementia (27.1% and 18%); Harrison and associates (1988) reported that 29% of their patients had dementia, 29% major depressive episodes, 19% delirium, 10% schizophrenia, and 8% other psychoses including acute manic episodes; Conwell and associates (1989) reported that 76% of their 168 patients had a primary affective disorder (19 were bipolar), and organic brain syndrome was the second most common diagnosis: 24.5% with dementia and 10.1% with delirium.

The population treated on inpatient units may vary according to the selectivity of each facility's admission criteria and availability of alternative treatment facilities for major diagnostic categories such as alcoholism and organic mental disorders. However, based on available data, one can say that staff working on these units should be prepared to treat patients who suffer from the following:

- Mood disorders, mostly major depressive and manic episodes.
- Dementia with significant behavioral complications such as wandering, agitation, aggressive behavior, paranoid behavior and delusions, or depression.
- Other organic mental disorders such as severe organic mood disorders, delirium secondary to prescribed psychotropic medications (most other patients with delirium are admitted to acute care medical units), and organic delusional syndromes.
- Paranoid psychoses of late life, including decompensated schizophrenia.
- Substance abuse—most commonly, abuse of alcohol, sedatives, hypnotics, anxiolytics, and analgesics.
- Personality disorders, which may complicate any of the foregoing diagnoses or prompt admission.

Sex Distribution

On psychiatric wards of general hospitals and private psychiatric facilities, elderly women account for 63.6% of the geriatric admissions, a ratio of almost 2 females for 1 male. On wards of state and county hospitals, however, where the average length of stay is longer, men outnumber women. There is, therefore, an overrepresentation of women in the more acute care facilities—according to demographic surveys, they should account for only 58% of admissions (Redick and Taube 1980). Spar and associates (1980) found the sex distribution of their sample (75% female and 25% male) to be very similar to one other study (Baribeau-Brown et al. 1979); Harrison and colleagues (1988) had 65% female and 35% male in their sample; Spar and associates (1980) had 73% female and 27% male, without significant difference in sex distribution in each 5-year increment of age.

Types of Units

In general hospitals, a geriatric psychiatry unit can be either part of the general psychiatric unit, with specific staff and programming for the elderly population, or a separate, additional (usually small) unit. Advantages of mixed (or age-integrated) acute care wards are that elderly patients can benefit from the interactions and physical assistance sometimes provided by the younger population. The disadvantages are the risk of injury from acutely ill younger patients and being frightened by their language and behavior. It is also more difficult to create a therapeutic milieu that actively addresses the problems related to aging unless there are staff, programming, and rooms provided specifically for the elderly. In age-segregated wards, it may be easier to create a milieu that encourages patients to deal with issues related to aging, and to recruit staff who have a specific interest in working with the elderly. Sexually integrated wards seem to encourage better grooming and manners, and problems of improper behavior toward members of the opposite sex are infrequent (Pitt 1982).

Geriatric psychiatry units sometimes are located in proximity to geriatric medicine units with part of the staff having joint appointments to both units to facilitate cross-consultation and joint teaching. Such "joint units," described by Arie and Jolley (1982), can come under one department (such as the Department of Health Care of the Elderly at Nottingham University, which combines geriatric medicine and psychiatry) or under separate geriatric medicine and psychiatry departments in which there is agreement on the basic principles of joint care. Joint care can even be provided by physicians who have their primary assignments in different hospitals.

In psychiatric hospitals (short-term or long-term care facilities), acute care psychogeriatric units are sometimes called admission or assessment wards. Patients are assessed and treated for a period of 1 to 3 months, and then discharged to the community (e.g., day hospital, nursing home facility with outpatient follow-up) or transferred to a rehabilitation or long-term care ward. For completeness it may be mentioned that there are other types of geriatric psychiatry inpatient units: rehabilitation wards for chronically psychotic individuals who have grown old in institutions or for those who need an intermediate stay in the hospital; and continuing care wards for those who show progressive mental deterioration and need a supportive, humane, and protective environment. Data comparing the efficacy of these various types of acute care units are not available.

Design of Units

Wandering and Agitation

Because wanderers and agitated patients are often admitted to geriatric psychiatry units, the optimal design of the unit allows for safe wandering and adequate exercise levels. Designs that allow the patient to walk around a square or loop, and covered walkways with an attractive view and landscaping can be used to contain wanderers within a designated area yet let them walk freely, decreasing the need for medication for agitated behavior.

Sensory Deficits

Visual impairment dictates good lighting throughout the unit with lots of natural light where possible; night lights to reduce falls "on the way to the bathroom"; large-print reading material; large clocks; easy-to-read signs; and the use of color coding, for example, using the same distinctive color for all bathroom doors. Because hearing impairment is common, sound-amplifying electronic systems facilitate individual and group therapy. Minimizing extraneous noises that tend to be amplified by hearing aids is also important.

Falls

Falls are frequent in the geriatric population, possibly because of the higher incidence of balance and coordination problems with age (Akhtar et al. 1973). Falls are associated with decreased mobility of the lower extremities, general weakness, sleeplessness, incontinence or urgency, confusion, depression, and substance abuse (Janken et al. 1986). Some data suggest that at least one of these risk factors is present in most admissions (Rivard unpublished data): arthritis or debilitating neurological illnesses such as Parkinson's disease often limit patients' mobility; depression contributes to general weakness and sleeplessness; organic brain disorders are associated with much confusion; and the frequent use of diuretics may contribute to urgency. In addition, psychotropic medications are widely used and contribute to falls through orthostatic hypotension, parkinsonism, or cerebellar toxicity.

Building and room type are important environmental factors related to falling (Janken et al. 1986). The design of the unit aims to minimize falls by location of wards at ground level; the absence of stairs; nonskid floors without thresholds or doorsteps; doors that open automatically; wide corridors with handrails; uncluttered rooms that allow easy access for wheelchairs and walkers; bathrooms with easy access to showers and tubs; and, in particular, an adequate number of well-located and properly lit washrooms to help reduce incontinence and urgency.

Safety Considerations

For safety, the unit may need to be locked periodically for patients who are acutely suicidal or psychotic and for wanderers who present a high risk of elopement. With recent technology, electronic and remote control locks can contribute to making the locks as unobtrusive as possible. One example of such technology is a system in which a transmitter worn in a bracelet emits unique encoded signals that are detected by alarm receivers; the receivers are located in strategic areas beyond which the patient should not wander, such as exits or stairs. A signal alerts staff and displays the patient's code through a central monitoring unit. The system may also be set up to trigger a lock on a door, thereby preventing the patient from leaving the facility. Short of a unit that can lock, wandering patients may have to be confined to a small area where they can be easily observed or need costly individual supervision until they no longer present an elopement risk. Suicide risks require environmental safeguards. Hooks and bars are eliminated to reduce the risk of patients hanging themselves; windows are designed so they cannot be easily opened or broken; and the use of sharp objects, scissors, and razor blades is monitored. Fire may be a hazard when patients smoke or use kitchen facilities. Five retardants, proper choice of building material, smoke detectors and sprinklers, and clear, well-rehearsed plans for evacuation are important considerations.

Space for Treatment

To allow optimal treatment, the unit is designed with sufficient space for various forms of therapy to take place. Interview rooms that provide privacy, examination and treatment rooms, space for physiotherapy, group therapy rooms, and activity rooms should be available in addition to lounges to encourage socialization and kitchen facilities to allow for functional assessments. A number of private rooms should be available for patients who need intensive nursing care or are too agitated to be reasonable roommates.

Comfort of Patients

The air temperature and humidity is controlled and adjusted to the needs of the patient. The elderly are often uncomfortable in cold environments and also tolerate excessive heat and humidity poorly, especially if they suffer from cardiac problems or are being treated with phenothiazines or other anticholinergic drugs that interfere with temperature regulation (Skeet 1983). Equipment that encourages patients to maintain their everyday skills and personal appearance enhances the therapeutic effort (e.g., full-length mirrors, washer and dryer, sewing machine, kitchen, and hairdressing facilities).

Staffing

Staffing ratios are very difficult to establish. There are few guidelines available for inpatient psychiatric care of the elderly. The Royal College of Psychiatrists in England has recommended that for each district of 200,000 to 250,000 population, geriatric psychiatrists spend a minimum total of 54 hours per week for the psychiatric care of elderly patients in their sector. In teaching districts, at least twice this minimum is recommended (Arie and Jolley 1982). There are no specific guidelines regarding the proportion of time that should be spent on geriatric inpatient units.

The same guidelines suggest 1 nurse or attendant per 1.20 patients in acute treatment wards, but higher ratios may be needed if the population served has a high rate of concurrent physical problems or particularly acute and severe psychiatric problems, or if the length of stay has to be kept particularly short because of economic pressures or shortage of beds.

Guidelines for staffing ratios related to social workers, psychologists, occupational therapists, and physiotherapists do not seem to be available. Overall, staffing should ensure that adequate evaluations take place and that a variety of treatment programs are available to respond to the needs of the inpatient population.

Indications for Inpatient Treatment

Whanger (1989) has provided a review of indications for inpatient treatment. While prescribing the treatment setting, the physician should keep alternatives in mind such as day hospital and intensive outpatient crisis intervention, which can be used to prevent many psychiatric admissions. Indications for inpatient treatment may be grouped into the following three broad categories.

First, imminent danger to self or others:

- Suicidal and potentially harmful behavior such as self-neglect, refusing essential medical care, or self-mutilating behavior.

- Homicidal, violent, or aggressive behavior; serious threatening behavior in the presence of acute psychosis; or behavior potentially harmful to others, such as fire setting (intentional or through neglect).
- Imminent and serious physical impairment through a lack of competence to care for oneself or to meet basic activities of daily living because of severe agitation, psychomotor retardation, or confusion and disorientation; imminent danger associated with wandering behavior, acute psychiatric reactions to medications, or impending delirium tremens—none of which requires hospitalization on a medical service.

These patients may require seclusion, restraint, or isolation because of agitated or destructive states and may need to be admitted against their will, following local regulations for civil commitment.

Second, need for intensive evaluation and/or treatment that cannot be provided in outpatient settings, including day hospitals:

- Difficult diagnostic issues where close observation over a few days is required for proper diagnostic assessment. These include organic brain syndromes when hospitalization can lead to identification and treatment of a reversible cause or amelioration of secondary psychiatric disturbances.
- Addiction to alcohol or drugs mixed with other psychiatric diagnoses where control and supervision are needed to ensure proper detoxification and safe withdrawal.
- Acutely psychotic patients with unpredictable behavior due to preoccupations with bizarre delusions or hallucinations (including acute decompensations of schizophrenia).
- Patients who need intravenous feedings or frequent intramuscular psychotropic medications.
- Patients who require electroconvulsive therapy.
- Patients whose multiple medical problems or drug sensitivities require close regulation of oral medication and close medical and nursing monitoring.
- Patients with psychiatric problems likely to improve with active and intensive treatment such as can be provided only on an inpatient unit.

Third, failure of the caregiving system:

- Principal caregiver dies, leaves, or needs temporary relief to keep from becoming totally exhausted or disorganized.
- Depletion of funds or care resources without alternatives.

This failure of the health care system is often due to the lack of responsive community resources or respite care beds in less intensive treatment settings. When the absence of alternative treatment settings places patients and/or others seriously at risk, acute hospitalization may become necessary.

Inappropriate Admissions

Whanger and Busse (1975) considered as inappropriate acute psychiatric admissions the following: patients who are physically sick and require urgent admission to a medical hospital; patients who are comatose or moribund; patients who have mild to moderate irreversible organic brain syndrome or other disorders and could live effectively in other group care facilities if they can no longer be maintained in their own homes; and patients who are basically in need only of adequate living accommodations or other economic, nutritional, or social support services. In addition, one may consider inappropriate the admission of patients who could have been treated easily in less intensive, less expensive settings that do not take them away from home and do not impose the financial burden and stigma of a psychiatric hospitalization.

Applications of Inpatient Treatment

Assessment and Diagnosis

It is axiomatic that a thorough medical, psychiatric, and functional assessment should be part of every admission. Inpatient admission is useful in allowing more accurate observation of sleep patterns, appetite and dietary intake, diurnal variation, psychomotor agitation or retardation, quality and quantity of interactions with others, energy levels, intensity of somatic complaints such as constipation or pain, presence of hallucinatory or paranoid behavior, ability to carry on activities of daily living independently, confusion, memory loss and disorientation, repetitive (perseverative) behavior, and circumstances leading to catastrophic reactions or aggressive behavior. These observations are particularly useful for patients who tend to exaggerate or minimize their difficulties and patients with mild to moderate dementia who demonstrate their deficits more clearly in unfamiliar surroundings.

Multidisciplinary, multiaxial evaluation according to the biopsychosocial model is necessary, and each team member contributes to the assessment according to his or her expertise. Instruments such as the Older American Resources and Services Research (OARS) or other multidimensional structured assessment tools can help ensure a thorough assessment and clear communication among team members. Typically, the treating physician focuses the initial assessment on the medical and psychiatric problems of the patient, taking a careful history, and getting appropriate medical and laboratory investigations done. Nurses, occupational therapists, and physiotherapists usually focus on the functional assessment, identifying problem areas and encouraging patients to use their abilities or accessory tools to compensate for their deficits. One of the standard instruments developed to assess instrumental activities of daily living in the elderly will provide useful information about the patient's baseline level of functioning and may be a useful measure of improvement at discharge. Social workers provide much needed detail on the patient's familial and social resources, identifying problem areas that need to be addressed urgently during hospitalization. Psychologists help document the cognitive abilities and deficits of the patients as well as adding perspective on the patient's potential to respond to specific forms of psychotherapy. They can do so through formal individual evaluations or through observation of the patients in group setting.

Treatment Modalities

Each patient should have an individualized treatment plan that takes into account physical, psychiatric, and social problems and makes optimal use of abilities. The goals of the admission are set clearly, according to the treatability of the patient's psychiatric-medical illnesses and best previous level of functioning. As much as possible, both the patient and the caregivers are included in formulating the treatment plan—formally, by inviting the patient and caregivers to participate in multidisciplinary patient conferences, or informally, by discussing the treatment plan with patient and family, with due and appropriate regard for confidentiality.

Many of the treatment modalities used on the inpatient unit are described in detail in other sections of this book and are briefly mentioned here only to highlight how they may need to be adjusted to the inpatient setting. A major important component of treatment in an inpatient setting is the possibility of creating a milieu that will, in itself, have therapeutic value to the patient.

Milieu

The general aim of milieu therapy is to provide a reasonably stable and coherent social organization that facilitates the development and implementation of an individualized treatment plan for each patient, based on realistic and specific therapeutic goals. Group and ward meetings serve to facilitate communication, address problems that affect the ward population, and give a sense of community. Activity groups provide opportunities for the observation of specific skills and social interactions. In general, a mixture of therapy groups, ward meetings, and activity groups contributes to the daily schedule of the unit. Therapeutic milieus serve to support individuals, provide structure and containment, apply prevailing social norms in such a way as to inhibit behavior that is antitherapeutic to the patient or the group, and encourage appropriate social interactions (Leeman 1986).

On a geriatric psychiatry unit, the milieu is conducive to dealing with problems common to its population, such as losses (including loss of health or youthfulness), adjustment to retirement, difficulties in finding worthwhile activities and maintaining self-esteem, adapting to changes in family relationships or changes in residence, and dealing with increased dependency needs.

Milieu also has to be conducive to an eventual return home or to good integration in one of the community facilities. Wearing one's own clothes, having to get dressed as one would at home, using kitchen facilities, planning and preparing meals (at least snacks), using appliances such as clothes washer and dryer, and carrying on responsibilities for self-care are important to prepare the patient who will be discharged home. Implementing a schedule of ward activities and regulations similar to those the patient will have to follow when discharged to a nursing home or extended care facility is also important.

While many writers emphasize the need of a stimulating environment on psychiatric units for the elderly, this literature has largely focused on long-term care units to demonstrate that custodial care of elderly patients with psychiatric illnesses fosters further regression. On acute care units, it is assumed that active treatment will be provided even for patients who have chronic psychiatric illnesses. Although stimulation through activities is the norm, one has to remember that the treatment plan for manic or agitated patients on acute care wards calls for decreased stimulation.

Individual Psychotherapy

Individual psychotherapy using such modalities as cognitive, insight-oriented, and supportive psychotherapy is an integral part of treatment on inpatient units. Although many inpatients are near discharge before they become suitable candidates for insight-oriented psychotherapy, the treatment team should have a sufficient understanding and familiarity with psychodynamic therapeutic interventions to provide empathic listening, gentle confrontation (e.g., pointing out obvious avoidance), and clarification to help patients recognize feeling states they may be unaware of, links between current events and personal history, and reasons for avoidance (fears). Interpretation of unconscious process is a rare intervention on most short-term treatment units, however, because it usually takes time before the therapist is certain of the accuracy of the interpretation and the patient is ready to hear it and tolerate the emotional impact of the revealed thought or feeling (Rogoff 1986). Cognitive psychotherapy, which uses higher-level defense mechanisms such as intellectualization and rationalization, is probably a useful component of the treatment of depressed, nonpsychotic inpatients, but studies on its efficacy with geriatric populations have been done in outpatient rather than inpatient settings (Steuer 1982).

Behavior Therapy

Various techniques of behavior therapy and behavior modification can be useful for selected inpatients. They have been studied mostly in long-term care or outpatient settings but can be applied to a limited extent to the inpatient, acute care population. The most commonly used forms of behavior therapy are relaxation training and desensitization for anxiety-related disorders, habit retraining (mostly used for incontinence), and biofeedback, which may be helpful in the management of chronic pain or incontinence. Behavior modification techniques, which can be applied by staff in the overall approach to the patient, include positive reinforcement of adaptive behavior (sometimes following the Premack principle, whereby already frequently occurring behavior is used as a reinforcement); removal of reinforcements for maladaptive behavior; counterconditioning; and reciprocal inhibition (Yates 1975).

Group therapy is fully discussed in Chapter 27.

Family Therapy

Common tasks of family therapy on the inpatient unit include involving and evaluating families in order to negotiate appropriate goals for family intervention. Common goals as described for families of inpatients (Glick and Clarkin 1986) include the following:

- Accepting the reality of the illness and understanding the current episode.
- Identifying the stresses that precipitated the current episode.
- Identifying likely future stressors, both within and outside the family, that will impinge on the patient.
- Elucidating the family interaction sequences that stress the identified patient and seem to trigger current symptoms, providing them with better ways to relate to the patient.
- Planning strategies for managing and/or minimizing future stresses.
- Accepting the need for continued treatment following discharge from the hospital.

Fears and anxiety can be reduced by keeping the family properly apprised of progress and supporting them in their efforts to help. When family problems are present, it is important to determine whether they are mostly related to the current illness of the patient or a reflection of more serious ongoing problems that will need to be addressed with formal therapy. Although patients often report stressful family relationships as a contributing factor to their illness, one has to keep in mind that the illness of the patient has often contributed greatly to the strained relations. In a recent study of elderly psychiatric inpatients (Liptzin et al. 1988), relatives of depressed and demented patients reported similar levels of burden (measured by the Burden Interview and the Memory and Behavior Problem Checklist of Zarit) at admission and follow-up (2 to 4 months after discharge). This finding reinforces that 1) depression severe enough to warrant admission and dementia produce great stress for relatives and caregivers, and 2) the treatment team can help reduce this stress through appropriate family interventions.

Physical Therapy

Because medical illnesses and physical disabilities are common among geriatric psychiatry inpatients, physical therapy is part of their care. Physical therapy usually includes individual and group exercise programs (e.g., walking, exercises to music); physiotherapy; and supervision or teaching on the appropriate use of physical aids to deal with decreased vision, decreased hearing, mobility and

balance problems, parkinsonism, and weakness following strokes
or fractures.

Occupational and Recreational Therapy

The occupational therapist can provide individual and group
therapeutic activities to provide structure and good contact with
reality for the confused patient, applying the principles of reality
orientation; improve self-esteem and remotivate depressed patients; develop interactional and social skills; encourage patients
to maintain or resume their usual activities; develop vocational interests; and increase patients' awareness of community resources.
This therapy is done through a variety of activities tailored to
match the abilities of the patients and their previous interests.

Recreational activities provide an opportunity to assess the patient's strengths, weaknesses, and customary modes of adapting.
Frequent themes addressed in recreation therapy include adjustment to retirement, finding worthwhile activities such as volunteer work or hobbies, setting personal goals in areas such as personal fitness, and learning about community activities or
resources available to seniors. The recreation therapist provides
information and encourages patients to experience some of the
suggested leisure activities by organizing exercise groups, community outings, music groups, card games, crafts, or parties that
stimulate socialization and provide pleasure and satisfaction.

Outcome

Costs of acute inpatient care can vary widely in different countries
or geographical areas. For example, per diem cost exclusive of physicians' fees but including overhead and support services is $400
per day in an acute care geriatric psychiatry unit in Seattle (Raskind 1990) and $275 in a Canadian acute care geriatric psychiatry
unit in Ottawa (Tourigny-Rivard 1990). Despite its high cost, inpatient care will continue to be required for a proportion of patients
with psychiatric disorders and cannot be avoided.

The cost of a psychiatric admission is usually higher for a geriatric patient than for the younger population because of increased
length of stay. Papers that describe geriatric psychiatry acute care
units report variable lengths of stay: 32 days (Harrison et al. 1988),
44.5 days (Spar et al. 1980), 59 days (Weingarten et al. 1982), and
53.3 days (Conwell et al. 1989). These geriatric units clearly pro-

vided assessment and enough treatment to allow the majority of their patients to be discharged home with almost no transfer to other inpatient facilities. Although length of stay can certainly be shorter, one has to evaluate the possible costs of premature discharge such as inability to return to independent living, need for adjunct services, or institutionalization and stress on the patient and family. These costs have not been systematically studied.

Also contributing to high costs are the characteristics of geriatric inpatients that make them an expensive "case mix." Case mix is usually evaluated on the basis of the following variables: complicated versus uncomplicated case; good prognosis versus poor prognosis for illness; presence versus absence of supportive resources (including family, day hospital, nursing homes, and community residences for patients with treatment resistant illness); presence versus absence of community treatment resources and well-established aftercare programs; and need for postdischarge placement. It is clear that the elderly are likely to have complicated chronic illnesses with guarded prognosis (such as dementia and treatment-refractory depression), fewer resources, and increased need for placement, all contributing to longer average lengths of stay and higher costs. On the other hand, rapid diagnosis and treatment on short-term geriatric inpatient units can result in a decreased rate of entry into state hospitals and a return home in the majority of cases (Brody et al. 1971); avoiding long-term hospitalization or institutionalization is associated with substantial savings that can easily offset the cost of a short-term admission.

A brief case example will illustrate this point.

> Mrs. X was a 77-year-old caregiver to her legally blind husband at the time of her admission for treatment-refractory depression. Both she and her husband had applied to go to a nursing home, for she was no longer able to care for herself or her husband. A 6-week inpatient admission allowed successful treatment of her depression and full recovery. Maintenance medication and minimal follow-up treatment have allowed this woman and her husband to stay home during the past 4 years rather than go to the nursing home. Their quality of life is much better at home, and the saving in government subsidies for the nursing home has long covered the cost of the admission.

A study on the effect of the creation of a geriatric psychiatry team in a long-term care hospital showed a decrease in waiting lists, increase in discharges to the community, decreased number of deaths, and a decreased proportion of patients staying more than 1 year in hospital. Readmission rates increased from 30% to 40%, but there was still an excess of patients who were discharged and did not need to return to hospital (Pitt 1982). This finding indicates that having a specialized team that takes an active interest in the care of the elderly can contribute to lower health care costs and improved quality of life. Unfortunately, there seem to be no published data on the evaluation of the cost-effectiveness of acute care geriatric psychiatry inpatient units, although a recent paper by Conwell and associates (1989) did attempt to evaluate the outcome of treatment on a 3-point scale (good, partial response, no response), length of stay, and characteristics of their patients.

To properly evaluate the cost-effectiveness of a geriatric psychiatry inpatient unit, one has to consider the average cost of admission (average per diem cost for the unit multiplied by the average length of stay), the number of patients treated (taking into account readmission rates), and the outcome with and without admission. Outcome measures should include measures of psychopathology, functional capacity, level of distress, quality of life, suicide rates, and need for placement or admission to a long-term care facility (which possibly could have been avoided or postponed with a timely admission). A highly cost-effective unit would be one that allowed significant reduction in distress and psychopathology with substantial improvements in functional capacity at a reasonable cost while the prognosis without inpatient treatment would be deterioration or ongoing distress, severe functional decline, and/or inevitable need for institutionalization. In addition, units with comparable case mix should be compared in cost-effectiveness studies. It is clear that much research remains to be done to develop realistic methods of calculating cost-effectiveness of inpatient psychiatric treatment (English and McGarrick 1986), starting with reliable appraisal of case mix, objective measures of improvement, and likely morbidity without treatment.

Limited Accessibility of Geriatric Psychiatry Inpatient Treatment

Elderly Canadians and Americans face different accessibility problems because of the vastly different methods of funding in the United States and Canada. In the United States, accessibility is limited to a great extent by one's personal financial resources and limited coverage of Medicare and private insurance plans. Elderly Canadians have Universal Health Coverage, paid through the income tax system and administered by each province. Accessibility to psychiatric inpatient treatment is limited by the number of beds funded by each province for psychiatric care and their uneven distribution in different regions. Where geriatric psychiatry inpatient services exist, there is usually an excess of needs in comparison to the supply, forcing the teams who run these units to establish priorities for admission and use ambulatory services as much as feasible. However, because geriatric psychiatry inpatient units are relatively rare, most geriatric patients who need psychiatric inpatient care are admitted to general psychiatry or medical units. Taxpayers and governments are currently reluctant to fund additional beds because of their high operational costs and rapidly rising health expenditures. As a result, elderly Canadians compete for a limited supply of services and inpatient beds, but personal finances neither limit nor facilitate access.

References

Akhtar AJ, Broe DA, Crombie A, et al: Disability and dependence in the elderly at home. Age and Aging 2:102–110, 1973

Arie T, Jolley D: Making services work: organisation and style of psychogeriatric services, in The Psychiatry of Late Life. Edited by Levy R, Post F. Oxford, Blackwell Scientific Publications, 1982, pp 222–251

Baribeau-Brown J, Goldstein S, Braun C: A multivariate study of psychogeriatric readmissions. J Gerontol 34:351–357, 1979

Becker PM, Cohen HJ: The functional approach to the care of the elderly: a conceptual framework. J Am Geriatr Soc 32:923–929, 1984

Brody EM, Kleban MH, Lawton MP, et al: Excess disabilities of mentally impaired aged: impact of individualized treatment. Gerontologist 11:124–133, 1971

Conwell Y, Nelson JC, Kim KL, et al: Elderly patients admitted to the psychiatric unit of a general hospital. J Am Geriatr Soc 37:35–41, 1989

English JT, McCarrick RG: The economics of inpatient psychiatry, in Inpatient Psychiatry: Diagnosis and Treatment, 2nd Edition. Edited by Sederer LI. Baltimore, MD, Williams & Wilkins, 1986, pp 367–382

Fillenbaum G, Smyer M: The development, validity, and reliability of the Older American Resources and Services Research (OARS): The Duke Multidimensional Functional Assessment Questionnaire. J Gerontology 36:428–434, 1981

Glick ID, Clarkin JF: The family, in Inpatient Psychiatry: Diagnosis and Treatment, 2nd Edition. Edited by Sederer LI. Baltimore, MD, Williams & Wilkins, 1986, pp 296–307

Harrison AW, Kernutt GJ, Piperoglou MV: A survey of patients in a regional geriatric psychiatry inpatient unit. Aust N Z J Psychiatry 22:412–417, 1988

Janken JK, Reynolds BA, Swiech K: Patient falls in the acute care setting: identifying risk factors. Nurs Res 35:215–219, 1986

Leeman CP: The therapeutic milieu and its role in clinical management, in Inpatient Psychiatry: Diagnosis and Treatment, 2nd Edition. Edited by Sederer LI. Baltimore, MD, Williams & Wilkins, 1986, pp 228–229

Liptzin B, Grob MC, Eisen SV: Family burden of demented and depressed elderly psychiatric inpatients. Gerontologist 28:397–401, 1988

Pitt B: Psycho-Geriatrics: An Introduction to the Psychiatry of Old Age. Edinburgh, Churchill Livingstone, 1982

Raskind M: Evaluation of the per diem cost of an American geropsychiatry acute care unit, unpublished data, 1990

Redick RW, Taube CA: Demography and mental health care of the aged, in Handbook of Mental Health and Aging. Edited by Birren JE, Sloane RB. New York, Prentice-Hall, 1980, pp 57–71

Rogoff J: Individual psychotherapy, in Inpatient Psychiatry: Diagnosis and Treatment, 2nd Edition. Edited by Sederer LI. Baltimore, MD, Williams & Wilkins, 1986, pp 240–262

Skeet M: Protecting the Health of the Elderly. Copenhagen, World Health Organization Regional Office for Europe, 1983

Spar JE, Ford CV, Liston EH: Hospital treatment of elderly neuropsychiatric patients, II: statistical profile of the first 122 patients in a new teaching ward. J Am Geriatr Soc 28:539–543, 1980

Steuer J: Psychotherapy with the elderly. Psychiatr Clin North Am 5:195–210, 1982

Tourigny-Rivard M-F: Evaluation of a Canadian geriatric psychiatry inpatient unit, unpublished data, 1990

Weingarten CH, Rosoff LG, Eisen SV, et al: Medical care in a geriatric psychiatry unit: impact on psychiatric outcome. J Am Geriatr Soc 30:738–743, 1982

Whanger AD: Inpatient treatment of the older psychiatric patient, in Geriatric Psychiatry. Edited by Busse EW, Blazer DG. Washington, DC, American Psychiatric Press, 1989, pp 593–633

Whanger AD, Busse EW: Care in hospital, in Modern Perspectives in the Psychiatry of Old Age. Edited by Howells JG. New York, Brunner/Mazel, 1975, pp 450–485

Williamson J, Stokoe IH, Gray S, et al: Old people at home, their unreported needs. Lancet 1:1117–1120, 1964

Yates AJ: Theory and Practice in Behavior Therapy. New York, John Wiley, 1975

CHAPTER 30

Allan Steingart, M.D.

Day Programs

Isolation is the worst possible counsellor.
—Unamuno, Civilization is civism

Overview

Most elderly individuals are able to partake of the same entertainments, services, and sins available to all, but some find themselves cut off. Friends and family are lost through death. The activity and social contact of employment are replaced by the ambiguous role of retirement. Physical illness can limit mobility. Psychiatric symptoms and syndromes such as depression, dementia, and paranoia can result in a tragic cycle of isolation for the elderly living at home. Day programs can offer caring, treatment, and support without institutionalization.

Day programs can be considered to span a continuum from the purely social or recreational seniors center, to the structured and protective adult day care or day hospital that functions on a nursing or medical model. In contrast to the usual outpatient department or recreational activity, which may require an hour or two of the patient's time, day programs occupy a substantial portion of the waking day, including one or more meals. Thus, overlapping programs exist: day centers, adult day care, and partial hospitals.

Thanks are due to Rhoda Kopstein for assisting the review of the social day care model, and to Katherine Steirman for the review questions.

Psychiatry day hospitalization has been described as "one of psychiatry's gifts to medicine" (Arie 1975). Psychiatry is credited with inventing partial hospitalization in Moscow in 1933, and programs were later established in Montreal and London in the 1940s. The first dedicated geriatric day hospital was established at the United Oxford Hospital in London (Cosin et al. 1958). A comprehensive overview of psychiatric partial hospitalization and day treatment was provided by Dibella and associates (1982).

Indications

Day care and day hospitals should be distinguished from day centers or senior citizens clubs. Seniors centers usually offer a variety of social, recreational, and cultural activities. They are occasionally located on the same premises as a residential or retirement home and may offer luncheons. Medical or nursing care is never provided. Seniors centers are usually organized by nonprofit religious or social institutions and rarely cater to the geriatric psychiatry patient, instead servicing the relatively robust and extroverted. The revelance of these types of programs to psychiatric care is that they represent a community resource following recovery from functional psychiatric illness. Although attendance at these programs cannot be "prescribed," involvement can be highly recommended in order to reduce risk of relapse if social isolation played a factor in the onset of illness. The role of skilled consulting clinicians such as a psychiatrist, social worker, psychologist, or other mental health professional can include assisting in program development, educating staff about the special problems of the elderly, and helping staff to identify clients in need of mental health services.

The terms "day care," "day hospital," and "partial hospitalization" have been used interchangeably to describe programs for the elderly with psychiatric and/or physical disorders (Tate and Brennan 1988). The National Institute on Adult Daycare (1984) defined day care as

> a community-based group program designed to meet the needs of impaired adults through an individual plan of care. It is a structured, comprehensive program that provides a variety of health, social and related support services in a protective setting during any part of the day but less than 24-hour care. Adult day care assists its participants to remain in the community, enabling families and

other caregivers to continue caring for an impaired member at home.

Diverse services are provided under the rubric of day care or day hospital, depending on the model of care. Although the ideal program offers multiple approaches to care, most day hospitals offer one of three models: 1) social, 2) active treatment, and 3) maintenance (see Table 30-1).

Social Model

Social day care emphasizes supervised and structured group recreational activities. Physicians are not a part of this model, but pa-

Table 30-1. Day program models of care

Model	Patients	Cost	Services	Discharge disposition
Social	"Clients" isolated, frail, cognitively impaired	Low	Social work Structured recreational and Social activities Protective environment Caregiver support	None planned
Active treatment	Functional and Organic psychiatric disorders Posthospital Post-nursing home	High	Multidisciplinary team Interconnected group therapies within a therapeutic milieu	Home; prevention of institutionalization
Maintenance	Chronic (dementia, functional psychiatric, and personality disorders)	Moderate	Multidisciplinary team[a] Long-term placement alternative Caregiver support	Prevention of institutionalization (hospital, nursing home)

[a]May include occupational therapy, physiotherapy, nursing, social work, psychology, and a physician.

tients are expected to continue to receive medical care from their personal physician in the community.

As the definition indicates, the programs provide essential supervision for frail and cognitively impaired clients. Admissions are based on family, nursing, or social work definitions of "need." In most instances a lay board of directors defines the criteria for membership. Participants do not require a particular diagnosis, and care plans address such issues as personal care, nutrition, and social and leisure activities as well as family support. Benefits to be derived from participating are summarized in Table 30-2. Specific days or locations of activities may be arranged for groups of individuals with differing capacities to participate in programming.

Programs usually operate 5 days a week, and the hours of operation are meant to accommodate the schedule of a working caregiver. All programs offer meals and transportation is usually included. Typical programming might include craft projects, sing-alongs, exercise, and community outings.

Strictly speaking, participants are never discharged, although dropouts are not infrequent. Common reasons for discontinuation are listed in Table 30-3. Most of these reasons involve inability to maintain the minimum level of autonomous functioning set by a particular program.

Social day care programs can be located by contacting community information services, the social work office of a nearby hospital, or United Way offices. Costs for clients are determined by the type of funding provided and can vary widely. A sliding fee scale is

Table 30-2.   Benefits of social day care services

Supervision and assistance with activities of daily living
Socialization
Support and respite for caregiver
Prevention or delay of institutionalization

Table 30-3.   Reasons for discontinuation of social day care

Dangerousness to self or others
Inability to toilet self, or urinary or fecal incontinence (additional staff and shower required)
Wandering (secure environment required)
Transfer to institution
Move away from transportation catchment area

usually offered, but day care in the United States is not covered by Medicare and is only rarely reimbursable by private insurance.

Problems and Pitfalls

The absence of on-site physicians directly affiliated with the program represents the most serious potential weakness of the social model. Reversible or treatable illnesses may be missed in the assessment and admission process. The participants have a high likelihood of physical and psychiatric comorbidity, which may go undetected. Even in the facilities where nursing staff is available, medication can usually only be monitored, and the absence of a prescribing physician on the premises precludes medication management. This problem can be partially overcome by developing a close collaborative relationship with the client's physician.

Recently, increased levels of staffing and a new emphasis on specialized nursing has eroded the social component of the programming. These changes have occurred in response to a trend toward clients who are older, sicker, and more frail. Units specializing in individuals with Alzheimer's disease and other dementing illnesses are appearing with increasing frequency, and more attention is being focused on supporting the family caregiver.

Active Treatment Model

This approach emphasizes the medical and restorative model. The terms "day hospital" and "partial hospitalization" are particularly appropriate when applied to these programs. Typically, a full range of physician-supervised ambulatory medical and/or psychiatric treatments is offered or prescribed to patients attending during weekdays (Dibella et al. 1982). Day hospitals are used as an alternative to inpatient care and to expedite discharge from the hospital.

Active treatment programs usually consist of carefully coordinated, interconnected group therapies within a therapeutic milieu. Treatment consists of biological interventions (e.g., pharmacotherapy or electroconvulsive therapy), psychological interventions (e.g., individual and group psychotherapy), and social interventions. Usually a psychiatrist—but sometimes another mental health professional—leads a multidisciplinary team including occupational therapy, social work, and nursing staff. There is an expectation that patients will improve sufficiently to be discharged from the day program.

Programs are generally located on hospital premises, providing access to specialized medical and diagnostic services. Costs are generally significantly higher in this type of program than in the social model, although direct patient costs depend on funding and financing arrangements. Transportation represents a significant barrier to access if not organized by the program. Finally, active treatment day hospitals are often promoted as cost-effective alternatives to inpatient care.

A variety of descriptive papers indicates that the full range of psychiatric disorders of the elderly can be effectively treated in day hospitals (Aronson 1976; Bergmann et al 1978; Brocklehurst 1979; Brocklehurst and Tucker 1980; Goldstein et al. 1968; Greene and Timbury 1979; McDonald et al. 1971; Woodford-Williams et al. 1962).

Inpatient treatment may be required for patients thought to be an imminent danger to themselves or others, and patients unwilling or unable to attend require more intensive supervision than is available in active day treatment.

Providing active treatment in the context of a day hospital has several advantages over inpatient admission. First and foremost, a patient's ties to the community are supported rather than severed. Day hospitals provide a "model" of the real world, where problem solving and coping strategies can be learned and practiced. Some of the advantages of treatment in day hospitals are listed in Table 30-4.

Table 30-4.   Advantages of active treatment in day hospitals

Other care	Day hospital
Usual outpatient	Intense exposure to therapeutic milieu and range of therapies
	"Real life" fit
	Crisis intervention possible
	Team shares responsibility for care
Inpatient	Less stigma
	Decreased risk of institutionalization, regression, and extreme dependency
	Less costly
	Maintenance of social network and avoidance of social breakdown syndrome
	Maintenance of community functioning

Source. Modified from Dibella et al. 1982, pp. 34–35.

Problems and Pitfalls

Although there are a number of excellent descriptions of individual programs, issues of efficacy and effectiveness are rarely addressed, and there have been no controlled studies (Hodkinson 1980). Little attention has been paid to the possibility of differential effectiveness by diagnostic categories. The therapeutic consequences of mixing patients with a variety of functional and dementing illnesses remain unclear.

The issue of cost-effectiveness also is not settled (Anand et al. 1982). When the costs of a well-staffed treatment program and transportation are considered, the cost differential with inpatient hospital treatment begins to narrow, suggesting that issues of cost should be considered secondary to the consideration of benefit and effectiveness.

Most active treatment programs are pressured to serve as placement alternatives for patients with irreversible dementing illnesses or other chronic psychiatric conditions (Arie 1975). Several descriptive papers (Goldstein et al. 1968; Greene and Timbury 1979; McDonald et al. 1971) have outlined the natural history of geriatric psychiatry day hospitals, documenting the shift from what Greene and Timbury (1979) termed the "optimistic view" of therapeutic efficacy, to the role of custodial facility. Even the possibility of providing active treatment has been questioned by Arie (1975, p. 34), when he stated, "The main function of day care in geriatric psychiatry is as a long term—indeed one might say a permanent—supportive facility." When a program becomes filled with chronic patients who have poor prognoses and are undischargeable from the program, the possibility of active treatment is diminished and staff expectations and morale may decline. This problem highlights the need for complementary and coexisting models of care, in the same catchment area, that can be offered to patients with differing requirements.

Maintenance Model

This approach represents a combination of the social and treatment models. Patients at high risk for institutional care are provided with long-term day care in order to delay and even prevent institutionalization. These patients represent a diverse group of frail individuals who may be suffering from chronic psychiatric disorders including schizophrenia, treatment-resistant affective disorders, and personality disorders as well as dementing illnesses. As in the other models, services are usually offered 5 days per week and provision is made to provide relief to family caregivers. This approach overlaps with respite care.

Referral to this type of program is usually initiated by a physician. The treatment team is multidisciplinary, usually including a psychiatrist in a leadership or consultative role.

Maintenance programs usually make some provision for active treatment of a small proportion of patients, but for most patients there is no expectation of improvement to the point of discharge. When discharge occurs it is almost always to a more intensive level of care such as a hospital or nursing home.

Problems and Pitfalls

The most serious criticism of this approach is that it represents an expensive use of potentially rehabilitative or curative therapeutic resources (Irvine 1980). Furthermore, active treatment becomes unlikely or even impossible if this model is applied.

Although it is often assumed that keeping an individual at home is preferable to institutionalization, in some situations quality of life may be optimized by institutional placement. Finally, increasing efforts are being made to bring services to the patient in the home rather than to bring the patient to the services. Homemakers, visiting nurses, and physicians as well as volunteer or paid companions may be preferable, for some patients, to long-term day care programs.

Summary

Social factors such as isolation and loneliness seem to contribute to the onset of psychiatric illness in the elderly. Day programs offer an organized social network that can reverse or prevent social isolation and provide opportunities for social interaction.

Social day centers include social and recreational activities with minimal support and structure. Day care and day hospitals offer varied programs of support, supervision, and treatment. Day care approaches can be classified according to three models of care: 1) social, 2) treatment, and 3) maintenance. Social and maintenance programs are specifically designed to provide relief and support to the caregivers of frail or cognitively impaired patients.

Day treatments can theoretically include all of the modalities available to inpatients without the necessity of removing a patient from familiar surroundings in the community. Special transportation arrangements are a critical factor in determining accessibility to these services.

Day programs are an important component of any comprehensive geriatric psychiatry service.

References

Anand KB, Thomas JH, Osborne KL, et al: Cost and effectiveness of a geriatric day hospital. Journal of the Royal College of Physicians of London 16:53–56, 1982

Arie T: Day care in geriatric psychiatry. Gerontologia Clinica 17:31–39, 1975

Aronson R: The role of an occupational therapist in a geriatric day hospital setting. Am Occup Ther 30:290–292, 1976

Bergmann K, Foster EM, Justice AW, et al: Management of the demented elderly in the community. Br J Psychiatry 132:441–449, 1978

Brocklehurst JC: The development and present status of day hospitals. Age and Ageing 8:76–79, 1979

Brocklehurst JC, Tucker JS: Progress is Geriatric Day Care. London, Pitman Press, 1980

Cosin LZ, Mort M, Post F, et al: Experimental treatment of persistent senile confusion. Int J Soc Psychiatry 4(2):24–42, 1958

Dibella GAW, Weitz GW, Poynter-Berg D, et al: Handbook of Partial Hospitalization. New York, Brunner/Mazel, 1982

Goldstein S, Sevriuk J, Grauer H: The establishment of a psychogeriatric day hospital. Can Med Assoc J 98:955–959, 1968

Greene JG, Timbury GC: A geriatric psychiatric day hospital service: a five-year review. Age and Ageing 8:49–53, 1979

Hildick-Smith M: Geriatric day hospitals—changing emphasis in costs. Age and Ageing 13:95–100, 1984

Hodkinson HM: A need for evaluation. Br Med J 281:100, 1980

Irvine RE: Geriatric day hospitals: present trends. Health Trends 12:68–71, 1980

McDonald RD, Neulander A, Holbod O, et al: Description of a nonresidential day-care facility. Gerontologist 11:322–328, 1971

National Institute on Adult Day Care: Standards for Adult Day Care. Washington, DC, National Council on the Aging, 1984

Ross DN: Geriatric day hospital: counting the cost compared with other methods of support. Age and Ageing 5:171–175, 1976

Tate AL, Brennan CM: Adult Day Care: A Practical Guidebook and Manual. New York, Haworth Press, 1988

Woodford-Williams E, McKeon JA, Trotter IS, et al: The day hospital in the community care of the elderly. Gerontology Clinics 4:241–256, 1962

Chapter 31

Carl Cohen, M.D.

Integrated Community Services

Overview

Psychiatric treatment of the geriatric patient generally cannot be conducted in isolation. Consequently, the psychiatrist may be called on to orchestrate the various components of the treatment plan. Even if the psychiatrist does not assume a coordinating role, it is nevertheless incumbent on the clinician to assist the patient, family, and other health professionals in identifying services that will help optimize the patient's level of functioning. The descriptions of services provided in this chapter are designed to provide the geriatric psychiatrist with the basic information that is critical to educating patients, families, and other health professionals about the types of support services available in the community.

In addition to helping patients negotiate the formal support system, clinicians often work with the patient's and family's informal support network, which is comprised of relatives, friends, clergy, storekeepers, letter carriers, and so forth. The importance of informal social supports cannot be overestimated. Gurland and associates (1983) developed the concept of "personal time dependency" to characterize the state of dependency that requires time-consuming help from another person. They found that 30% of persons aged 65 and older, living in the community, fulfilled criteria for personal time dependency. In 80% of the cases, the primary caregiver was a member of the informal network, usually a spouse or daughter. These members of the informal network may be important informants as well as providing, or helping to secure, crucial support for the patient in such matters as food, household chores, and shopping. In recent years, community outreach efforts have spawned the development of network techniques—that is, teaching persons to better use their existing networks or encouraging them to broaden their support system to obtain additional emotional and material support (Biegel et al. 1984; Collins and Pancoast 1976; Gottlieb 1983).

There has been increased interest in determining what factors inhibit or facilitate access to services. A variety of structural and individual barriers to obtaining services have been identified. Structural barriers thought to be important are 1) inconvenient locations for services; 2) a relative lack of services in a community; 3) the financial cost of obtaining services; 4) negative professional attitudes and behaviors; 5) bureaucratic orientation of programs; and 6) the lack of any real coordination, integration, or organization within and between agencies servicing the elderly (Krout 1985; Reed 1980). Impediments to obtaining help at the individual patient level include 1) fear for personal safety, 2) poor health, 3) lack of knowledge about the availability of services, 4) negative attitudes toward services, and 5) fear of becoming too dependent on such services (Krout 1985). Finally, sources of information may play a significant role. Silverstein (1984) found that information that the elderly obtained through formal sources (e.g., seniors centers or medical facilities) was the best predictor of service use. Most respondents, however, learned of services through media or informal sources such as neighbors, family, and friends.

Gerontological practitioners, planners, and researchers are frequently required to impose some order on the myriad services and facilities available to community elderly (Goland and McCaslen 1979). Although there is no consensus or well-accepted rationale for any existing classification schema, Table 31-1 is a synthesis of a classifying schema proposed by Goland and McCaslen (1979) and Cantor and Little (1985). On the vertical axis is a measure of independence and self-functioning divided into three categories—well, moderately impaired, and frail or severely impaired. On the horizontal axis services are organized in three broad levels of needs: the basic level consisting of physical and mental health needs; an intermediate level of self-maintenance needs such as dressing, grooming, cooking, transportation, cleaning, and handling money; and a complex level of social needs such as work roles, friendship, intimacy, and education. Services described in this chapter have been inserted into the categorical schema of Table 31-1. Thus, for example, a comparatively well, older person who recently lost several close friends might be helped by referrals to social and voca-

Table 31-1. Types of services available

Function level	Physical and mental health needs	Self-maintenance needs	Social needs
Well (60% of population)	Mutual help groups Consumer health education Health insurance Health screening	Shared housing Converted boarding homes "Granny" flats Section 8 and Section 202 housing and parents Elderly apartment complexes Retirement community Congregate Meals Program Nutrition education Brown Bag Program	Seniors centers Voluntary associations Retired seniors Volunteer programs Foster Grandparents Senior Companions Service Corps of Retired Executives Green Thumb Senior Aides Adult education
Moderately impaired (30% of population)	Outreach services Visiting nurse Crisis intervention teams	Case management Home care services Domiciliary care Foster care Vocational rehabilitation Board and care homes Congregate housing Meals on Wheels Transportation Escort services Chore services	Friendly visiting Telephone reassurance Strengthen informal social support network
Frail or severely impaired (10% of population)	Mutual help groups for family Outreach services Visiting nurse Crisis intervention teams Inpatient psychiatric and medical care	Day care Respite care Home care services Hospice Nursing home Meals on Wheels Protective services Case management	Friendly visiting Telephone reassurance Strengthen informal social support network

Sources. Modified from Goland and McCaslen (1979) and Cantor and Little (1985).

tional services listed in the upper right-hand corner of Table 31-1. Similarly, a moderately impaired person with Alzheimer's disease might benefit from the self-maintenance and social services contained in the center and right-hand cells of the middle row of Table 31-1.

Community Services

In this section, an overview of the principal geriatric community services is provided. More detailed descriptions are available elsewhere (Huttman 1985). The intensity and level of services vary from those that are primarily aimed at clinical populations (e.g., day care, nursing homes) to those that are psychosocially supportive (e.g., mutual aid groups, volunteer groups). The latter may serve a preventive function by assuring that the elderly do not become socially isolated and, if disease develops, that they are already part of a network that makes clinical care accessible.

Table 31-2 summarizes the principal governmental programs relevant to the community services described in the text. One should also be aware that in recent years a variety of private health insurance policies have emerged that may cover home care and nursing homes. Moreover, some health maintenance organizations may provide home and institutional care in their prepaid plans. In a few regions, social health maintenance organizations are being tested. They offer prepaid health and long-term care services specifically for older persons (Skolnick and Warrick 1985). Finally, elderly veterans may be eligible for a variety of long-term care services (for example, nursing home, domiciliary care) provided by the U.S. Department of Veterans Affairs.

Assistance and Protection

Information and Referral Services. These resources are frequently the initial contact point for clients, family, and professionals to learn about available entitlements and services for the elderly. State "units on aging" are required by law to offer information and referral services at no cost (American Association of Retired Persons 1986a). The states are divided into smaller areas (usually by county) called "area agencies on aging" (AAAs). There are 662 AAAs throughout the country. State units can refer persons to the appropriate area agency. Other important resource services include social service departments, seniors centers, family service

Table 31-2. Summary of principal Government programs relevant to community services

Program	Service	Eligibility
Old Age Survivors and Disabled Insurance (OASDI) (1935)	Social security benefits	All persons age 65 and older, disabled workers, and dependent survivors when worker dies. Reduced amounts for retirees aged 62, widows aged 60, disabled aged 50.
Supplemental Security Income Program (1972)	Supplemental payments to bring persons to poverty threshold. States have option to pay for domiciliary care homes and personal home care.	Indigent persons 65 and older, disabled, and blind.
Title XVIII of the Social Security Act (1965)	Medicare, which includes hospital costs, physicians' fees, skilled nursing facility (limited), home health care, and hospice care.	Persons 65 and older and those under 65 who receive Social Security disability.
Title XIX of the Social Security Act (1965)	Medicaid, which includes medical services, skilled nursing care (unlimited), and home health care. Optional by state: adult day care, drugs, intermediate care facility.	Indigent aged, disabled, blind.
Social Services Block Grant (1981) (formerly Title XX of the Social Security Act 1975)	Varying levels by state: chore services, congregate meals, home-delivered meals, homemaker, seniors centers, protective services.	Indigent persons (all ages) up to 115% of state median income.
Older Americans Act (OAA) (1965)— Title III	Services vary by state: congregate meals, home-delivered meals, home health care, chore services, seniors centers, friendly visiting.	All persons 60 and older. Low-income persons are special targets.

Table 31-2. *Continued*

Program	Service	Eligibility
Older Americans Act (OAA) (1965)— Title V	Community employment (e.g., senior aides, Green Thumb).	Indigent persons 55 and older.
ACTION (1971)	Federal agency established to coordinate volunteer programs. Programs for aged include Foster Grandparents, RSVP, Senior Companions.	Some programs open only to indigent.
Section 202 Housing (1959)	Low-interest loans for construction of low-rent housing.	Nonprofit sponsors.
Section 8 (1974)	Rent subsidies to cover difference between fair market rent and 30% of participants' income.	Low-income elderly.
Food Stamp Program (1964)	Department of Agriculture program to purchase foods at lower prices.	Low-income persons.

Sources. Huttman 1985; Maddox 1987; Skolnick and Warrick 1985.

facilities, and mental health associations. The local telephone directory is also an excellent source to locate agencies such as the Social Security Administration, home care services, mayor's or governor's office on aging, and various religious social services organizations. The Silver Page Directory, a nationwide directory for persons aged 60 or older, also contains lists of services offered by local agencies.

Case Management. The primary aim of case management is to help clients and families deal with a fragmented and complex system by locating and coordinating existing resources through a process that includes screening, assessment, case planning, linkage to services, advocacy, monitoring, and in some instances, therapeutic counseling (Huttman 1985). Case management may be provided by public agencies, in which case eligibility may depend on medical or psychiatric history and being insured by Medicaid. A growing number of professionals are offering private case management.

Private case management organizations are listed in the Yellow Pages under social services, social workers, aging services, senior citizens services, and home health organizations. Fees generally vary from $50 to $100 for an initial consultation (American Association of Retired Persons 1986a).

White (1987) observed that the popularity and success of case management is evidenced by its proliferation in all types of health and social service settings, especially in programs serving long-term care populations. Several studies have demonstrated that case management services for the elderly can be cost-effective (Eggert and Brodows 1984; Zawadski and Ansak 1983). An important but unresolved issue concerns the most appropriate functions and background of case managers (Huttman 1985). Should they include therapeutic counseling? Should case managers be specially trained paraprofessionals or should they be primarily persons with a background in psychiatric social work?

Protective Services.   These services aid persons who are 1) incapable of performing functions necessary to meet basic physical and health requirements; 2) incapable of managing finances; 3) dangerous to self or others; or 4) exhibiting behavior that brings them into conflict with the community. Such agencies may facilitate hospitalization or assist with various legal actions. In general, these services have been provided by public departments of social services and legal service centers (Beattie 1976).

The effectiveness of the protective casework model, in use since the 1960s, has been questioned (Zborowsky 1985); in several demonstration projects this model was found to be no more effective than the usual community control services (Blenkner et al. 1974). Studies of elder abuse programs have also raised questions about the ability of professionals to resolve the abuse problem successfully (Zborowsky 1985). Despite the controversy that exists over these findings (Berger and Piliavin 1976), Zborowsky (1985) argued that there needs to be a continued search for more effective protective social services.

Community Treatment

Geriatric Day Care.   These programs are designed for at-risk persons who are mentally, physically, or socially impaired and who need day services to maintain or improve their level of functioning so that they can remain in, or return to, their own homes. Such programs also provide some respite for families. Weissert (1976) categorized two broad types of day care centers: health oriented and social services oriented. More recently, such centers have been subdivided into three models (Weissert et al. 1989). Model 1 is situated in nursing homes and rehabilitation centers and provides services to physically dependent, older populations; services include nursing, physical, occupational, and speech therapies and health and social services. Revenues come primarily from philanthropic and self-pay sources, with some Medicaid reimbursement. Model 2 is situated in a general hospital or in a social service or housing agency. Most patients can perform activities of daily living, but more than 40% have mental disorders. Services include case management, professional counseling, transportation to and from centers, nutrition, education, and health assessment. Revenues come heavily from governmental sources, particularly Medicaid. Model 3 involves special-purpose centers to serve a single type of clientele such as the blind, the mentally ill, or veterans. When not reimbursed by Medicaid, out-of-pocket daily costs range from $10 to $105, with a median of $30 (Weissert et al. 1989).

Research on adult day care has been generally positive, although its cost-effectiveness has been more equivocal (Weiler 1987). Compared with a community control group, day care participants showed higher levels of physical and emotional functioning (Weiler et al. 1976). The costs are lower than for nursing homes (Capitman and Gregory 1984; Rathbone-McCuan and Elliot 1976/77), and day care compares favorably with the cost of a home visit from a home health nurse ($40) or a 4-hour visit from a homemaker ($25 or more). Nevertheless, for persons less at risk for nursing home placement, the cost benefits of day care are thought to be modest (Skellie et al. 1982).

Respite Care. Respite is temporary relief (usually several hours to several weeks) for caregivers from the demands of providing care (Tanner and Shaw 1985). Respite can be provided in the home, in the community, in institutions caring for the elderly, or in hospitals. Services may be organized by churches and synagogues, nursing homes, home health agencies, and volunteer agencies. Funding is primarily from Medicaid or out of pocket; Medicare does not reimburse.

Respite care has not been subjected to thorough evaluation (George 1987). One study (Scharlach and Franzel 1986) found that respite care contributed to the caregiver's improved physical and mental health, better relationships, and increased confidence in their ability to continue the caregiving role, but did not improve patients' physical or mental functioning. Contrary to expectations, respite care did not affect rates of institutionalization. Several areas require further study: the most effective models for delivery care (e.g., comparison of care in home vs. institution, and determination of the degree of training required for respite workers); the variables in the effects of respite care for different types of caregivers and/or patients; and financing and reimbursement issues (George 1987).

Home Health Care. Included is a wide variety of services offered at home, usually under a physician's supervision. Home health care may include medical services provided by nurses or physical therapists, and personal care and chore services such as assistance with dressing and grooming provided by homemaker aides or home health aides (American Association of Retired Persons 1986b). Home health care services must be provided by a home health agency that is certified by the state health department. Four types of organizations exist: government-sponsored agencies (e.g., local departments of social service), nonprofit agencies (e.g., visiting nurse service), proprietary agencies, and hospital-based programs.

Although home care services are gaining ardent supporters, their cost-effectiveness is unclear because it depends on which factors are included in the equation (Ellis 1984). There is general consensus that home care is more humane and improves the older person's quality of life. A study comparing community elderly in New York City and London found that, despite the considerably higher levels of professional home health care services in London, rates of institutionalization were comparable (Gurland et al. 1983). The authors of this study proposed that home care services could be more effective if the family, rather than the disabled person, were the primary focus of intervention and if the capacity to provide emotional support for the family and the dependent elderly were included in the repertoire of home care skills in addition to more material services.

Home Care. This category includes a variety of nonmedical services provided at home: friendly visiting, telephone reassurance, emergency response systems, and chore services. Because they do not include medical services, these programs are generally not reimbursable by Medicaid, Medicare, or private insurance. However, the Older Americans Act (OAA) provides funding for some services such as meal programs, home chores, and home-

maker health aides. Everyone aged 60 and older is eligible for services provided by OAA. There is no charge, but contributions are
sometimes accepted. Because each state receives a block grant
under OAA, the level of services varies considerably. AAAs provide
services directly or through contracts with local agencies, religious
organizations, or firms (American Association of Retired Persons
(1986a). The principal home care programs are described in this
section. The meal programs that fall under this category (e.g.,
"Meals on Wheels") are described in the "Nutritional Services" section.

With *friendly visiting,* a volunteer visits the home usually one or
two times per week for general conversation, to inquire about
needs, to help with errands, and so forth. There is no charge for this
service, which is usually offered by a volunteer group or religious
organization. A few studies have examined the effectiveness of
friendly visiting programs in the community. Muligan and Bennett
(1977), comparing a group of elderly persons participating in such
services with a nonvisited control group, concluded that their
friendly visiting program had a positive impact on the mental status, grooming, and apartment upkeep of visited clients. However,
Calsyn and associates (1984) found no differences in clients' life
satisfaction when comparing elderly receiving face-to-face visiting
versus phone visiting and a no-treatment control group. In a second study, the authors found friendly visits that involved more reciprocal client-visitor interaction to be more effective than interactions in which the client maintained a more passive role. They
suggested that friendly visiting can be made more effective by increasing reciprocity in the client-visitor relationship (Calsyn et al.
1984).

In *telephone reassurance* programs, clients are given a number
to call if they feel lonely or have a request for help. Volunteers also
call to check on the client.

Emergency response systems provide a reliable contact by telephone or electronic device to police or rescue squads in the event
of an emergency.

In *chore services* programs, minor household repairs, household
cleaning, and yard work are offered. Costs average $4 an hour, plus
materials (American Association of Retired Persons 1986b).

Seniors Centers.   These are generally multipurpose centers that
may provide nutritional programs, recreation, education, socialization, health services, friendly visiting, religious services, social
services, information, and referrals. There have been several stud-

ies suggesting that use of seniors centers varies in the elderly population. For example, seniors centers tend to attract women (Harris and Associates 1975; Vickery 1972), the mentally healthy (Tissue 1971), people from blue collar backgrounds (Kent 1978; Tissue 1971), and people who have recently experienced the death of a spouse (Demko 1979). "Lack of interesting activities" was cited as a major obstacle to seniors center use, particularly among middle-class elderly (Ralston and Griggs 1985). In addition, minority elderly reported lack of transportation as a major impediment (Brown and O'Day 1981). Although blacks often lack opportunities to use centers, they appear significantly more committed than whites to attending programs when they are available (Ralston and Griggs 1985). Ralston and Griggs (1985) concluded that practitioners need to examine the fit between the needs of elderly subgroups and the types of programs planned in seniors centers.

Social Network Interventions and Mutual Aid (Self-Help) Groups. A growing number of community mental health programs have begun to experiment with a variety of social network techniques including 1) helping clients expand their networks; 2) assisting individuals to increase the support and exchange within existing networks; 3) identifying natural helpers and gatekeepers (e.g., clergy, letter carriers, and physicians) who can assist clients; and 4) teaching service personnel to work with existing networks (Pancoast et al. 1983). Although most reports have been descriptive and anecdotal, the more systematic studies have tended to be favorable and to make several important stipulations. For example, in an experimental study in a midtown Manhattan, single-room-occupancy hotel in which social workers were instructed to attempt to service clients only through network interventions, it was found that one-third of the clients had one successful intervention (Cohen and Adler 1984). However, only 16% of all presenting problems could be addressed through a network procedure. The authors concluded that network interventions are neither for every problem nor for everybody. It is no surprise that transactions that have long been part of a population's cultural world are most likely to yield successful network outcomes. In other words, service workers should not expect to undertake network tasks with which clients are not already familiar. The authors also cautioned that use of natural supports should not be used to justify public policies that might result in the withholding of professional services.

Self-help or mutual help groups are one of the most popular network modalities. These groups provide mutual assistance by creating a personal, intimate, face-to-face environment where elderly persons with similar experiences can exchange ideas and coping techniques. Examples include caregiver support groups such as those for Alzheimer's disease and political action groups such as the Gray Panthers. The fluidity of membership and the difficulty in controlling the number of complex variables has limited the scope of evaluative research (Lieberman and Borman 1979). Evaluation of self-help groups has been sparse, especially with respect to hard data (Gartner and Riessman 1977; Maddox 1987). According to Spiegel (1982), the widespread acceptance and apparent effectiveness of self-help groups stem from commonality of experience, mutual support, receiving of help through giving it, collective willpower, information sharing, and goal-directed problem solving. Self-help groups provide assistance to individuals who may have never availed themselves of professional help.

Mental Health Crisis Intervention Services. The aim of these services is to provide rapid restabilization of a person's psychiatric symptoms and social adjustment (Phipps and Liberman 1988). Crisis services are often hospital based or tied to community mental health centers. Services may be delivered in the patient's home or at a designated place outside the home. Mobile units or home treatment teams may visit the home or maintain daily phone contact. Alternatively, the patient may receive crisis care in the hospital or emergency room, or leave her or his home to live in a respite home or in crisis lodging. A number of innovative programs provide care, as well as crisis intervention, by using mobile teams to seek out patients in the community rather than seeing them in offices and clinics.

Most reports of geriatric mobile units and community outreach programs have been descriptive or have measured success based on new cases that they have uncovered or treated. For example, an elderly outreach program in Iowa identified and treated 420 patients during its first 2 years of operation. Cost per patient was approximately one-half the cost of mental health services provided by psychologists and psychiatrists in private practice. Similarly, Parish and Landsberg (1984) found that their outreach efforts in a rural community reduced psychiatric hospitalizations by 60%.

Psychiatric Vocational Rehabilitation. Although older patients are underserved by psychiatric vocational rehabilitation programs, these programs should be considered a treatment option for aging psychiatric patients. Two basic types of programs exist:

first, "sheltered employment" (also known as sheltered workshops or compensated work therapy programs) provides work opportunities for individuals who are not ready for competitive employment. Workdays may be decreased, tasks simplified and structured, and on-the-job pressures reduced. Some programs are based in psychiatric treatment centers, but most are managed by nonprofit agencies such as Goodwill Industries or Jewish Vocational Services. Patients receive either piecework pay or hourly pay according to their abilities and the specific contract (Jacobs 1988). Second, "transitional employment" provides real-work jobs with commercial establishments that are supervised by psychiatric or rehabilitation professionals. The vocational rehabilitation program contracts with local businesses for jobs and assumes responsibility for their completion. Patients earn the same pay as regular workers. These programs are operated by various nonprofit agencies (e.g., Fountain House in New York City, and Thresholds in Chicago). Assistance in identifying these programs can be obtained from state divisions of vocational rehabilitation or local AAAs.

Residential Programs

Long-Term Care Facilities

These facilities provide medical and psychosocial care to individuals who have relatively severe chronic impairments.

Domiciliary Care Residences. These facilities are also known as personal care residences, custodial care, homes for the aged, rest homes, sheltered care facilities, and adult homes. These are nonmedical institutions for persons with no major health problems or injuries but who need supervision. Services include food, some personal care, and usually recreational and social work. They are often used to provide the chronically mentally ill with a protective environment. These facilities must be licensed by state departments of social services. No Medicare or Medicaid benefits are available; however, qualified residents may receive additional reimbursement from Supplemental Security Income. With respect to efficacy, one study found elderly participants in a Pennsylvania domiciliary program to be more optimistic, engaged in more social activities, and expressive of greater satisfaction with living conditions, all at lower costs than a matched community control group (Vandivort et al. 1984).

Nursing Homes. These institutions can be divided into two broad categories: 1) skilled nursing facilities that provide 24-hour nursing care and medical coverage for persons who require extensive care (reimbursement is provided by Medicaid, and time-limited coverage by Medicare); and 2) intermediate care facilities, which provide health-related care for persons who are more stabilized but require some medical and nursing supervision (not full-time; costs are covered by Medicaid but not Medicare). Nursing home care is discussed in detail in chapter 27.

Specially Designed Housing for the Elderly

The aim of this type of housing is to include a variety of supportive services to help older persons compensate for physical decline and deal more effectively with special health problems of advanced age (Huttman 1985).

Congregate Housing. Congregate housing includes apartment houses or group accommodations that provide limited health services and other support services (e.g., meals in a central dining room, heavy housekeeping, social services, recreational activities) to functionally impaired, older persons to enable them to continue to live an independent lifestyle. These facilities are somewhat less institutionalized than domiciliary care residences. These institutions may include a "life care" arrangement with a congregate wing adjacent to an apartment complex (U.S. Department of Health and Human Services 1986). These facilities are usually operated by government agencies or nonprofit groups, and many receive funding for construction from federal housing programs. Costs vary widely. Ruchelin and Morris (1987) reported that monthly service costs were $563 per tenant, which they considered cost-effective in comparison to nursing home placement.

Elderly Apartment Complexes. These include public, nonprofit, and privately owned buildings for the elderly, many of which have been built with Section 202 federal funds. These do not routinely provide health care. Section 8 housing allowances—a federally subsidized program administered by local housing authority for low-income elderly—has frequently been a rent supplement to Section 202 housing.

Retirement Communities. These are nonlicensed, age-segregated communities of apartments or freestanding homes. Services are generally of a social nature (e.g., clubhouses, tennis courts) and do not routinely include health services.

Life Care Facilities. These are a special type of congregate living in which users must pay a large sum of money to buy into the development. Residents live in apartments or townhouses and there is usually a continuum of services including comprehensive medical care, meals, housekeeping, and recreational programs. The complex usually has a well-staffed infirmary and, in some instances, a full-scale nursing home. Users are guaranteed more intensified care when more supports are needed. Because a number of private facilities have gone bankrupt, states have issued regulations to ensure that developers meet their obligations.

Alternate Housing

Many types of housing for older people do not fit into traditional categories. Several representative alternative housing types are presented here. For a comprehensive survey of residential alternatives for older persons, the reader is referred to Lawton's review (1981).

Foster Care. For older persons (particularly those with chronic mental illness) in need of care and protection in a substitute family, foster care can provide socialization, stimulation, support, and protection. The number of paying residents is usually limited to four. Evaluations of foster care programs have been favorable. One study (Newman and Sherman 1979) found that elderly participants interacted to a moderate degree with family and community, and several investigators (Braun and Rose 1986; Oktay and Volland 1981; Vandivort et al. 1984) have reported higher levels of well-being and equal improvements in activities of daily living functions versus nursing home patients. It is worth noting that the cost of foster care was approximately three-fifths that of nursing homes.

Board and Care Facilities. This term describes a variety of facilities and is sometimes used interchangeably with domiciliary care facilities; the latter are licensed, but board and care are generally unlicensed. Commonly, these homes are privately owned; they are unlocked, residents share rooms, three meals per day are served, medications are dispensed, and minimal staff supervision is provided. The number of residents ranges from 1 to more than

100. These facilities have been a popular placement for discharged mental patients. Costs and quality of care vary widely. The Supplemental Security Income Program may provide supplementary case payments.

Granny Flats and Second-Unit Ordinances. These are special ordinances that permit elderly to live in mobile minihouses or in attached units on their children's land.

Shared Housing ("Senior Matching"). A social service agency matches occupants (owner or renter) with renters, or an agency buys or rents units and then rents them to others. Results have been favorable. One study of apartment- or house-sharing elderly found that two-thirds of these arrangements were still functioning after 1 year (Lawton 1981).

Hospice. This setting provides comfort, friendship, familiar possessions, and relief from pain in a person's last weeks of a terminal illness. Hospices may be found in hospital units, freestanding facilities, outpatient units for counseling and medical visits, or home care programs. The duration of care averages about 1 month. Medicare provides benefits to those who are diagnosed as having 6 months or less to live. Benefits under Medicaid vary by state. Some private insurance policies also provide reimbursement.

Nutritional Services

Congregate Meals Program. Begun under Title III of the OAA, the Congregate Meals Program provides to all persons aged 60 and older inexpensive meals at nearby centers such as churches, seniors centers, and schools. The original legislation also provided for nutrition education, information and referral, social service counseling, and recreational activities.

Home Delivery Program ("Meals on Wheels"). Also funded under OAA, nonprofit agencies prepare, package, and deliver midday meals and occasionally cold suppers or snacks to persons aged 60 and older who are homebound (according to accepted medical criteria).

Nutrition Education Program. Also funded under OAA, this program is designed to provide nutrition education either as part of a meal program or separately.

"Brown Bag" Program. Various community groups provide volunteers who fill shopping bags for low-income elderly.

Food Stamp Program. Started in 1964 by the Department of Agriculture, the program allows low-income Americans of all ages to purchase, at less than face value (or if very indigent, obtain for free) food stamps that substitute for cash in buying specified kinds of food at grocery stores. Applications can be obtained by mail or at local Social Security offices. A large proportion of elderly who are eligible do not use the program.

In 1969, the original thrust of the national program on nutrition was not only to provide older persons with meals, but also to offer outreach and services such as education, counseling, and recreation. Austin (1987) argued that because of insufficient funding, the focus over time has been primarily on serving meals, and the other goals have largely evaporated. Moreover, even the goal of serving meals has been elusive in that the average program participant receives seven meals per 10-week period—a level of participating that can barely contribute to the client's nutritional status (Austin 1987). Since 1983, budgetary cutbacks at the federal level have further weakened these programs.

Transportation and Escort Services

Transportation Services. Generally funded by the Urban Mass Transportation Act and OAA, communities provide three modes of transport to assist elderly to get to doctors and do errands: subsidized taxis, minibuses, and private cars.

Escort Services. Community agencies and police provide escorts to assist frail elderly to do errands and other activities.

Shopping Assistance. Seniors centers and other seniors organizations provide transport service to help the aged get to shopping centers.

Adult Education, Volunteer, and Employment Programs

Adult Education. Various colleges, junior colleges, public schools, museums, libraries, and seniors centers offer courses and matriculation for seniors. Elder Hostel, Inc., provides short courses on campus for many out-of-state seniors.

Retired Seniors Volunteer Program (RSVP).   This program originated under OAA, but is now funded through ACTION, the same organization that runs the Peace Corps. Volunteers aged 60 and older work in hospitals, nursing homes, and seniors centers. Local seniors centers sponsor a variety of RSVP programs such as friendly visiting. RSVP also works with children and delinquents.

Foster Grandparents.   Subsidized through ACTION, this program provides a small stipend to low-income seniors to work with youths in need of supportive and affectionate adults. It is conducted in various settings including schools, care centers, and hospitals.

Senior Companions.   This is another ACTION-supported program that provides a stipend for low-income older persons to assist other elderly in nursing homes and hospitals, and to provide visits to the homebound.

Service Corps of Retired Executives.   This program gives retired professionals an opportunity to assist small-business owners who lack funds to pay for such services.

Green Thumb.   Funded under the Senior Community Service Employment Program (SCSEP) of OAA, the program employs retired farmers and other low-income rural elderly to work part-time in parks and in beautification programs.

Senior Aides.   Another program of SCSEP, Senior Aides offers small stipends for part-time work in such community service jobs as homemaker, home health aide, and assisting with food programs.

Several studies have demonstrated that older participants in volunteer work derive substantial benefits. Hunter and Linn (1980–1981) found aged volunteers to have greater life satisfaction and to have fewer somatic and depressive symptoms than those who did not volunteer. Similarly, Friedman (1975) and Fengler and Goodrich (1980) observed positive experiences when aged volunteers worked with institutionalized and disabled elderly. Cutler (1976) noted that the type of organization in which the older person volunteered was important. Of 33 organizations examined, Cutler found that only those older persons volunteering in church-related organizations reported significantly higher levels of well-being. Although volunteerism appears to benefit older persons, one study (Carp 1968) found that increased happiness and self-esteem were highest among elderly who were in paid, rather than in volunteer, activities.

Summary

Because treatment of the geriatric patient, particularly the moderately or severely impaired, requires a comprehensive array of services, it is important that geriatric psychiatrists familiarize themselves with the principal community services described in this chapter. Moreover, as outlined in Table 31-1, the psychiatrist should be able to match services with the patient's level of functioning, and then link the patient to the appropriate services. Assistance with linking is usually available from the local AAAs and/or through the services of a social worker. There has been a relative dearth of evaluative studies of community programs. Although cost-effectiveness has not always been demonstrated, community programs generally have been judged to be at least clinically equivalent to institutional programs and considerably more humane. Future studies must identify older persons who are inadequately served by current programs, develop methods for overcoming barriers to services, and refine existing programs to maximize their clinical benefits and reduce costs.

References

American Association of Retired Persons: Miles Away and Still Caring. Washington, DC, AARP, 1986a

American Association of Retired Persons: Making Wise Decisions for Long Term Care. Washington, DC, AARP, 1986b

Austin C. Nutrition programs, in The Encyclopedia of Aging. Edited by Maddox GL. New York, Springer, 1987, pp 495–496

Beattie WM: Aging and social services, in Handbook of Aging and the Social Sciences. Edited by Binstock RH, Shanas E. New York, Van Nostrand Reinhold, 1976

Berger RM, Piliavin I: The effect of casework: a research note. Social Work 21:205–208, 1976

Biegel DE, Shore BK, Gordon E: Building Support Networks for the Elderly. Beverly Hills, CA, Sage, 1984

Blenkner M, Bloom M, Nielsen M, et al: Final Report: Protective Services for Older Adults. Cleveland, OH, Benjamin Rose Institute, 1974

Braun KL, Rose CL: The Hawaii geriatric foster care experiment: impact, evaluation, and cost analysis. Gerontologist 26:516–524, 1986

Brown C, O'Day M: Services to the elderly, in Handbook of Social Services. Edited by Gilbert N, Specht H. Englewood Cliffs, NJ, Prentice Hall, 1981

Calsyn RJ, Munson M, Peaco D, et al: A comparison of various approaches to visiting isolated community elderly. Journal of Gerontological Social Work 7:29–42, 1984

Cantor M, Little V: Aging and social care, in Handbook of Aging and the Social Sciences, 2nd Edition. Edited by Binstock RH, Shanas E. New York, Van Nostrand Reinhold, 1985

Capitman JA, Gregory KL: Supplemental Report in the Adult Day Health Care Program in California: A Comparative Cost Analysis. Sacramento, CA, Department of Health Services, 1984

Carp F: Differences among older workers, volunteers, and persons who are neither. J Gerontol 23:497–501, 1968

Cohen C, Adler A: Network Interventions: Do They Work? Gerontologist 24:16–22, 1984

Collins AH, Pancoast DL: Natural Helping Networks. Washington, DC, National Association of Social Workers, 1976

Cutler SJ: Membership in different types of voluntary associations and psychological well-being. Gerontologist 16:335–339, 1976

Demko D: Utilization, attrition, and the senior center. Journal of Gerontological Social Work 2:87–93, 1979

Eggert GM, Brodows BS: Five years of ACCESS: what have we learned? in Community-Based Systems of Long-Term Care. Edited by Zawadski RT. New York, Haworth Press, 1984, pp 27–48

Ellis NB: Sustaining frail disabled elderly in the community: an innovative approach to in-home services. Journal of Gerontological Social Work 7:3–15, 1984

Fengler AP, Goodrich N: Money isn't everything: opportunities for elderly handicapped men in a sheltered workshop. Gerontologist 20:636–641, 1980

Friedman S: The resident welcoming committee: institutionalized elderly in volunteer services to their peers. Gerontologist 15:362–367, 1975

Gartner A, Riessman F: Self-Help in Human Services. San Francisco, CA, Jossey-Bass, 1977

George LK: Respite care, in The Encyclopedia of Aging. Edited by Maddox GL. New York, Springer, 1987, pp 576–577

Goland SM, McClaslen R: A functional classification of services for older people. Journal of Gerontological Social Work 1:187–209, 1979

Gottlieb BH: Social Support Strategies. Beverly Hills, CA, Sage, 1983

Gurland B, Copeland J, Kuriansky J, et al: The Mind and Mood of Aging. New York, Haworth Press, 1983

Harris L, et al: The Myth and Reality of Aging in America. Washington, DC, National Council on the Aging, 1975

Hunter KI, Linn MW: Psychosocial differences between elderly volunteers and non-volunteers. International Journal of Aging and Human Development 12:205–213, 1980–1981

Huttman ED: Social Services for the Elderly. New York, Free Press, 1985

Jacobs HE: Vocational Rehabilitation, in Psychiatric Rehabilitation of Chronic Mental Patients. Edited by Liberman RP. Washington, DC, American Psychiatric Press, 1988, pp 245–284

Kent D: The how and why of senior centers. Aging May/June: 2–6, 1978

Krout JA: Service awareness among the elderly. Journal of Gerontological Social Work 9:7–19, 1985

Lawton MP: Alternative housing. Journal of Gerontological Social Work 3:61–80, 1981

Lieberman M, Borman L: Self-Help Groups for Coping With Crisis. San Francisco, CA, Jossey-Bass, 1979

Maddox GL: Mutual support groups, in The Encyclopedia of Aging. Edited by Maddox GL. New York, Springer, 1987, p 465

Muligan M, Bennett R: Assessment of mental health and social problems during multiple friendly visits: the development and evaluation of a Friendly Visitor Program for the isolated elderly. International Journal of Aging and Human Development 8:43–65, 1977

Newman ES, Sherman SR: Community integration of the elderly in foster family care. Journal of Gerontological Social Work 1:175–186, 1979

Oktay JS, Volland P: Health and Social Work. Washington, DC, National Association of Social Workers, 1981

Pancoast DL, Parker P, Froland C: Rediscovering Self-Help. Beverly Hills, CA, Sage, 1983

Parish B, Landsberg G: Developing a geriatric mental health outreach unit in a rural community. Journal of Geriatric Social Work 7:75–82, 1984

Phipps C, Liberman RP: Community support, in Psychiatric Rehabilitation of Chronic Mental Patients. Edited by Liberman RP. Washington, DC, American Psychiatric Press, 1988, pp 285–311

Ralston PA, Griggs MB: Factors affecting utilization of senior centers: race, sex, and socioeconomic differences. Journal of Gerontological Social Work 9:99–111, 1985

Rathbone-McCuan E, Elliot MW: Geriatric day care in theory and practice. Social Work in Health Care 2:153–170, 1976–1977

Reed WL: Access to services by the elderly: a community research model. Journal of Gerontological Social Work 3:41–52, 1980

Ruchelin HS, Morris JN: The Congregate Housing Services Program: an analysis of service utilization. Gerontologist 27:87–91, 1987

Scharlach A, Franzel C: An evaluation of institution-based respite care. Gerontologist 26:77–82, 1986

Silverstein NM: Informing the elderly about public services: the relationship between sources of knowledge and service utilization. Gerontologist 24:37–40, 1984

Skellie AF, Mobley GM, Goan RE: Cost-effectiveness of community-based long-term care: current findings of Georgia's alternative health services project. Am J Public Health 72:353–358, 1982

Skolnick B, Warrick P: The Right Place at the Right Time: A Guide to

Long-Term Care Choices. Washington, DC, American Association of Retired Persons, 1985

Spiegel D: Self-Help and Mutual Support Groups: A Synthesis of the Recent Literature in Community Support and Mental Health. Edited by
Biegel D, Naparstek A. New York, Springer, 1982

Tanner F, Shaw S: Caring: A Guide to Managing the Alzheimer's Patient
at Home. New York, New York City Department for the Aging, 1985

Tissue T: Social class and the senior center. Gerontologist 11:196–200,
1971

U.S. Department of Health and Human Services: Age Words: A Glossary
of Health and Aging. Washington, DC, National Institutes of Health,
1986

Vandivort R, Kurren G, Braun K: Foster family care for frail elderly: a
cost-effective quality care alternative. Journal of Geriatric Social Work
7:101–114, 1984

Vickery FE: Creative Programming for Adults. New York, Association
Press, 1972

Weiler PG: Adult day care, in The Encyclopedia of Aging. Edited by Maddox GL. New York, Springer, 1987, p 8

Weiler PG, Kim P, Pickard LS: Health care for elderly Americans: evaluation for an adult day health care model. Med Care 14:700–708, 1976

Weissert WG: Two models of geriatric day care: findings from a comparative study. Gerontologist 16:420–427, 1976

Weissert WG, Elston JM, Bolda EJ, et al: Models of adult day care: findings
from a national survey. Gerontologist 29:640–649, 1989

White M: Case management, in The Encyclopedia of Aging. Edited by
Maddox GL. New York, Springer, 1987, pp 92–96

Zawadaski RT, Ansak MK: Consolidating community-based long-term
care: early returns from the On Lok demonstration. Gerontologist
23:364–369, 1983

Zborowsky E: Developments in protective services: a challenge for social
workers. Journal of Geriatric Social Work 8:71–83, 1985

SECTION 5

Medical-Legal, Ethical, and Financial Issues

CHAPTER 32

Robert L. Sadoff, M.D.

Medical-Legal Issues

The law is generally divided into broad classifications of administrative law, civil law, and criminal law. Medical-legal issues in geriatric psychiatry may fall within the scope of any or all of these three areas.

Administrative aspects of law include patients' rights, the right to treatment, the right to refuse treatment, involuntary commitment, informed consent, confidentiality, privacy, and competency. The administrative or regulatory matters involving older patients are discussed in this chapter in order to provide a full understanding of the medical-legal issues that affect all patients, with special reference to geriatric patients.

Confidentiality

Confidentiality is an ethical matter until it is breached, and then it becomes a legal issue. The American Medical Association's Principles of Medical Ethics as Applied to Psychiatry, Section 9 (1973, p. 1063) state: "A physician may not reveal the confidences entrusted to him in the course of medical attendance, or the deficiencies he may observe in the character of patients, unless he is required to do so by the law, or unless it becomes necessary in order to protect the welfare of the individual or of the community." Thus confidentiality is not absolute secrecy; communications between patient and physician may be disclosed under appropriate circumstances. There are limitations to confidentiality that must be recognized by the therapist. However, if confidentiality is breached inappropriately, and that improper disclosure leads to damage to the patient, a lawsuit may follow.

Privileged communication is a legal matter (as opposed to an ethical one) that is developed by legislation and affects physicians and patients. The privilege—which belongs to the patient, not to the therapist—prohibits the therapist from disclosing information about the patient in court without the patient's consent. In some cases, the patient may waive the privilege, allowing the doctor to testify. These conditions of waiver include criminal or civil matters in which patients raise their mental state as an issue for the court to determine. Examples of privileged communication include communications between attorney and client, priest and penitent, husband and wife, and physician and patient. It should be noted that in most jurisdictions, the physician-patient privilege is not as strong as the attorney-client privilege. Thus, physicians may be forced to testify about their patients if the court orders such disclosure of information.

Right to Privacy

Right to privacy is the right of patients to protect the privacy of information obtained about them in the course of treatment. This right pertains primarily to patients' records that may be sought in a legal case. Psychiatrists may receive requests for patient records from attorneys by letter or subpoena, or by court order.

If the request is through a letter by an attorney, the psychiatrist should first consult the patient to obtain consent and permission to release the records. The physician should record in a patient's chart the receiving of that permission. It is not sufficient to receive a release of records that is signed by the patient but is not dated and time limited. All release forms requesting patient records should be current, that is, dated and time limited. It is also wise for the psychiatrist to check with the patient before releasing the records, to determine whether the patient wants the records sent. In the event that the patient is incompetent (e.g., cognitively impaired and unable to give consent), it is wise to consult the patient's family to determine the best course of action for the patient.

If the request is by subpoena, the psychiatrist should respond to the subpoena, but may do so by questioning the patient regarding the release of records. On occasion, patients, who are represented by their own attorneys, may wish that the records not be released and may have the attorney resist the subpoena. The psychiatrist should adhere to the wishes of the patient or the family before responding with a "knee jerk" release of records.

In cases in which the subpoena is resisted, the court makes a determination following a proper hearing at which arguments are presented by both sides. The court may quash the subpoena and thereby disallow the release of the records; or the court may order release of records. A subpoena is a demand for records; a court order is a command for records. The subpoena may be quashed, but the court order must be obeyed. The physician should remember that responding to a court order ensures immunity in the event of damage to the patient by the disclosure of information in the records. A psychiatrist who does not respond to a court order faces the risk of contempt of court; thus, there can be no double jeopardy before the psychiatrist in such circumstances.

Right to Refuse Treatment

The patient's right to privacy is also a key element of a patient's right to refuse treatment. There are two major areas of the patient's right to refuse: one involves psychiatric patients refusing psychiatric treatment; the other involves patients refusing general medical treatment. In the former case, courts have ruled that involuntarily committed patients have the right to refuse neuroleptic medications that may have long-term harmful side effects (American Psychiatric Association 1968). The courts' decisions in these cases do not include other types of medication such as antidepressants, anxiolytics, or lithium; more intrusive forms of treatment such as electroconvulsive therapy or psychosurgery require the patient's informed consent. Psychotherapy, milieu therapy, and other forms of noninvasive treatments are not included in the patient's right to refuse.

Competency

The issue of competency is the essential feature in numerous situations involving geriatric patients. Therefore, it is essential to understand the general concept of competency and its application to specific clinical situations. Competency is defined as the ability of individuals to know and understand the nature and consequences of the legal proceedings in which they are involved, or the medical situations confronting them (Appelbaum et al. 1987).

Competency implies a cognitive ability to know and understand the proceedings and their consequences. This ability is determined by specific questions posed by the evaluator of competency, which include questions about patients' awareness of their surroundings and the purpose of the legal or medical procedure. Specific questions asked refer to the intent and the consequences of the proceedings, for example, does the patient know that he or she is about to have an operation on a lower limb that will save his or her life? Is the patient aware of other possible treatment procedures and their consequences? There are specific questions for each particular situation in which competency is assessed. Thus geriatric patients who show evidence of cognitive impairment may not have the capacity to fully understand or appreciate a contemplated medical procedure. Patients may forget what was said to them in the course of the physician's explanation of the operation or procedure. Furthermore, at a subsequent time, impaired geriatric patients may accuse physicians of never explaining the procedure and claim that they were not fully informed and therefore did not give informed consent.

Psychiatrists often are asked to consult to determine whether patients are incompetent to refuse critical medical procedures and if guardians should be appointed so life-threatening conditions can be treated. These cases are not unusual, and psychiatrists should be aware of the means by which competency is assessed. As with patients of any age, infirm older adults may be resistant to change and to undergoing procedures that they do not or cannot understand. It behooves the consulting psychiatrist to spend time establishing rapport with patients in order to develop an environment in which the patients will be receptive to communication and information. Patients may refuse lifesaving treatment as a matter of course, and they may be considered incompetent as a result. However, spending time with patients and explaining carefully the proposed procedures in the context of their lives improves the psychiatrist's understanding of the reasons for reluctance or refusal. In addition, clarity of explanation and more detailed discussion may improve the likelihood of compliance.

Emergency situations require a different approach. The consulting psychiatrist may agree with the surgeon that unless the operation is performed immediately, the patient will die. The psychiatrist, upon examining the patient, may be able to determine that the patient is incompetent to give consent to the procedure. In that event, the family is consulted and consent obtained from them for the procedure on their elderly relative. Following the emergency, proper court proceedings may occur. It is unwise to operate on an incompetent person without consent of family or court, because a criminal charge of assault and battery may be brought against a physician who operates without proper consent. Assault and battery are legal terms for improper touching of patients without informed consent. An incompetent person cannot give informed consent, and operating on such a person may result in a charge of improper touching of the person's body, that is, assault and battery.

Emergency situations, properly documented, usually protect against such lawsuits. It is important for the primary physician and the consulting psychiatrist to indicate the urgency and nature of the emergency in the medical record. Courts usually uphold the opinions of the physicians in such emergency situations (Kayser-Jones and Kapp 1989). Saving the patient's life is accepted by most courts as the highest priority in these situations (McGarry 1973). However, competent geriatric patients who refuse surgery, for example, may be supported in their refusal by a court of law, even if such refusal could be life threatening (Meisel and Roth 1981). Courts refer to living wills as establishing patients' competent decisions regarding their treatment, even if they have become incompetent by the time a decision is required.

The ultimate issue is competency: if patients are competent, physicians must adhere to the wishes of patients. If patients are not competent, it is wisest to proceed medically in the patients' best interest, while pursuing guardianship, when feasible.

Informed Consent

Informed consent is the keystone of any treatment procedure in medicine (Brakel et al. 1985). Patients must have a clear understanding of what is to be done to or for them, and must be able to voluntarily consent to the procedure. The issue of voluntariness is essential to prevent subsequent accusation of coercion. The difference between persuasion and coercion may be slight, but it must be distinct: physicians must not exploit patients or coerce them into procedures that are not accepted voluntarily. Physicians or psychiatrists may give patients the benefit of the physician's experience in recommending a particular treatment course. However, physicians must also explain potential adverse effects as well as the benefits of the procedure. Benefits and advantages of alternative methods of treatment, or no treatment at all, must also be discussed with patients. Thus, for patients to give informed consent, they must have ability to understand the procedures contemplated and must be able to give voluntary consent. When patients cannot understand or make voluntary choices, they may be considered incompetent to give informed consent. Psychiatrists then may discuss treatment options with the family in order to obtain proper substitute consent to proceed. If patients are incompetent to give informed consent, they may require a guardian or conservator to make the decision for the operation or the medical procedure.

Guardianship

Guardians may be appointed to act over patients' persons or estates. Some states differentiate between these two types of guardians. Decisions about patients' assets ensure that patients do not inappropriately and incompetently squander their assets or become victims of designing persons. Guardians of such patients are appointed by the court in order to make medical decisions for patients about their persons, including medical procedures, research procedures, and where and with whom the patients live. In some jurisdictions, guardians represent the interests of both the patients and the state. In some jurisdictions conservators are appointed instead of guardians. Generally, conservators and guardians have similar functions with respect to patients (Brooks 1974).

Petitions for guardianship are usually initiated by the family, at the request of the physician. In the event that no family exists, the physician, social worker, or hospital administrator may initiate the petition for guardianship. The hearing regarding incompetency is usually quite formal, and judges are very concerned about depriving persons of the ability to make decisions about their lives. Testimony must be clear and convincing to the judge that the patients are not able to make decisions regarding their estates or their persons. Psychiatrists may be called on to testify about assessment of competency of the patient and about why a guardian is required for that particular person at that time. Physicians may provide evaluations of mental status and function and opinions about the patient's incompetency; however, only judges can declare a person to be legally incompetent. Alternatively, the court may make a patient a ward of the court, thus allowing the court or judge to make decisions for the patient, rather than appointing an independent guardian.

Guardians are usually selected from among close family members, trusted friends, or attorneys. Occasionally, a coguardian is appointed in matters of financial concern. A banker or an attorney may be appointed to oversee the estate as a trustee. This step may be required in order to prevent family members from abusing the privilege of guardianship and inappropriately depriving patients of their estates. Guardians are appointed by the court and are beholden to the court for fiduciary responsibility (i.e., proper management) of patients' estates.

Involuntary Hospitalization

Even in apparent emergencies, geriatric patients often have difficulty obtaining appropriate psychiatric care. Many may be considered "only senile" and therefore inappropriate for commitment to mental institutions. Most state laws exclude senility as a basis for involuntary hospitalization (Monahan 1984). Thus, psychiatrists must look for and determine whether mental illness accompanies "senility." The law excludes senile persons from involuntary commitment, because senility is not considered a mental illness. Some have equated "dementia" with senility, but it is not so in the law. Dementia implies an organic brain syndrome, which is properly classified as a mental illness and can be considered for involuntary commitment, especially if accompanied by bizarre behavior and unusual thinking. Memory loss alone is not sufficient for involuntary commitment, for that is seen as a sign of "senility." Memory loss may also be a sign of dementia, but without other features such as bizarre behavior or psychotic thinking, individuals with memory loss alone are not connsidered mentally ill. If demented individuals require institutional care, they are usually sent to a nursing home or other community care facility rather than to a state psychiatric hospital.

It is unwise and unethical to label a person mentally ill in order to effect a commitment, when no mental illness exists. Commitment laws are a written order to protect patients from unwarranted paternalism by psychiatrists and other physicians.

Some patients require transfer from nursing homes to psychiatric hospitals when their condition deteriorates. Commitment papers may be prepared by the treating physician in a nursing home, but delays in transport may occur, necessitating continued treatment at the nursing home. Reassessment on a regular basis must occur for those patients in nursing homes awaiting transfer to psychiatric hospitals. If the patient's condition improves, the transfer may be cancelled, while if the condition of the patient deteriorates more rapidly, an accelerated transfer may be appropriate. It is important to manage these cases on an individual basis, depending on the condition of the patient. The physician's certificate for transfer to a psychiatric hospital may be time limited in some jurisdictions. Therefore, it is also important to reassess the patient to determine whether a new certificate must be presented after a period of delay in transporting the patient. The physician should consult the laws in individual jurisdictions.

The rules and guidelines for involuntary commitment have changed in the past two decades (Romano 1974). Whereas previously, persons could be involuntarily hospitalized because they required hospitalization, currently that concept has been deemed unconstitutionally vague by the courts (Sadoff 1973). All states now require that patients have a diagnosable mental illness, and that as a result of that mental illness, they are "a clear and present danger of harm to self or others" (Sadoff 1978). Thus, patients must be both "mentally ill and dangerous" in order to be committed involuntarily. The concept of "dangerousness" has caused difficulty for psychiatrists, because courts have insisted that psychiatrists can predict dangerousness in patients, even when no clear definition of that concept has been offered (Sadoff 1974). It is true that psychiatrists can predict, in a limited fashion, potential violence under certain situations, especially if the patient has a history of previous violence under similar clinical conditions (Shah 1975). However, psychiatrists cannot accurately predict general aspects of dangerousness when there is no clinical correlation.

Nevertheless, elderly patients can be committed involuntarily to hospitals if they are mentally ill and present a clear and present danger of harm to themselves or to others. Involuntarily committed patients have the right to refuse treatment (e.g., neuroleptic medication) unless they are incompetent to refuse or unless their condition represents an emergency situation (Usdin 1957). The right adheres to those who are involuntarily committed, because of the limitation on their constitutional right to freedom. Voluntary patients who refuse medication may choose to leave the hospital, whereas involuntary patients cannot. It is usually the physician's determination of the clinical nature of the emergency situation that is held to be important in assessing the need for neuroleptic medication. The incompetency in such matters, however, may be either the assessment of the psychiatrist or, in many states, only the determination of the court (Appelbaum et al. 1987).

Documentation

In all cases, it is essential for psychiatrists to document properly the assessment of patients and the recommendations. The assessment of competency includes the questions asked and the responses given, if any. Examples of questions to be asked include the orientation of patients and their understanding of the procedures involved or the medication to be given. Specific questions regarding specific aspects of competency should be asked, and the responses noted. Conclusory statements alone are not sufficient when others review and evaluate the means by which a psychiatrist has determined that a patient is incompetent. Psychiatrists have at their disposal the elements of the mental status examination and the particular behavior of the patient, either before commitment or after hospitalization. The psychiatrist includes all aspects of the assessment of competency, including the specific questions regarding the particular issues of treatment or research. When an assessment is made to give treatment to a patient refusing treatment, it is wise to have a second independent opinion by a respected colleague, who then documents the evaluation and conclusions on the patient's record.

Civil Cases

Civil-legal cases involving geriatric patients may include issues of competency, especially in writing a will, or damages in a personal injury or malpractice case. There are several types of competency in civil matters. The most common assessment for competency is in managing one's affairs. In that situation, the questions asked include whether patients know what assets they have, in what form, and how they may spend their money appropriately. They must be able to make reasonable decisions about the money they have accumulated and to whom they wish to leave this money. Psychiatrists may need to check with objective sources to determine whether patients' recollections of their assets are accurate.

Psychiatrists assessing geriatric patients involved in personal injury cases obtain a preaccident evaluation, if it exists, in order to compare the postaccident condition of patients with baseline functioning. Injuries of the head, especially, are assessed carefully by examining psychiatrists, because even slight blows to the head may cause profound disturbances of cognition and behavior in the vulnerable elderly. Use of neuropsychological testing, as well as electroencephalogram, computed tomography scans, and neurological examination, should be included in the total assessment.

Posthumous evaluation of individuals is often performed in cases involving will contests. The retrospective assessment of individuals at the time they prepared a will is a difficult but important task when the validity of the will is challenged. In these cases, it is the assumed competency of the testator that is assessed. The person who wrote the will may not only have been incompetent, but also may have been the subject of undue influence of others. In these cases, the behavior of testators has to be examined for impaired cognition and judgment and/or a dependent relationship on others who may have exploited them through undue influence. Such assessment after death is conducted by review of available documents and materials. Depositions and sworn statements of those who knew the testator prior to and at the time of the signing of the will are also examined.

In order to avoid challenges after death, an attorney may wish to have elderly clients evaluated by a psychiatrist at the time wills are prepared and signed. In these cases, the psychiatrist asks specific questions of the elderly persons to determine testamentary capacity. The psychiatrist wants to know if testators know the extent of their bounty, that is, how much they have in various assets and to whom they can leave their assets (i.e., their heirs or "natural objects of [their] bounty and affection"). The psychiatrist assesses testamentary capacity by asking particular questions and noting the responses. All of these questions and answers are recorded so that future reviewers may evaluate the examination by the psychiatrist at the time the will is signed, in the event the will is challenged. Again, conclusory statements are not sufficient and must be attended by data supporting those conclusions.

Among the most important evaluations in civil law is the assessment of elderly patients' competency to manage their affairs. Typically, psychiatrists may be asked to evaluate older persons living alone in their own homes or in assisted-living situations. The children of such patients may become concerned that their parents have impaired memory for recent events and cannot properly manage their property or affairs. Often, one of the children will indicate that he or she has been managing the patient's daily activities over the past several years, possibly using a power of attorney (an informal agreement that the child has the power to pay bills and handle a parent's affairs). The children's attorney may have advised them that an incompetency proceeding should be formally initiated and a guardian properly appointed to protect the estate and interests of the elderly patient.

The questions asked by the examining psychiatrist in this circumstance are different from those in will contests. Here, the psychiatrist asks patients if they know how much money they have, in what form, and how it may be obtained. Questions of general information are also asked with respect to patients' orientation, such as time, place, and person, and prices of various items on the market, such as food, clothing, or automobiles. Judges often allow latitude for error about some matters, but not errors in knowledge about gross financial assets. For example, patients who have $250,000 estates may not be considered competent if they believe they have only $5,000. Patients must know where their money is (i.e., in which banks or in which accounts, or in what form—stocks, bonds, or real estate). The assessing psychiatrist, of course, must have corroborating information from the family or from the attorney in order to determine the accuracy of the patient's statements. Whenever possible, the psychiatrist should give a specific diagnosis and indicate how or if that diagnostic condition interferes with the patient's competency. Special testing, such as neuropsychological assessment, may be required and is used whenever necessary.

Criminal Law

In criminal-legal procedures, the elderly individual may be a victim, a perpetrator, or a witness. Geriatric patients who are the accused in criminal matters may be evaluated for competency to proceed, competency to waive their rights, competency to confess, and competency to be incarcerated if found guilty. They may also be evaluated for criminal responsibility. Competency in criminal matters is similar to that in civil cases in that the definition involves the capacity of individuals to know the nature and consequences of the current legal situation in which they are involved. Competency also involves evaluating the ability of defendants to work with their attorneys in preparing a rational defense (Brakel et al. 1985). If patients are suffering from dementia or serious medical problems that affect their ability to understand their situation, they may be incompetent to stand trial.

The different levels of competency in the criminal justice system begin with the competency of persons to make confessions or statements to the police. Under current law, the police must give Miranda warnings to defendants or individuals they are questioning and accusing (Brakel et al. 1985). Elderly patients may have difficulty understanding the warnings given, because of the speed with which they are read; patients may have difficulty hearing or difficulty incorporating the information into their cognitive awareness and in making a reasoned judgment to confess at the time of arrest.

Cognitively impaired defendants may also have difficulty understanding their rights in the criminal system even after the rights have been explained by an attorney. Such defendants may not be competent to waive their rights with respect to pleading guilty or to testifying in court.

There are a number of areas of competency in the criminal justice system that require understanding by the defendant at various levels of the proceedings. Psychiatrists may be called on to assess defendants at any stage of the criminal proceedings from the initial accusatory stage through the pretrial stage, the trial phase, and posttrial proceedings. Elderly patients may have difficulty in working with attorneys, in providing witnesses, or in helping in the preparation of a defense. Patients may not understand the concept of insanity as presented by their attorneys, and they may refuse the option of pleading insane, which would be the most effective defense. Again, psychiatrists may be called on to assess patients at various stages of the proceedings in order to help patients and their attorneys determine competency to proceed and to work effectively with counsel.

Elderly patients found guilty of crime may be at risk if they serve time in prison, where they may be victims or targets of the hostility of younger, stronger, and more aggressive prisoners. They may also be given the equivalent of a death sentence if sentenced to a long prison term. Many elderly defendants have multiple medical problems requiring hospital treatment, rather than a prison environment.

Special considerations for the elderly regarding the insanity defense include the more likely presence of delirium, dementia, or chronic medical problems such as diabetes, congestive heart failure, emphysema, or other system illnesses that affect patients' mental abilities. All of these issues must be considered when assessing geriatric patients' competency to participate in a criminal proceeding.

Often, geriatric individuals are victims of criminal behavior, particularly homicide. Most often, it is within the family, as one spouse may kill another, or an adult child may kill an elderly parent. Several cases have emerged in which elderly individuals killed their spouses in the spirit of euthanasia. The healthy spouse feels sorry for the ill one, who is demented or crippled, and puts the loved one "out of his or her misery." In trials of these cases, defendants have been found guilty and sentenced to long terms in prison. In other cases, defendants have pled guilty to a lesser charge as part of a negotiated plea agreement.

In other cases, caregivers have killed their spouses because they could no longer endure the stress of caring for a disabled elderly person. Special consideration is often given to elderly persons who kill within the family, especially when there is evidence of organic brain damage, paranoid syndromes, or dementia.

The use of medication, illegal drugs, or alcohol may complicate the picture in criminal cases involving elderly defendants, and elderly defendants should be examined after all such substances are eliminated, except those that are essential for health maintenance.

Elderly persons who are witnesses in criminal cases may also require evaluation by a psychiatrist. Elderly prosecution witnesses may be challenged by defense attorneys for competency to testify or for general competency, because of apparent or assumed infirmity or sensory impairment. Specialists may evaluate visual or hearing acuity, but mental state is examined by psychiatrists. The issue here is testimonial capacity, that is, the competency of individuals to serve as witnesses in criminal cases. Do the elderly individuals know the nature and consequences of the situation in which they are involved, and can they testify truthfully and accurately within the limits of their ability? These points are assessed by psychiatrists by asking specific questions of the individuals regarding the particulars of the situations and their understanding of their roles in the situations.

Elder Abuse

The elderly are subject to multiple abuses by family members, other individuals, institutions, and agencies. Estimates of the prevalence of elder abuse are likely to be inaccurate because of underreporting. Clarke (1984) suggested that 10% of the elderly (aged older than 65) were subject to abuse, and it seemed to be a frequently recurring act (in up to 80% of cases) when it did occur (O'Malley et al. 1983). The abuser was most often a relative (in 86% of O'Malley's cases) who lived with the elderly person. Caregivers who were more likely to be abusers of the elderly were characterized by isolation, stress (from internal or external sources), substance abuse, previous family violence, and refusal of outside services despite frustration in dealing with the elderly person. Risk factors for abuse that characterized the victims include age over 75, mental and/or physical impairment, inability to meet daily self-care needs, and care needs that exceed the caretaker's ability to respond (O'Malley et al. 1983). Most of the abuse appeared to come from family members who could not tolerate the problems generated by an elderly parent or family member. Victims may be restrained, restricted, neglected, or beaten. Sometimes, as in child abuse cases, the abuse may lead to death and charges of murder are brought against family members. More often, the charges are physical or emotional abuse.

The abuse may be financially motivated, the family member wanting privileges or money from an unwilling older adult. This conflict may be particularly acute when a family member who has been appointed guardian of his or her parents' estate attempts aggressively to preserve the estate for his or her own inheritance rather than spend it appropriately for the parents' well-being.

Occasionally, groups of individuals exploit or abuse an elderly person. Con artists may trick elderly persons out of their money by promising trips or safe homes in which to live. There are many reports of cases of elderly people being bilked out of their life savings.

Neglect and starvation are not uncommon, but the most common way families reject their elderly members is by physically "dumping" them into hospitals, nursing homes, or other facilities. The elderly who are dependent on their family members may not remember or may not reveal the physical abuse, because of fear or memory problems. It is important for emergency room physicians, assessing bruises in the elderly, to determine the origin of the injuries.

Recent cases of abuse of elderly impaired patients in institutions raises the question of legal advocacy for the mentally impaired elderly. Who speaks for the elderly who are unable to speak for themselves? What legal facilities or institutions can be developed to protect the welfare of geriatric patients?

Conclusion

The relationship between geriatric psychiatry and forensic psychiatry has many interfaces. Generally, the psychiatrist is called on to assess competency of geriatric patients for medical and legal purposes. Elderly patients may also require guardianship, assessments, and evaluation for testamentary capacity. Involuntary commitment statutes have excluded many geriatric patients on the basis of diagnosis of dementia alone. The rights of the elderly are also in need of further development and protection. Geriatric advocates will continue to assume the role of protecting elderly patients, as have the mental health advocates for psychiatric patients in general. Elderly patients will assume a greater proportion of the population of psychiatric patients and will require further care and protection as they become an increasingly vulnerable group within psychiatric care.

References

American Medical Association: Principles of Medical Ethics as Applied to Psychiatry, Official Actions. Am J Psychiatry 130:1063, 1973

American Psychiatric Association: Position Statement on Confidentiality and Privilege With Special Reference to Psychiatric Patients. Am J Psychiatry 124:1015, 1968

Appelbaum PS, Lidz CW, Meisel A: Informed Consent: Legal Theory in Clinical Practice. New York, Oxford University Press, 1987

Brakel SJ, Parry J, Weiner BA: The Mentally Disabled and the Law, 3rd Edition. Chicago, IL, American Bar Foundation, 1985

Brooks AD: Competency, in Law, Psychiatry, and the Mental Health System. Edited by Brooks AD. Boston, MA, Little, Brown, 1974

Clarke CB: Geriatric abuse—out of the closet. J Tenn Med Assoc 77:440–471, 1984

Kayser-Jones J, Kapp MB: Advocacy for the mentally impaired elderly: a case study analysis. Am J Law Med XIV:353–376, 1989

McGarry AL: Competency to Stand Trial and Mental Illness. Rockville, MD, National Institute of Mental Health, 1973

Meisel A, Roth LH: What we do and do not know about informed consent. JAMA 246:24–73, 1981

Monahan J: The prediction of violent behavior: toward a second generation of theory and policy. Am J Psychiatry 14:10–15, 1984

O'Malley TA, Everitt DE, O'Malley HC, et al: Identifying and preventing family-mediated abuse and neglect of elderly persons. Ann Intern Med 98:998–1005, 1983

Romano J: Reflections on informed consent. Arch Gen Psychiatry 30:129–135, 1974

Sadoff RL: The importance of informed consent. J Leg Med, May-June 1973, pp 25–27

Sadoff RL: Informed consent, confidentiality, and privilege in psychiatry: practical applications. Bull Am Acad Psychiatry Law 2:101–106, 1974

Sadoff RL: Indications for involuntary hospitalization: dangerousness or mental illness? in Law and Mental Health Professionals. Edited by Barton WE, Sanborn CJ. New York, International Universities Press, 1978

Shah SA: Dangerousness and civil commitment of the mentally ill: some public policy considerations. Am J Psychiatry 132:502–505, 1975

Usdin GL: The psychiatrist and testamentary capacity. Tulane Law Review, 32:89–100, 1957

CHAPTER 33

Spencer Eth, M.D.

Ethical Issues in Clinical Care

Geriatric psychiatrists face a wide array of ethical challenges, perhaps more than any of their psychiatric colleagues. This phenomenon is largely a function of having a patient population that is typically medically and cognitively impaired. In this chapter I will survey a broad range of compelling ethical issues that are relevant to geriatric psychiatry, while focusing on those that significantly affect clinical decision making.

Historical Overview

Ethics has been the province of academic study from the time of Socrates, but only since World War II have its practical applications captured broad professional and public attention. Certainly, physician involvement in the Nazi concentration camp experiments provoked widespread moral outrage. Later revelations of analogous research practices in American teaching hospitals (Beecher 1966; Rothman 1987) led directly to the creation of the National Commission for the Protection of Human Subjects of Biomedical and Behavioral Research and to the establishment of a formal ethics infrastructure through local institutional review boards.

Another factor promoting medical ethics has been the implementation of innovative technologies. The development of hemodialysis, for example, forced painful decisions about precisely who should receive this scarce, expensive, life-extending treatment (Abrams 1968; Fox and Swazey 1979). A generation later the same questions are being asked about the totally implantable artificial heart (Caplan 1987). A different, but no less difficult, set of moral problems arise in the context of abortion, and the resulting intensely emotional debate has repeatedly placed medical ethics on the front page of American newspapers (Goldstein 1988).

Allocation of Scarce Resources

Ethical dilemmas occur whenever conflicts arise between competing sets of moral values. In geriatric psychiatry these difficulties may be encountered from the first diagnostic intervention through to the conclusion of all treatment and research efforts. Consider the initial evaluation of an elderly patient presenting with a mild memory impairment. The importance of establishing a definitive diagnosis is the foundation of quality patient care, especially when the list of diagnostic possibilities includes a treatable dementia. From this perspective, the diagnostic workup should be comprehensive, given that the procedures themselves carry little risk of harm and great potential benefit to the individual patient. However, although modern brain imaging is, for example, safe and useful, it is also quite expensive. Providing such costly studies to every forgetful elderly patient would, in aggregate, represent a sizable financial investment. Because the health care budget is finite, society is already being forced to priorize its allocation of resources (Evans 1983). It is conceivable that a low-yield diagnostic procedure for geriatric patients would be sacrificed in favor of a large-scale preventive intervention such as a prenatal nutrition program. Such policy decisions would be based on a balancing of macrolevel social needs (Jecker and Perlman 1989).

Physicians may be pressured to ration diagnostic services in advance of any future policy constraints. Medicare-imposed reimbursement constraints have already caused the costs of diagnostic tests to be weighed against their hypothetical value for patients whose care demands many expensive procedures and lengthy hospital stays. This analysis must also be employed each time the use of intensive care facilities is considered for elderly patients (Callahan 1988). No longer does the sanctity of the doctor-patient relationship protect medical care from the intrusion of social and financial pressures that accent value conflicts.

Truth Telling

Over the last half-century, conventional wisdom regarding honesty in the doctor-patient relationship has changed radically. Formerly, a policy of deception about catastrophic diagnoses was considered to be in the patient's best interest. For example, Oliver Wendell Holmes argued, "It is no kindness for science to reveal what Nature is kindly concealing" (Worcester 1935). Accordingly, the benevolent physician would conceal very disturbing information, lest the unsuspecting patient be harmed by such disclosure. The situation has reversed itself; it is generally accepted that lying is morally wrong (Bok 1978). Physicians, regardless of motive, are not exempt from the duty to tell the truth. This position respects the importance of the patient's standing as an independent agent deserving of all relevant personal information in order to preserve moral autonomy. Further, empirical evidence increasingly confirms the supposition that patients want to learn the truth no matter how distressing it may be. For example, one survey of adult outpatients aged younger than 60 found that 97.5% would want to be told of the diagnosis of Alzheimer's disease (Erde et al. 1988). Presumably, armed with this critical information, the patient would then be better able to plan for the increasing disability associated with this illness.

Naturally, the process of disclosure varies with individual patient needs. A delirious patient should not be confronted immediately with cognitive material too complex to be understood. Similarly, patients with dementia present with characteristic fragility of ego defenses. Should they be challenged with an overwhelming cognitive task, they may respond with a catastrophic reaction of agitation and helpless panic. Under these circumstances, the discretionary withholding of information that would be frankly harmful to patients is legally and ethically permissible under the rubric of therapeutic privilege. However, the physician has an obligation to confide the diagnosis when and if it is safe to do so: "One must at least inform the patient that significant cognitive problems have been detected and that these may progress in time to the extent that the individual's ability to make decisions for himself or herself and the family may be impaired" (Overman and Stoudemire 1988, p 1496).

Confidentiality

From the Hippocratic oath's pledge to silence on professional secrets to the current Principles of Medical Ethics guideline to safeguard patient confidences within the constraints of the law, the rule of confidentiality has always been fundamental to patient care (American Psychiatric Association 1989). However, strict confidentiality is not an absolute value. Relevant patient information may be ethically released at the patient's request, as necessary to protect life, or as required by law. Statutes have been passed in several states mandating the formal reporting of elder abuse to protective services, and of Alzheimer's disease to the motor vehicles department; these statutes are examples of instances in which the physician has the responsibility to notify the authorities of possible injury, regardless of the patient's instructions on the matter. Psychiatrists may also need to document certain confidential clinical data in order to institute civil commitment or conservatorship proceedings. In these instances, the decision to overrule a patient's insistence on secrecy is consonant with local law and the desire to preserve life.

Major disagreements about privacy often surface in the context of involvement with the geriatric patient's family. The importance of sharing clinical impressions and prognosis with concerned relatives may clash with the patient's wish that this material remain confidential. Even in the first session the psychiatrist may need to question family members in order to augment an incomplete or confusing history elicited from an organically impaired patient. In the case of a progressive dementia, the role of a supportive family expands as the patient becomes increasingly disabled. It is therefore wise to obtain early in the treatment, while the patient is still competent, written consent for sharing information. Unfortunately, such permission is not always granted. Some cognitively impaired patients may insist on strict confidentiality as a means of exerting a measure of control over their lives. This dynamic may operate with greater force when adult children have assumed a care-providing role for their own parents.

Interpretation by the therapist of these unconscious themes may promote resolution of the conflict. But if the patient persists in the refusal to reveal the diagnosis or prognosis, the psychiatrist is morally bound to comply until the patient relents or a conservator is appointed. A particularly painful dilemma confronts the psychiatrist whose patient suffers from a hereditary illness such as Huntington's disease. Even in this extreme case the patient's desire for secrecy ought to be honored, despite the children's vital interest in being told of the diagnosis. Helping the patient work through the shame and guilt associated with this illness would be a treatment priority designed to facilitate disclosure. After a patient's death, the constraints of confidentiality are eased and appropriate medical information may be divulged to concerned family members (American Psychiatric Association 1987).

Consent

Unlike confidentiality, the primacy of consent has evolved only in this century. Historically, physicians were afforded considerable discretion in discharging their duty to care for the sick (Jonsen et al. 1986). Because doctors were expected to use their expertise to benefit the patient, any infringement on their actions could result in harm to the patient. Doing good by helping others is a powerful justification for unfettered freedom to deliver medical care dictated solely by the patient's condition. The model for beneficent paternalism is predicated on the loving parent who nurtures and protects a child without waiting for permission. Case law has irrevocably shattered the presumption that the physician is the final decision maker by replacing medical paternalism with patients' rights (Katz 1984).

Consent refers to the patient's specific right to information and to choose among the available treatment options. The ethical priority ascribed to consent derives from the profound importance of retaining control over one's own body. Thus, the patient can accept or refuse any medical intervention, even if the denial of consent for that procedure results in death. Many physicians are uncomfortable with the limitations on their therapeutic actions imposed by their patient's wishes. Not infrequently a referral for psychiatric consultation is provoked by a competent patient's behavior that is noncompliant or uncooperative with the physician's direction (Perl and Shelp 1982). Exercising self-determination according to one's personal set of values may or may not reflect an underlying psychiatric diagnosis. But as long as the patient is competent to consent, that choice must be respected (Eth and Robb 1986).

Competence

Every adult is presumed competent under the law. However, many illnesses, in particular dementia and delirium, affect mentation and render the patient less able to perform the task at hand. If an elderly patient experiences difficulty comprehending the risks and benefits associated with treatment, then the question of competency must be explored. The physician is responsible for the rigorous, detailed assessment of the patient's mental status. The court is empowered to rule on whether the patient's cognitive deficits satisfy that jurisdiction's definition of incompetence. If the court so rules, it will appoint a substitute decision maker.

In general, patients are usually deemed competent if they are capable of appreciating the elements of the consent process. That is, they should have the capacity to understand information, consider relevant alternatives, and express a clear decision about medical care. It is usually necessary that the patient acknowledge that a diagnosis has been made and that a judgment about accepting or refusing treatment is needed. Under this minimum standard a patient may be demented, psychotic, or severely depressed and still be found competent to consent (Applebaum and Grisso 1988). From an ethical perspective, it has become apparent that our society has placed an extraordinary premium on individual liberty, daring to allow even patients with major mental illness the right to select the treatment of their choice or to reject treatment entirely.

Nursing Home Placement

Many of our senior citizens live in the community, either alone or with family. However, when infirmity or behavioral disturbance interferes with the activities of daily living, institutional placement may become desirable. The decision to admit a relative or patient to a long-term care facility is often difficult. Although the intention is to secure appropriate treatment and to preserve function, the actual result can be iatrogenic morbidity and mortality. Perhaps as many as one-third of the persons entering nursing homes succumb in the first year, and the surviving residents are likely to experience the negative impact of institutionalization (Butler and Lewis 1982). The seemingly arbitrary rules and loss of privacy in nursing homes produce feelings of frustration, powerlessness, hopelessness, and loss of self-confidence and self-esteem (Mercer 1982). Two consequences of institutionalization are increased dependence and diminished efficacy. The effects further compromise the nursing home resident's capacity to exercise self-determination. The result may be the frank loss of adult status as a morally autonomous agent. The harm associated with erosion of personhood should be weighed against whatever benefits may accrue from the physical care and convenience offered in this setting.

Because the nursing home resident's family and physician are instrumental in effecting placement, they are uniquely responsible for attending to ethical issues as integral to the decision-making process. While confined in nursing homes, two-thirds of all patients exhibit some form of behavioral disturbance, frequently related to their cognitive impairment. In addition, many demented patients develop secondary psychiatric disorders (Rovner and Rabins 1985). Ideally, a psychiatrist would be called on to diagnose and treat the mental disorders found in this captive population. Unfortunately, treatable conditions such as depression may go unrecognized, especially when the psychiatrist is summoned to manage a disruptive patient. In such instances the patient may fall victim to an inadequate evaluation, if the psychiatrist prematurely focuses on the troubling behavior rather than on the exhibiting of a behavioral symptom in the context of institutional placement.

If the consulting psychiatrist is also employed by the facility, there exists the danger that the patient's interests will be subordinated in favor of promoting efficiency in the operation of the institution. This role conflict, in which the psychiatrist is contending with a dual allegiance, has been termed the "double agent dilemma" (Mersky 1978). Nursing home staff also struggle to balance the competing clinical needs of an individual patient with the desire to maintain a quiet and orderly routine. However, the problem of chronic understaffing of these facilities often forces the use of excessive psychotropic medication with little medical supervision or understanding by staff of possible side effects (Avorn et al. 1989).

The prevailing conditions of many nursing homes may confer an ethical agenda on our profession. Psychiatrists are morally bound to ensure that each geriatric patient receives the benefit of all available community resources before placement is considered. The guiding principle is that the patient is to remain in the least restrictive environment for as long as possible to maximize autonomy and protect personhood. Some have advocated social and political activism to improve patient care in long-term care facilities (Cassel and Jameton 1981). Such a call to action is consonant with Section 10 of the Principles of Medical Ethics: "The honored ideals of the medical profession that the responsibilities of the physician extend not only to the individual, but also to society, [and to] activities which have the purpose of improving both the health and the well-being of the individual and the community" (American Psychiatric Association 1989, p 9).

Death and Dying

No discussion of ethics in geriatric psychiatry is complete without serious attention to the issues of death and dying. Patients suffering from primary degenerative dementia and other catastrophic diseases can become progressively and severely incapacitated. Depending on their underlying medical condition, these patients eventually enter a terminal phase of their dementing illness, during which time their level of function will have markedly deteriorated. The question of exactly what type of care is appropriate for such patients is being asked with great urgency. Ultimately, the decision must be made about whether to initiate, continue, or withdraw the variety of life support measures sustaining the patient (Wanzer et al. 1989). Hospital staff quickly realize that their actions in initiating or withdrawing a necessary treatment, such as mechanical ventilation, would be the proximate cause of death (Miles et al. 1989). The issue is perhaps most painfully faced when the targeted treatment is the administration of fluid and nutritional support (i.e., food and water).

Until recently, a critical distinction was drawn between ordinary and extraordinary care. The physician was deemed to be morally bound to deliver all ordinary forms of care to patients, befitting their status as human beings. Extraordinary care, however, was indicated only when there was a compelling reason to provide such treatment. With our escalating technical sophistication, it becomes increasingly difficult to distinguish into which category a particular procedure should be placed. For example, should cardiopulmonary resuscitation (CPR) be considered ordinary care because it is commonly taught by the Red Cross in the community? If so, then it would be obligatory to begin CPR in all cases, regardless of whether the result would be "a blessing or a curse" (Podrid 1989). Moreover, is the distinction between ordinary and extraordinary meaningful, no matter how difficult it may be to make? In place of the largely arbitrary and nonindividualized decision about what is ordinary versus extraordinary, medical ethics has come to recognize the overwhelming importance of the patient's personal sense of the value of a proffered treatment (Jonsen 1983). Further, patients may have their own views on what is ordinary, which may be in contrast to the accepted norm.

The salient factor may simply be the extent to which any treatment offers benefits or burdens to a particular patient. This concept, termed "proportionality," was convincingly articulated by the President's Commission for the Study of Ethical Problems in Medicine and Biomedical and Behavioral Research (1983). Proportionate care has at least a reasonable likelihood of providing benefits that outweigh the detriment associated with the treatment, whereas in disproportionate care the ratio is reversed. Thus, an ordinary treatment that briefly prolongs the life of a patient in agony is disproportionate care and ought to be avoided. But an extremely painful and intrusive procedure that is curative may be proportionate and highly desirable. This form of patient-centered analysis is directly applicable to the geriatric population (Wikler 1988).

An ethical consensus is forming around several policy positions affecting geriatric psychiatry. Authority for medical care rests with competent patients who must offer their consent for treatment to commence or continue. For patients who have been adjudicated as incompetent, their legal surrogate is empowered to make the relevant medical decisions for them. The surrogate should, in all possible instances, follow the patient's previously communicated instructions with regard to appropriate care. In the absence of a clear notion of the patient's preferences, the surrogate should choose a course consistent with the patient's best interests (Suber and Tabor 1982). In instances in which medical care imposes unacceptable burdens—as would be the case for irreversibly comatose, terminally ill patients—all such efforts may ethically cease (Ruark et al. 1988). Disproportionate treatment of no benefit would not be provided, including fluid and nutritional support, although prudence may dictate consultation with legal counsel. Hospital staff who hold religious or moral objections to an agreed-upon course of treatment may be replaced by staff comfortable with the definitive care plan.

Several issues in terminal care remain open. Murphy (1988) has suggested that CPR for severely demented patients in long-term care settings is not indicated regardless of the wishes of the patient's family or surrogate. He contends that the substitute decision maker's refusal to accept "do not resuscitate (DNR)" status may be influenced by guilt or misinformation. Accordingly, the physician should unilaterally withhold a CPR procedure that is usually futile and always cruel for patients who cannot possibly understand its intent. This argument is admittedly paternalistic and intensely controversial. The traditional view is expressed by the American Medical Association Council on Ethical and Judicial Affairs (1989, para. 2.21): "Unless it is clearly established that the patient is terminally ill or permanently unconscious, a physician should not be deterred from appropriately aggressive treatment of a patient."

In cases of extreme suffering, the psychiatrist may be asked to directly assist the patient in achieving death. Active, voluntary euthanasia is the deliberate ending of the life of a terminally ill patient at his or her own request (Pellegrino 1989). A number of medical institutions in Holland have developed procedures to enable physicians to participate in active euthanasia in an "acceptable and controllable manner" (deWachter 1989). However, in the United States active euthanasia is "illegal in all jurisdictions" and "violates the ethical standards of medical practice" (American College of Physicians 1989).

Research Concerns

The importance of clinical research in geriatric psychiatry cannot be overstated. Without such studies, advancement in the understanding and treatment of mental disorders afflicting the elderly will be stifled. Although there is no dispute about the need for research involving geriatric patients, there are major obstacles to its performance. Consider the problem of research on Alzheimer's disease. As a function of their cognitive deficits, these patients, especially if they reside in long-term facilities, are vulnerable to exploitation by overzealous investigators. The best means of safeguarding the process of patient recruitment is through scrupulous attention to the requirement for voluntary informed consent. Voluntary informed consent is internationally recognized as prerequisite for the inclusion of human subjects in medical research (World Psychiatric Association 1989). Informed consent is also the mechanism that permits patients to participate as subjects in studies regardless of the likelihood of personal benefit. Our society allows altruistic adults to submit to the risks of basic research in accord with the rights and privileges of autonomy.

Patients who "volunteer" may have been exposed to unintended coercion. Nursing home residents who are poor and powerless may be fearful of offending their doctors by refusing to enter their protocols. Patients' reluctance to assert the wish to refuse or withdraw from a study is intensified when the treating physician is eager to conduct research on a convenient sample of patients whose environment and diet can be controlled and who are readily available for testing and measuring. It is unethical to offer inequitable incentives of significantly better care exclusively to those patients enrolled in a study or to threaten loss of care for those patients who decline to participate (Rothman 1982). "Voluntary" means just that: no rewards for patients who join, and no reprisals for patients who do not.

Informed consent implies that the patient has the mental ability to comprehend the study procedures with their attendant risks and benefits, and the capacity to offer consent. Incompetent patients lack the ability to give informed consent for both treatment and research endeavors. However, it is these very patients—those with pronounced Alzheimer's disease, for instance—who may be the most valuable subjects. Although the patient's surrogate can offer substitute consent for treatment, some restraints must be placed on a surrogate's decision to expose another person to the research situation. One approach has been to separate therapeutic from nontherapeutic research. In this framework, surrogate decision makers may freely approve research projects in which there is the intent and reasonable probability of improving the health or well-being of the subject, such as an experimental drug study. In the matter of nontherapeutic studies, representatives of incompetent patients would be limited to approving only those studies that carry minimal risk. It is unethical to place an incompetent patient in danger of harm in order to further scientific progress. That decision to sacrifice bodily integrity for the sake of others ought to be made only by the individual in jeopardy (Eth and Mills 1989).

Perhaps rules designed to protect incompetent patients have had a chilling effect on clinical research. One study has found that family members serving as proxies for nursing home patients often refuse to allow relatives to participate in even innocuous research, often for irrational reasons (Warren et al. 1986). Alternatives to conventional surrogate consent have been proposed that could facilitate dementia research (Schneiderman and Arras 1985). Competent patients could be asked to consent in advance to future studies that will be performed when they are no longer competent. Perhaps specially trained advocates or community representatives can be appointed to serve as special research surrogate consentors. Collaboration among physicians, investigators, and ethicists may help resolve the dilemma of encouraging participation in needed clinical research while simultaneously protecting vulnerable patients.

Conclusion

Geriatric psychiatrists are inescapably embedded in a health care system that demands scientific competence and ethical sensitivity.

Patients and their families are increasingly sophisticated and assertive in articulating their particular wishes about medical care. They expect to be informed and insist on a full partnership in selecting a course of treatment from the time of diagnosis until the end of life. The challenge remains to deliver compassionate care while respecting patient autonomy in an era of diminishing resources and expanding knowledge. Never has being a physician been more vexing or more exhilarating.

References

Abrams HS: The psychiatrist, the treatment of renal failure, and the prolongation of life. Am J Psychiatry 124:1351–1358, 1968

American College of Physicians: Ethics Manual. Ann Intern Med 111:245–252, 327–335, 1989

American Medical Association Council on Ethical and Judicial Affairs: Current Opinions. Chicago, IL, American Medical Association, 1989

American Psychiatric Association: Guidelines on Confidentiality. Am J Psychiatry 144:1522–1526, 1987

American Psychiatric Association: Principles of Medical Ethics. Washington, DC, American Psychiatric Association, 1989

Appelbaum PS, Grisso T: Assessing patients' capacities to consent to treatment. N Engl J Med 319:1635–1638, 1988

Avorn J, Dreyer P, Connelly K, et al: Use of psychoactive medication and the quality of care in rest homes. N Engl J Med 320:227–232, 1989

Beecher HK: Ethics and clinical research. N Engl J Med 274:1354–1360, 1966

Bok S: Lying: Moral Choice in Public and Private Life. New York, Panthean, 1978

Butler RN, Lewis MI: Aging and Mental Health, 3rd edition. St. Louis, MO, CV Mosby, 1982

Callahan D: Allocating health resources. Hastings Center Report 18(2):14–20, 1988

Caplan AL: Equity in the selection of recipients for cardiac transplants. Circulation 75:10–19, 1987

Cassel CK, Jameton AC: Dementia in the elderly: analysis of medical responsibility. Annals Internal Med 94:802–807, 1981

deWachter MAM: Active euthanasia in the Netherlands. JAMA 262:3316–3319, 1989

Erde EL, Nadal EC, Scholl TO: On truth telling and the diagnosis of Alzheimer's disease. J Fam Pract 26:401–403, 1988

Eth S, Mills MJ: Ethical issues, in Treatments of Psychiatric Disorders, Vol 2. Edited by Karasu TB. Washington DC, American Psychiatric Association, 1989, pp 994–1008

Eth S, Robb JW: Informed consent, in Ethics in Mental Health Practice. Edited by Kentsmith DK, Salladay SA, Miya PA. Orlando, FL, Grune & Stratton, 1986

Evans RW: Health care technology and the inevitability of resource allocation and rationing decisions. JAMA 249:2047–2053, 2208–2219, 1983

Fox RC, Swayze JP: Courage to Fail: Social View of Organ Transplantation and Dialysis, 2nd Revised Edition. Chicago, IL, University of Chicago Press, 1979

Goldstein RD: Mother-Love and Abortion. Berkeley, CA, University of California Press, 1988

Jecker NS, Perlman RA: Ethical constraints on rationing medical care by age. J Am Geriatr Soc 37:1067–1075, 1989

Jonsen AR: A concord in medical ethics. Ann Intern Med 99:261–264, 1983

Jonsen AR, Siegler M, Winslade WJ: Clinical Ethics, 2nd Edition. New York, Macmillan, 1986

Katz J: The Silent World of Doctor and Patient. New York, Free Press, 1984

Mercer SO: Consequences of institutionalization of the aged, in Maltreatment of the Elderly. Edited by Kosberg JI. Boston, John Wright, 1982

Mersky H: In the service of the state: the psychiatrist as double agent. Hastings Center Report 8:1–24, 1978

Miles SH, Singer PA, Siegler H: Conflicts between patients' wishes to forgo treatment and the policies of health care facilities. N Engl J Med 321:48–50, 1989

Murphy DJ: Do-not-resuscitate orders: time for reappraisal in long-term care institutions. JAMA 260:2098–2101, 1988

Overman W, Stoudemire A: Guidelines for legal and financial counseling of Alzheimer's disease patients and their families. Am J Psychiatry 145:1495–1500, 1988

Pellegrino ED: Ethics. JAMA 261:2843–2845, 1989

Perl M, Shelp EE: Psychiatric consultation masking moral dilemmas in medicine. N Engl J Med 307:618–621, 1982

Podrid PJ: Resuscitation in the elderly: a blessing or a curse? Ann Intern Med 111:193–195, 1989

President's Commission for the Study of Ethical Problems in Medicine and Biomedical and Behavioral Research: Deciding to Forego Life-Sustaining Treatment. Washington, DC, U.S. Government Printing Office, 1983

Rothman DJ: Were Tuskegee and Willowbrook studies of nature? Hastings Center Report 12:5–8, 1982

Rothman DJ: Ethics and human experimentation. N Engl J Med 317:1195–1199, 1987

Rovner BW, Rabins PV: Mental illness among nursing home patients. Hosp Community Psychiatry 36:119–128, 1985

Ruark JE, Raffin, TA: The Stanford University Medical Center Committee on Ethics: Initiating and withdrawing life support. N Engl J Med 318:25–30, 1988

Schneiderman LJ, Arras JD: Counseling patients to counsel physicians on future care in the event of patient incompetence. Ann Intern Med 648–693, 1985

Suber DG, Tabor WJ: Withholding of life-sustaining treatment from the terminally ill, incompetent patient. JAMA 248:2250–2251, 2431–2432, 1982

Wanzer SH, Federman DD, Adelstein SJ, et al: The physician's responsibility toward hopelessly ill patients. N Engl J Med 320:844–849, 1989

Warren JW, Sobal J, Tenney JH, et al: Informed consent by proxy: an issue in research with elderly patients. N Engl J Med 315:1124–1128, 1986

Wikler D: Patient interests: clinical implications of philosophical distinctions. J Am Geriatr Soc 36:951–958, 1988

Worcester A: Care of the Aged, the Dying, and the Dead. Springfield, IL, Charles C Thomas, 1935

World Psychiatric Association Bulletin: Declaration of Hawaii/II. World Psychiatric Association 1:23–24, 1989

CHAPTER 34

Gary L. Gottlieb, M.D., M.B.A.

Financial Issues

Introduction

Financing strategies have shaped the development of psychiatric services for older adults (Goldman et al. 1987; Goldman and Frank, in press). Payment mechanisms and associated policy influence the identification of patient populations, the organization of services, the site of service delivery, the type and behavior of providers, and the process of evaluation and treatment.

For the most part, government has driven the economic priorities and incentives of geriatric mental health care. As financial responsibility shifted from local to state government, older adults who were cared for in the almshouses and asylums of the 19th century helped to fuel the growth of the state hospital systems of the early and middle 20th century (Grob 1983). In 1965, the implementation of Medicare and Medicaid shifted a substantial proportion of the financial responsibility for the psychiatric care of the elderly from the states to the federal government. The fee-for-service framework of these programs and the growth of private indemnity insurance stimulated the rapid growth of private and general hospital psychiatric settings (Goldman et al. 1987). Simultaneously, deinstitutionalization and the combined federal and state support provided by Medicaid fostered the expanded use of nursing homes for the care of the chronically mentally ill (Goldman et al. 1986). Similarly, limited reimbursement of outpatient specialty mental health services by Medicare and other third parties has helped to fortify the general health care sector as the dominant source of psychiatric services, particularly for the elderly (Regier et al. 1978;

Schurman et al. 1985). Prospective payment and nursing home reform, implemented in the 1980s, are already affecting the process and content of psychiatric care for older adults (English et al. 1986; Goldman et al. 1987).

Providers of care and policymakers who seek to optimize the psychiatric well-being of the elderly require an understanding of the economic context of aging in late 20th-century America. In addition, a working knowledge of the organization of the geriatric mental health delivery system and mechanisms for payment for health and mental health services for the elderly is fundamental to this effort. In this chapter I will highlight key financial issues that affect the psychiatric care of older adults. Essential details specific to reimbursement of geriatric psychiatric services are provided, and recent changes in third-party payment schemes are described. An understanding of the terminology and subtleties of this system should help providers to cope with some of the barriers to the care of this exceptionally needy population.

Economic and Health Policy Issues

The size, need, and diversity of the aging population shape the economic environment of geriatric mental health care. Just 30 years ago, only 1 of every 11 Americans was aged older than 65. Today, slightly less than 1 in 8 Americans is over 65. The U.S. Bureau of the Census (1987) expects to find that the elderly population grew by 23% to nearly 31 million during the 1980s. This increase is somewhat smaller than the 28% growth experienced during the 1970s. As a result of relatively small Depression-era birth rates, the older population should grow by only about 10% in the 1990s and by 12% in the first decade of the next century. This rate of projected expansion will yield about 39 million older Americans by 2010. Shortly thereafter, the aging of the post-World War II baby boom cohort will cause dramatic growth in the over-65 population segment: by the year 2030, about one-fourth of the population (66 million people) will be in this age group.

Sex differences in life expectancy and the distribution of minorities among the elderly have important economic consequences. There are approximately 1.5 women for every man over age 65 and about 2.5 women for every man over age 85 (U.S. Bureau of the Census 1987). Traditional work roles and Social Security and pension provisions affect surviving women adversely. In general, continued earning potential from work and from pension income in late life is less for women than it is for men. Generally, older women have more limited financial assets. Inasmuch as they usually live longer than their spouses, they are more likely to become dependent on adult children and on the health care establishment to meet social and medical needs (Soldo and Agree 1988).

Ethnic minorities comprise a growing segment of the older population. In 1980, about 10% of persons aged older than 65 were nonwhite. However, by the year 2025, about 15% of the elderly are projected to be from minority groups (National Center for Health Statistics 1987). Although life expectancy at birth for whites now exceeds that for blacks by about 8%, at age 75 mortality rates for black people are lower than for whites (National Center for Health Statistics 1988). However, very old blacks have considerably higher rates of poverty and illness than whites in the same age group (Soldo and Agree 1988). Economic and social discrimination and underprivilege associated with minority status in the United States are exacerbated by the socioeconomic realities of older age: accrued social and financial resources are limited; barriers to preventive and acute health care are more substantial; and the need for non-health care governmental services including housing, transportation, meals, and income maintenance is greater (Furino and Fogel, in press; Markides and Mindel 1987). Cultural differences may also affect the expression of illness and the ways in which American health care, designed for a predominantly white population, is accessed (Hazzard 1989).

The distribution of wealth and income among older adults is highly variable. The degree of this variability has impeded the development of rational policy, thereby affecting reimbursement and delivery of health and mental health services to older adults.

Retirement is generally associated with a one-third to one-half reduction in personal income (Soldo and Agree 1988). Many individuals retire in their late fifties or early sixties. In 1986, nearly 90% of men in their early fifties participated in the labor force while only about 45% of men between the ages of 62 and 64 were still working (Schulz 1988). This rate declines remarkably with age; after age 70, only about 10% of men and 4% of women are in the labor force. Elimination of a mandatory retirement age and the shift of the American economy from heavy industry to less physically demanding service and technology production may extend the working longevity of the population in the near future. In addition to the emotional consequences of retirement, leaving the work force may affect health insurance premium costs, the type of insurance available, and the possibility of participating in some health delivery systems (e.g., some health maintenance organizations [HMOs] and other managed systems).

The reduction of income associated with retirement may affect standard of living adversely. Most older adults derive postretirement income from a combination of Social Security benefits, public and private pensions, and income from savings or investments (Soldo and Agree 1988). Of course, the magnitude of these earnings depends almost entirely on preretirement income. For many, these relatively fixed sources may be inadequate and older adults may suffer the consequences of poverty for the first time in their lives (Furino and Fogel 1990). In 1986, 1 in 8 people aged older than 65, or about 3.5 million Americans, had income below the established poverty level. About 10% of the younger population were in that income category. Indigence appears to increase with age: about one-fifth of people who live past the age of 85 had incomes at or below the poverty level. These rates are even more dramatic for women and for minorities. For example, a remarkable 60% of black women aged older than 65 and not living with their families were below the poverty level in 1986 (Soldo and Agree 1988).

Poverty and aging are not synonymous, however. More than 10% of households headed by an individual aged older than 65 have annual incomes over $40,000, and almost 13% of these households have net assets in excess of $250,000 (Gottlieb 1988).

This disparity in distribution of wealth and income has an important effect on health and welfare policy. Lawmakers frequently do not recognize the socioeconomic heterogeneity of the older population. Therefore, programs like Social Security and Medicare do not address completely the financial and health care needs of *all* older adults. Resulting gaps are filled unevenly by programs for the indigent. These inequities are particularly important in mental health and in long-term care, where out-of-pocket payments comprise a substantial component of costs to consumers (Gottlieb 1988).

In the past 20 years, the older population has grown twice as rapidly as the rest of the population. In addition, the older population is aging at an extraordinary rate: by the year 2000, 45% of the older population will be at least 75 years old, with the number of people older than 85 growing at a faster rate than any other segment of the population (Soldo and Agree 1988). Growth in the absolute number of older people continues to augment demand for the products that elderly individuals are likely to consume. Because many of the programs that benefit older adults depend on contributions from the younger population, the growing ratio of older Americans to younger persons may affect society's ability to supply the goods, services, and costs necessary to meet this expanding demand. There are currently about 19 Americans older than 65 per 100 people aged 18 to 64. This so-called dependency ratio is expected to double by 2050 (U.S. Bureau of the Census 1987). Therefore, emerging policy is likely to require the older generation to support its own needs.

The first government program requiring older adults to support financially the increased medical needs of their own generation was the Catastrophic Coverage Act (CCA) of 1988. This legislation provided compulsory insurance against catastrophic health care costs for Medicare beneficiaries. CCA required beneficiaries (predominantly individuals aged older than 65) to pay an additional premium to cover the cost of increased coverage. Among other factors, the shifting of financial responsibility to potential recipients made CCA unacceptable politically, and the program was repealed in 1989. Despite the current political environment, growth in the dependency ratio will influence policy strategy long into the future and it will affect the labor market and national productivity. Therefore, medical and psychiatric interventions that promote the health and productivity of older workers may have social benefits that mirror individual improvements in function and quality of life (Furino and Fogel 1990; Hazzard 1989).

The Medicare System

Enacted in 1965 and initiated on July 1, 1966, under Title XVIII of the Social Security Act, Medicare is a social insurance program first designed to provide medical care benefits for Americans aged older than 65 (Cutler and Fine 1985; Gottlieb 1988; U.S. Senate 1978). The program was developed in response to years of debate regarding national health insurance policy and to data derived from comprehensive evaluation of the needs of the elderly provided by the Senate Select Committee on Aging. In 1972, the program was expanded to include younger disabled individuals and older adults who are not eligible for Social Security but who are willing to pay a monthly premium for coverage. In 1973, Medicare coverage was extended to provide medical coverage for individuals suffering end-stage renal disease. More than 32 million people are now covered by Medicare, and 90% of these individuals are elderly (U.S. Congress, Committee on Ways and Means 1989).

Despite aggressive efforts to contain costs, expenditures for health care have grown remarkably, and Medicare outlays have made an important contribution to this expansion. In 1988, total health care expenditures accounted for about 11% of the U.S. gross national product (GNP). The nearly $88 billion of federal spending for Medicare in 1988 accounted for approximately 7.6% of the federal budget and about 1.7% of the GNP (Physician Payment Review Commission [PPRC] 1989). Adjusted for inflation and age, the average annual growth rate for Medicare expenditures per beneficiary was 5% during the 1970s and more than 5.5% for most of the 1980s (Long and Welch 1988). During the same time periods, health care costs for the general population grew at rates of 3.6% and 4.3%, respectively.

Specialty mental health services for older adults account for only a tiny fragment of Medicare expenditures. Outlays for treatment of psychiatric disorders are about 2.5% of total Medicare spending. In contrast, between 7% and 18% of private insurers' reimbursements are for psychiatric services (Morrison et al. 1984). These data are more striking when one considers that more than half of all Medicare-covered psychiatric hospitalizations are for nonelderly, disabled individuals (Goldman et al. 1987). The relative underuse of specialty mental health services by older Medicare beneficiaries results from the reinforcement of long-standing provider- and patient-induced barriers to care by economic disincentives and systematic stigmatization.

Medicare benefits are designed to cover acute care services primarily. Preventive services, long-term care, and dental services are excluded. Some services, including mental health care, are subject to limitations in coverage and substantial copayments. Under current conditions, Medicare covers only about 75% of elderly hospital care, 2% to 3% of nursing home care, and about 58% of physician services, totaling slightly less than half of geriatric health care costs (PPRC 1989; Waldo and Lazenby 1984).

Medicare has two components: Part A, the hospital insurance program, covers inpatient hospitalization, limited home care, skilled nursing facility (SNF) services, and hospice care. Part B, the supplemental medical insurance (SMI) program, covers physician services and provides additional benefits for clinical laboratory tests, durable medical equipment, and some outpatient hospital care.

Hospital Insurance (Part A)

By virtue of participation in the Social Security system, most Americans aged older than 65 are entitled to Part A coverage. The Part A hospital insurance trust fund is underwritten through Social Security payroll taxes paid by employers and employees.

Part A hospital coverage is intentionally limited to coverage of relatively brief inpatient stays, presumably for stabilization of acute conditions. Regulations provide coverage for "spells" of illness. A spell is defined as an inpatient episode that begins with inpatient admission and ends with the close of the first period of 60 consecutive days after discharge. It is possible for a patient to be discharged and readmitted on several occasions during a given episode of illness and still be considered to be in the same spell, as long as 60 days have not elapsed between discharge and admission. For admission to general hospitals, there is no limit on the number of spells or "total lifetime" days covered. However, the maximum number of covered days during a single spell is 150 days.

The first 60 days of coverage for each episode are fully paid after a deductible equal to the average cost of 1 day of hospitalization ($560 in 1989) has been met. The next 30 inpatient days are subject to a daily coinsurance payment equal to 25% of the hospital deductible, and the last 60 days of covered hospitalization require a daily copayment equal to half of the deductible amount. These last 60 days of a spell of illness (days 91–150) are designated as "lifetime reserve" days. Coverage for these days may be used electively during any episode, but it may be used only once. For example, a patient who requires three hospitalizations totaling 110 days with no period of discharge between hospitalizations as great as 60 days would have 40 reserve days of remaining coverage in his or her lifetime for subsequent spells lasting more than 90 days. Patients may elect to save these days for future prolonged hospitalizations and use other financial resources for payment of any part of the costs of days 91 to 150. Medicare regulations require that a hospital or SNF notify a beneficiary of this right at least 5 days prior to the end of coverage. If a facility is not informed that an individual has exhausted all coverage, including lifetime reserve days, Medicare regulations guarantee payment for up to 6 days of hospitalization (American Psychiatric Association Office of Economic Affairs 1986; Gottlieb 1988).

Although there is no limit on the total number of hospitalizations or inpatient days covered for medical or surgical diagnoses or for psychiatric care in general hospitals, coverage for inpatient psychiatric care in facilities recognized by the Health Care Financing Administration as freestanding psychiatric hospitals is limited to a total of 190 days during an individual's lifetime. In addition, if an individual becomes Medicare eligible during the course of a first episode of psychiatric hospitalization, Medicare's local intermediary may elect to cover fewer than the full 150 benefit days of that spell of illness. This provision is designed to restrict Part A psychiatric benefits to the active component of treatment and to prevent full reimbursement for a person who may have been institutionalized for long periods of time.

Part A also provides limited coverage for care in SNFs. Services provided by domiciliary personal care and intermediate care facilities are not reimbursable by Medicare. In order to obtain SNF benefits, an individual must have been hospitalized for at least three consecutive days and admission must occur within 30 days of hospital discharge. Part A covers up to 100 days of SNF care. The need for continued skilled care must be reassessed and documented regularly. Similarly, home health services are limited and must be related to acute and remediable conditions (APA Office of Economic Affairs 1986; Gottlieb 1988; Waldo and Lazenby 1984).

From 1966 until late 1983, Part A of Medicare paid for all inpatient care through a retrospective cost-based reimbursement system. In an effort to prevent depletion of the Hospital Insurance Trust Fund, Congress and the Reagan administration enacted the Tax Equity and Fiscal Responsibility Act (TEFRA) of 1982. TEFRA emphasized cost containment, provided for limits on all inpatient operating costs, and established target rates for cost increases. Incentives were developed providing for reduced hospital reimbursement if targets were not met and extra payments if limits were not exceeded. Reimbursement limits were adjusted to reflect patient mix, geographic location, and training costs. TEFRA mandated legislation to replace cost-based reimbursement with a prospective payment system (PPS) (APA Office of Economic Affairs 1986; English et al. 1986; Frazier et al. 1986; Scherl et al. 1988).

Public Law 98-21 (the Social Security Amendments of 1983) established a PPS for Medicare. PPS is based on a patient-discharge classification system using diagnosis-related groups (DRGs) to cluster patients who presumably require similar care. The DRG system categorizes patients into 23 relatively general, major diagnostic categories and then assigns the discharge to one of 468 DRGs derived from principal and secondary diagnoses; procedures rendered; and (to a lesser degree) age, sex, comorbidity, complications, and discharge status. Hospitals are paid a predetermined amount for each case according to the DRG assigned. This sum is independent of actual costs incurred. Therefore, payment is considered to be an incentive for efficient use of resources. If patients consume extraordinary resources or require prolonged inpatient care, they are classified as "outliers," and Medicare will provide additional payments to the hospital at a rate considerably less than actual cost.

Fourteen of the DRGs apply to discharges related to treatment of psychiatric disorders. Concerns regarding the ability of DRGs to predict resource consumption accurately for psychiatric disorders led to a temporary exemption from this payment method for freestanding psychiatric hospitals and for distinct psychiatric units in general hospitals. However, treatment of primary psychiatric patients in "scatter" beds on general medical and surgical units are reimbursed through the DRG system. In 1984, discharges from scatter beds accounted for nearly 46% of psychiatric cases reimbursed by Medicare (Goldman et al. 1987).

Research regarding the application of DRGs to treatment of patients with principal psychiatric diagnoses has substantiated the inaccuracy of DRGs in predicting resource consumption. DRGs have been shown to account for only a limited proportion of the variation in individual lengths of stay for all diagnoses (16%–40%). Moreover, they are considerably less accurate in predicting psychiatric use, generally accounting for less than 8% of the variance (English et al. 1986; Frank and Lave 1985; Goldman 1988). The APA's comprehensive assessment of DRG data (English et al. 1986) suggested that the similarity among patients in a given psychiatric DRG is extremely limited. Patients who require very brief hospitalizations are frequently clustered with individuals in need of much longer hospital stays. Analysis of study data indicates that DRGs favor less severely ill patients and settings that provide short-term evaluation and limited treatment.

Freestanding psychiatric hospitals and exempted psychiatric units in general hospitals continue to be paid retrospectively by Medicare. However, TEFRA modified and substantially limited these reimbursements. Medicare reimbursement for treatment in these sites is "capped" at a target rate established for each facility based on resource use during a "base" year (the first full fiscal year of operation after October 1, 1983). If the actual cost per case exceeds the target rate, the hospital must absorb the loss. If the cost is less than the TEFRA-capped rate, the hospital may retain 50% of the difference up to 5% of the target rate. For hospitals that care for a substantial number of complicated geriatric patients, this payment scheme is even more arbitrary than DRGs. As geriatric psychiatry expands as a field, recognition and aggressive treatment of acute mental disorders in Medicare recipients are also growing. This situation will likely translate into greater resource consumption in acute care settings. Therefore, the employment of relatively old utilization experience (which may derive from a base year of 1984 or 1985) to set payment limits can easily become de facto per-case reimbursement at a rate that has nothing to do with the patient—or even with the diagnosis!

The nature of psychiatric disorder in the elderly makes these incentives worrisome. Incomplete evaluation of complicated patients in settings that are discouraged from employing expensive, but often necessary, diagnostic technologies may add unnecessary disability and ultimately generate substantially greater costs (Fogel et al. 1990). In addition, the high prevalence of medical disorders among older adults with psychiatric diagnoses makes both DRGs and TEFRA caps inoperable. Patients with active medical diagnoses treated by psychiatric personnel in scatter beds and/or in exempt units have not been considered in research assessing these payment mechanisms.

A number of alternative mechanisms have been proposed to allow implementation of a PPS for psychiatry. Although several methods substantially improve predictability of length of stay and other measures of resource consumption, no system has been tested with adequately large data sets in a way that reflects the extremely differentiated nature of the mental health care delivery system (Goldman 1988). Research in this area remains active, and potential improvements in policy are possible in the near future.

Supplemental Medical Insurance (Part B)

The SMI benefit program of Medicare Part B is voluntary. Subscription requires payment of a monthly premium ($27.90 in 1989). About 97% of Medicare Part A recipients elect to purchase SMI benefits. The Part B trust find is financed by general revenues from the federal treasury, trust fund interest, and these premiums. The Part B premium is set by law at 25% of the average monthly benefit per enrollee, and premiums cover about one-fourth of program expenditures (PPRC 1989).

Medicare pays for physician services through a system called customary, prevailing, and reasonable (CPR). The payment rate or reasonable allowed charge for a specific service is the lowest of the following charges: the actual charge, a physician's usual charge for similar services (customary), the charge in the community for similar services provided by other physicians (prevailing), and the fiscal intermediary's usual reimbursement for comparable services to its own policyholders under comparable circumstances. The fiscal intermediary updates CPR rates annually, and revisions during a fiscal year are not permitted (Gottlieb 1988; PPRC 1989).

Part B benefits are subject to an annual deductible ($75 in 1990) and a copayment. For nonpsychiatric physician services and psychiatric inpatient services, a 20% copayment is required. Coverage of medical and surgical visits has never been limited by number of visits or costs of resources consumed. However, when Part B psychiatric benefits were designed, mental illness was depicted as "lacking precise diagnostics and established treatment protocols expected to lead to specified outcomes within a defined period of time" (Cutler and Fine 1985, p. 20). Therefore, coverage for outpatient psychiatric treatment was limited severely. From the initiation of Medicare in 1966 through early 1988, total annual reasonable charges were set at $500 and the law required that the maximum annual Medicare reimbursement for outpatient psychiatric services was $312.50 or 62.5% of reasonable charges, whichever was lower. The 80% federal share, which was the maximum amount paid by Medicare to the psychiatrist, was only $250 per year.

The Omnibus Budget Reconciliation Act of 1987 (OBRA-87; Public Law 100-203) recognized, in part, the discrimination against services for mental disorders inherent in the SMI benefit. Coverage for outpatient psychiatric services was increased to $2,200 annually by 1989. However, the 50% copayment remained. In addition, services for the medical management of psychiatric disorders were exempted from the $2,200 limit and are subject to the same 20% copayment as nonpsychiatric outpatient services. The Omnibus Budget Reconciliation Act of 1989 (OBRA-89; H.R. 3299, Report 101-386) provided further improvement of the psychiatric benefit. Effective July 1, 1990, the annual dollar limit for outpatient mental health services was eliminated. However, the discriminatory 50% copayment and 190-day lifetime psychiatric hospital utilization limit were unaffected by the new law.

OBRA-89 was also revolutionary in its expansion of coverage provided by nonphysician providers. Until the enactment of this legislation, necessary services delivered by psychologists, social workers, therapists, nurses, and aides were reimbursable only under the "direct supervision" of a physician. "Direct supervision" is defined as immediate availability to provide assistance at the time of service. Exceptions to this rule included psychological testing and services provided by psychologists in some community mental health settings. The new law provided for direct reimbursement of psychologists in all settings. Direct reimbursement of clinical social worker services at the rate of 80% of the lesser of the actual charge or 75% of the amount paid to a psychologist is also provided except when they are provided to an inpatient of a hospital or SNF as required for the facility's participation in Medicare.

OBRA-89 also described criteria regarding consultation with a physician for these nonphysician providers. These criteria are vague and somewhat superficial: the provider must document that the patient has been informed of the desirability of consultation with the patient's primary care physician to consider potential medical conditions that may contribute to the patient's condition. In addition, the provider must document written or verbal communication with the primary physician regarding the patient's treatment, unless the patient specifically refuses such contact. The law makes no provision for assessment or consultation with a psychiatrist. Reimbursement of services provided by psychiatric nurses and other therapists continues to require direct physician supervision.

For the most part, direct patient treatment or evaluation is required in order to bill Medicare. Services rendered by telephone, and patient contacts purely for the purpose of renewing a prescription that do not involve evaluation of patient status, are not reimbursable. However, charges for obtaining treatment information from relatives or close associates of a patient who is unreliable or uncommunicative are allowable. Family counseling services are covered only when the purpose of counseling is to facilitate treatment of the identified patient.

There are currently two procedures available for Medicare beneficiaries to receive benefits for provider services under Part B. First, a provider may agree to *accept assignment* from SMI and thereby accept the Medicare reasonable charge as payment in full. The fiscal intermediary pays the approved amount, less copayment and deductible, to the provider directly. The coinsurance and deductible must be collected from the patient. Second, a provider may elect not to accept assignment. In this arrangement, the beneficiary must present an itemized bill from this provider to the fiscal intermediary in order to receive reimbursement at the CPR-determined level. Providers who choose not to accept assignment also face limits in the fees that they may charge to Medicare recipients. The maximum allowable actual charge (MAAC) is based on a physician's profile of charges and adjustments made to his or her fee schedule for services rendered in the second quarter of 1984 or during his or her first year of practice if it began after the second quarter of 1984 (PPRC 1989). The MAAC is the highest fee that a nonparticipating provider may charge to a Medicare recipient. The nonparticipating physician must collect the entire fee directly from the patient.

OBRA-89 will phase out MAAC limits and replace them with new ceilings on balance billing while creating new incentives to accept assignment. Nonparticipating providers will continue to be paid 95% of the Medicare-approved charge. In 1991, nonparticipating providers fees will be limited to the lesser of the physician's MAAC or 125% of the Medicare payment for nonparticipating providers. In 1992, this limit will fall to 120% of the payment for nonparticipating providers, and in 1993 and thereafter the limit will be 115% of the Medicare payment amount for these providers. In addition, as of April 1, 1990, all providers are required to accept assignment from indigent Medicare beneficiaries who are also recipients of Medicaid. By 1992, assignment will be required for all Medicare recipients who are at or below the federal poverty level (OBRA-89 Physician Payment Reform Summary Draft).

Since the initiation of PPS for hospital services, the annual growth rate for costs of physicians' services has been more than twice the rate of growth for inpatient hospital services (Roper 1988). Rising prices for services and increases in the number of services consumed per beneficiary are the greatest contributors to this growth. Part B expenditures grew about 17% per year during the 1980s, and they now account for about a third of Medicare expenditures—nearly $35 billion in 1988 (PPRC 1989). This growth has concerned policymakers and, in addition to the aforementioned expansion of coverage for mental health services, OBRA-89 stipulated the implementation of significant reform in methods of physician payment under Medicare.

OBRA-89 provided for the development of expenditure targets or volume performance standards (VPS) to control growth in physician services. The Secretary of Health and Human Services is mandated to recommend to Congress an overall VPS growth rate before the beginning of each fiscal year. The VPS should be related to fee increases, growth in the size of the Medicare population, changes in service volume and intensity, and a volume performance factor ($-.5$% for fiscal year (FY) 1990, -1% for FY 1991,

− 1.5% for FY 1992, and − 2% thereafter). At the end of the year the Secretary will compare actual growth in outlays with the VPS and will use those data to determine if and by how much fees should be increased or decreased (Psychiatric News 1989; Summary of OBRA 1989 Medicare Physician Payment Reform).

In addition, OBRA-89 provided for the development of a uniform Medicare fee schedule to replace the CPR payment system. The new fee schedule will be based on a resource-based, relative-value scale (RBRVS), developed after extensive research led by Hsiao and his colleagues (1988) at Harvard and substantial input from the PPRC (1989) and professional groups nationally. The RBRVS will be used to determine the relative values of about 7,000 physician services. The relative value for each procedure will have three measurable components: 1) the work required to perform the procedure, 2) associated practice expenses, and 3) malpractice expenses. These proportions will be based on a weighted average of specialty-specific practice expense and malpractice data. Approximately 60% of each fee will be adjusted for geographic variations in cost (Psychiatric News 1989). The product of each relative value and a monetary conversion factor will determine the fee for each service.

The transition to the new fee schedule began in 1990 with reductions in payments for "overvalued procedures." Existing fee schedules for anesthesia and radiology were adjusted to conform to the RBRVS fee schedule. For most other specialties, the RBRVS fee schedule will be phased in gradually from 1992 to 1996.

In an effort to correct for perceived overvaluation of noncognitive procedures, the RBRVS emphasizes cognitive assessment, patient management, and caring activities performed by providers (Hsiao et al. 1988). The work component of relative values is based largely on time, intensity, and stress associated with delivery of services. Case vignettes are assessed by provider panels in each specialty so that appropriate values can be assigned. Procedure codes from the American Medical Association's (1990) Common Procedural Terminology are then employed to describe the procedure performed.

Unfortunately, preliminary efforts to apply the RBRVS to psychiatry have been seriously flawed. The vignettes employed were simplistic and unrepresentative of psychiatric practice. Measurements of clinical work performed and of practice costs were inconsistent, and efforts to develop work scenarios comparable to those encountered in other specialties considered the circumstances of psychiatric care poorly. Furthermore, the CPT codes for psychiatry are extremely broad and therefore difficult to map onto the activities associated with specific vignettes (Sharfstein 1990). Therefore, Hsiao and his colleagues have reconvened a technical consulting group for RBRVS in psychiatry and will undertake development of new vignettes and a new technical survey.

Medicaid

Medicaid is a social insurance program enacted in 1965 to pay for medical care for indigent Americans by providing matching funds to the states. Although minimum basic benefits are required for these matching funds, the program allows states to impose some restrictions on the types of services funded and the level of reimbursement for specific services. Therefore, Medicaid services for mental health care and for specific services for indigent older adults vary substantially by state. Overall, it is estimated that Medicaid pays for as much as 25% of psychiatric care in the United States (English et al. 1984; Gottlieb 1988; Medicare and Medicaid Data Book 1982).

Between 3 million and 4 million individuals aged older than 65 receive Medicaid benefits annually. Older adults represent about 16% of all Medicaid beneficiaries, and they account for about 40% of program expenditures (Waldo and Lazenby 1984). Most older Medicaid recipients also have Medicare. Additionally, many state Medicaid programs have Part B buy-in provisions, which allow these states to reduce their risk for payment of physician services by paying for Medicare SMI on behalf of their older Medicaid recipients. Therefore, Medicaid is principally a coinsuror for many older adults. The program covers Medicare deductibles, copayments, uncovered physician services, and other services after Medicare benefits have been exhausted (Waldo and Lazenby 1984). Fees for all Medicaid services are set at the state level, and they are generally unrelated to prevailing or reasonable charges.

State governments have some discretionary power in the development of local Medicaid programs. Local needs often influence the nature of services offered. Numerous programs that are not covered by Medicare may be available to indigent older adults. These include day treatment programs (often longer term and broader than Medicare's hospital-based partial hospitals), home mental health services, and prescription drugs.

The Medicaid program is most important in its role as payor for long-term care services. Medicaid pays for about 42% of skilled and intermediate level nursing home care, whereas Medicare pays for only 2% of all long-term care costs. The balance of these expenses is borne out of pocket by patients and their families. Most states require that individuals spend down their assets below an established level before they become eligible for Medicaid benefits (Levit et al. 1985).

The nursing home is probably the most important site of care for older adult psychiatric patients, particularly those with severe and chronic disorders like dementia, depression associated with medical illness and disability, and schizophrenia (Goldman et al. 1986). Deinstitutionalization has left the nursing home as the last resort for care of many chronically, psychiatrically ill younger and older adults. From the federal government's perspective, this phenomenon has effectively shifted costs from the states (i.e., from state hospitals) to federally supported Medicaid nursing home beds. In the nursing home reform provisions of OBRA-87, the federal government required preadmission screening of nursing home applicants for psychiatric illness. Referral is required for "active treatment" if it cannot be provided in the nursing home. (The specifics of the nursing home reform provisions of OBRA-87 are detailed in Chapter 27.) These requirements may simultaneously improve psychiatric care for disabled, indigent, older adults in nursing homes while creating significant barriers to admission for others.

Private Insurance and Out-of-Pocket Expenditures

Out-of-pocket expenditures are those health care costs that older adults must pay from personal or family income or savings. Out-of-pocket expenses include premiums for SMI and private "medigap" policies; copayments and deductibles for Parts A and B; charges that exceed Medicare-approved limits imposed by providers who do not accept assignment; and charges for uncovered services, including much of long-term care. The average out-of-pocket health care cost per Medicare beneficiary, excluding long-term care, was nearly $1,700 in 1988. Long-term care costs affect about 5% of older adults and average about $20,000 per year (Moon 1987; PPRC 1989). Older adults spend about 15% of their income on medically related expenses. Older adults with psychiatric disorders are affected even more adversely, for copayments are higher, total psychiatric hospital days are limited, and the ability to continue to work to provide income may be even more impaired.

In order to reduce risk related to out-of-pocket expenditures, 71% of older adults purchase private medigap policies designed to cover deductibles and copayments. Some of these policies also provide coverage for some nursing care, physicians' charges in excess of Medicare-approved charges, and prescription drug costs. Nursing home care not approved by Medicare is usually excluded from these policies. Most medigap policies add only 12.5% of approved charges to the 50% Medicare payment for outpatient psychiatric services, leaving a 37.5% copayment even if the provider accepts assignment (Gottlieb 1988). The average medigap premium is between $500 and $700 annually (PPRC 1989). Therefore, poor Medicare beneficiaries without Medicaid—the least able to afford the costs of major illness—are the least likely to have private supplemental insurance.

A small number of employed older adults are required to retain the group private insurance of their employing companies as their primary coverage and use Medicare as a secondary insurer. These individuals are subject to the usual limitations on psychiatric benefits pervasive in insurance for younger adults.

TEFRA contains a provision that facilitates the use of HMOs by elderly Medicare recipients (Iglehart 1985). This policy allows qualified managed care programs to contract directly with Medicare. Each month Medicare pays the contractor a premium equal to 95% of estimated fee for service payments to provide the complete Medicare benefit to subscribers. The program allows HMOs to earn normal profit margins. However, cost savings above a predetermined rate must be used to provide extra services for elderly members.

The market for long-term care insurance has exploded in the past 5 years. This market has been poorly regulated, and prices and products vary remarkably. Policies frequently cover 2 to 3 years of institutionalization in a variety of facilities. Some also cover home care services. Many of these policies exclude patients with psychiatric disorders while including coverage for patients with dementia. Premiums are often five times higher than those for medigap policies, and deductibles and copayments can be substantial.

Conclusion

The economic and health care needs of older adults are extensive and diverse. Health and mental health policy for the elderly has been a patchwork that has left extraordinary gaps despite massive and growing expenditures. For nearly 25 years, Medicare policy has been the most important force in the organization and delivery of geriatric psychiatric services. Stigmatization and discrimination, reflected in exceptionally poor reimbursement of services and perverse incentives to employ expensive inpatient services, have reinforced existing barriers to care for this important and needy population.

Recent legislation has provided small incremental steps to improved access to mental health services for older adults. Simultaneously, innovative cost containment methods may potentially reward the cognitive and caring activities of psychiatric providers. However, the greatest challenges in this dynamic environment lie ahead. It is hoped that proactive policy development will facilitate the delivery of higher-quality services to this population as it grows.

References

American Medical Association: Common Procedural Terminology, 4th Edition. Chicago, IL, American Medical Association, 1990

American Psychiatric Association Office of Economic Affairs, The Coverage Catalog. Washington, DC, American Psychiatric Press, 1986, pp 403–420

Cutler J, Fine T: Federal health care financing of mental illness: a failure of public policy, in The New Economics of Psychiatric Care. Edited by Sharfstein SS, Beigel A. Washington, DC, American Psychiatric Press, 1985, pp 17–37

English JT, Kritzler ZA, Scherl D: Historical trends in the financing of psychiatric services. Psychiatric Annals 14:321–331, 1984

English JT, Sharfstein SS, Scherl DJ, et al: Diagnosis-related groups and general hospital psychiatry: the APA study. Am J Psychiatry 143:131–139, 1986

Fogel BS, Gottlieb GL, Furino A: Present and future solutions, in Mental Health Policy for Older Americans: Protecting Minds at Risk. Edited by Fogel BS, Furino A, Gottlieb GL. Washington, DC, American Psychiatric Press, 1990, pp 257–277

Frank RG, Lave JL: The psychiatric DRGs: are they different? Med Care 23:1148–1155, 1985

Frazier SH, Goldman H, Taube CA: Psychiatry, Medicare, and prospective payment (editorial). Am J Psychiatry 143:198–200, 1986

Furino AF, Fogel BS: The economic perspective, in Mental Health Policy for Older Americans: Protecting Minds at Risk. Edited by Fogel BS, Furino A, Gottlieb GL. Washington, DC, American Psychiatric Press, 1990, pp 23–36

Goldman HH: Overview of studies on psychiatric hospital care under a prospective payment system, in Prospective Payment in Psychiatric Care. Edited by Scherl DJ, English JT, Sharfstein SS. Washington, DC, American Psychiatric Association, 1988, pp 81–89

Goldman HH, Frank RG: Division of responsibility among payors, Mental Health Policy for Older Americans: Protecting Minds at Risk. Edited by Fogel BS, Furino A, Gottlieb GL. Washington, DC, American Psychiatric Press, 1990, pp 85–95

Goldman HH, Feder J, Scanlon W: Chronic mental patients in nursing homes: reexamining data from the National Nursing Home Study. Hosp Community Psychiatry 37:269–272, 1986

Goldman HH, Taube CA, Jencks SJ: The organization of the psychiatric inpatient services system. Med Care 25(9 suppl):S6–S21, 1987

Gottlieb GL: Financial issues affecting geriatric psychiatric care, in Essentials of Geriatric Psychiatry. Edited by Lazarus L. New York, Springer, 1988, pp 230–248

Grob GN: Mental illness and American society, 1875–1940. Princeton, NJ, Princeton University Press, 1983

Hazzard WR: Geriatric medicine: life in the crucible of the struggle to contain health care costs, in The Medical Cost Containment Crisis. Edited by McCue JD. Ann Arbor, MI, Health Administration Press, 1989, pp 263–264

Hsiao WC, Braun P, Dunn D, et al: Resource-based value scale. JAMA 260:2347–2353, 1988

Iglehart JK: Health policy report: Medicare turns to HMOs. N Engl J Med 312:132–136, 1985

Levit KR, Lazenby H, Waldo DR, et al: National health expenditures, 1984. Health Care Financing Review 7:731–734, 1985

Long SH, Welch WP: Are we containing costs or pushing on a balloon? Health Affairs 7(4):113–117, 1988

Markides KS, Mindel CH: Aging and ethnicity. Newburg Park, CA, Sage, 1987, pp 31–35

Medicare and Medicaid Data Book. Washington, DC, Health Care Financing Administration, 1982

Moon M: The elderly's access to health care services: the crude and subtle impacts of Medicare changes. Social Justice Research 1:361–375, 1987

Morrison L, Janssen T, Motter L: Evaluation of the Medicare mental health demonstration. Silver Spring, MD, Macro Systems, 1984

National Center for Health Statistics: Health statistics in older persons; United States, 1986. Vital and Health Stat, Series 3, no 25 (DHHS Pub. No. (PHS) 87-1409). Washington, DC, U.S. Government Printing Office, 1987

National Center for Health Statistics: Health, United States, 1987. (DHHS Pub. No. (PHS) 88-1232). Washington, DC, U.S. Government Printing Office, 1988

Omnibus Budget Reconciliation Act 1989, Medicare Physician Payment

Reform: Annual Report to Congress. Washington, DC, U.S. Government Printing Office, 1989

Physician Payment Review Commission: Annual Report to Congress. Washington, DC, U.S. Government Printing Office, 1989, pp 7–28

Psychiatric News: New Medicare fee schedule gets Congressional approval. Psychiatric News 24(24):2, 1989

Regier DA, Goldberg ID, Taube CA: The de facto U.S. mental health services system. Arch Gen Psychiatry 35:685–693, 1978

Roper WL: Statement before the Committee on Ways and Means. Washington, DC, U.S. Congress, House of Representatives, September 29, 1988

Scherl DJ, English JT, Sharfstein SS: Preface to Prospective Payment of Psychiatric Care. Washington, DC, American Psychiatric Association, 1988, pp xv–xxii

Schulz J: Economics of Aging, 4th Edition. Dover, MA, Auburn House Publications, 1988

Schurman RA, Kramer PD, Mitchell JB: The hidden mental health network. Arch Gen Psychiatry 42:89–94, 1985

Sharfstein SS: Payment for services: a provider's perspective, in Mental Health Policy for Older Americans: Protecting Minds at Risk. Edited by Fogel BS, Furino A, Gottlieb GL. Washington, DC, American Psychiatric Press, 1990, pp 97–107

Soldo BJ, Agree EM: America's elderly population. Population Bulletin 43(3):1–53, 1988

U.S. Bureau of the Census: An aging world. International Population Reports, Series P-95, no 78. Washington, DC, U.S. Government Printing Office, 1987

U.S. Congress, House of Representatives, Committee on Ways and Means: Background material and data on programs within the jurisdiction of the Committee on Ways and Means. Washington, DC, U.S. Government Printing Office, 1989

U.S. Senate Committee on Finance: Background material on health insurance. Washington, DC, U.S. Government Printing Office, 1978

Waldo DR, Lazenby HC: Demographic characteristics and health care use by the aged in the United States: 1977–1984. Health Care Financing Review 6:1–29, 1984

Self-Assessment Section

Chapter 1: Introduction

Choose the one best response

1. Which of the classic psychoanalysts wrote the following: "With persons who are too advanced in years, it [psychoanalytic methods] fails because, owing to the accumulation of material, so much time would be required so that the end of the cure would be reached at a period of life in which much importance is no longer attached to nervous health":
   a. Freud
   b. Abraham
   c. Jung
   d. Ferenczi

2. Which of the following is true regarding Alois Alzheimer?
   a. His famous monograph was written in 1923.
   b. He was a psychiatrist.
   c. His contribution is in describing the signs and symptoms of multi-infarct dementia.
   d. His primary psychiatric interest was personality disorders.

3. Following World War II clinical research in geriatric psychiatry was most notable in which of the following countries?
   a. The Federal Republic of Germany
   b. The United States of America
   c. United Kingdom
   d. France

4. Which of the following journals was being published before 1970?

   a. The Journal of Geriatric Psychiatry
   b. The Journal of Gerontology
   c. The Journal of the American Geriatric Society
   d. All of the above

5. All of the following organizations emphasize geriatric psychiatry except:

   a. The APA
   b. AAGP
   c. AOA
   d. IPA

6. The first director of the National Institute on Aging was

   a. Robert Butler
   b. Carl Eisdorfer
   c. Eric Pfeiffer
   d. Gene Cohen

Chapter 2: Epidemiology of Psychiatric Disorders

Answer a if only 1, 2, 3 are correct
          b if only 1 and 3 are correct
          c if only 2 and 4 are correct
          d if only 4 is correct
          e if all are correct

1. The prevalence of a psychiatric disorder is the frequency

   1. of new cases counted over a period of time.
   2. of all cases counted at a single point in time.
   3. of the total number of cases counted during one year.
   4. of all cases counted over a period of time.

2. Epidemiologic data on Alzheimer's disease and related dementias indicate that

   1. most cases are in nursing homes, not in the community.
   2. the prevalence is about 50% or more for nursing-home residents.
   3. the incidence is 4% annually.
   4. the prevalence is about 7½% of all elderly (age 65 +).

3. The combined incidence of schizophrenia and paranoid disorders or related conditions among the elderly (age 65⁺) is
   1. 30%–60% of long-stay inpatients in state psychiatric hospitals.
   2. 5%–10% of first admissions to psychiatric hospitals.
   3. 1%.
   4. higher in those with long-standing deafness.

4. As a person grows older (beyond age 65) the risk of developing
   1. alcohol abuse becomes negligible.
   2. mania remains present.
   3. major depression increases.
   4. any type of depression secondary to physical illness increases.

5. Epidemiologic findings in old age populations suggest that preventive efforts might be successful in reducing the incidence of
   1. deliria, by use of sedatives to minimize fear of hospital admission.
   2. late-onset paranoid states, by treating certain types of hearing impairment in middle age.
   3. Alzheimer's disease, by maintaining an active intellectual life.
   4. depression, by reducing the number of potent medications taken by the elderly medical patient.

Choose the one best response

6. The prevalence of depression among the whole population age 65 and over is
   a. less than 1% for all DSM-III-R subtypes of depression.
   b. 2%–4% for major depression.
   c. less than 5% for all depressions requiring clinical attention.
   d. less than 5% for elderly psychiatric outpatients.
   e. None of the above.

7. The lifetime risk of Alzheimer's disease or related dementias for men who survive to 85 or older is
   a. well over 50%.
   b. 7½%.
   c. 1 in 3.
   d. 4% annually.
   e. None of the above.

8. Depression (any type defined by DSM-III-R criteria) in the elderly person is prolonged by

a. continuing physical illness.
b. poor quality rather than small size of the social network.
c. lack of a confidant.
d. the omission of early treatment.
e. All of the above.

Chapter 3: Genetics of Geriatric Psychopathology

Choose the one best response

1. The incidence of which one of the following dementing illnesses is most clearly age related?

a. Pick's disease
b. Huntington's disease
c. Alzheimer's disease
d. Wilson's disease
e. Multi-infarct dementia

2. A fragment length polymorphism is

a. a segment of DNA.
b. a gene with known function.
c. a gene whose function is unknown.
d. an RNA transcript.
e. a regulatory protein.

3. A healthy man whose mother died of Huntington's chorea
wants to know his risk for developing the disease. He knows
that by his age, 43, about half of the children of persons with
Huntington's disease have themselves developed the disease.
Using that information, and the fact that the disease appears
only in females in his family, he reasons that his risk is now
close to zero. Approximately, what is his actual risk?

a. 50%
b. 33%
c. 25%
d. 12.5%
e. zero

Answer a if only 1, 2, and 3 are correct
  b if only 1 and 3 are correct
  c if only 2 and 4 are correct
  d if only 4 is correct
  e if all are correct

4. Which of the following statements about DNA are correct?
  1. Thymidine is one of the nucleotides/bases in DNA.
  2. Nuclear DNA is mirrored by DNA.
  3. DNA itself provides binding sites for regulation.
  4. DNA is the template on which proteins are constructed.

5. What information about a family constitutes the minimum needed for genetic counseling based on fragment length polymorphisms?
  1. DNA must be available on at least two persons, one known gene carrier and one likely not a gene carrier.
  2. DNA must be available from at least two generations.
  3. Phase must be determinable.
  4. The family history of disease must be known for at least two generations.

6. Which of the following statements about Alzheimer's disease are correct?
  1. Amyloid is coded for by DNA on chromosome 21.
  2. DNA coding for amyloid is linked to DNA coding for Alzheimer's disease.
  3. In all populations studied, the incidence of Alzheimer's disease is about 1% per year after age 75.
  4. Alzheimer's neuropathology is found only in Alzheimer's disease.

Chapter 4: Biological Aspects

Answer a if only 1, 2, 3 are correct
  b if only 1 and 3 are correct
  c if only 2 and 4 are correct
  d if only 4 is correct
  e if all are correct

1. Neurons may degenerate or change their configuration. They may exhibit "down" regulation in surface receptors, synthesize

less transmitter or metabolize it more slowly. Selective cell loss disrupts the delicate homeostatic balance among the array of neurotransmitters maintaining nervous system function. Which of the following are associated with non-disease-related normative variations in function noted in the elderly?

1. ACH levels remain unchanged reflecting no changes in synthesis but decreased release and metabolism.
2. DA synthetic rates and thus serum levels decline selectively as a result of cell loss.
3. Circulating NE increases with age because of receptor downregulation and slowed clearance.
4. Beta receptors in non-nervous tissues show declines in responsiveness with downregulation.

2. Which of the following statements about age-related sensory changes are false?
   1. Social isolation can be caused by hearing and vision loss.
   2. Taste discrimination declines significantly at puberty.
   3. Presbyopia is related to loss of the ability to accommodate.
   4. Retinal degeneration is a sign of normal aging in the eye.

3. Which of the following statement(s) is (are) true?
   1. Most cell growth stops at puberty though a fraction of prenatal mitotic activity continues in all tissues into late adulthood.
   2. Most enzymatic activities drop off slowly due to decreasing rates of synthesis as well as clearance.
   3. Aging and sun exposure accelerate the migration of melanocytes in the exposed skin.
   4. The musculoskeletal system, gonads, and heart show gender-specific aging patterns whereas the kidneys, skin, and lungs do not.

4. With the redistribution of body fat in the elderly, the following can be seen:
   1. Increased incidence of hypothermic-related disease.
   2. Increased incidence of hemorrhage and vascular accidents with heparin therapy.
   3. Increased wrinkling of the face and extremities.
   4. Decreased sensitivity to insect bites.

5. In the absence of significant arteriosclerotic disease, the following functional changes are evidence of the aging of the cardiovascular system:

1. Ventricular walls thicken and the ventricles dilate to increase cardiac output.
2. Heart rate slows because of decreases in circulating levels of epinephrine.
3. Hypertension is inevitable as collagen is deposited, along with calcium in the walls of large vessels in areas of medial necrosis.
4. Women have slower rates of vascular degeneration because of the protective effects of estrogens prior to menopause.

6. Aerobic exercise
   1. improves conditioning as measured by increased VO_2 and anaerobic threshold.
   2. is of questionable value because of the risk of fracture and the frequency of degenerative joint disease.
   3. can lead to lower levels of total and LDL cholesterol and elevations in HDL levels.
   4. is effective in elevating systolic and diastolic blood pressure responses.

7. An 85-year-old man was brought to a geriatric assessment center because of a 6-month history of weight loss, early morning wakefulness, general anhedonia, and mild forgetfulness. On questioning, he stated that food didn't taste good and he had some mild difficulty in swallowing and increasing numbness and pain in the feet.
   1. His systems are classic for depression in the elderly.
   2. He has pathognomonic symptoms of pancreatic cancer.
   3. He may be malnourished with early symptoms of pernicious anemia.
   4. He has a typical presentation for early dementia.

8. Hypothalamus–anterior pituitary–end organ feedback loops show minimal changes over time except when disease is present. However, aging does occur in some parts of the endocrine system. Which of the following phenomena are common in older individuals?
   1. TSH is elevated in males over the age of 60.
   2. There is a decreased blood level of estrogen in women beginning around age 35 and elevated levels of LH.
   3. There is complete cessation of progesterone production in anovulatory women producing, via negative feedback, elevations in serum FSH levels.

    4. Slow decrease in measurable circulating testosterone levels occurs in 50-year-old men.

9. The immune system is complex, intimately tied to the endocrine and nervous systems. Which of the following statements best describe normal immunological aging?
   1. There are increased E receptors on aging OKT4 helper lymphocytes and NK cells.
   2. Less vigorous responses to immunization occur with some elderly mounting no response.
   3. B-lymphocytes increase in total number and have enhanced function.
   4. Thymic hormones are present until late into the 60's despite involution of the thymus in adolescence.

10. Aging of the peripheral nervous system may be confounded by the stigmata of chronic diseases. Examples of functional losses that may be exaggerated by other illnesses include the following:
    1. Tandem stepping
    2. Rising from a chair
    3. Hand dexterity
    4. Fine touch discrimination

11. Current understanding of pharmacokinetics in the elderly predicts that:
    1. It is reasonable to generalize about medication tolerance from one elderly individual to another because of the heterogeneity of the elderly population.
    2. Lipid-soluble drugs are likely to have a relatively lower volume of distribution than water-soluble drugs.
    3. Efficacy of drug clearance dependent on aging-associated impaired renal function is not apparent from serum creatinine levels.
    4. Drug absorption is generally decreased among the elderly to a clinically significant degree.

Chapter 5: Psychosocial Aspects

Choose the one best response

1. Biological theories of aging include
   a. Continuity theory.

    b. Activity theory.

    c. Integrity theory.

    d. Eversion theory.

    e. None of the above.

2. Internal continuity according to Atchley is

    a. easily disrupted by external events.

    b. characterized by stability of skills and roles.

    c. a normative preparation for death.

    d. a foundation for day-to-day decision making.

    e. All of the above.

3. The major psychological tasks of aging include

    a. achieving psychological integrity.

    b. reworking adolescent trauma.

    c. mourning liberation.

    d. coping with omni-convergence of events.

    e. All of the above.

4. Self-concept and self-image

    a. are disrupted by environmental change in old age.

    b. remain stable with advancing age.

    c. are disrupted by interpersonal losses.

    d. are independent of early-life experiences.

    e. None of the above.

5. The reminiscence process in old age

    a. very accurately describes past life events and relationships.

    b. is associated with greater degrees of life satisfaction.

    c. is always associated with working through of internal conflict.

    d. is accepted by everyone as a universal phenomenon in the aged.

    e. All of the above.

6. The experience of narcissistic loss in the elderly

    a. is less profound if selfobject ties are maintained.

    b. is modified by environmental support for the individual.

    c. is modified by the individual's capacity to experience gratitude.

    d. may be compensated for through idealization of one's children.

    e. All of the above.

7. Thoughts of death in the elderly

   a. are overt and pervasive.

   b. do not appear on projective testing.

   c. are generally associated with anxiety.

   d. are generally well-contained and controlled.

   e. All of the above.

8. Sociological theories about aging include

   a. Error theory.

   b. Continuity theory.

   c. Free radical theory.

   d. Mourning liberation theory.

   e. All of the above.

9. Mourning losses

   a. is a life-long process.

   b. is an essential capacity for late-life adaptation.

   c. releases otherwise blocked creativity.

   d. protects against the trauma of interpersonal loss.

   e. All of the above.

Chapter 6: Neuroimaging

Choose the one best response

1. Which of the following is a structural imaging technique:

   a. Positron emission tomography (PET)

   b. Single-photon emission computed tomography (SPECT)

   c. Magnetic resonance imaging (MRI)

   d. Computerized electroencephalography (CEEG)

2. The imaging technique that has the best spatial resolution is

   a. MRI

   b. PET

   c. SPECT

   d. CEEG

3. The most widely accessible type of scan is

   a. PET

   b. CEEG

   c. CT

   d. MRI

4. Advantages of MRI over X-ray computed tomography (CT) include all of the following except:

   a. MRI is more easily tolerated by patients.
   b. MRI has better penetration of the skull.
   c. Images can be acquired in planes other than the transverse.
   d. More than anatomical information can be gained.

5. The best MRI image type for detecting white matter pathology is

   a. T1-weighted.
   b. T2-weighted.
   c. MR spectroscopy.
   d. Inversion recovery.

6. Advantages of PET over SPECT include all of the following except:

   a. PET is quantitative.
   b. PET is more widely accessible.
   c. PET can image a wider variety of physiological processes.
   d. PET has better spatial resolution.

7. PET and SPECT findings in multi-infarct dementia include

   a. isolated frontal lobe hypermetabolism/blood flow.
   b. bilateral parietal lobe hypometabolism/blood flow.
   c. flow or metabolism reductions in the infarcted areas.
   d. interictal hypometabolism with ictal increase.

8. Commonly reported types of white matter lesions on MRI include all of the following except:

   a. Periventricular hyperintensity.
   b. Discrete deep white matter focal hyperintensity.
   c. Focal decreases in intensity on T2-weighted images.
   d. Confluent patches of increased signal in the deep white matter.

9. Common dementing disorders diagnosable by neuroimaging include those due to

   a. folate deficiency.
   b. brain tumors.
   c. drug intoxication.
   d. subdural hematoma.

For the following questions, match the best lettered item. Each lettered item can be used once, more than once, or not at all.

    a. Bilateral parietal lobe decrease in metabolism (hypometabolism)
    b. Caudate hypometabolism
    c. Frontal lobe atrophy and localized frontal hypometabolism
    d. Interictal hypometabolism

10. Huntington's disease

11. Pick's disease

Answer a if only 1 and 3 are correct
         b if only 2 and 4 are correct
         c if only 1, 2, and 3 are correct
         d if only 4 is correct

12. Reasons why functional imaging might be better than structural imaging in psychiatric disorders include:
    1. Functional tissue disturbances occur earlier than structural disturbances.
    2. Most psychiatric disorders don't have obvious associated structural abnormalities.
    3. The pathophysiology of major psychiatric disorders includes physiological dysfunctions amenable to functional neuroimaging.
    4. Functional neuroimaging is so much less expensive than structural imaging that it is a cost-effective screening tool.

Chapter 7: Psychological Aspects

Choose the one best response

1. The study of cognitive processes includes all *except*
    a. visual acuity
    b. memory
    c. problem solving
    d. reasoning
    e. decision making

2. The locus of age-related differences in memory capacity is in

    a. sensory memory
    b. primary memory
    c. secondary memory
    d. tertiary memory
    e. text memory

3. The following are true statements about intellectual functioning *except:*

    a. Research on intellectual functioning has one of the most productive records in the psychology of aging.
    b. Crystallized intelligence is a measure of knowledge acquired in the course of the socialization process.
    c. Fluid intelligence involves the ability to solve novel problems.
    d. Crystallized intelligence tends to remain stable over the adult life span.
    e. Fluid intelligence tends to improve from young to old adulthood.

4. In examining the cognitive functioning of the older person, the literature found that

    a. the level of education and verbal intelligence could account for a significant portion of age effects on text recall performance.
    b. older persons cannot compensate for peripheral hearing loss by taking advantage of word-sentence context.
    c. older persons can perform at the same level as young adults in problem solving situations.
    d. training in fluid abilities for older persons cannot significantly improve their performance.
    e. None of the above.

5. The literature on patterns of personality development over the life span found that

    a. greater stability in personality across the adult life cycle is found with subjective measures of personality.
    b. self-esteem is not maintained at adult levels in late life.
    c. different personality typologies adapt or respond differently to life events.
    d. gender differences are generally not found.
    e. All of the above.

6. Vaillant, in his study of adult development, found

a. no specific age linkages to achievement of life stages.

b. adult development was relatively dependent on social status.

c. adult development was not observed in an ordered sequence.

d. positive relationship between level of adult development and socioeconomic status.

e. None of the above.

7. Studies on the role of social support as a moderating variable in the lives of middle-aged and older persons found

a. a strong relationship between the presence of social support and health.

b. middle-aged persons tend not to pay as much attention to their health.

c. social support has little to do with the well-being of middle-aged and older persons.

d. the size of the social support network increases with the adult age span.

e. All of the above.

8. In studies of health and behavior, the literature consistently found that

a. hospitalization accounts for the economic decline of the aged.

b. there is minimal relationship between health and behavior in middle-aged adults.

c. variations in health, rather than age, are responsible for a large portion of expected age difference in behavior.

d. older adults who tend to stay healthy have a difficult time in being financially solvent.

e. None of the above.

9. Behavioral treatments applied to nursing home populations found

a. no effects on the behavior of its residents.

b. increases in psychosocial competence among residents after short-term group therapy.

c. patients generally do not like the treatment.

d. resentment among the nursing home staff.

e. None of the above.

Chapter 8: History and Mental Status Examination

Answer a if only 1, 2, 3 are correct
b if only 1 and 3 are correct
c if only 2 and 4 are correct
d if only 4 is correct
e if all are correct

1. Ideomotor apraxia:
   1. is detected by observing how a patient uses a key.
   2. is indicative of nondominant parietal lobe dysfunction.
   3. is detected with commands involving both limbs simultaneously.
   4. is suggested by the patient's use of body parts as objects.

2. According to Lawton, physical activities of daily living include all of the following *except*
   1. bathing.
   2. going to toilet.
   3. dressing.
   4. ability to tell time.

3. In the psychogeriatric mental status examination, the cognitive assessment
   1. helps guide the choice of more elaborate laboratory and psychological testing.
   2. should be organized such that higher order cognitive functions are tested prior to more basic functions.
   3. should help to describe the quantity and quality of cognitive impairment.
   4. can be omitted if cognitive impairment is not detected during the history taking.

4. In order to perform the cognitive assessment, the clinician will need to
   1. introduce the procedure to the patient with a a brief explanation.
   2. be flexible in the choice of tests administered.
   3. provide an atmosphere that helps to maximize a patient's performance.
   4. disregard the patient's premorbid intellectual abilities and level of education.

5. Paraphasias
   1. are specific errors of speech.
   2. include problems in the melodic expression of speech.
   3. include semantic and phonemic errors.
   4. cannot be elicited in spontaneous speech.

6. Constructional apraxia
   1. can be elicited by asking the patient to copy figures.
   2. can suggest disability of the nondominant parietal lobe.
   3. can be elicited by asking a patient to draw a clock.
   4. can be indicative of subtle changes in overall cognition.

7. In frontal brain systems tasks,
   1. impairment can be indicative of extrapyramidal disorders.
   2. performance is rarely impaired in Pick's disease.
   3. tests include multiple loops and alternating sequences.
   4. higher-order functions such as abstraction and insight are not involved.

8. The following types of delusions are seen in dementia:
   1. misidentification syndrome
   2. delusional jealousy
   3. reincarnation of lost relatives
   4. stealing delusions

9. A comprehensive geriatric psychiatric assessment includes the following:
   1. the history of presenting illness
   2. frontal lobe tasks
   3. family psychiatric history
   4. assessment of activities of daily living

Chapter 9: Medical Evaluation and Common Medical Problems

Choose the one best response

1. During screening evaluation on admission to an outpatient psychiatric clinic, an otherwise well older woman is found to have a microcytic anemia. Which one of the following statements is *true:*
   a. Anemia in older patients is common and does not warrant further evaluation.

b. Anemia in older patients is common and does not warrant further evaluation, but oral iron therapy should be started.

c. If stools for occult blood are negative, no further investigation is necessary.

d. Initial investigation should focus on documenting iron deficiency and gastrointestinal evaluation.

e. None of the above.

2. An older patient is admitted to the psychiatric ward for depression. Screening thyroid function tests reveal the following: T_4 = 13.5 ug/dl (normal = 5–12.0), FTI = 10.0 (normal = 6–10.5), TSH = 3.0 μU/ml (normal = 0.5–4.0). The most appropriate initial management would be:

a. Treat with radioactive iodine.

b. Treat with propylthiouracil.

c. Treat with propylthiouracil and a beta-blocker.

d. Observe the patient and repeat the thyroid function tests within a couple of months.

e. None of the above.

3. An older patient is referred to the psychiatrist for a progressive dementia and delusions. On exam the patient has generalized weakness with hyperreflexia and pupils that react to accommodation but not to light. Serum VDRL is negative, but serum FTA-ABS is positive. The patient has never been treated for syphilis. The most appropriate step would be:

a. lumbar puncture

b. repeat VDRL monthly

c. repeat FTA-ABS monthly

d. benzathine penicillin 2.4 million units as a single dose

e. All of the above

4. Antihypertensive agents that have been commonly associated with sedation and depression in older patients include all of the following *except:*

a. reserpine

b. methyl-dopa

c. clonidine

d. calcium-channel blockers

5. Which *one* of the following statements regarding psychiatric symptoms in patients with diabetes mellitus is *not* true:

a. Mental status changes accompanying hyperglycemic hyperosmolar nonketotic coma always resolve rapidly when serum glucose returns to normal.

b. Chronic hyperglycemia may cause nonspecific constitutional symptoms.

c. Hypoglycemia may present with a variety of psychiatric symptoms, ranging from subtle dullness to coma.

d. It is safer for elderly patients to have slightly elevated blood sugars rather than run the risk of hypoglycemia.

6. Clues which should prompt a search for causes of joint pain other than osteoarthritis in an older patient include

a. markedly elevated sedimentation rate.

b. weight loss.

c. destructive bone lesions on plain X-ray films.

d. All of the above.

e. None of the above.

7. Which of the following statements is true:

a. The older patient with diarrhea may have a fecal impaction as the cause.

b. Substantial increase in fiber intake is not as important in older as in younger patients.

c. Chronic stimulant laxatives or oral mineral oil is recommended as treatment for chronic constipation in the majority of older patients.

d. Soap suds or hydrogen peroxide enemas are well tolerated and safe in older patients.

e. None of the above.

8. Which of the following is a contraindication to electroconvulsive therapy in older patients

a. osteoporosis

b. increased intracranial pressure

c. past history of myocardial infarction

d. pacemaker

e. All of the above

9. With regard to electroconvulsive therapy in older patients, which of the following is correct:

a. ECT is medically dangerous for many older patients.

b. No special precautions are necessary in patients with pacemakers.

    c. Pretreatment atropine is dangerous in patients at risk for developing post-ECT bradycardia.

    d. Evidence does not suggest that electrode placement influences the risk of memory loss.

    e. None of the above.

10. The evaluation of older patients prior to beginning a tricyclic antidepressant should include

    a. orthostatic blood pressure measurements.

    b. electrocardiogram.

    c. inquiry about urinary retention.

    d. All of the above.

11. Changes in the electrocardiogram prior to instituting tricyclic antidepressant therapy that warrant caution include

    a. bifascicular block.

    b. second degree heart block.

    c. QT prolongation.

    d. All of the above.

Chapter 10: Neurological Evaluation

Answer a if only 1, 2, 3 are correct
           b if only 1 and 3 are correct
           c if only 2 and 4 are correct
           d if only 4 is correct
           e if all are correct

1. Neurological changes that may be seen in normal aging include

    1. loss of ankle jerks.

    2. spontaneous bucco-lingual dyskinesias.

    3. dysmetria on finger-to-nose testing.

    4. impaired lateral gaze.

2. Hearing deficits in the aged have been associated with

    1. conductive loss.

    2. sensorineural loss.

    3. paranoia.

    4. hallucinations.

3. There is evidence that normal aging involves
   1. increased cerebral blood flow.
   2. some demyelination in the peripheral nervous system with sparing of axons.
   3. loss of cortical neurons with relative sparing of white matter.
   4. increase in monoamine oxidase.

4. Clinically
   1. amyotrophic lateral sclerosis may be associated with upper motor neuron signs and depression.
   2. amyotrophic lateral sclerosis may be associated with lower motor neuron signs and depression.
   3. subacute combined degeneration produces absent reflexes and positive Babinski signs.
   4. olivopontocerebellar atrophy may be associated with Parkinsonism and depression.

Choose the one best response

5. Frontal release signs
   a. reveal frontal lobe pathology.
   b. are often found in the healthy aged.
   c. include patellar hyperreflexia.
   d. do not occur with frontal lobe pathology.
   e. can distinguish basal ganglia from frontal lobe pathology.

6. Olivopontocerebellar atrophy, progressive supranuclear palsy, and idiopathic Parkinson's disease have all been associated with
   a. rigidity and preserved cognition.
   b. corticospinal tract impairment and cognitive impairment.
   c. rigidity and impaired cognition.
   d. dysmetria and impaired cognition.
   e. dysmetria and preserved cognition.

7. Which of the following statements is correct:
   a. Unilateral resting tremor is seen in idiopathic Parkinson's disease.
   b. Brain tumors usually produce papilledema in the elderly.
   c. Gait disorders affect less than 5% of the elderly.
   d. Unilateral temporal lobe pathology usually produces bilateral anosmia.

e. Alcoholic cerebellar degeneration produces more appendicular than truncal ataxia.

Chapter 11: Neuropsychological Evaluation

Choose the one best response

1. Patients' learning ability can be assessed in the course of interviewing by
   a. asking them how they would find their way to a familiar location.
   b. observing if they keep their mind on the conversation.
   c. asking them to interpret a common proverb.
   d. asking them to describe their favorite recipe.
   e. discussing current events.

2. Patients who are non-fluent
   a. in almost all cases have difficulty with comprehension.
   b. have the most difficulty with small connective words such as "if" or "and."
   c. have the most difficulty with no verbs.
   d. have halting speech but do not have a preferential impairment with any particular part of speech.
   e. in almost all cases substitute sounds incorrectly in a word.

3. Dysnomia can most easily be assessed by
   a. asking the patient to perform a single command.
   b. listening to the fluency of the patient's speech.
   c. asking the patient to read a complex sentence.
   d. asking the patient to name common objects.
   e. asking the patient to write a sentence.

4. The most commonly used mental status screening tests all assess
   a. conceptualization.
   b. figure copying.
   c. naming.
   d. verbal fluency.
   e. memory.

5. Persons with low educational achievement who are administered a mental status screening test

    a. can perform below cut-offs for impairment even when they have not declined in cognitive ability.

    b. are rarely identified as being impaired when they are not.

    c. are as frequently misidentified as showing impairment as well educated persons.

    d. are likely to refuse some of the items.

    e. are less likely to fail than well-educated persons.

6. A dementing disease that is known for its rapid rate of progression is

    a. Alzheimer's disease.

    b. Pick's disease.

    c. Creuzfeldt-Jacob disease.

    d. Progressive Supranuclear Palsy.

    e. Binswanger's disease.

7. A dementing disease that has been associated with early evidence of personality change is

    a. Pick's disease.

    b. Alzheimer's disease.

    c. Wilson's disease.

    d. Etat Lacunaire.

    e. Normal pressure hydrocephalus.

8. In most cases, fewer cognitive tasks can be performed well if there is an impairment in

    a. memory.

    b. spatial ability.

    c. conceptualization.

    d. attention.

    e. language.

9. The language dimension that is most commonly assessed when dementia is suspected is

    a. comprehension.

    b. repetition.

    c. reading.

    d. writing.

    e. naming.

10. The most important thing to include in the assessment of memory for the differential diagnosis of dementia is

    a. immediate recall.

b. the difference between immediate and delayed recall.

c. remote memory.

d. procedural memory.

e. None of the above.

11. The examination of conceptualization includes tasks that evaluate

a. concept formation.

b. set shifting.

c. abstraction.

d. set maintenance.

e. All of the above.

12. If patients have difficulty learning new information, then

a. they will, in most cases, have difficulty remembering things from the remote past.

b. they will, in most cases, have lost the ability to carry out well-learned skills.

c. they can still have the ability to carry out well-learned skills.

d. they will, in most cases, have attentional deficits.

e. they will, in most cases, have language deficits.

13. Neuropsychological testing can assist in

a. the initial diagnosis of a patient.

b. the development of a treatment plan.

c. assessing change in function over time.

d. measuring response to treatment.

e. All of the above.

Chapter 13: Electroencephalography

Choose the one best response

1. The EEG in the elderly

a. does not differ at all from that of young adults.

b. may be used to diagnose dementia.

c. may be used to "rule out" seizures.

d. may normally show temporal slow waves.

e. should be routinely performed in depressed patients.

2. Common "normal" findings in the EEG of the elderly include
   a. a posterior dominant rhythm of less than 9 Hz.
   b. isolated temporal slow waves.
   c. spike-and-wave foci.
   d. All of the above.
   e. a and b only.

3. In the evaluation of confusion, an EEG should be performed
   a. only when delirium is suspected.
   b. whenever there are focal neurologic signs.
   c. to document the presence of an organic mental disorder.
   d. only to rule out possible seizures.
   e. even when the diagnosis of dementia is clear.

4. A normal EEG in an elderly patient is
   a. inconsistent with the presence of dementia.
   b. rules out the presence of an encephalopathy.
   c. seen rarely after the age of 90.
   d. frequently of lower voltage than that in a young adult.
   e. usually lacks an alpha rhythm.

5. The EEG in delirious patients
   a. is almost invariably abnormal.
   b. often shows slowing that is proportional to the level of con-
      fusion.
   c. may appear similar to that of a demented patient.
   d. All of the above.
   e. b and c only.

6. Normal EEGs may be seen in
   a. dementia.
   b. delirium.
   c. aging.
   d. seizure disorders.
   e. All of the above.

Answer a if only 1, 2, and 3 are correct
            b if only 1 and 3 are correct
            c if only 2 and 4 are correct
            d if only 4 is correct
            e if all are correct

7. A seizure disorder may be diagnosed
   1. on the basis of clinical symptoms.
   2. on the basis of spike-and-wave complexes in the EEG.
   3. in the absence of any EEG abnormalities.
   4. with certainty when occipital spikes are detected.

8. Spikes or spike-and-wave complexes
   1. may be seen in patients with Alzheimer's disease.
   2. indicate an increased risk of seizures when seen very frequently in the temporal regions.
   3. are commonly seen as a result of strokes in the elderly.
   4. are never seen in patients who have been seizure free.

9. In the healthy elderly, the EEG
   1. is identical to that of a young adult.
   2. does not attenuate in amplitude.
   3. does not show any temporal slow waves.
   4. always has an alpha rhythm above 8 Hz.

Chapter 14: The Dementias

Choose the one best response

1. With current demographic trends, by the year 2040 the number of severely demented patients in the United States is expected to increase by
   a. 100%
   b. 200%
   c. 300%
   d. 400%
   e. 500%

2. Dementia is a primary feature of all the following *except*
   a. amyotrophic lateral sclerosis
   b. Huntington's disease (Chorea)
   c. Jakob-Cruetzfeldt Disease
   d. normal pressure hydrocephalus
   e. Pick's disease

3. Which of the following psychiatric disorders is most commonly implicated in mistaken diagnosis of dementia?
   a. Conversion disorder.

    b. Major depressive episode.

    c. Acute mania.

    d. Schizophrenia.

    e. Anxiety disorders.

4. Dopamine deficiency has been implicated primarily in

    a. Alzheimer's disease.

    b. Huntington's disease.

    c. Pick's disease.

    d. Parkinson's disease.

    e. All of the above.

5. The most consistently deficient neurotransmitter in Alzheimer's disease is

    a. acetylcholine.

    b. norepinephrine.

    c. dopamine.

    d. GABA.

    e. None of the above.

6. The following is contraindicated when treating depression that accompanies dementia:

    a. MAO inhibitors.

    b. ECT.

    c. Tricyclic antidepressants.

    d. Group psychotherapy.

    e. None of the above.

7. All of the following tend to increase brain acetylcholine levels *except*

    a. physostigmine

    b. lecithin

    c. tetra-hydro aminoacridine (THA)

    d. scopolamine

8. Degeneration of the caudate nucleus characterizes which of the following?

    a. Alzheimer's disease

    b. Parkinson's disease

    c. Huntington's disease

    d. Jakob-Creutzfeldt disease

    e. None of the above

9. Degeneration of the substantia nigra characterizes which of the following?

a. Alzheimer's disease
b. Parkinson's disease
c. Huntington's disease
d. Jakob-Creutzfeldt disease

Answer a if only 1, 2, and 3 are correct
b if only 1 and 3 are correct
c if only 2 and 4 are correct
d if only 4 is correct
e if all are correct

10. Symptoms typical of Huntington's disease include
    1. psychosis.
    2. tremor.
    3. chorea.
    4. myoclonus.

11. Delirium is almost always characterized by
    1. abnormal EEG.
    2. distractibility.
    3. inattention.
    4. amnesia.

12. Which of the following is/are not coded separately in DSM-III-R as a subsyndrome of dementia?
    1. Depression.
    2. Anxiety.
    3. Delusions.
    4. Aggression.

13. The presence of which of the following supports a diagnosis of dementia?
    1. Aphasia.
    2. Amnesia.
    3. Apraxia.
    4. Personality change.

14. The following statements about dementia and depression are true:
    1. Depression occurs in primary degenerative dementia.
    2. Depression can mimic primary degenerative dementia.
    3. Depression is common in caregivers of dementia patients.
    4. Depression complicating dementia is untreatable.

15. Which of the following are characteristic of the pathology of Alzheimer's disease?

    1. Neurofibrillary tangles.
    2. Caudate degeneration.
    3. Senile plaques.
    4. Microvascular infarction.

16. Which of the following should be considered in the long-term management of dementia patients?

    1. Location of residence.
    2. Driving privileges.
    3. Delegation of legal authority (guardianship).
    4. Family support systems.

17. Which of the following typically does *not* involve early motor system disability?

    1. Multi-infarct dementia.
    2. Pick's disease.
    3. Parkinson's disease.
    4. Alzheimer's disease.

18. Which findings can contribute to a pathological diagnosis of multi-infarct dementia?

    1. White matter degeneration.
    2. Large arterial vessel infarction.
    3. Hypertensive lacunae.
    4. Micro-vascular amyloid.

19. Which of the following support a DSM-III-R diagnosis of multi-infarct dementia?

    1. Sudden onset.
    2. Focal neurological findings.
    3. "Patchy" deficits.
    4. Myoclonus.

20. Which of the following conditions may be etiologically related to multi-infarct dementia?

    1. Atrial fibrillation.
    2. Aortic valve sclerosis.
    3. Carotid atherosclerosis.
    4. Hypertension.

Chapter 15: Delirium and Other Organic Mental Disorders

Choose the one best response

1. Which of the following is *not* categorized as an organic mental disorder in DSM-III-R?
   a. Delirium
   b. Organic mood syndrome
   c. Posttraumatic stress disorder
   d. Amnestic syndrome
   e. Organic personality syndrome

2. Common causes of delirium in the elderly include all of the following *except*
   a. Infections
   b. Postoperative status
   c. Toxic effect of drugs
   d. Cardiac failure
   e. Hypoparathyroidism

3. Which of the following is *not* included in the diagnostic criteria for delirium (DSM-III-R):
   a. Reduced ability to maintain attention to external stimuli
   b. Disorganized thinking
   c. Memory impairment
   d. Labile affect
   e. Perceptual disturbances

4. The high-risk period for the development of post-stroke depression is approximately
   a. 6 months.
   b. 1 year.
   c. 2 years.
   d. 4 years.
   e. 7 years.

5. According to Robinson et al., depression is most likely to develop following a stroke involving the
   a. anterior right hemisphere.
   b. anterior left hemisphere.
   c. posterior right hemisphere.
   d. posterior left hemisphere.
   e. brain stem.

6. Which of the following is *not* one of the common causes of organic anxiety syndrome?
   a. Hypoglycemia
   b. Hypercortisolism
   c. Hypothyroidism
   d. Caffeine
   e. Sympathomimetic agents

7. According to Erkinjuntti et al., what percentage of patients with dementia were suffering from delirium on admission to hospital?
   a. 5%
   b. 9%
   c. 18%
   d. 28%
   e. 40%

8. Which of the following is most likely to help a patient with Wernicke's encephalopathy?
   a. Niacin (Vitamin B_3)
   b. Ascorbic acid (Vitamin C)
   c. Thiamine (Vitamin B_1)
   d. Cyanocobalamin (Vitamin B_{12})
   e. Pyridoxine (Vitamin B_6)

Answer a if only 1, 2 and 3 are correct
          b if only 1 and 3 are correct
          c if only 2 and 4 are correct
          d if only 4 is correct
          e if all are correct

9. The clinical features of Wernicke's encephalopathy include
   1. ophthalmoplegia.
   2. anosmia.
   3. ataxia.
   4. cardiac failure.

10. Diagnostic criteria for organic personality syndrome include
    1. affective instability.
    2. recurrent outbursts of aggression or rage.
    3. impaired social judgment.
    4. apathy and indifference.

11. Which of the following can cause mania (organic mood syndrome) in the elderly?

    1. Thyroxine
    2. Hydrochlorothiazide
    3. Levodopa
    4. Propranolol

Chapter 16: Mood Disorders

Choose the one best response

1. Suicide rates are

    a. higher among white females over 65 than among white males over 65 in the United States.
    b. higher among females over 65 than males over 65.
    c. higher among white males over 65 than black males over 65.
    d. affected by age but not cohort.
    e. have steadily increased among the elderly in the United States since the beginning of the 20th century.

2. The most prevalent of the following depressive disorders in late life is

    a. bipolar disorder, depressed type.
    b. single episode of major depression in unipolar depression.
    c. recurrent episodes of major depression in unipolar depression.
    d. dysthymic disorder.
    e. major depression with psychotic features.

3. The following are correct statements regarding the symptoms of major depression in the elderly over 65 *except*

    a. Older people frequently complain of difficulty concentrating and memory problems.
    b. Older people are more likely to complain of suicidal ideation than middle-aged adults.
    c. Older people are less likely to complain of guilt than middle-aged adults.
    d. Sleep problems are a frequent complaint.
    e. Weight loss is more common than weight gain as a symptom of depression.

4. The following are correct statements regarding electroconvulsive therapy in the elderly *except*
   a. It is effective in treating major depression with psychotic features.
   b. It is effective in treating major depression with melancholia.
   c. Cardiotoxic effect is less than for tricyclic antidepressants.
   d. It does not produce memory difficulties when pulse unilateral nondominant treatments are prescribed.
   e. It is contraindicated with mass lesions in the brain.

5. Psychotherapy for the treatment of late-life depression
   a. has not proven effective in controlled trials.
   b. should be limited to cognitive/behavioral therapies.
   c. is poorly tolerated by older adults.
   d. can be effective for nonmelancholic depressive disorders.
   e. requires effective termination in order to be successful.

6. Major depression in the elderly is more frequent in
   a. women than men.
   b. the oldest old than the young old.
   c. cognitively intact than cognitively impaired.
   d. blacks than non-blacks.
   e. None of the above.

7. The following lesions on magnetic resonance imaging (MRI) scanning have been found more prevalent among the elderly suffering major depression than age-matched controls:
   a. Cortical infarcts
   b. Subcortical white matter lucencies
   c. Atrophy of the locus ceruleus
   d. Shrinkage in ventricular size
   e. Temporal lobe atrophy

Answer a if only 1, 2, and 3 are correct.
          b if only 1 and 3 are correct.
          c if only 2 and 4 are correct.
          d if only 4 is correct.
          e if all are correct.

8. An elderly patient with Parkinson's disease is at increased risk for developing the following disorders:
   1. Schizophrenia

2. Dementia
3. Bipolar disorder
4. Major depression

9. In the elderly suffering from major depression, which antidepressants are least likely to result in postural hypotension?
   1. Nortriptyline
   2. Amitriptyline
   3. Desipramine
   4. Thioridazine

10. To prevent recurrence of mania or depressive episodes, the following drugs have been demonstrated effective in controlled trials:
    1. Valproic acid
    2. Lithium carbonate
    3. Carbamazepine
    4. Phenytoin

11. The following is true of depression in the elderly:
    1. Familial or genetic contribution is less likely in late life.
    2. Increased monoamine oxidase levels have been hypothesized to produce age-related biologic vulnerabilities to depression.
    3. Leukoencephalopathy is observed in late-life depression.
    4. Impaired social support predicts onset but not outcome of late onset depression.

12. The following conditions are associated with depression in the elderly:
    1. Cushing's disease
    2. Hypothyroidism
    3. Subdural-hematoma
    4. Right-sided stroke

Chapter 17: Psychoses

Choose the one correct response

1. Auditory hallucinations
   a. occur more often than delusions in patients with Alzheimer dementia.

    b. are pathognomonic of "paranoia," as defined by Kraepelin.

    c. may be inferred from the behavior of an Alzheimer patient.

    d. do not occur in late-onset schizophrenia.

    e. None of the above.

2. A 67-year-old man with dementia is given thioridazine to reduce his agitation. Which of the following statements is true, concerning this medication:

    a. The medication may cause delirium to worsen.

    b. The patient will likely require higher doses of the drug than would a 30-year-old woman.

    c. The drug produces extrapyramidal symptoms in the majority of patients.

    d. The drug is likely to improve cognitive functioning.

    e. None of the above.

3. All of the following are true statements about late-onset schizophrenia *except*

    a. Onset can be after age 55.

    b. Premorbidly schizoid personality may be associated with this disorder.

    c. Patients may respond to low doses of neuroleptics.

    d. Men are more likely than women to develop this disorder.

    e. None of the above.

4. Prevalence of schizophrenia in first-degree relatives of probands with late-onset schizophrenia is

    a. the same as that in families of normal controls.

    b. greater than that in families of normal controls.

    c. the same as that in families of earlier-onset schizophrenics.

    d. greater than that in families of earlier-onset schizophrenics.

    e. None of the above.

Answer a if 1, 2, and 3 are correct

           b if 1 and 3 are correct

           c if 2 and 4 are correct

           d if 4 is correct

           e if all are correct

5. Delusional disorder

    1. usually presents in middle to late adulthood.

    2. occurs in about 8%–15% of the psychiatric population.

3. has a somewhat earlier age of onset in men than in women.
4. is characterized by the presence of bizarre delusions.

6. Regarding the elderly delusional patient and neuroleptic medications,
   1. the elderly usually require lower doses.
   2. a relatively high risk of tardive dyskinesia may be expected.
   3. noncompliance is a common problem.
   4. the low-potency neuroleptics are superior to high-potency neuroleptics.

7. Schneiderian first-rank symptoms characterize
   1. late-onset schizophrenia.
   2. Alzheimer dementia.
   3. early-onset schizophrenia.
   4. delusional disorder.

8. Duration of psychotic symptoms of 2 months is *inconsistent* with a diagnosis of
   1. delusional disorder.
   2. brief reactive psychosis.
   3. schizophreniform disorder.
   4. schizophrenia.

9. Aging of schizophrenic patients taking a neuroleptic is usually accompanied by
   1. increased severity of positive symptoms.
   2. appearance of visual hallucinations.
   3. development of new types of delusions.
   4. remission of illness in one-third of patients.

Chapter 18: Anxiety and Personality Disorders

Answer a if only 1, 2, and 3 are correct
        b if only 1 and 3 are correct
        c if only 2 and 4 are correct
        d if only 4 is correct
        e if all are correct

1. Based on recent epidemiologic data, which one of the following statements about anxiety disorders is correct?
   1. Phobic disorders usually emerge in the mid-thirties.

2. The mean age for onset of panic disorder is in the mid-twenties.
3. Men and women over 65 have the same prevalence of anxiety disorders.
4. The prevalence of anxiety disorders declines by age 65.

2. Treatment of anxiety disorders in geriatric patients
   1. is mainly pharmacologic.
   2. is characterized mostly by the use of low-dose neuroleptic medications.
   3. is sometimes successfully achieved by treatment of concurrent major depression.
   4. is prescribed mostly by psychiatrists.

3. According to the maturation hypotheses of personality disorders,
   1. DSM-III-R personality disorders can be divided into mature and immature categories.
   2. impulsiveness and suicide in patients with antisocial personality disorder decline over time.
   3. immature personality disorders tend to have earlier onset than mature personality disorders.
   4. florid borderline symptomatology usually remains stable over many years.

4. Which of the following syndromes are commonly associated with personality disorders or dysfunctional personality traits in the elderly?
   1. Dysthymia
   2. Double depression
   3. Masked depression
   4. Pseudodementia

5. The following statement(s) characterize personality disorders in the elderly:
   1. They invariably emerge in adolescence or young adulthood.
   2. Symptoms of the personality disorder must reflect the individual's recent and long-term functioning.
   3. They must be present continuously from young adulthood to old age to meet DSM-III-R criteria.
   4. Their course may be affected by major depression, organic brain changes, or reactions to age-related life events.

Chapter 19: Alcohol and Drug Dependence

Choose the one best response

1. According to DSM-III-R criteria, alcohol and drug dependence are defined, in part, by the elements of addiction, which are
   a. preoccupation with acquisition.
   b. compulsive use of alcohol and drugs.
   c. pattern of relapse.
   d. All of the above.

Answer a if only 1, 2, and 3 are correct
      b if only 1 and 3 are correct
      c if only 2 and 4 are correct
      d if only 4 is correct
      e if all are correct

2. The bimodal distribution for the onset of alcoholism proposes which of the following:
   1. A common onset of alcoholism is in early adulthood.
   2. Remission from alcoholism occurs in middle age and relapses in later ages.
   3. A second common onset of alcoholism arises de novo in individuals over the age of 60.
   4. Early-onset alcoholism is diagnosed by different criteria.

3. The data support which of the following statements about the use of legal drugs by the elderly:
   1. The elderly are the largest users of legal drugs.
   2. The elderly account for 30% of all prescriptions.
   3. At least one drug is prescribed at two-thirds of all office visits for patients over age 65.
   4. Twenty-five percent of all individuals of geriatric age use psychoactive drugs.

4. Regarding the prevalence of alcohol and drug dependence among inpatients, which of the following has been found:
   1. Ten to twenty percent of general medical geriatric patients are alcohol and drug dependent.
   2. Twenty-five to fifty percent of general medical geriatric patients are alcohol and drug dependent.
   3. Twenty-five to fifty percent of general psychiatric patients are alcohol and drug dependent.

4. Fifty to seventy-five percent of general psychiatric patients are alcohol and drug dependent.

5. Regarding drug dependence among the elderly, which of the following has been established:
   1. The physician is the largest source of drugs.
   2. The consequences of drug dependence are similar for the elderly and the young.
   3. The lifetime prevalence rate for illicit drugs is less than 1%.
   4. Surgical complications account for the majority of the risk for developing drug dependence.

6. Among the reasons for the high prevalence of use of over-the-counter medications are which of the following:
   1. Many are psychotropic medications.
   2. The cost is similar to prescribed medications.
   3. The elderly commonly have ailments that correspond to the available medications.
   4. The elderly have less pharmacological sensitivity to medications in general.

7. The consequences of alcohol and drug dependence may be different for the elderly in comparison to younger adults in which of the following ways:
   1. The elderly suffer from interpersonal and intrapsychic problems.
   2. The elderly have alcohol-related legal problems.
   3. The elderly have family problems.
   4. The elderly are often not employed.

8. Which of the following statements are characteristic of tolerance and dependence to alcohol and drugs in the elderly:
   1. Marked tolerance and dependence develop.
   2. The definitions for tolerance and dependence are different for the elderly than the young.
   3. Tolerance increases with increasing age.
   4. Tolerance and dependence are not essential criteria for the diagnoses of alcohol and drug dependence.

9. The sensitivity to alcohol and drugs is increased in the elderly because:
   1. The intravascular volume is increased.
   2. The neuroreceptors have increased sensitivity.

3. The alcohol and drug concentrations are decreased.
4. The lean muscle mass is less.

10. The development of alcohol dependence depends on which major variables according to the genetic and environment models:

    1. The existence of an additional psychiatric disorder.
    2. The presence of a family history of alcoholism.
    3. The origin of birth near the equator.
    4. The exposure to alcohol.

11. Chronic administration of benzodiazepines may lead to

    1. tolerance and dependence.
    2. anxiety.
    3. insomnia.
    4. depression.

12. In the diagnosis and treatment of alcohol and drug dependence in the elderly,

    1. the elderly may require inpatient detoxification because of concurrent medical problems.
    2. effective treatment is not available.
    3. adequate diagnosis is not possible in geriatric patients.
    4. similar treatments are effective in the elderly and the young but special considerations may be necessary.

13. Which of the following statements regarding diagnosis of alcohol and drug dependence have been documented in geriatric populations:

    1. Alcohol and drug dependence are underdiagnosed.
    2. Denial is a prominent obstacle to diagnosis.
    3. Alcohol and drug dependence are primary disorders.
    4. Direct confrontation of the patient is never indicated.

14. Stimulants and depressants have which of the following pharmacological characteristics:

    1. Both produce depression with chronic use.
    2. Only stimulants produce hallucinations.
    3. Both induce tolerance and dependence.
    4. Only depressants produce anxiety.

Chapter 20: Sleep Disorders

Choose the one best response

1. Age effects on sleep include all the following *except*
   a. decreasing stages 3 and 4 sleep with increasing sleep.
   b. increasing stage 1 sleep with advancing age.
   c. decreasing percentage of REM sleep with increasing age.
   d. increasing numbers of arousals after sleep onset with increasing age.
   e. relative age stability of sleep latency.

2. The electroencephalographic sleep characteristics of major depression in elderly adults include all of the following *except*
   a. short REM sleep latency.
   b. increased amounts of stages 3 and 4 relative to normals.
   c. shift of REM sleep time and rapid eye movement activity into the first half of the night.
   d. difficulty maintaining sleep and early morning awakening.
   e. increased total sleep time in the depressed phase of manic-depressive illness.

3. Which *one* of the following is *not* characteristic of obstructive sleep apnea?
   a. Complications include first and second degree heart block.
   b. Morning headache, confusion, depression, and impotence.
   c. NREM apneas longer than REM apneas.
   d. More common in men than in women and in the elderly than in the young.
   e. May respond to protriptyline, progestational agents, or tracheotomy.

4. All of the following characterize sleep changes in Alzheimer's dementia *except*
   a. decreased phasic activity (spindles, K-complexes) during NREM sleep.
   b. increased phasic rapid eye movements during dream sleep.
   c. increased prevalence of sleep apnea.
   d. loss of sleep-wake consolidation, i.e., polyphasic sleep-wake patterns.
   e. relatively normal circadian temperature rhythmicity.

5. For the long-term management of chronic insomnia in late life, all of the following should be considered as having a definite role in the treatment armamentarium *except*

   a. stimulus control
   b. temporal control
   c. sleep restriction therapy
   d. enhanced aerobic fitness
   e. short-acting benzodiazepine

6. Agitated behavior at sundown or at night is frequently associated with

   a. dementia.
   b. recent relocation or room shift.
   c. sleeping pill prescription.
   d. sleep apnea or partial arousals from REM sleep.
   e. All of the above.

7. All of the following statements about the pharmacotherapy of late-life insomnia are true *except*

   a. A sedating phenothiazine probably has less behavioral toxicity than a benzodiazepine in an agitated demented patient.
   b. Long-acting benzodiazepines probably have less behavioral toxicity than shorter-acting benzodiazepines.
   c. Benzodiazepines may exacerbate sleep apnea.
   d. Low-dose sedating antidepressant medication probably retains its sedating efficacy longer and has less behavioral toxicity than a benzodiazepine.
   e. Some nonpsychotropic drugs such as alpha-methyldopa or diphenhydramine can cause daytime sedation and disrupt sleep/wake rhythms.

8. Approximately what proportion of patients with major or endogenous depression improve transiently after all-night sleep deprivation?

   a. 10%
   b. 30%
   c. 50%
   d. 70%
   e. 90%

9. Approximately what proportion of spousally bereaved individuals will report ongoing sleep disturbance 13 months after their loss?

   a. 10%
   b. 30%

c. 50%
d. 70%
e. 90%

10. Snoring has been shown to be a risk factor for which of the following:
    a. Sleep apnea
    b. Hypertension
    c. Ischemic heart disease
    d. Stroke
    e. All of the above

11. The proportion of community-resident elderly with five or more apneas per hour of sleep is approximately
    a. 5%
    b. 18%
    c. 24%
    d. 40%
    e. 65%

Answer a if only 1, 2, and 3 are correct
           b if only 1 and 3 are correct
           c if only 2 and 4 are correct
           d if only 4 is correct
           e if all are correct

12. True statements about the age-dependent changes in the structure and circadian distribution of sleep include
    1. Elderly men sleep less deeply and have more arousals from sleep than elderly women.
    2. The major sleep period is frequently shifted earlier in time in the elderly (i.e., phase advanced).
    3. The frequency of arousals after sleep onset increases with age, due partly to the increased prevalence of sleep apnea and nocturnal myoclonus with advancing age.
    4. While the percentage of REM sleep is usually maintained until old age, the percentage of time spent asleep in slow-wave sleep increases in old age.

13. Physiological differences between REM and non-REM sleep include the following:
    1. During REM sleep, heart rate, respiratory rate, and blood pressure tend to decrease.

2. The onset of REM sleep is mediated by the firing of cholinergic cells in the pontine tegmentum.
3. Ventilatory response to increased concentrations of inhaled CO_2 is enhanced during REM sleep compared to non-REM sleep.
4. The occurrence of REM sleep is more likely near the nadir or throughout the circadian temperature rhythm.

14. Which of the following has (have) antidepressive efficacy in melancholia?
    1. whole-night sleep deprivation.
    2. REM-sleep deprivation.
    3. deprivation of sleep during the second half of the night.
    4. deprivation of sleep during the first half of the night.

Chapter 21: Sexuality

Answer a if only 1, 2, and 3 are correct
            b if only 1 and 3 are correct
            c if only 2 and 4 are correct
            d if only 4 is correct
            e if all are correct

1. Erectile disorders
   1. may occur transiently at any age.
   2. may be related to alcohol excess.
   3. may be related to anxiety, conflict, depression, divorce, grief.
   4. may be psychogenic, but organic causes must be ruled out since both may co-exist.

2. Orgasmic disorders in women over the age of 65
   1. rarely occur.
   2. are not uncommon.
   3. are always due to urinary infections.
   4. are responsive to brief sex therapy.

3. The following ingested substances may cause reversible impotency and/or ejaculatory difficulties:
   1. ethanol
   2. antihypertensives

    3. propranolol
    4. antibiotics

4. A man, 53 years old, is being discharged after coronary bypass surgery. He asks about resuming sex relations. The physician's best response(s) is/are:

    1. He should forget sex because of danger to his heart.
    2. He may have sex as soon as he can walk up two flights of stairs comfortably.
    3. He should instead jog every evening to avoid sex.
    4. His physical reaction during masturbation is slightly more intense than during coitus.

5. Psychosexual dysfunctions include

    1. recurrent problems with obtaining erection or ejaculation.
    2. concerns about body image.
    3. recurrent problems with orgasm or sexual desire.
    4. teen pregnancy.

6. Brief sex therapy for sexual dysfunction includes

    1. a brief sex history of symptom duration, relationship to illness, medications, stress, and interpersonal conflict.
    2. a thorough physical examination plus sex education.
    3. suggestions of home reading and specific home body-massage exercises.
    4. analysis of transference and personality restructuring.

7. Premature ejaculation

    1. is a common sexual dysfunction that sometimes is followed by erectile disorder.
    2. is highly responsive to brief sex therapy.
    3. is related to high anxiety about sexual performance.
    4. usually improves physiologically after age 50 years.

8. Management of erectile disorder includes

    1. genital examination: vascular, blood hormone/glucose profile.
    2. invasive techniques: penile injections or surgical implants.
    3. noninvasive techniques: brief sex therapy, mechanical external vacuum devices.
    4. referral for group therapy.

9. Dyspareunia in women over 50 years
   1. is unknown in those with children.
   2. may relate to menopausal atrophic vaginitis.
   3. is usually due to unconscious rejection of males.
   4. responds to local or systemic estrogen and lubrication for coitus.

10. Libido differences at any age
    1. are common when either partner has a higher sex drive than the other.
    2. are usually neurotic.
    3. are not considered a diagnostic category.
    4. rarely become a medical complaint.

Chapter 22: Psychopharmacology

Choose the one best response

1. Decreased renal function with age results in
   a. increased hepatic metabolism of neuroleptics.
   b. decreased volume of drug distribution of lipid-soluble drugs.
   c. decreased excretion of hydroxylated TCA metabolites.
   d. increased gastrointestinal absorption of lithium.

2. Secondary amine TCAs, as contrasted with tertiary amine TCAs, are characterized by
   a. greater orthostatic hypotensive effects.
   b. less anticholinergic effect.
   c. higher plasma concentrations per milligram dose.
   d. less efficacy in the elderly.

3. Very low plasma concentration of TCA in depressed nonresponders suggests
   a. rapid hepatic metabolism.
   b. poor compliance.
   c. slow hepatic metabolism.
   d. either a or b.

4. Pharmacodynamics can be altered by all of the following *except*
   a. drug interactions at tissue level.

   b. diseases.
   c. aging.
   d. decreased absorption.

5. High-potency neuroleptics, compared to low-potency neuroleptics, produce
   a. fewer extrapyramidal side effects.
   b. greater sedation.
   c. less orthostatic hypotension.
   d. greater anticholinergic effect.

6. Risks of benzodiazepine use in the elderly include
   a. cognitive dysfunction.
   b. manic states.
   c. quinidine-like cardiac effects.
   d. hypertension.

7. Assessment of blood pressure in antidepressant and neuroleptic treatment should always include
   a. exercise stress values.
   b. sitting values only.
   c. orthostatic measurement.
   d. bedtime measurement.

8. Changes in plasma proteins in the elderly lead to
   a. increased albumin with decreased free benzodiazepine con-
      centrations.
   b. altered binding of lithium salts.
   c. increases in total plasma TCA concentrations.
   d. both a and b.

9. Adequate drug treatment of delusional depression most often
   requires
   a. neuroleptic treatment alone.
   b. antidepressant drug treatment alone.
   c. combined lithium and antidepressant treatment.
   d. combined neuroleptic and antidepressant treatment.

10. Use of anticholinergic agents can be associated with
    a. urinary retention.
    b. bradycardia.
    c. altered thyroid function.
    d. All of the above.

11. Compliance with drugs in the elderly can be facilitated by
    a. divided dose regimens.
    b. cognitive impairment.
    c. using the fewest drugs.
    d. None of the above.

12. Congestive heart failure is associated with
    a. decreased risk of orthostatic hypotension.
    b. increased hepatic drug metabolism.
    c. decreased renal drug clearance.
    d. a + b.

13. The following statements are true of quinidine-like prolonged conduction time *except*
    a. It is a toxic effect of TCAs.
    b. It is exacerbated by type I antiarrhythmics used with TCAs.
    c. It is correlated with plasma TCA and hydroxylated metabolite concentrations.
    d. It occurs more often with MAO inhibitors than TCAs.

14. Neuroleptic side effects that occur frequently in the elderly include all of the following *except*
    a. dystonia.
    b. pseudoparkinsonism.
    c. tardive dyskinesia.
    d. akathisia.

15. Which of the following statements is true about monoamine oxidase inhibitors:
    a. They produce orthostatic blood pressure effects within a few days if they are likely to occur at a given dose.
    b. They are clinically useful in combination with fluoxetine.
    c. They are effective in maintaining symptom remission in major depression.
    d. They have potent anticholinergic effects.

16. In patients with degenerative dementia,
    a. abnormalities of catecholaminergic as well as acetylcholinergic systems are found in postmortem brain tissue.
    b. depressive syndromes are responsive to TCAs.
    c. neuroleptics can decrease cognitive performance.
    d. All of the above.

17. In using lithium salts, which of the following drug interactions are relevant to the elderly:

a. Benzodiazepine increases volume of distribution.
b. Antidepressants decrease absorption.
c. Diuretics decrease clearance.
d. Nonsteroidal antiinflammatory drugs increase clearance.

18. All of the following have been useful in treating agitation in elderly patients with dementia *except*
   a. stimulants
   b. neuroleptics
   c. benzodiazepines
   d. lithium salts

19. Steady-state plasma concentrations of a drug are
   a. inversely proportional to volume of distribution.
   b. achieved after 5–6 half-lives.
   c. inversely proportional to absorbed dose.
   d. a and b.

Chapter 23: Electroconvulsive Therapy

Answer a if only 1, 2, and 3 are correct
            b if only 1 and 3 are correct
            c if only 2 and 4 are correct
            d if only 4 is correct
            e if all are correct

1. Indications for ECT in the elderly include
   1. major depressive disorder.
   2. schizoaffective disorder.
   3. bipolar disorder.
   4. severe organic affective psychosis.

2. ECT may be especially effective for elderly patients with symptoms of
   1. delusional depression.
   2. nondelusional depression with somatic preoccupation.
   3. depressive pseudodementia.
   4. major depression with neuroleptic-induced movement disorders.

3. The clinical features that frequently indicate a better outcome from ECT in the depressed elderly include

1. situational stress.
2. guilt feelings.
3. death of a spouse.
4. delusions.

4. When comparing ECT in the elderly with ECT in young adult populations,
   1. efficacy of ECT diminishes with age.
   2. safety and possible complications from ECT become of greater concern with age.
   3. the higher incidence of memory problems in the elderly make ECT much less suitable for this population.
   4. elderly patients tend to have a higher seizure threshold than young patients.

5. ECT has been successfully used in the elderly to treat
   1. major depression.
   2. Alzheimer's disease.
   3. affective disorder with coexistent neuroleptic-induced parkinsonism.
   4. dysthymia.

6. ECT in the treatment of major depression in the elderly has been shown to be as effective if not more effective than
   1. tricyclic antidepressants.
   2. monoamine oxidase inhibitors (MAOI).
   3. sham ECT.
   4. combination neuroleptic/tricyclic.

7. Absolute contraindictions to ECT include
   1. recent myocardial or cerebral infarction.
   2. severe hypertension.
   3. age over 90 years.
   4. None of the above.

8. Pre-ECT evaluation of the mouth of the elderly patient is important to determine
   1. number, location, and stability of existing permanent teeth.
   2. identification of any dentures (full or partial).
   3. if dental consult is necessary to evaluate safety for patient.
   4. strength of masseter muscle.

9. Medical problems of elderly patients who often can be treated successfully with ECT as long as special observation and precautions are taken include

    1. severe degenerative joint disease.
    2. hypertension.
    3. angina.
    4. remote stroke with ongoing anticoagulation therapy.

10. Various premedications to prevent the development of danger-
    ous hypertension, tachycardia, rebound hypotension, brady-
    cardia, and bradyarrhythmias include
    1. labetalol.
    2. esmolol.
    3. propranolol.
    4. succinylcholine.

11. Total relaxation of the patient after administration of succi-
    nylcholine can be evaluated by observing for
    1. cessation of fasciculations.
    2. loss of deep tendon reflexes.
    3. loss of facial, radial, or other nerve reflex (by nerve stimu-
    lator).
    4. abdominal relaxation.

12. Older patients treated with ECT for primary affective dis-
    orders may have temporary (or longer) improvement in the fol-
    lowing movement disorders
    1. idiopathic Parkinson's disease.
    2. neuroleptic-induced parkinsonism.
    3. dystonias.
    4. tardive dyskinesia.

13. Lithium administration coincident with ECT
    1. may pose a hazard because it prolongs the muscular block-
    ade of succinylcholine.
    2. has been shown to improve outcome of ECT in the elderly.
    3. has been implicated in producing acute confusional states.
    4. may work synergistically to lessen the symptoms of depres-
    sion.

Choose the one best response

14. Treatment of patients with arrhythmias with ECT may include
    a. pre-ECT lidocaine.
    b. pre-ECT verapamil.

    c. post-ECT digitalis.

    d. post-ECT lidocaine or verapamil.

15. Most studies indicate that the least memory loss in patients treated with ECT is associated with

    a. sine-wave with bilateral electrode placement.

    b. sine-wave with unilateral electrode placement.

    c. brief pulse with bilateral electrode placement.

    d. brief pulse with unilateral electrode placement.

16. Patients on anticoagulation therapy

    a. should not have ECT.

    b. should be switched from warfarin to heparin just prior to ECT.

    c. can be maintained on warfarin throughout ECT series.

    d. are at a greater risk for cardiovascular problems with warfarin during ECT.

17. Regarding maintenance ECT in the elderly,

    a. coexistent use of maintenance lithium should always be employed if possible.

    b. the frequency of maintenance ECT should gradually be decreased and the interval treatments be increased over time and then discontinued when possible.

    c. the pre-ECT workup including laboratory and other testing should be current to the prior 12 months.

    d. maintenance ECT should be employed subsequent to all series of ECT.

18. ECT is most often implemented as a first choice treatment for elderly patients

    a. with severe symptoms of delusional depression.

    b. who are on multiple cardiac medications.

    c. who have had previous ECT.

    d. who have bipolar disorder and obsessive-compulsive traits.

19. Post-ECT treatment for the elderly usually includes

    a. maintenance heterocyclic antidepressants and/or maintenance ECT.

    b. psychoanalytic psychotherapy.

    c. benzodiazepines.

    d. L-tryptophan.

Chapter 24: Individual Psychotherapy

Choose the one best response

1. In psychodynamic psychotherapy with the elderly,
    a. transference should not be interpreted.
    b. the normative elderly cannot tolerate regression.
    c. psychoanalysis is contraindicated for those over age 70.
    d. significant adult relationships of the patient appear in the transference.
    e. All of the above.

2. Regarding cognitive therapy with the elderly,
    a. depressed patients with endogenous signs respond better than those without endogenous signs.
    b. cognitive therapy does not have to be modified to the special problems of the elderly.
    c. cognitive therapy is especially efficacious for the depressed, cognitively impaired patient with a concomitant personality disorder.
    d. cognitive therapy with the elderly has the advantages of being time limited and easily integrated with other treatment modalities.
    e. None of the above.

3. In the elderly patient with a dramatic (Cluster B) personality disorder, which of the following signs are often observed:
    a. clinging behavior
    b. somatization
    c. apathetic withdrawal
    d. reacting to others as all-good or all-bad
    e. All of the above

4. Treatment of the elderly patient with a personality disorder may include
    a. behavior modification.
    b. psychodynamically oriented psychotherapy.
    c. psychotropic medication.
    d. milieu therapy.
    e. All of the above.

Answer a if only 1, 2, and 3 are correct
b if only 1 and 3 are correct
c if only 2 and 4 are correct
d if only 4 is correct
e of all are correct

5. Pyschotherapy with the elderly
   1. should be predominantly supportive.
   2. is effective in treatment of depression.
   3. is most effective if family interview does not contaminate the transference.
   4. should only involve the family of the competent elderly patient with the permission of the patient.

6. In the initial psychotherapy sessions with the frail elderly, the therapist
   1. maintains a neutral reflective attitude.
   2. conveys the therapist's acceptance and desire to help.
   3. maintains a distant, reserved attitude.
   4. actively explores and works through resistances to treatment.

7. Developmental tasks of later-life include
   1. adapting to biopsychosocial losses.
   2. accepting shifts in traditional masculine/feminine roles.
   3. maintaining self-esteem and a sense of continuity with one's past.
   4. returning to adolescent modes of coping.

8. Psychotherapy with the elderly
   1. rarely includes cognitive/behavioral techniques.
   2. can engender in the therapist grandiose wishes to conquer death.
   3. should rarely terminate because of the patient's powerful dependency.
   4. often induces feelings of sadness and pity that impede accurate empathy.

9. In treating the cognitively impaired elderly,
   a. psychodynamic issues are often of practical importance.
   b. behavioral techniques are most effective if used in conjunction with other verbal or environmental interventions.
   c. the aim is often to reduce excess disability.

   d. aggressive introduction of reality helps the paranoid, cog-
     nitively impaired patient to give up his/her delusion.

Chapter 25: Family Therapy

Choose the one best response

1. Indications for family therapy in geriatrics include
   a. intrafamilial diversity of perceptions of the elderly rela-
      tive's impairments.
   b. relocation decision-making.
   c. abuse, neglect, or exploitation.
   d. caregiver stress.
   e. All of the above.

2. Demographic data of those over 65 include the following:
   a. 80% have surviving children.
   b. 20% have never been married.
   c. 50% have a surviving sibling.
   d. 25% of women had one or more children.
   e. 5% of first marriages reach the 50th anniversary.

3. Stress in caregivers of the elderly
   a. is statistically unassociated with elder abuse.
   b. is associated with social isolation.
   c. generates little conflict in the nuclear family.
   d. leads to symptoms of depression in the majority of care-
      givers.
   e. None of the above.

4. The family therapist can improve communications between
   family members of the elderly by
   a. reducing conflict by seeing identified patient and children
      in separate sessions.
   b. focusing on reminiscence as the primary intervention.
   c. focusing on the identified patient.
   d. focusing attention on the "identified" primary caregiver.
   e. None of the above.

Answer a if only 1, 2, and 3 are correct
           b if only 1 and 3 are correct
           c if only 2 and 4 are correct
           d if only 4 is only correct
           e if all are correct

5. Models of family therapy for the elderly
   1. have research-proven outcomes.
   2. are widely practiced by psychiatrists.
   3. have Medicare procedure codes.
   4. can include determination of individual defense mechanisms.

6. The family therapist can effectively contribute by
   1. overcoming familial resistance to use of appropriate extra-familial resources.
   2. helping families of the elderly monitor medications.
   3. being patient advocate when needed community resources are unavailable.
   4. primarily advocating for the victimized family member.

7. Family therapy models include
   1. network therapy.
   2. focus on "justice" and "loyalty."
   3. home support services.
   4. modeling of roles.

8. Goals of family therapy include
   1. enhancing the identified patient's sexual experience.
   2. dealing with death anxiety in the identified patient.
   3. enhancing split transference.
   4. multigenerational conflict resolution.

Chapter 26: Group Therapy

Answer a if only 1, 2, and 3 are correct
b if only 1 and 3 are correct
c if only 2 and 4 are correct
d if only 4 is correct
e if all are correct

1. Important components of effective group psychotherapy with the cognitively impaired elderly include
   1. active reinforcement of interpersonal and cognitive skills.
   2. therapist modeling of activities and exercise.
   3. ongoing reality orientation on the ward.
   4. therapist interpretation of group dynamics and process.

2. Obstacles to the effective utilization of group psychotherapy with the elderly may include

    1. culturally derived resistances to self-disclosure.
    2. therapist countertransference.
    3. patient's physical disability and sensory deficits.
    4. interdisciplinary competition within institutional settings.

3. Factors associated with poor outcome in the group psychotherapy of the depressed elderly include

    1. presence of severe physical illness.
    2. chronicity of depression.
    3. irregular attendance.
    4. age of patient.

4. Common manifestations of therapist countertransference in
the group psychotherapy of elderly patients include

    1. feelings of pessimism and demoralization.
    2. feelings of specialness.
    3. boredom.
    4. therapist level of activity increased relative to psychody-
namic psychotherapy groups with younger adults.

Choose the one best response

5. Regarding group composition, it is most important that the
group members be homogeneous in terms of

    a. level of physical functioning.
    b. age.
    c. level of cognitive functioning.
    d. marital status.
    e. gender.

6. Resocialization and remotivation therapy groups for the cognitively impaired elderly generally emphasize all of the following *except*

    a. reality orientation.
    b. insight.
    c. sensory stimulation.
    d. memory.
    e. interpersonal interaction.

7. Therapeutic aspects of life-review group therapy include

    a. restoration of self-esteem.
    b. grief work.
    c. stimulation of group cohesion.

    d. linkage of reminiscence to the here-and-now group process.

    e. All of the above.

8. The treatment objectives of group therapy with the elderly include

    a. reduction of feelings of isolation.

    b. acquisition of interpersonal skills.

    c. restoration of self-esteem.

    d. grieving of losses.

    e. All of the above.

Chapter 27: Psychiatric Aspects of Long-Term Care

Choose the one correct response

1. The proportion of Americans older than 65 who reside in long-term care facilities is

    a. 1%.

    b. 5%.

    c. 12%.

    d. 20%.

    e. 25%.

2. What percentage of Americans can now expect to spend part of their lives in a nursing home?

    a. 1%

    b. 5%

    c. 12%

    d. 20%

    e. 25%

3. The prevalence of DSM-III-R psychiatric disorders among residents of long-term care facilities is

    a. ≤2%.

    b. 10%.

    c. 25% to 40%.

    d. 50%.

    e. ≥75%.

4. Psychotic symptoms have been reported in what percentage of patients with a primary dementing illness?

    a. 3–10%

b. 10–20%
c. 25–50%
d. 55–75%
e. 75–90%

5. What percentage of residents of long-term care facilities receive psychotropic medications?

a. 5%
b. 25%
c. 50%
d. 75%
e. 90%

6. The two most commonly prescribed classes of psychotropic medications for residents of long-term care facilities are

a. neuroleptics and lithium.
b. barbiturates and benzodiazepines.
c. neuroleptics and antidepressants.
d. neuroleptics and benzodiazepines.
e. antidepressants and benzodiazepines.

7. The majority of psychiatric consultations requested in long-term care settings are for the evaluation and treatment of

a. depression.
b. delirium.
c. behavioral disturbances.
d. schizophrenia.
e. cognitive impairment.

Answer a if only 1, 2, and 3 are correct
b if only 1 and 3 are correct
c if only 2 and 4 are correct
d if only 4 is correct
e if all are correct

8. The psychiatric diagnoses most commonly reported in residents of nursing homes are

1. generalized anxiety disorder.
2. depression.
3. schizophrenia.
4. dementia.

9. The risks of mechanical restraints are
   1. increased risk of falls and other injuries.
   2. skin breakdown.
   3. physiological effects of immobilization stress.
   4. disorganized behavior.

10. The Omnibus Budget Reconciliation Act (OBRA) and Health Care Financing Administration (HCFA) regulations require
    1. that residents of long-term care facilities who display psychosocial adjustment difficulties receive appropriate treatment and services.
    2. that residents of long-term care facilities must not be administered psychotropic medications or placed in physical restraints for the purpose of convenience or discipline.
    3. that an independent, external consultant must review, at least annually, the appropriateness of psychopharmacological treatment of residents in long-term care facilities.
    4. that psychopharmacological medications can only be administered to a resident in a long-term care facility on the orders of a physician and only as part of a documented treatment plan.

Chapter 28: Consultation-Liaison in the General Hospital

Answer a if only 1, 2, and 3 are correct
   b if only 1 and 3 are correct
   c if only 2 and 4 are correct
   d if only 4 is correct
   e if all are correct

1. Among patients age 60 and over referred for psychiatric consultation in a general hospital,
   1. there is a pattern of under-referral in comparing the percentage of geriatric cases referred for consultation versus the percentage of geriatric cases admitted to the medical-surgical wards.
   2. a recent trend is for the treating medical-surgical physician to refer early in the hospital course.
   3. a recent trend is for the treating medical-surgical physician to refer more severe cases in terms of psychiatric disorder compared to referrals of younger patients.
   4. there is a trend to refer only those elderly patients who are in need of transfer to an inpatient psychiatric ward.

2. Patients seen in consultation for behavioral or psychiatric complications of dementia such as confusion, agitation, or psychosis

   1. are more likely to be admitted from the ER than are patients representing other diagnostic categories.
   2. are less likely to be admitted from the ER than are patients representing other diagnostic categories.
   3. represent the greatest percentage of geriatric patients seen in emergency consultation.
   4. contribute to the overutilization of the ER by geriatric patients.

3. The elderly suffer a disproportionate amount of disease and constitute a significant proportion of patients in general hospitals. Facts supportive of this statement include:

   1. A higher incidence of nonorganic mental or "functional" syndromes, compared to younger adults.
   2. A higher incidence of organic mental syndromes compared to younger adults.
   3. A higher incidence of hypochondriasis or other cases assigned "somatoform disorder" on DSM-III-R compared to younger adults.
   4. A lower incidence of cases assigned a "no diagnosis" diagnosis on DSM-III-R compared to younger adults.

4. Psychiatric liaison services geared especially to the hospitalized elderly have been shown to

   1. improve medical-surgical physicians knowledge of organic brain syndromes, late-life mood disorder, and other prevalent psychiatric disturbance seen in medical-surgical patients.
   2. decrease length of hospital stay significantly.
   3. lead to the development of psychiatry-medicine inpatient units.
   4. improve concordance between the consultant and treating physician with recommendations and follow-up plans.

5. Delirium occurring in an elderly hospitalized medical-surgical patient

   1. is not associated with an increased risk of mortality in the months following its onset.
   2. may represent an iatrogenic disorder.

3. does not usually represent a medical emergency.

4. is not likely to result from a single etiologic factor.

6. Manifestations of depression in medical-surgical patients in the general hospital

1. occur in about 5% of the medical-surgical population.

2. can be confirmed by identifying vegetative disturbances.

3. usually remit spontaneously when the underlying medical problems are successfully treated.

4. may represent a pathologic or prolonged form of grief.

7. Consultation requests to assess competency of medical-surgical patients

1. must seek to address the specific area of competency in question.

2. should render a global and comprehensive assessment of competency.

3. should respect and preserve the patient's fullest possible autonomy over life-style and body.

4. do not usually need to consider the patient's life-style or current living situation in addressing more specific questions of competency.

8. Geriatric patients in general hospitals on medical-surgical wards represent

1. approximately half of all beds and half of all expenditures for health care in general hospitals.

2. approximately 20% or more of consultation requests referred to a consultation-liaison service.

3. an overutilization problem in the emergency department with respect to the current percentage of population over 65 years of age.

4. the vast majority of patients assigned a DSM-III-R diagnosis of delirium.

9. The ability of the medical-surgical physician to diagnose and treat depression among the hospitalized elderly

1. has not improved significantly with the increased awareness of the epidemiology of depression in the general hospital.

2. is often impeded by contraindications or relative contraindications for antidepressant medication.

3. could be improved by carefully questioning the patient for

core symptoms and obtaining a history from an ancillary source.
4. has been shown to be improved through psychiatric liaison activity.

10. Increased mortality in geriatric patients referred for psychiatric consultation have been shown to be associated with
    1. delirium.
    2. depression.
    3. functional disability.
    4. Axis II disorders.

11. Delirium in the hospitalized elderly is associated with
    1. increased hospital length of stay.
    2. high rates of mortality.
    3. high rates of morbidity from falls, pulmonary embolism, or infection.
    4. transfer to a psychiatric inpatient unit when seen in psychiatric consultation.

Choose the one correct response

12. Regarding diagnosis assigned in consultation to the geriatric medical-surgical patient,
    a. hypochondriasis is more prevalent than in younger patients referred for psychiatric consultation.
    b. competency evaluations frequently result in a "no diagnosis" assignment.
    c. mood disorders occur with a greater frequency than do organic mental disorders.
    d. organic mental syndromes occur with a greater frequency than do mood disorders.
    e. None of the above.

13. Geriatric patients referred for psychiatric consultation in the general hospital
    a. suffer from chronic medical illness more often than do nongeriatric patients.
    b. are more likely to receive an Axis II diagnosis.
    c. suffer less often from severe psychiatric illness than nongeriatric patients.
    d. are seen more quickly than nongeriatric patients.
    e. All of the above.

14. Elderly medical-surgical patients receiving psychiatric consultation are likely
    a. to be suffering from an organic mental syndrome in one-third to one-half of cases.
    b. to be suffering depression in about one-fifth to one-third of cases.
    c. to give history of past psychiatric disturbance including alcohol abuse in about one-third or more of cases.
    d. to have been referred for symptoms of confusion or altered mental status.
    e. All of the above.

Chapter 29: Acute Care Inpatient Treatment

Answer a if only 1, 2, and 3 are correct
b if only 1 and 3 are correct
c if only 2 and 4 are correct
d if only 4 is correct
e if all are correct

1. When elderly patients are admitted to acute care inpatient units, discharge planning should start at admissions with
    1. a good understanding of the patient's living situation.
    2. identifying potential obstacles to discharge.
    3. maintaining community resources.
    4. encouraging patients and families to look for a supervised facility *immediately* in case it will be needed.

2. Statistics related to the diagnosis responsible for admission of elderly patients to private psychiatric hospitals and psychiatric units of general hospitals reveal that
    1. depression is responsible for approximately one-third of the admissions.
    2. dementia is responsible for the majority of admissions.
    3. alcohol-related disorders account for less than 3% of admissions.
    4. schizophrenia accounts for less than 15% of admissions.

3. Which of the following statements are true about the staffing of acute-care geriatric psychiatry inpatient units:
    1. British guidelines for staffing recommend 1 nursing full-time equivalent per 1.2 patients.

    2. A geriatrician or internist with special interest in the elderly should be available for regular visits.

    3. Staffing almost always includes physicians, nurses, social workers, occupational therapists, and psychologists.

    4. Physicians and nurses often have to give significant amounts of physical care in addition to the psychiatric care.

4. In addition to patients who present an imminent danger to themselves or others, elderly patients who may be appropriate candidates for inpatient admission include

    1. acutely psychotic patients.

    2. patients who have multiple non-acute medical problems requiring close monitoring.

    3. patients addicted to alcohol or painkillers who require treatment for significant psychiatric symptoms.

    4. patients with uncomplicated dementia who need a higher level of care than can be provided in their current residence.

5. Problems that are more common in the geriatric population and call for particular attention on the part of architects when they design inpatient units are

    1. falls.

    2. sensory deficits.

    3. wandering.

    4. aggressive behavior.

6. When we look at the population of inpatient psychiatric units,

    1. there is an overrepresentation of women in the acute-care geriatric psychiatry inpatient unit population.

    2. there is an overrepresentation of women in the long-term care geriatric psychiatry inpatient unit population.

    3. Men and women should be admitted to the same units as it is normal for men and women to live side by side.

    4. The majority of patients admitted to acute-care geriatric psychiatry units suffer from dementia.

7. Which of the following patients would appropriately be admitted to a geriatric psychiatry inpatient unit?

    1. Elderly patient who suffers from an episode of psychotic agitated depression.

    2. Demented patient who has become a fire hazard in her apartment due to poor memory and poor judgment and refuses placement in a supervised facility as a result of paranoid ideation.

3. Elderly schizophrenic patient living in a group home who suddenly becomes agitated and aggressive.

4. Elderly patient known to your psychiatric service for major recurrent depressive episodes who presents with a new complaint of chest pain and shortness of breath.

8. Which factors may influence the number of falls on a geriatric inpatient unit:

1. Aging effects on balance and blood pressure.
2. Psychotropic medications.
3. Environmental factors such as location of washrooms.
4. Prevalence of medical disorders such as arthritis and parkinsonism.

9. Risk factors for falls include

1. decreased mobility.
2. sleeplessness.
3. incontinence or urgency.
4. confusion.

Chapter 30: Day Programs

Choose the one correct answer

1. Social day care emphasizes

   a. supervised and structured group recreational activities.
   b. unstructured and unsupervised recreational activities.
   c. unsupervised luncheons and tea time.
   d. supervised luncheons and tea time.
   e. active medical treatment.

2. The active treatment model for geriatric psychiatric day hospital implies

   a. a place to rest during the day and return home in the evening.
   b. a preliminary phase prior to entering the hospital inpatient unit.
   c. a place where a full range of physician supervised ambulatory medical and/or psychiatric treatments are offered or prescribed to patients attending during weekdays.

d. a place to attend so that inpatient hospital admission is prevented.

e. a program for inpatient treatment of difficult cases.

3. Which disorders are particularly amenable to active treatment in a day care facility?

a. Depressive and anxiety disorders
b. Psychotic disorders
c. Personality disorders
d. Dementia
e. All of the above

4. Discharge from a maintenance model program is usually to

a. another community program.
b. the client's home with follow-up by a family physician.
c. a more intensive level of care facility such as a hospital or nursing home.
d. social and recreational clubs.
e. None of the above.

Answer a if only 1, 2, and 3 are correct
b if only 1 and 3 are correct
c if only 2 and 4 are correct
d if only 4 is correct
e all are correct

5. The active treatment day care model is

1. an alternative to inpatient care.
2. an alternative to the day center.
3. a therapeutic intervention to expedite discharge from the hospital.
4. a custodial facility.

6. Studies clearly show that a day hospital treatment center has advantages over an inpatient unit because

1. there is exposure to a therapeutic milieu and a range of therapies.
2. a model of the real world is provided so that problem solving and coping strategies can be learned and practiced.
3. a patient's ties to the community are supported rather than severed.
4. None of the above.

7. Which models of day programs are specifically designed to provide caregiver relief?

1. Social day hospital.
2. Active treatment/day hospital.
3. Maintenance day care.
4. Senior citizen's clubs.

Chapter 31: Integrated Community Services

Answer a if only 1, 2, and 3 are correct
b if only 1 and 3 are correct
c if only 2 and 4 are correct
d if only 4 is correct
e if all are correct

1. Case managers provide which of the following services:
   1. Assessment
   2. Vocational training
   3. Advocacy
   4. Linkage

2. Which of the following services might be suitable for a moderately impaired person with Alzheimer's disease?
   1. Domiciliary care
   2. Volunteer program
   3. Home care service
   4. Mutual help group

3. Which of the following are sources of information about services for the elderly?
   1. Area Agencies on Aging (AAA)
   2. Social service departments
   3. Senior centers
   4. Silver Page Directory

4. Which of the following is/are true about protective services?
   1. Provides respite care.
   2. Serves persons who exhibit dangerous behavior.
   3. Provides day treatment services.
   4. Serves persons who are incapable of performing functions necessary for daily survival.

5. Which of the following are generally considered long-term care facilities?

1. Domiciliary care
2. Section 8 programs
3. Intermediate care facilities
4. Foster care

6. Which of the following is/are generally true about home health care?
   1. It provides nursing care.
   2. It provides personal care services.
   3. It requires physician supervision.
   4. It must be provided by a state certified agency.

Choose the one best response

7. Which of the following is *not* one of the principal models of geriatric day care:
   a. A health-oriented model for physically dependent persons.
   b. A model that consists of special purpose centers to serve a single type of clientele.
   c. A psychosocial-oriented model that often serves those with mental disorders.
   d. A vocational model for those requiring work-skill training.

8. Which of the following is *not* a senior volunteer or vocational program?
   a. Green Thumb
   b. Service Corps of Retired Executives
   c. Retired Seniors Volunteer Program
   d. American Association of Retired Persons
   e. Foster grandparents

9. Home health care services and long-term care services may *not* be provided under:
   a. Title III of the Older American Act
   b. The Social Services Block Grant (formerly Title XX of the Social Security Act)
   c. Title XIX of the Social Security Act (Medicaid)
   d. Title XVIII of the Social Security Act (Medicare)

Chapter 32: Medical-Legal Issues

Choose the one best response

1. Competency of a geriatric patient is determined by

  a. psychiatric assessment of the patient.
  b. neuropsychological testing of the patient.
  c. judicial determination of incompetency.
  d. the disorientation of the patient.
  e. the patient's marital status.

2. Confidentiality within the doctor-patient relationship means
  a. absolute secrecy.
  b. never divulging any information about the patient under any circumstances.
  c. never recording in the patient's chart any sensitive information given by the patient.
  d. divulging information about the patient only when mandated by court or in order to protect the patient or the community.
  e. divulging information when the psychiatrist believes it is appropriate.

3. Privacy
  a. refers to the patient's right to restrict flow of information about him/her to others.
  b. is the right of the patient to keep the physician from revealing information without his/her consent.
  c. is the right of the patient to protect his/her bodily integrity.
  d. All of the above.
  e. None of the above.

4. The concept of informed consent means
  a. the patient has been given sufficient information about the procedure contemplated.
  b. the patient has given voluntary permission to perform the procedure.
  c. alternative procedures have been explained to the patient.
  d. the patient understands the information given.
  e. All of the above.

5. In order for a geriatric patient to be involuntarily committed to a psychiatric hospital,
  a. the patient must be mentally ill and in need of hospitalization.
  b. the patient must be mentally ill and a clear and present danger of harm to self or others.
  c. the patient must be senile.

    d. the patient must have been hospitalized before.

    e. the patient must have no other place to live.

6. Abuse of the elderly may occur at the hands of

    a. family members.

    b. institutions.

    c. agencies.

    d. strangers.

    e. All of the above.

7. In order for a patient to be competent to write a will, the patient must know

    a. how much money he/she has.

    b. who his/her lawyer is.

    c. who his/her parents were.

    d. not have a diagnosable mental illness.

    e. All of the above.

8. In order for an elderly patient to be competent to refuse medication in a psychiatric hospital, the patient

    a. must not have a diagnosable mental illness.

    b. must not be legally insane.

    c. must know what the medication will do for him/her, and its side effects.

    d. All of the above.

    e. None of the above.

9. An incompetent elderly patient may have a guardian

    a. of the person.

    b. of his/her estate.

    c. who makes decisions about his/her treatment.

    d. who can spend his/her money.

    e. All of the above.

10. In order to assess the incompetency of an elderly individual, the psychiatrist must

    a. do a battery of psychological tests.

    b. get a neurological examination.

    c. spend time with the patient.

    d. get a CAT scan.

    e. determine whether the patient knows the nature and consequences of his/her current situation.

11. In assessing a testator's testamentary capacity, the psychiatrist must

    a. examine the patient.

    b. determine how much money the patient has.

    c. determine whether the patient knows the nature and extent of the objects of his/her bounty and affection.

    d. determine whether the patient has a mental illness.

    e. determine whether the patient can work with his/her attorney.

12. In criminal cases, the elderly patient may be

    a. the victim of a violent crime.

    b. the perpetrator of a violent crime.

    c. the witness to a violent crime.

    d. All of the above.

    e. None of the above.

Chapter 33: Ethical Issues in Clinical Care

Choose the one best response.

1. Unethical medical experimentation involving human subjects has been documented in

    a. Nazi concentration camps.

    b. American chronic care facilities.

    c. American teaching hospitals.

    d. All of the above.

2. Ethical dilemmas involve

    a. disagreements over facts.

    b. conflicts over values.

    c. illegal acts.

    d. None of the above.

3. Rationing of health care

    a. attempts to balance competing needs.

    b. may impose strict limitations on diagnostic procedures.

    c. may limit the availability of ICU beds for geriatric patients.

    d. All of the above.

4. Regarding doctor-patient confidentiality,

    a. confidentiality must be maintained in *all* circumstances.

    b. information sharing with immediate, concerned family member is permissible.

    c. sensitive information may be released as required by law.

    d. None of the above.

5. The concept of consent

    a. refers to the patient's right to information.

    b. refers to the patient's right to choose among available treatment options.

    c. permits the refusal of life-saving treatment.

    d. All of the above.

6. Concerning competency,

    a. its determination is the responsibility of the physician.

    b. its determination is the responsibility of the court.

    c. our society has generally disregarded the liberty interest of patients.

    d. None of the above.

7. Regarding the use of patients as research subjects,

    a. voluntary informed consent is generally viewed as a prerequisite for participation.

    b. competent patients may consent to studies in which the risks exceed the benefits.

    c. rewarding patients in research studies with better care is unethical.

    d. All of the above.

Chapter 34: Financial Issues

Choose the one best response

1. Which of the following are associated with retirement?

    a. 30–50% reduction in income.

    b. Increased dependence on fixed income sources.

    c. Increased probability of living below the poverty level.

    d. Reduced access to some health care delivery systems.

    e. All of the above.

2. The "dependency ratio" refers to

    a. the likelihood that older adults will require public assistance payments.

    b. the relationship between function in the activities of daily living (ADL) and financial autonomy.

c. the relative number of older adults requiring in-home services and long-term care.

d. the number of people over age 65 per 100 people ages 18–64.

e. the number of older retirees per 100 older workers.

3. The percentage of black women over age 65 not living with their families who live at or below the poverty level is

a. 20%.

b. 40%.

c. 10%.

d. 60%.

e. 90%.

4. The highest billable fee for a provider who does not participate in Part B of Medicare (does not accept assignment) is

a. the Medicare approved CPR fee.

b. the MAAC.

c. the provider's usual charge.

d. 50% of the provider's usual charge.

e. 62.5% of the approved Medicare fee.

5. DRGs

a. have no application to psychiatry.

b. affect payment for psychiatric hospitalization in general hospital "scatter" beds.

c. apply to payment of all psychiatric hospitalizations.

d. explain a substantial proportion of the variance in psychiatric inpatient resource consumption.

e. are used to calculate all physicians' inpatient fees.

6. "Medigap" policies

a. generally cover all Medicare psychiatric copayments and deductibles.

b. generally cover inpatient psychiatric deductibles and co-payments and one-fourth of the copayment for approved psychiatric outpatient charges.

c. usually provide extensive long-term care and in-home services coverage.

d. are extremely low cost.

e. provide the primary insurance coverage for Medicare recipients who choose to purchase them.

7. The resource-based relative value scale (RBRVS)

a. will be used to further correct overpayment for institutional services.
b. will be key in the development of physician payment reform.
c. will be used to assess work by physicians in rendering care to Medicare patients.
d. will reinforce the use of procedures as a principal source of income for physicians.
e. b and c.

8. The largest combined source of payment for long-term care (nursing home) costs are

a. Medicare and Medicaid.
b. Medicaid and out-of-pocket payments.
c. Medicare and long-term care insurance.
d. Private commercial insurance policies.
e. None of the above.

Answers to Self-Assessment Section

Ch. 1	1. a	2. b	3. c	4. c	5. c	6. a					
Ch. 2	1. c	2. c	3. c	4. c	5. c	6. e	7. c	8. e			
Ch. 3	1. c	2. a	3. b	4. b	5. a	6. b					
Ch. 4	1. b	2. d	3. e	4. a	5. d	6. b	7. b	8. a	9. c	10. e	11. d
Ch. 5	1. d	2. d	3. e	4. b	5. b	6. e	7. d	8. b	9. e		
Ch. 6	1. c	2. a	3. c	4. a	5. b	6. b	7. c	8. c	9. b	10. b	11. c
	12. c										
Ch. 7	1. a	2. c	3. e	4. a	5. c	6. a	7. a	8. c	9. b		
Ch. 8	1. d	2. d	3. b	4. a	5. b	6. e	7. b	8. e	9. e		
Ch. 9	1. d	2. d	3. a	4. d	5. a	6. d	7. a	8. b	9. e	10. d	11. d
Ch. 10	1. a	2. e	3. d	4. e	5. b	6. c	7. a				
Ch. 11	1. e	2. b	3. d	4. e	5. a	6. c	7. a	8. d	9. e	10. b	11. e
	12. c	13. e									
Ch. 13	1. d	2. e	3. c	4. d	5. d	6. e	7. a	8. a	9. d		
Ch. 14	1. d	2. a	3. b	4. d	5. a	6. e	7. d	8. c	9. b	10. b	11. a
	12. c	13. e	14. a	15. b	16. e	17. c	18. e	19. a	20. e		
Ch. 15	1. c	2. e	3. d	4. c	5. b	6. c	7. e	8. c	9. b	10. e	11. b
Ch. 16	1. c	2. d	3. b	4. d	5. d	6. a	7. b	8. c	9. b	10. a	11. a
	12. a										
Ch. 17	1. c	2. a	3. d	4. b	5. b	6. a	7. b	8. c	9. d		

Ch. 18   1. d   2. c   3. a   4. a   5. b

Ch. 19   1. d   2. b   3. e   4. b   5. b   6. b   7. a   8. d   9. c   10. c   11. e
12. d   13. a   14. b

Ch. 20   1. c   2. b   3. c   4. b   5. e   6. e   7. b   8. c   9. c   10. e   11. c
12. a   13. c   14. a

Ch. 21   1. e   2. c   3. a   4. c   5. b   6. a   7. e   8. e   9. c   10. b

Ch. 22   1. c   2. b   3. d   4. d   5. c   6. a   7. c   8. c   9. d   10. a   11. c
12. c   13. d   14. a   15. c   16. d   17. c   18. a   19. d

Ch. 23   1. e   2. e   3. c   4. c   5. b   6. e   7. d   8. a   9. e   10. a   11. e
12. e   13. b   14. d   15. d   16. c   17. b   18. a   19. a

Ch. 24   1. d   2. d   3. e   4. e   5. c   6. c   7. a   8. c   9. a

Ch. 25   1. e   2. e   3. b   4. e   5. d   6. a   7. c   8. d

Ch. 26   1. a   2. e   3. a   4. a   5. c   6. b   7. e   8. e

Ch. 27   1. b   2. e   3. e   4. c   5. c   6. d   7. c   8. c   9. e   10. e

Ch. 28   1. a   2. b   3. c   4. c   5. c   6. d   7. b   8. c   9. a   10. a   11. a
12. d   13. a   14. e

Ch. 29   1. a   2. d   3. e   4. a   5. a   6. b   7. a   8. e   9. e

Ch. 30   1. a   2. c   3. a   4. c   5. b   6. d   7. b

Ch. 31   1. a   2. b   3. e   4. c   5. b   6. e   7. d   8. d   9. e

Ch. 32   1. c   2. d   3. d   4. e   5. b   6. e   7. a   8. c   9. e   10. e   11. c
12. d

Ch. 33   1. d   2. b   3. d   4. d   5. c   6. d   7. b   8. d

Ch. 34   1. e   2. d   3. d   4. b   5. b   6. b   7. e   8. b

INDEX

Abstract thinking, 166
Acetylcholine, 69, 295
Activity-centered groups, 535, 540–541
  See also Group therapy
Adaptation, 85, 492–493
Adjustment disorder, 344, 502
Adolescence, 88–89
Adult education, 629–631
Aerobic exercise, 59
Affective disorders, 261–262
  See also name of individual disorder
Age Discrimination in Employment Act,
  126
Agnosia, 289
Akathisia, 459
Alcoholism
  age of onset, 387–388
  and anxiety, 373–374
  course, 392
  diagnosis, 391–392
  epidemiology, 387
  etiology, 395
  genetics, 395
  medical complications, 394
  medical history, 154
  prognosis, 399–400
  psychiatric complications, 393
  and sexual dysfunction, 427
  treatment, 396–400
Aluminum, 296
Alzheimer's disease
  course, 230–232, 300–301
  and delusions, 364–366
  and depression, 34
  diagnosis, 298–299
  electroencephalography, 275–276
  etiology, 295–298
  genetics, 50–51, 295–296
  laboratory tests, 299–300
  neuroimaging, 255–257
  pathology, 299
  sleep disorders, 410
  tests, 231–232
  treatment, 301, 449, 458
  See also Dementia, 34
Amnestic syndrome, 321–323
Anemia, 180–181
Anesthesia and electroconvulsive therapy,
  477
Anomia, 163
Antidepressants, 452–456
  and electroconvulsive therapy, 480
  side effects, 191–192

as sleep medication, 413–414
  See also name of individual drug
Anxiety
  cognitive vs. somatic, 371–372
  and depression, 370–371
  diagnosis, 371–374
  epidemiology, 27, 369–376
  sex differentiation, 369
  and sleep disorders, 410
  treatment, 374–376
Anxiolytics, 375–376, 460–461
Aphasia
  cognitive assessment, 162
  dementia, 289
  neuropsychological testing, 225
Appearance and psychiatric evaluation,
  156
Apraxia, 289
Area agencies on aging, 616–618
Arthritis, 175
Attention, 162, 224–225
Atypical psychosis, 364
Axis I disorders and physical illness, 376

Bed sores, 185–186
Behavioral medicine, 134–137
Behavior changes
  physical illness, 200–201, 332–333
  reflexes, 213
Behavior problems
  mechanical restraints, 556–557
  in nursing homes, 553–554
  treatment, 499, 532, 558–559, 596
Benzodiazepines
  for acute withdrawal, 392
  for delirium, 320
  and electroconvulsive therapy, 480
  in nursing homes, 555
  side effects, 460–461
  for sleep disorders, 413, 414
Bereavement and sleep disturbances, 405
Bibliography, 118
Biochemical changes, 199
Blood-flow and Alzheimer's disease, 297
Blood pressure, 447
Board and care facilities, 627–628
Brain disorders, 443
  affecting coordination, 212–213
  electroencephalography, 273
  neuroimaging, 253–254
  neuron loss, 199
  See also name of individual disorder